NURSING TODAY

TRANSITIONS and TRENDS

TENTH EDITION

NURSING TODAY

TRANSITIONS and TRENDS

JoAnn Zerwekh, EdD, RN

President/CEO
Nursing Education Consultants
Chandler, AZ;
Nursing Faculty
Upper Iowa University Online Campus
Mesa, Arizona

Ashley Zerwekh Garneau, PhD, RN

Nursing Faculty
GateWay Community College
Phoenix, Arizona

ELSEVIER

Elsevier
3251 Riverport Lane
St. Louis, Missouri 63043

NURSING TODAY: TRANSITIONS AND TRENDS, TENTH EDITION   ISBN: 978-0-323-64208-8

Notice

Practitioners and researchers must always rely on their own experience and knowledge in evaluating and using any information, methods, compounds or experiments described herein. Because of rapid advances in the medical sciences, in particular, independent verification of diagnoses and drug dosages should be made. To the fullest extent of the law, no responsibility is assumed by Elsevier, authors, editors or contributors for any injury and/or damage to persons or property as a matter of products liability, negligence or otherwise, or from any use or operation of any methods, products, instructions, or ideas contained in the material herein.

Previous editions copyrighted 2018, 2015, 2012, 2009, 2006, 2003, 2000, 1997, 1994.

Library of Congress Control Number: 2019955927

Senior Content Strategist: Sandra Clark
Senior Content Development Manager: Lisa Newton
Publishing Services Manager: Catherine Jackson
Senior Project Manager: Kate Mannix
Designer: Patrick Ferguson

Printed in India

Last digit is the print number: 9   8   7   6   5   4   3

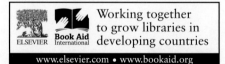

*To the memory of my husband, John
Masog, who left this world and departed
from our lives way too early. I cherish the
wonderful years that we had together.
I love and miss you dearly.* ~ JoAnn

CONTRIBUTORS

Peggy J. Black, MSN, RN, NE-BC
Assistant Professor of Nursing
Upper Iowa University
West Des Moines, Iowa
Chapter 10: Challenges of Nursing Management and Leadership

Mary Boyce, MSN, RN, CCRN, CNE
Faculty–Nursing Division
Mesa Community College
Mesa, Arizona
Chapter 25: Workplace Issues

Julie V. Darmody, PhD, RN, ACNS-BC
DNP Program Director
College of Nursing
University of Wisconsin Milwaukee
Milwaukee, Wisconsin
Chapter 16: Economics of the Health Care Delivery System

Alice E. Dupler, MSN, JD, ANP-BC, Esq.
Professor, School of Health Professions
University of Providence
Great Falls, Montana
Chapter 20: Legal Issues

Michael L. Evans, PhD, RN, NEA-BC, FACHE, FAAN
Dean and Professor
UMC Endowed Chair for Excellence in Nursing
Texas Tech University Health Sciences Center
School of Nursing
Lubbock, Texas
Chapter 17: Political Action in Nursing

Ashley Zerwekh Garneau, PhD, RN
Faculty–Nursing Division
GateWay Community College
Phoenix, Arizona
Chapter 1: Role Transitions
Chapter 3: Mentorship, Preceptorship, and Nurse Residency Programs
Chapter 7: Nursing Education
Chapter 8: Nursing Theories
Chapter 12: Effective Communication, Team Building, and Interprofessional Practice
Chapter 21: Cultural and Spiritual Awareness

Ruth I. Hansten, MBA, PhD, RN, FACHE$_R$
Hansten Healthcare PLLC
Santa Rosa, California
Chapter 14: Delegation in the Clinical Setting

Peter G. Melenovich, PhD, RN, CNE
Faculty–Nursing Division
GateWay Community College
Phoenix, Arizona
Chapter 24: Using Evidence-Based Practice and Nursing Research

Cheryl D. Parker, PhD, RN-BC, CNE, FHIMSS
Clinical Assistant Professor and Educational Technology Specialist
The University of Texas at Tyler School of Nursing
Tyler, Texas
Chapter 23: Nursing Informatics

Jessica Maack Rangel, MS, RN, ASPPS
University of North Texas Health Science Center
Institute for Patient Safety
Senior Fellow, Nurse Executive
Fort Worth, Texas
Chapter 11: Building Nursing Managements Skills

Karin J. Sherrill, RN, MSN, CNE, ANEF, FAADN
Faculty–Nursing Division
GateWay Community College
Phoenix, Arizona
Chapter 19: Ethical Issues

Susan Sportsman, PhD, RN, ANEF, FAAN
Managing Director
Collaborative Momentum Consulting
Forestburg, Texas
Chapter 15: The Health Care Organization and Patterns of Nursing Care Delivery

Christa L. Steffens, EdD, MSN, RN
Director and Department Chair, Nursing
Upper Iowa University-Cedar Rapids Center
Cedar Rapids, Iowa
Chapter 9: Professional Image of Nursing

Stephanie Tippin, RN, MSN, NP-C
Assistant Professor
Department of Nursing
Upper Iowa University-Mesa Center
Mesa, Arizona
Chapter 22: Quality Patient Care

Jennifer Wing, MSN, RN

Assistant Professor and Academic
   Advisor
Upper Iowa University
West Des Moines, Iowa
Chapter 18: Collective Bargaining:
   Traditional (Union) and
   Nontraditional Approaches

JoAnn Zerwekh, EdD, RN

President/CEO, Nursing Education
   Consultants
Chandler, Arizona;
Nursing Faculty
Upper Iowa University Online
   Campus
Mesa, Arizona
Chapter 1: Role Transitions
Chapter 2: Personal Management:
   Time and Self-Care Strategies
Chapter 4: Employment
   Considerations: Opportunities,
   Resumes, and Interviewing
Chapter 5: NCLEX-RN® Exam and the
   New Graduate

Chapter 6: Historical Perspectives:
   Influences on the Present
Chapter 12: Effective Communication,
   Team Building, and Interprofessional
   Practice
Chapter 13: Conflict Management
Chapter 26: Emergency Preparedness

**Tyler Zerwekh, BA, MPH, DrPH,
REHS**

Epidemiologist III–Invasive and
   Respiratory Infectious Disease
   Team
Emerging and Acute Infectious
   Disease Branch
Texas Department of State Health
   Services
Austin, Texas;
Adjunct Faculty
School of Public Health
University of Memphis
Memphis, Tennessee
Chapter 26: Emergency Preparedness

REVIEWERS

Jean Conlon-Yoo, DMHc, MSN, RN, APN
Adult Psychiatric Mental Health
    Clinical Nurse Specialist
Instructor–Prelicensure Nursing
    Program
Felician University
Lodi, New Jersey

Elizabeth Ann Delaney, RN, BSN, MSN, APRN
Associate Professor of Nursing with
    Tenure
Center for Nursing Education
Ohio University, Southern Campus
Ironton, Ohio

Ruth Gladen, MS, RN
Assistant Professor, Nursing
North Dakota State College of
    Science
Wahpeton, North Dakota

Jennifer L. Grobe, PhD, RN, CNE
Associate Dean
Nursing and Allied Health
Highland Community College
Freeport, Illinois

Shirley MacNeill, MSN, RN, CNE
Allied Health Department Chair
LVN to ADN Program Coordinator
Allied Health
Lamar State College Port Arthur
Port Arthur, Texas

Denise Marie McEnroe-Petitte, PhD, MSN, BSN, AS, RN
Associate Professor, Nursing
Kent State University Tuscarawas
New Philadelphia, Ohio

PREFACE

Nursing Today: Transitions and Trends evolved out of the authors' experiences with nursing students in their final semester and the students' transition into the realities of nursing practice. With the changes in health care and the practice of nursing, there is even more emphasis on the importance of assisting the new graduate through the transition from education to practice. Nursing education and the transition process are experiencing a tremendous impact from changes in the health care delivery system.

In this tenth edition, we provide several new features that we feel are vital to the professional development and success of our future generation of nurses. For the soon-to-be nurse, we have added information about incorporating mindfulness into your practice as well as offered several mindfulness exercises that you can begin practicing right now! We have also provided tips for studying effectively in groups, strategies for maximizing your time effectively, online resources for improving your time-management skills, and popular apps for organizing documents in Chapter 2, *Personal Management: Time and Self-Care Strategies*. We have provided information on dedicated education units as a clinical teaching model for assisting nursing students' transition to practice, along with helpful tips for transitioning from mentee to mentor, in Chapter 3, *Mentorship, Preceptorship, and Nurse Residency Programs*. Additionally, we have added communication techniques for promoting an effective mentee-mentor relationship. We have also updated information on transition programs and characteristics of effective transition programs. We have continued to provide the graduate nurse with information on nursing informatics and management and have continued to increase the focus on the use of information technology for the transitioning graduate by including new content on cybersecurity, patient engagement through online technologies, and the use of robotics and artificial intelligence in patient care delivery. We have updated information on how technology such as cloud computing, clinical decision support systems (CDSSs), and point-of-care electronic documentation can provide data tracking and analysis for improving workflow processes and patient care. The enhanced nurse licensure compact (eNLC) program's influence on telehealth services provided by nurses is elaborated on in Chapter 17, *Political Action in Nursing*. Chapters related to current issues in health care, such as Chapter 15, *The Health Care Organization and Patterns of Nursing Care Delivery*; Chapter 16, *Economics of the Health Care Delivery System*; Chapter 18, *Collective Bargaining: Traditional (Union) and Nontraditional Approaches*; Chapter 19, *Ethical Issues*; Chapter 20, *Legal Issues*; Chapter 21, *Cultural and Spiritual Awareness*; Chapter 22, *Quality Patient Care*; Chapter 25, *Workplace Issues*; and Chapter 26, *Emergency Preparedness*, have been expanded. We kept the same easy reading style to present timely information, along with updated information on the 2019 NCLEX-RN® Detailed Test Plan and samples of the alternate-item format test items appearing on the NCLEX-RN® Exam. One of our goals with this book is to provide graduating nurses with practical guidelines that can be implemented in their transition from nursing students to effective entry-level nursing practice. Additionally, we have provided foundational content that will serve as a resource for graduating nurses continuing their nursing education.

For these reasons, we have introduced key differences among evidence-based practice, research utilization, and nursing research using relevant patient case scenarios to highlight the steps involved in each process in Chapter 24, *Using Evidence-Based Practice and Nursing Research*. Compassion fatigue and strategies for preventing burnout through practicing mindfulness are introduced in Chapter 2, *Personal Management: Time and Self-Care Strategies*. Recognizing the need for new graduate nurses to develop effective management skills to navigate and practice in the rapidly changing healthcare setting, we have updated information on the change process and have offered strategies for adapting to change in Chapter 10, *Challenges of Nursing Management and Leadership*. Content on interprofessional collaborative practice, group dynamics and group member roles, and strategies for communicating in the workplace have been updated and can be found in Chapter 12, *Effective Communication, Team Building, and Interprofessional Practice*. Updated information on TeamSTEPPS as a tool for improving interprofessional communication has also been added to Chapter 11, *Building Nursing Management Skills*.

The classic findings and experience of Marlene Kramer and her research on reality shock and Patricia Benner's work on performance characteristics of beginning and expert nurses continue to affect the need for transition courses in nursing education programs. These courses focus on trends and issues to assist the new graduate to be better prepared to practice nursing in today's world. With the increased demands and realities of the health care system, it is necessary for the new graduate to make the transition rapidly to an independent role. We have written this book for use in these transition courses and to assist individual students in anticipating encounters in a rapidly changing, technologically oriented work environment.

We have revised and updated each chapter to reflect the changes in the health care delivery system and have maintained recommendations from the 2010 Institute of Medicine *Future of Nursing* report. To illustrate this, the results of initiatives based on the recommendations from the *Future of Nursing* (2010) report have been included in Chapter 15, *The Health Care Organization and Patterns of Nursing Care Delivery*; health equity initiatives focusing on providing culturally and linguistically appropriate services to diverse populations and improving the health needs of the lesbian, gay, bisexual, and transgender community are explored in Chapter 21, *Cultural and Spiritual Awareness*; methods for evaluating patient care, patient satisfaction, and quality outcome measures in today's redesigned health care system have been highlighted in Chapter 22, *Quality Patient Care*; issues in emergency preparedness education and training and patient triage have been expanded in Chapter 26, *Emergency Preparedness*. Some of the lengthy tables and figures have been moved to Evolve Resources to keep the material intact and to make the reading easier. We have maintained and added additional cartoons drawn by C.J. Miller, BSN, RN. We feel they add a smile and perhaps make the difficult information a little easier to comprehend.

Each chapter begins with Learning Objectives and a quote as an introduction to the content. Within each chapter, there is a practical application of the concepts discussed. Critical Thinking boxes in the text highlight information to facilitate the critical thinking process. Using a question approach, material is presented in a logical, easy-to-read manner. There are also opportunities to respond to thought-provoking questions and student exercises to facilitate self-evaluation. Research for Best Practice boxes have been incorporated to provide implications for nursing practice and opportunities for discussion on how to incorporate the information into the practice setting. We have continued to provide online resources and relevant websites for each chapter.

The student receives an overall view of the nursing profession from historical events that influenced nursing to the present-day image and also the legal, ethical, political, and on-the-job issues confronting today's professional nurse. Communication and delegation in the workplace, time management, how to write an effective resume, interviewing tips, guidelines for using social media as a professional, employee benefits, attaining certification in a nursing specialty, and self-care strategies are among the sound career advancement tools provided.

FOR NURSING FACULTY

Our key goal in developing this book has been to provide timely information that is applicable to current practice and is fun to read. An Instructor's TEACH for Nurses lesson plan manual, which is web-based, is available from the publisher on the Evolve website to assist faculty in planning and promoting a positive transition experience. This valuable website contains suggestions for classroom and clinically based student activities. Additionally, we have included the 2017 Accreditation Commission for Education in Nursing (ACEN) Standards throughout each TEACH for Nurses lesson plan manual among other curriculum standards (i.e., QSEN, BSN Essentials).

At the request of nursing faculty using our book, we have continued to provide a secure, updated, web-based Test Bank and have more than 300 questions, with detailed rationales included on higher order level test questions; text page references indicating where the correct answer can be obtained in the chapter have been provided for all test items. Additional alternate-format test items have also been added to the Test Bank. We have provided students with more than 100 NCLEX-style questions that test their knowledge of the chapter content. We have also provided suggested responses for selected critical thinking questions threaded throughout each chapter. We have included accompanying textbook appendices and have expanded the content within Evolve, which supports the textbook, that includes PowerPoint presentations with audience-response questions, sample NCLEX-style questions, including alternate-format items, and case studies. The Evolve website will continue to provide updated information as new trends and issues affect the practice of nursing.

Please consult your local Elsevier representative for more details.

JoAnn Zerwekh
Ashley Zerwekh Garneau

ACKNOWLEDGMENTS

The success of previous editions of this book is a result of the contributions and efforts of our chapter contributors, who provided their expertise and knowledge, and our book reviewers, who provided their insights and suggestions on pertinent issues in nursing practice. This new edition is no exception. We thank the staff at Elsevier for their assistance and guidance during the revision of the 10th edition: Sandy Clark, Senior Content Strategist, and Lisa Newton, Senior Content Development Manager. We also extend our gratitude to Kate Mannix, Senior Project Manager, for monitoring the production of this book to ensure its delivery on schedule; a special thank you to Patrick Ferguson, Design Direction, for the overall book layout and design.

I would like to thank my children, Tyler and Ashley (my coauthor!); their significant other and spouse (Julie Goehring and Brian Garneau); and my grandchildren (Maddie and Harper Zerwekh; Ben Garneau; Alexis and Brooklyn Parks; Owen, Emmett, and Cole Masog) for putting a smile on my face and coaxing me to step away from the computer during those challenging times in the revision process. I would also like to thank my stepchildren, Carrie Parks and Matt Masog, for their support and great friendship and also for blessing me with more grandchildren. For my husband, John Masog, in memoriam.

The end is nothing; the road is all. —Willa Cather

— **JoAnn**

To my husband, Brian, for your unwavering support, unconditional love, wittiness, and patience during the manuscript revision. Thank you for keeping me grounded and balanced. To our son, Ben, who amazes us every day with how he sees the world around him. And to my little kitties Eva and Louie, who always let me know when it was time for a break from the computer by blocking my computer monitor! Last, I would like to thank my Mom, JoAnn, for her kindred spirit and for inspiring me to pursue the profession of nursing. You are my confidant, mentor, and the nurse I aspire to be.

— **Ashley**

CONTENTS

UNIT II: NURSING: A DEVELOPING PROFESSION

UNIT III: NURSING MANAGEMENT

UNIT IV: CURRENT ISSUES IN HEALTH CARE

UNIT V: CONTEMPORARY NURSING PRACTICE

Professional Growth and Transition

Role Transitions

JoAnn Zerwekh, EdD, RN and Ashley Zerwekh Garneau, PhD, RN

ⓔAdditional resources are available at http://evolve.elsevier.com/Zerwekh/nsgtoday/.

> *When you're finished changing, you're finished.*
> **Benjamin Franklin**

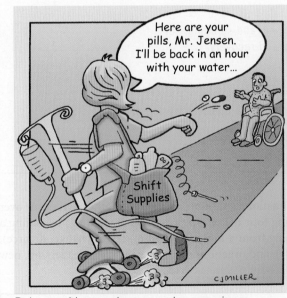

Role transition can be a complex experience.

After completing this chapter, you should be able to:
- Discuss the concept of transitions.
- Identify the characteristics of reality shock.
- Compare and contrast the phases of reality shock.
- Identify the stages of transition shock.
- Identify times in your life when you have experienced a reality shock or role transition.
- Describe methods to promote a successful transition.

Welcome to the profession of nursing! This book is written for nursing students who are in the midst of transitions in their lives. As a new student, you are beginning the transition to becoming indoctrinated into nursing, and sometimes it is not an easy transition. For those of you who are in the middle of nursing school, do you wonder if life even exists outside of nursing school? To the student who will soon graduate, hang on; you are almost there! For whatever transition period you are encountering, our goal is to help make your life easier during this period of personal and professional adjustment into nursing. We have designed this book to help you keep your feet on the ground and your head out of the clouds, as well as to boost your spirits when the going gets rough.

As you thumb through this book, you will notice that there are cartoons and critical thinking questions that encourage your participation. Do not be alarmed; we know you have been over-loaded with "critical thinking" during nursing school! These critical thinking questions are not meant to be graded; instead, their purpose is to encourage you to begin thinking about your tran-sition, either into nursing school or into practice, and to guide you through the book in a practical, participative manner. Our intention is to add a little humor here and there while giving information on topics we feel will affect your transition into nursing practice. We want you to be informed about the controversial issues currently affecting nursing. After all, the future of nursing rests with **you**!

Are you ready to begin? Then let's start with the real stuff. You are beginning to experience tran-sitions—for some of you, just getting into nursing school has been a long struggle—and you are there! For others, you can see the light at the end of the tunnel as graduation becomes a reality. Nursing is one of the most rewarding professions you can pursue. However, it can also be one of the most frustrating. As with marriage, raising children, and the pursuit of happiness, there are ups and downs. We seldom find the world or our specific situation the exact way we thought it would or should be. Often your fantasy of what nursing *should* be is not what you will find nursing to be.

You will cry, but you will also laugh.
You will share with people their darkest hours of pain and suffering, but
You will also share with them their hope, healing, and recovery.
You will be there as life begins and ends.
You will experience great challenges that lead to success.
You will experience failure and disappointment.
You will never cease to be amazed at the resilience of the human body and spirit.

TRANSITIONS

What Are Transitions?

Transitions are passages or changes from one situation, condition, or state to another that occur over time. They have been classified into the following four major types: developmental (e.g., becoming a parent, midlife crisis), situational (e.g., graduating from a nursing program, career change, divorce), health/illness (e.g., dealing with a chronic illness), and organizational (e.g., change in leadership, new staffing patterns) (Schumacher & Meleis, 1994).

Transitions are complex processes, and a lot of transitions may occur at the same time.

What Are Important Factors Influencing Transitions?

Understanding the transition experience from the perspective of the person who is experiencing it is important because the meaning of the experience may be positive, negative, or neutral, and the expectation may or may not be realistic. The transition may be desired (e.g., passing the NCLEX exam) or undesirable (e.g., the death of a family member, after which you have to assume a new role in your family).

Often, when you know what to expect, the stress associated with the change or transition is reduced.

BOX 1.1 STRESSES REPORTED BY NEW GRADUATES RELATED TO SIX CRUCIAL COMPETENCY AREAS

1. Communication
   - Calling or talking with a physician, completing shift reports, addressing patient requests, and resolving conflict
2. Leadership
   - Lack of delegating skills
   - Anxiety associated with collaborative teamwork
3. Organization
   - Lack of organizational and management skills to prioritize care
4. Critical thinking
   - Difficulty with clinical decision making
   - Feeling unprepared to meet the challenges of the workplace
   - Deficits in clinical knowledge
5. Specific situations
   - Lack of confidence when dealing with acutely ill patients, emergency situations, and end-of-life scenarios
6. Stress management
   - Unfamiliarity with stress management techniques
   - Lack of social support

From Theisen, J., & Sandau, K. (2013). Competency of new graduate nurses: A review of their weaknesses and strategies for success. *Journal of Continuing Education in Nursing, 44*(9), 406–414. https://doi.org/10.3928/00220124-20130617-38.

Another factor in the transition process is the new level of knowledge and skill required, as well as the availability of needed resources within the environment. Dealing with new knowledge and skills can be challenging and stressful and can lead to a variety of different emotions related to the expectation of the new graduate to be competent (Box 1.1). This will resolve as your confidence grows and you have more understanding of the concept of how to "think like a nurse."

Transitions are a part of life and certainly a part of nursing. Although the following discussions on role transition and reality shock focus on the graduate nurse experience, there are many applicable points for the new student as well. As you learn more about transitions, reality shock, and the graduate nurse experience, think about how this information may also apply to your transition experience into and through nursing school (Critical Thinking Box 1.1).

? CRITICAL THINKING BOX 1.1

What is your greatest concern about your transition? Is it personal or work transitions because you are a student nurse, or is it your transition from school to the practice setting?

Looking back, what transitions have you experienced? What transitions are occurring in your life now? Has your entry into, as well as progress through, nursing school caused transitions in your personal life? Has your anticipated job search caused transitions in your professional as well as personal life?

Transitions in Nursing

The paradox of nursing will become obvious to you early in your nursing career. This realization may occur during nursing school, but it frequently becomes most obvious during the first 6 months of your first job.

Health care organizations are very concerned about your transition experience and job satisfaction during that first 6 months of employment. Have you been hearing about "evidence-based practice?"

Well, it is working for you now! During the first 6 months of employment, new graduates need a period of time to develop their skills in a supportive environment. Employee retention and job satisfaction are key issues with the hospital; confidence in performing skills and procedures, nurse residency programs, and dependence versus independence are key graduate nurse issues driving this research. The well-being of the graduate nurse and the ability to deliver quality nursing care during the transition period have sparked research to validate the need for special considerations of the graduate nurse experiencing transition (Casey et al., 2004; Duchscher, 2008, 2009; Godinez et al., 1999; Lavoie-Tremblay et al., 2002; Spector, 2015a; Steinmiller et al., 2003; Varner & Leeds, 2012). With identification of the basic problems encountered by new graduates during this first 6 months, there is a concerted effort to begin to meet the special needs of the graduate nurse and assist him or her to "think like a nurse" (Research for Best Practice Box 1.1).

🔍 RESEARCH FOR BEST PRACTICE BOX 1.1
Role Transition: Think Like a Nurse

Practice Issue

Students report that when they first entered their nursing courses they were unaware of the complexity of thinking and problem solving that occurs in the clinical setting. They often are unable to "think on their feet" and change a planned way of doing something based on what is happening with a specific patient at any given moment. Research supports the finding that the beginning nursing graduate continues to have difficulty making clinical judgments (i.e., thinking like a nurse). Graduates with baccalaureate degrees in nursing were interviewed three times in 9 months to determine their perceptions of how they learned to think like nurses (Tanner, 2006). In a later simulation study by Ashley and Stamp (2014), thinking like a nurse was one of the major themes that emerged when comparing sophomore and junior students. During simulation, the sophomore student approached the clinical scenario more as a layperson than as a professional with specialized knowledge, which was exhibited by little preplanning and the expectation that the clinical problem would be self-evident and would require nothing more than common sense to achieve an outcome.

Implications for Nursing Practice
Clinical Judgments—Thinking Like a Nurse
- Nursing students and new graduates are often unaware of the level of responsibility required of nurses and lack confidence in their ability to make clinical judgments.
- The process of learning to think like a nurse is characterized by building confidence, accepting responsibility, adapting to changing relations with others, and thinking more critically.
- Multiple clinical experiences, support from faculty and experienced nurses, and sharing experiences with peers were critical in the transition from student nurse to beginning practitioner.
- Nursing education must assist nursing students to engage with patients and act on a responsible vision for excellent care of those patients and with a deep concern for the patients' and families' well-being. Clinical reasoning must arise from this engaged, concerned stance.

Considering This Information

What types of resources will you use as a nursing student to improve your clinical reasoning skills? What characteristics have you observed in staff members who effectively "think like a nurse"? How can you begin to incorporate these aspects into your practice as a new graduate nurse?

References

Ashley, J., & Stamp, K. (2014). Learning to think like a nurse: The development of clinical judgment in nursing students. *Journal of Nursing Education, 53*(9), 519–525. dx.doi.org/10.3928/01484834-20140821-14.

Etheridge, S. A. (2007). Learning to think like a nurse: Stories from new nurse graduates. *Journal of Continuing Education in Nursing, 38*(1), 24–30.

Tanner, C. A. (2006). Thinking like a nurse: A research-based model of clinical judgment in nursing. *Journal of Continuing Education in Nursing, 45*(6), 204–211.

The role transition process that occurs on entry into nursing school and the process from student to graduate nurse do not take place automatically. Having the optimal experience during role transition requires a great deal of attention, planning, and determination on your part. How you perceive and handle the transition will determine how well you progress through the process. It is important that you keep a positive attitude. The challenges and rewards of clinicals, tests, and work situations will cause your emotions to go up and down, but that is okay. It is expected, and you will be able to deal with it effectively. It is important that you keep a positive attitude. The wide range of emotions experienced during the transition process can often affect your *emotional and physical well-being;* check out the discussion of self-care strategies in Chapter 2.

So, let's get started. Reality shock is often one of the first hurdles of transition to conquer in your new role as a graduate nurse or registered nurse (RN or Real Nurse). ☺

REALITY SHOCK

What Is Reality Shock?

Reality shock is a term often used to describe the reaction experienced when one moves into the workforce after several years of educational preparation. The recent graduate is caught in the situation of moving from a familiar, comfortable educational environment into a new role in the workforce in which the expectations are not clearly defined or may not even be realistic. For example, as a student you were taught to consider the patient in a holistic framework, but in practice you often do not have the time to consider the psychosocial or teaching needs of the patient, even though they must be attended to and documented.

The recent graduate in the workplace is expected to be a capable, competent nurse. That sounds fine. However, sometimes there is a hidden expectation that graduate nurses should function as though they have 5 years of nursing experience. Time management skills, along with the increasing acuity level of patients, are common problems for the new graduate. This situation may leave you with feelings of powerlessness, depression, and insecurity because of an apparent lack of effectiveness in the work environment. There are positive ways to deal with the problems. You are not alone! Reality shock is not unique to nursing. It is present in many professions as graduates move from the world of academia to the world of work and begin to adjust to the expectations and values of the workforce.

What Are the Phases of Reality Shock?

Kramer (1974) described the phases of reality shock as they apply to nursing (Table 1.1). Although she identified this process in 1974, these phases remain the basis for understanding the implications of reality shock and successfully progressing through the process. In our current world of nursing, we are still dealing with this same process. Adjustments begin to take place as the graduate nurse adapts to the reality of the practice of nursing. The first phase of adjustment is the honeymoon phase (Fig. 1.1). The recent graduate is thrilled with completing school and accepting a first job. Life is a "bed of roses" because everyone knows nursing school is much harder than nursing practice. There are no more concept care maps to create, no more nursing care plans to write, and no more burning the midnight oil for the next day's examination. No one is watching over your shoulder while you insert a catheter or administer an intravenous medication. You are not a "student" anymore; now you are a nurse! During this exciting phase, your perception of the situation may feel unreal and distorted, and you may not be able to understand the overall picture.

HONEYMOON PHASE
I just can't believe how wonderful everything is! Imagine getting a paycheck—money, at last! It's all great. Really, it is.

TABLE 1.1 PHASES OF REALITY SHOCK		
HONEYMOON	**SHOCK AND REJECTION**	**RECOVERY**
Sees the world of nursing looking quite rosy Often fascinated with the thrill of "arriving" in the profession	Has excessive mistrust Experiences increased concern over minor pains and illness Experiences decrease in energy and feels excessive fatigue Feels like a failure and blames self for every mistake Bands together and depends on people who hold the same values Has a hypercritical attitude Feels moral outrage	Beginning to have sense of humor (first sign) Decrease in tension Increase in ability to be objective

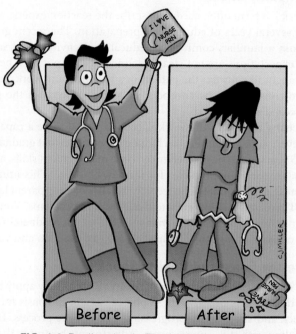

FIG. 1.1 Reality shock. The honeymoon's over.

The honeymoon phase is frequently short lived as the graduate begins to identify the conflicts between the way she or he was taught and the reality of what is done. Every graduate nurse will have a unique way of coping with the situations; however, some common responses have been identified. The graduate may cope with this conflict by withdrawing or rejecting the values learned during nursing school. This may mark the end of the honeymoon phase of transition. The phrase "going native" was used by Kramer and Schmalenberg (1977) to describe recent graduates as they begin to cope and identify with the reality of the situation by rejecting the values from nursing school and beginning to function as everyone else does.

SHOCK AND REJECTION PHASE

Mary was assigned 10 patients for the morning. There were numerous medications to be administered. It was difficult to carry all of the medication administration records to each room for patient identification. Because she "knew the patients" and because the other experienced nurses did not check identification, she decided she no longer needed to check a patient's identification before administering medication. Later in the day, she gave insulin to Mrs. James, a patient she "knew"; unfortunately, the insulin was for Mrs. Phillips, another patient she "knew."

With experiences such as this during transition, graduates may feel as though they have failed and begin to blame themselves for every mistake. They may also experience moral outrage at having been put in such a position. When the bad days begin to outnumber the good days, the graduate nurse may experience frustration, fatigue, and anger and may consequently develop a hypercritical attitude toward nursing. Some graduates become very disillusioned and drop out of nursing altogether. This is the period of shock and rejection.

I had just completed orientation in the hospital where I had wanted to work since I started nursing school. I immediately discovered that the care there was so bad that I did not want to be a part of it. At night, I went home very frustrated that the care I had given was not as I was taught to do it. I cried every night and hated to go to work in the morning. I did not like anyone with whom I was working. My stomach hurt, my head throbbed, and I had difficulty sleeping. It was hard not to work a double shift because I was worried about who would take care of those patients if I was not there.

A successfully managed transition period begins when the graduate nurse is able to evaluate the work situation objectively and predict the actions and reactions of the staff effectively. Prioritization, conflict management, time management, and support groups (peers, preceptors, and mentors) can make a significant difference in promoting a successfully managed transition period.

Nurturing the ability to see humor in a situation may be the first step. As the graduate begins to laugh at some of the situations encountered, the tension decreases and the perception increases. It is during this critical period of recovery that conflict resolution occurs. If this resolution occurs in a positive manner, it enables the graduate nurse to grow more fully as a person. This growth also enables the graduate to meet the work expectations to a greater degree and to see that she or he has the capacity to change a situation. However, if the conflict is resolved in a less positive manner, the graduate's potential to learn and grow is limited.

Kramer (1974) described four groups of graduate nurses and the steps they took to resolve reality shock. The graduates who were considered to be most successful at adaptation were those who "made a lot of waves" within both their job setting and their professional organizations. Accordingly, they were not content with the present state of nursing but worked to effect a better system. This group of graduates was able to take worthwhile values learned during school and integrate them into the work setting. Often, they returned to school—but not too quickly. Since Kramer's original work, students are now encouraged to go back to school fairly quickly, especially with the emphasis from the Institute of Medicine (IOM) report of encouraging more advanced degrees in nursing.

RECOVERY PHASE

I am really glad that I became a nurse. Sure, there are plenty of hassles, but the opportunities are there. Now that I am more confident of my skills, I am willing to take risks to improve patient care. Just last week my head nurse, who often says jokingly, "You're a thorn in my side," appointed me to the Nursing Standards Committee. I feel really good about this recognition.

Another group limited their involvement with nursing by just putting in the usual workday. Persons in this group seldom belonged to professional organizations and cited the following reasons for working: "to provide for my family," "to buy extra things for the house," and "to support myself." Typically, this group's negative approach to conflict resolution leads to burnout, during which time the conflict is turned inward, leading to constant griping and complaining about the work setting.

> I was so happy, at first. Gee, I was able to buy my son all those toys he wanted. But things here always seem to be the same—too many patients, not enough help. I get so upset with the staff, especially the nursing assistants, and the care that is given to patients. I wonder whether I will ever get the opportunity to practice nursing as I was taught. Well, I'll hang on until my husband finishes graduate school; then I'll quit this awful job!

Another group of graduates seemed to have found their niche and were content within the hospital setting. However, their positive attitude toward the job did not extend to nursing as a profession; in fact, it was the opposite. Rather than leave the organization during conflict, these "organization nurses" would change units or shifts—anything to avoid increasing demands for professional performance.

> During those first few months as I was just getting started, I sure had a tough time. It was difficult learning how to delegate tasks to the aides and practical nurses. But now that I have started working for Dr. Travis, everything is under my control. I just might go back to school someday.

The last group of graduates frequently changed jobs. After a short-lived career in hospital nursing, this group would pirouette off to graduate school, where they could "do something else in nursing" (meaning, "I can't nurse the way I've been taught, so I might as well teach others how to do things right"). Achieving a high profile in professional nursing organizations was common for these graduates, along with seeking a safer, more idealistically structured environment in which the values learned in school prevail.

> Finally, I got so frustrated with my head nurse that I just resigned. What did she expect from a recent graduate? I couldn't do everything! Cost containment; early discharge; no time for teaching; rush, rush, rush, all the time. Well, I've made up my mind to look into going back to school to further my career.

The job expectations of the hospital administration or the employing community agency and the educational preparation of the graduate nurse are not always the same. This discrepancy is considered to be the basis of reality shock. Relationships among the staff, nursing professionalism, job satisfaction, and employee alienation were studied by Casey and colleagues (2004), Roche and colleagues (2004), and Varner and Leeds (2012). Interestingly, the issues of reality shock and role transition described by Kramer in the early 1970s are still around. We (nurses) have entered the 21st century with many of the same issues we had in the 20th century.

It might seem to you right now, after reading all of this information, that reality shock is a life-threatening situation. Be assured, it is not. However, you may experience some physical and psychological symptoms in varying degrees of intensity. For example, you may feel stressed out or have headaches, insomnia, gastrointestinal upset, or a bout of post-student blues. Just remember that it takes time to adjust to a new routine and that sometimes, even after you have gotten used to it, you still may feel overwhelmed, confused, or anxious. The good news is that there are various ways to get through this critical phase of your career while establishing a firm foundation for future professional growth and career mobility. Try the assessment exercise in Critical Thinking Box 1.2.

CRITICAL THINKING BOX 1.2

Reality Shock Inventory

All students, as well as new graduates, experience reality shock to some extent or another. The purpose of this exercise is to make you aware of how you feel about yourself and your particular life situation.

Directions: To evaluate your views and determine your self-evaluation of your particular life situation, respond to the statements with the appropriate number.

1 Strongly agree	4 Slightly disagree
2 Agree	5 Disagree
3 Slightly agree	6 Strongly disagree

1. I am still finding new challenges and interests in my work.
2. I think often about what I want from life.
3. My own personal future seems promising.
4. Nursing school and/or my work has brought stresses for which I was unprepared.
5. I would like the opportunity to start anew knowing what I know now.
6. I drink more than I should.
7. I often feel that I still belong in the place where I grew up.
8. Much of the time my mind is not as clear as it used to be.
9. I have no sense of regret concerning my major life decision of becoming a nurse.
10. My views on nursing are as positive as they ever were.
11. I have a strong sense of my own worth.
12. I am experiencing what would be called a crisis in my personal or work setting.
13. I cannot see myself as a nurse.
14. I must remain loyal to commitments even if they have not proven as rewarding as I had expected.
15. I wish I were different in many ways.
16. The way I present myself to the world is not the way I really am.
17. I often feel agitated or restless.
18. I have become more aware of my inadequacies and faults.
19. My sex life is as satisfactory as it has ever been.
20. I often think about students and/or friends who have dropped out of school or work.

To compute your score, reverse the number you assigned to statements 1, 3, 9, 10, 11, and 19. For example, 1 would become a 6, 2 would become a 5, 3 would become a 4, 4 would become a 3, 5 would become a 2, and 6 would become a 1. Total the number. The higher the score, the better your attitude. The range is 20 to 120.

Modified from White, E. (April 23, 1986). Doctoral dissertation. *Chronicle of Higher Education* (p. 28). Reprinted with permission.

What Is Transition Shock?

More recently, based on research by Duchscher (2008) building on Kramer's seminal work, the process has been redefined as *transition shock* to describe the transition experience within a contemporary health care environment and according to Wakefield (2018), "penetrates beyond professional aspects of shock" (p. 47). Duchscher and Windey (2018) identify the stages of transition as a process of "becoming" that occur within the initial 12 months of nursing practice of the new graduate nurse and involves three stages: *doing, being, and knowing.* Box 1.2 summarizes the three stages.

The healthiest role transition experiences are influenced by support both personally and professionally, stability with assigned mentor and work schedule, consistency with feedback and assignments, familiarity with skills and procedures, predictability of experiences, reinforcement of effective behaviors, and reassurance about performance and learning.

BOX 1.2   STAGES OF TRANSITION

Doing

- Occurs during the first 3–4 months post orientation.
- Feelings of being overwhelmed with practice expectations.
- Find themselves within weeks after being hired working with full patient loads (often equal to senior nurse counterparts).
- Unable to set appropriate limits or boundaries related to work responsibilities.
- Experience a steep learning curve and feel stressed about everything.
- High anxiety associated with caring for unstable patients, multitasking (e.g., answering phones), processing health care provider orders, dealing with multiple family and patient issues concurrently, providing direct care to patients.
- Fear of missing something or doing something inadvertently or unintentionally that might bring harm to the patient, due to their ignorance or inexperience.
- Stages are learning, performing, concealing, adjusting, and accommodating.

Being

- Encompasses the next 4–5 months.
- Consistent and rapid advancement in thinking, knowledge level, and skill competency.
- Confronted with the inconsistencies and inadequacies within the health care system.
- Want to be surrounded by familiarity, consistency, and predictability.
- Around 5–7 months a crisis of confidence occurs characterized by moderate anxiety related to insecurities regarding practice competency and fear of failing with their patients, colleagues, and themselves.
- Toward the end of this stage, a rejuvenated spirit awakened and provided inspiration to seek out new challenges to their thinking and to also place themselves in new and unfamiliar practice situations and plan long-term career goals.
- Stages are searching, examining, doubting, questioning, and revealing.

Knowing

- Final stage focuses achieving a separateness from established nurses around them.
- Anxiety about leaving the new graduate/learner role.
- Ability to organize and prioritize complex clinical and relational situations with increasing confidence in skills.
- By 12 months, stable level of comfort and confidence noted in roles, responsibilities, and routines.
- Stages are separating, recovering, exploring, critiquing, and accepting.

Duchscher, J. B. (2008). A process of becoming: The stages of new nursing graduate professional role transition. *Journal of Continuing Education in Nursing*, *39*(10), 441–450.

Duchscher, J. B. (2009). Transition shock: The initial stage of role adaptation for newly graduated registered nurses. *Journal of Advanced Nursing*, *65*(5), 1103–1113.

Duchscher, J. B., & Windey, M. (2018). Stages of transition and transition shock. *Journal of Nurses Professional Development, 34* (4), 228–232. doi: 10.1097/NND.0000000000000461.

ROLE TRANSFORMATION

Remember when you first started nursing school? The war stories everybody told you? The changes that occurred in your family as a result of your starting nursing school? Are you in the midst of that now, or does it seem like a long time ago? Can you really believe where you are now and where you were when you first began nursing school, those first nursing courses, and clinicals? It has taken a lot of work and sacrifice to get to where you are now. Believe it or not, you have already experienced a role transition—you successfully transitioned to a student nurse. Now, as you draw nearer to the successful completion of that experience, you are ready to embark on a new one. Take a minute to read the thoughts of one of your peers about her transition into nursing. I'm sure you will smile at her satire (Critical Thinking Box 1.3).

CRITICAL THINKING BOX 1.3

Survival Techniques From One Who Has Survived

You finally did it; you have decided nursing is what you want to do for the rest of your life. After all, who would go through all this anguish if you only wanted to do this as a pastime? If you are taking this like everyone else, you are probably going to do this by trial and error, "war" stories, or by helpful hints from the nursing staff.

You need to prioritize your time. This is a familiar and much-used term that you will hear often. It is also easier said than done. If you are single, you have an advantage—maybe. You can decide right now that single is "where it's at" and stay that way for the duration. Of course, this means literally living the "single" life. There are no "dinners-for-two," no telephone conversations, no movies at the cinema (rarely any TV)—in other words, no physical contact with the opposite sex. I know you were not thinking about it anyway, but in case you are studying anatomy and physiology, and hormonal thoughts pervade your consciousness, dismiss them.

If you are married, I am not suggesting divorce, just abstinence. Hopefully, you kissed your spouse good-bye when you came to school for your first day of class because your next chance will be on your breaks or when you graduate.

If you happen to be a parent, do as I did. I put pictures of myself in all rooms of my house when I started school so that the kids would not forget me. My children, in return, helped me by plastering their faces in my fridge (they know I'll look there) or on my mirror (another sure spot). I have acquired a son-in-law, a daughter-in-law, and five grandchildren in the past 2{1/2} years, and I usually do not recognize them if I run into them on the rare occasions when I go to the store for essentials (like food) or out to pay our utility bills. Christmas is fun, though, because each year I get to spend a few days getting to know the family again. But we all must wear name tags for the first day!

If your children are small, buy them the Fisher Price kitchen and teach them how to "cook" nourishing "hot" cereal on the stove that does not heat up. For the infant, hang a TPN (hint: Total Parental Nutrition) of Similac with iron at 40 mL/h that the baby can control by sound! Crying should do it! Instead of a needle, use a nipple....

Diapers—what would we do without those disposable diapers that stay dry for 2 weeks at a time? You can even buy the kind that you touch the waistband, and Mickey Mouse and his friends jump off to entertain your baby.

Some of you may feel guilty about not fixing those delicious meals your family once enjoyed. Do not! We get two "breaks" a year, and during that time, fix barrels of nourishing liquid (you can add a few veggies). When your family gets hungry, just take out enough to keep fluids and lytes balanced. Remind them that this is only going to last another year or two.

Have I covered everything? Oh, I forgot dust.... Dust used to bother me but not anymore. I use it to write notes to my 17-year-old, to let him know what time I am going to be in the house, so he will not mistake me for a burglar, and to say "I Love You."

On a serious note, each semester you will get regrouped with new classmates. They will become your family, your support group. You will form a chain, and everyone is a strong link. This is a group effort. These are people who will laugh with you and cry with you. You will form friendships that will last a lifetime. Take advantage of these opportunities.

On a closing note, do not listen to all the "war stories" that go around—just to the credible ones like mine!

From Beagle, B. (May/June, 1990). Survival techniques. *AD Clinical Care* (p. 17). Reprinted with permission.

Give yourself a well-deserved pat on the back for what you have accomplished thus far. It is important to learn early in your practice of nursing to take time to reflect on your accomplishments. Now, back to the present. Let's look at the current role-transition process at hand, from student to graduate nurse RN.

When Does the Role Transition to Graduate Nurse Begin?

Does the transition begin at graduation? No. It started when you began to move into the novice role while in your first nursing course (Table 1.2). According to Benner (1984, p. 20):

Beginners have no experience of the situation in which they are expected to perform. To get them into these situations and allow them to gain experience also necessary for skill development, they are taught about the situation in terms of objective attributes, such as weight, intake/output, temperature, blood pressure, pulse, and other objective, measurable parameters of a patient's conditions—features of the task world that can be recognized without situational experience.

TABLE 1.2 FROM NOVICE TO EXPERT

STAGE	CHARACTERISTICS
Novice Nursing student Experienced nurse in a new setting	• No clinical experience in situation expected to perform • Needs rules to guide performance • Experiences difficulty in applying theoretical concepts to patient care
Advanced Beginner Last-semester nursing student Graduate nurse	• Demonstrates ability to deliver marginally acceptable care • Requires previous experience in an actual situation to recognize it • Begins to understand the principles that dictate nursing interventions • Continues to concentrate on the rules and takes in minimum information regarding a situation
Competent 2–3 years' clinical experience	• Conscientious, deliberate planning • Begins to see nursing actions in light of patients' long-term plans • Demonstrates ability to cope with and manage different and unexpected situations that occur
Proficient Nurse clinicians Nursing faculty	• Ability to recognize and understand the situation as a whole • Demonstrates ability to anticipate events in a given situation • Holistic understanding enhances decision making
Expert Advanced practice nurse clinicians and faculty	• Demonstrates an understanding of the situation and is able to focus on the specific area of the problem • Operates from an in-depth understanding of the total situation • Demonstrates highly skilled analytical ability in problem solving; performance becomes masterful

Modified from Benner, P. (2001). The Dreyfus model of skill acquisition applied to nursing. In *From novice to expert* (Commemorative Edition). Menlo Park, CA: Addison-Wesley.

For example, the instructor gives the novice or student nurse specific directions on how to listen for bowel sounds. There are specific rules on how to guide their actions—rules that are very limited and fairly inflexible. Remember your first clinical nursing experiences? Your nursing instructor was your shadow for patient care. As nursing students enter a clinical area as novices, they have little understanding of the meaning and application of recently learned textbook terms and concepts. Students are not the only novices; any nurse may assume the novice role on entering a clinical setting in which he or she is not comfortable functioning or has no practical experience. Consider an experienced medical-surgical nurse who floats to the postpartum unit; she would be a little uncomfortable in that clinical setting.

By graduation, most nursing students are at the level of advanced beginner. According to Benner (1984, p. 20):

Advanced beginners are ones who can demonstrate marginally accepted performance, ones who have coped with enough real situations to note (or to have pointed out to them by a mentor) the recurring meaningful situation components....

To be able to recognize characteristics that can be identified only through experience is the signifying trait of the advanced beginner. Thus, when directed to perform the procedure of checking bowel sounds, the students at this level are learning how to discriminate bowel sounds and understand their meaning. They do not need to be told specifically how to perform the procedure.

Let's look at what you and your nursing instructors can do to promote your well-being and success during the role-transition experience. These activities reinforce your progress and movement along the continuum from advanced-beginner to competent nurse (see Table 1.2).

How Can I Prepare Myself for This Transition Process?

During the last semester of nursing school, it is very advantageous to have as much clinical experience as possible. The most productive area for experience is a general medical-surgical unit, which will have a variety of patient cases. This will help you to ground your assessment and communication skills, as well as help you to apply principles that are most often tested on the NCLEX exam. This is also the area in which you will most likely be able to obtain some much-needed experience with basic nursing skills.

Begin Increasing Independence

It is time to have your nursing instructor cut the umbilical cord and allow you to function more independently, without frequent cueing and directing during the last semester of your clinical experience.

More Realistic Patient-Care Assignments

Start taking care of increasing numbers of patients to help you with time management, prioritization, and work organization. Evaluate the nursing staff's assignments to determine what a realistic workload is for a recent graduate.

Clinical Hours That Represent Realistic Shift Hours

Obtain experience in receiving shift reports, closing charts, completing patient care, and communicating with the oncoming staff and other health care professionals involved in providing patient care.

Perform Nursing Procedures Instead of Observing

Take an inventory of your nursing skills and be sure to have this available for potential employers so they can see what skills you are familiar with. If there are nursing skills you lack or procedures you are uncomfortable with, take this opportunity while you are still in school to gain the experience. Identify your clinical objectives to meet your personal needs. Request opportunities to practice from your instructor and staff nurses. Casey and colleagues (2004) identified skills that were challenging for the graduate nurses in the first year of practice, which are currently still applicable. These skills included code blues, chest tubes, intravenous skills, central lines, blood administration, and patient controlled analgesia (PCA). Although it is important for you to be proficient and safe in performing skills, Theisen and Sandau (2013) pointed out in their review that new graduate nurses lack competency in communicating with the health care team, delegating, resolving conflict during stressful situations (i.e., end-of-life care, deteriorating patient), prioritizing patient care, and critical decision making. Make an effort to gain experience in these areas while you are still in school; you will be more comfortable in your nursing care as a graduate.

More Truth About the Real Work-Setting Experience

Identify resource people with whom you can objectively discuss the dilemmas of the workplace. Talk to graduates: Ask them what they know now that they wish they had known the last semester of school.

Look for Opportunities to Problem Solve and Practice Critical Thinking

Actively seek out learning opportunities in both the clinical and classroom setting to exercise your critical thinking skills and decision making. Now is the time to stand on your own two feet while there is still a backup—your instructor—available. Look for opportunities to communicate with the interprofessional team.

Request Constructive Feedback From Staff and Instructors

Stop avoiding evaluation and constructive criticism. Find out now how you can improve your nursing care. Ask questions and clarify anything that is not understood. Evaluate your progress on a periodic basis. The consequences may be less severe now than later with your new employer.

Request Clinical Experience in an Area or Hospital of Interest

If you have some idea of where you would like to work, it is very beneficial to have some clinical experiences in that facility the last semester of school. This gives you the opportunity to become involved with staff nurses, identify workload on the unit, and evaluate resources and support people. It also gives the employing institution an opportunity to evaluate you—Are you someone that institution would like to have work for them?

> Attitude is the latitude between success and failure.

Think Positively!

Be prepared for the reality of the workplace environment, including both its positives and negatives. You may have encountered by now the "ol' battle ax" who has a grudge against new nursing graduates.

> I do not know why you ever decided to be a nurse. Nobody respects you. It's all work, low pay. I guess as long as you've got a good back and strong legs, you'll make it. Boy, do you have a lot to learn! I wouldn't do it over again for anything!

When you find these nurses, tune them out and steer out of their way! They have their own agenda, and it does not include providing supportive assistance to you. Eventually, you will learn how to work with this type of individual (see Chapter 13), but for now you should concentrate on identifying nurses who share your philosophy and are still smiling.

> Surround yourself with nurses who have a positive attitude and are supportive in your learning and growing transition.

Another way to keep a positive perspective is to focus on the good things that have happened during the shift rather than on the frustrating events. When you feel yourself climbing onto the proverbial "pity pot," ask yourself "Who's driving this bus?" and turn it around!

Anticipate small irritations and disappointments and keep them in perspective. Do not let them mushroom into major problems. Turn disappointments and unpleasant situations into learning experiences. Once you have encountered an unpleasant situation, the next time it occurs you will recognize it sooner, anticipate the chain of events, and be better able to handle it.

> Do not major in a minor activity.

Be Flexible!

Procedures, policies, and nursing supervisors are not going to be the same as those you experienced in school. Be prepared to do things differently from the way you learned them as a student. You do not have to give up all the values you learned in school, but you will need to reexamine them in light of the reality of the workplace setting. Flexibility is one of the most important qualities of a good nurse!

School-learned ideal. Sit down with the patient before surgery, and provide preoperative teaching.

Workplace reality. One of your home care patients is receiving daily wound care for an extensive burn. You receive a message that the patient has been scheduled for grafting in the outpatient surgery department and is to be a direct admit at 6 a.m. the next morning. You have two more home visits to make: one to hang an intravenous preparation of vancomycin and the other a new hospice admission, which you know will take considerable time.

Compromise. You delegate to one of the home care practical nurses to take the preoperative teaching and admission instructions to your patient. Later on, you make a telephone call to your preoperative patient and go over the preoperative care teaching information from the home care practical nurse. You make arrangements to meet this patient at home immediately after the grafting procedure is complete.

Get Organized!

Does your personal life seem organized or chaotic, calm or frantic? Sit back and take a quick inventory of your personal life. How do you expect to get your professional life in order when your personal life is in turmoil? For some helpful tips on organizing your personal life, check out the personal management chapter (see Chapter 2).

Stay Healthy!

Have you become a "couch potato" while in school? Are you too tired, or do you lack the time to exercise when you get home from work? Candy bars during breaks, pepperoni pizza at midnight, and Twinkies PRN? How have your eating habits changed during your time in school? Your routine should include exercise, relaxation, and good nutrition. Becoming aware of the negative habits that can have detrimental effects on your state of mind and overall physical health is important in developing a healthy lifestyle.

Find a Mentor!

Negotiating this critical transition as you begin your nursing career should not be done in isolation. Evidence suggests that close support relationships, mentors, and preceptors are key, if not essential, ingredients in the career development of a successful, happy graduate (Duchscher & Windey, 2018). For additional tips on finding a mentor as you begin your professional practice, take a look at the mentoring chapter (see Chapter 3). In addition to your family and close nursing school friends, it will be important to develop professional support relationships.

Find Other New Graduates!

Frequently, several new graduates are hired at the same time. Some of them may even be your classmates. Find them and establish a peer support group. Sharing experiences and problems and knowing that someone else is experiencing the same feelings you are can be a great relief!

Have Some Fun!

Do something that makes you feel good. This is life, not a funeral service! Nursing has opportunities for laughter and for sharing life's humorous events with patients and coworkers. Surround yourself with people and friends who are lighthearted and merry and who bring those feelings out in you. Remember, the return of humor is one of the first signs of a healthy role transition. Loosen up a little bit. Go ahead, have some fun! Check out the information in Chapter 3 for more on selection of mentors and preceptors.

Know What to Expect!

Plan ahead. Plan your employment interviews; ask to talk to nurses on the units and find out how nursing care is delivered in the institution. The length of orientation, staffing patterns, opportunity for internship, areas where positions are open, and resources for new graduates are all important to establish prior to employment. This helps you know what to expect when you go to work. Work satisfaction is a positive predictor of a successful role transition during the first year (Roche, 2004). Know what is expected of you on your work unit. How can you expect to do a job correctly if you do not know what the expectations are? Learn the "rules of the road" early. This may be in the hospital, doctor's office, or community setting. While still in school, you may find it helpful to interview nurse managers to determine their perspectives on the role of the graduate nurse during the first 6 months of employment. This will give you a base of reference when you interview for your first job. How do you measure up to some of the common expectations nurse managers may be looking for in a graduate nurse?

Are you:

1. Excited and sincere about nursing?
2. Open-minded and willing to learn new ideas and skills?
3. Comfortable with your basic nursing skills?
4. Able to keep a good sense of humor?
5. Receptive to constructive feedback?
6. Able to express your thoughts and feelings?
7. Able to evaluate your performance and request assistance?
8. Comfortable talking with your patients regarding their individual needs?

What Is the Future of Role Transition?

In 2008, the Practice and Education Committee of the National Council of State Boards of Nursing (NCSBN) reported there was adequate evidence to support a regulatory model for transitioning new graduates to practice (NCSBN, 2008). The committee noted that the need for a transition regulatory model has grown from the changes occurring in health care over the past 20 years, not from deficiencies in nursing education and/or unrealistic expectations of the workplace. In the

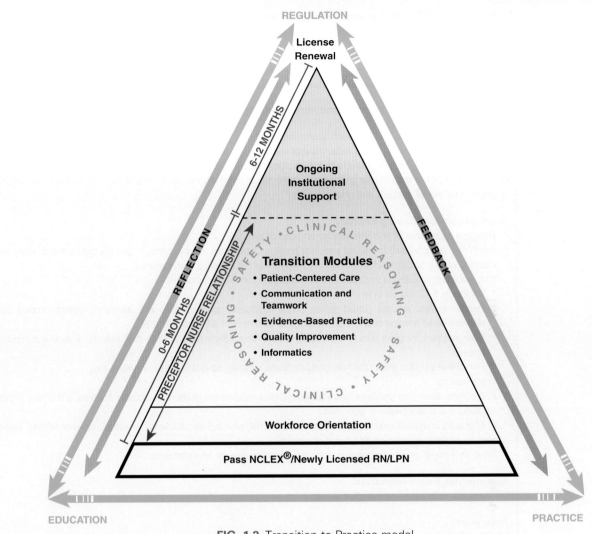

REGULATION

License
Renewal

6-12 MONTHS

Ongoing
Institutional
Support

REFLECTION

FEEDBACK

PRECEPTOR NURSE RELATIONSHIP

0-6 MONTHS

SAFETY • CLINICAL REASONING

Transition Modules
- **Patient-Centered Care**
- **Communication and Teamwork**
- **Evidence-Based Practice**
- **Quality Improvement**
- **Informatics**

CLINICAL REASONING • SAFETY • CLINICAL REASONING • SAFETY

Workforce Orientation

Pass NCLEX®/Newly Licensed RN/LPN

EDUCATION

PRACTICE

FIG. 1.2 Transition to Practice model.

report from the committee to the NCSBN, the goal for the transition to practice regulatory model is "to promote public safety by supporting newly licensed nurses in their critical entry and progression into practice" (NCSBN, 2008, p. 2). In 2009, the NCSBN finalized the design of an evidence-based "transition to practice" regulatory model (Fig. 1.2) that includes modules on communication and teamwork, patient-centered care, evidence-based practice, quality improvement, informatics, and an additional module of preceptor training.

The results from the national Transition to Practice (TTP) study in hospital settings conducted by the NCSBN have been reported (NCSBN, 2015), which addressed questions about the effectiveness of the NCSBN's TTP program and whether or not TTP programs make a difference in new graduate outcomes in terms of safety, competence, stress, job satisfaction, and retention (Research for Best Practice Box 1.2).

🔍 RESEARCH FOR BEST PRACTICE BOX 1.2

Role Transition

Practice Issue

With the increased complexity of the health care environment, new graduates struggle with the transition into clinical practice. This matter is related to several issues: sicker patients in an increasingly complex health care setting, the shortened gap between taking NCLEX and being licensed, variable transition experiences, increased patient workload due to the nursing shortage, high job stress and turnover rates in new graduate registered nurses (RNs) (approximately 25% of new nurses leave their position within the first year of practice), and practice errors.

Implications for Nursing Practice

- Transition experiences of new RNs vary across practice settings.
- Health care agencies with formalized transition programs have noted a marked drop in new graduate attrition, along with improved patient outcomes when a transition program has the following characteristics.
  - A preceptorship with the preceptor receiving education for the preceptor role.
  - Program is 9–12 months in length.
  - Program content includes patient safety, clinical reasoning, communication and teamwork, patient-centered care, evidence-based practice, quality improvement, and informatics (QSEN competencies).
  - New graduates are given time to learn, apply content, obtain feedback, and share their reflections about the transition process.
  - Programs are customized so the new graduate learns specialty content in the areas where they are working.
- At 6 months, when new graduates typically become more independent, there is an increase in errors, a decrease in job satisfaction, and an increase in work stress.
- At 12 months in practice, work stress and reported errors decrease and job satisfaction increases; research findings support need for ongoing support during first year of practice.
- The 6- to 9-month period of practice is the most vulnerable time for new graduates.

Considering This Information

What can you do to ease your transition process?

References

NCSBN. (2018). *Transition to practice.* Retrieved from https://www.ncsbn.org/transition-to-practice.htm.

Spector, N. (2015c). The National Council of State Boards of Nursing's transition to practice study: Implications for educators. *Journal of Nursing Education, 54*(3), 119–120. https://doi.org/10.3928/01484834-20150217-13.

Spector, N., Blegen, M. A., Silvestre, J., Barnsteiner, J., Lynn, M. R., Ulrich, B., et al. (2015a). *Transition to practice study in hospital settings.* Retrieved from https://www.ncsbn.org/Spector_Transition_to_Practice_Study_in_Hospital_Settings.pdf.

What is happening in your state regarding the Transition to Practice model?

The TTP model recommends a 9- to 12-month internship, so the new graduate receives continued support during the vulnerable period from 6 to 9 months. For the transition process to be effective, it should occur across all settings and at all education levels. This would include both the RN and the LPN/LVN. To promote safer nursing practice through a regulatory transition period, practice, education, and regulation all must work together on the development of a model that will effectively support the new nurse in his or her transition to safe practice (Spector, 2015c; Spector et al., 2015b).

The NCSBN Learning Extension (2017) offers an e-learning transition to practice course based on the NCSBN's evidence-based comprehensive research study, "Transition to Practice" that incorporates the recommendations from the Quality and Safety Education for Nurses (QSEN) project and the IOM. The program consists of five courses for new graduate nurses on the topics of communication and teamwork, patient- and family-centered care, evidence-based practice, quality improvement, and informatics, along with a preceptor course. It is a 6-month online program, which requires only 1 h/week of coursework with continuing education credit provided upon completion.

In response to the 2010 IOM report, the Robert Wood Johnson Foundation has developed the Initiative on the Future of Nursing (2011) to address the IOM recommendations for the nursing profession. One recommendation is to implement nurse residency programs for new graduate nurses to acquire skills and develop competency as nurses in providing care to today's complex and diverse health care population. Since the IOM report, state boards of nursing, nursing education programs, and health care institutions have joined together and developed nurse residency programs to prepare the future nurse—that's you! For additional resources and research on nurse residency programs, check out the mentoring, preceptorship, and nurse residency program chapter (see Chapter 3).

CONCLUSION

What will be the direction for role transition of graduate nurses? Has your state adopted the Transition to Practice model? How will preceptors be selected, and will they be credentialed? As you progress through the chapters in this book, you will find references to the IOM, The Joint Commission (TJC), and other health care resources concerned with the safety of patients, the reduction of errors, the economic impact of errors, retention of nurses, and cost of health care. These are key players and important considerations in the new nurse's transition to safe nursing practice.

As you progress through your own personal transition into nursing practice, the "rules of the road" for transition can be likened to traffic signs (Fig. 1.3). Check out the following signs that will help you to direct your transition experience. Fig. 1.4 gives additional advice from graduates who have successfully made the transition.

Look for the humor in each day, and take time to laugh. You will be surprised by how good it makes you feel!

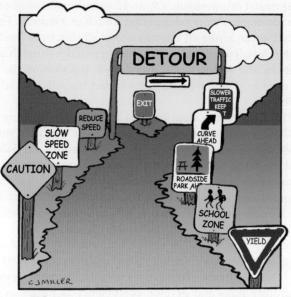

FIG. 1.3 "Rules of the road" for transition.

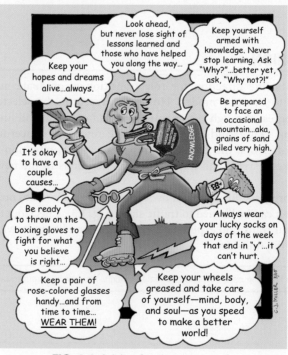

FIG. 1.4 Advice for the new grad.

RULES OF THE ROAD

 Stop. Take care of yourself. Take time to plan your transition. Get involved with other recent graduates; they can help you. Do not be afraid to ask questions, and do not be afraid to ask for help.

 Detour. You will make mistakes. Recognize them, learn from them, and put them in the past as you move forward. Regardless of how well you plan for change, there are always detours ahead. Detours take you on an alternate route. They can be scenic, swampy, or desolate, or they can bog you down in heavy traffic. Do not forget to look for the positive aspects—the detour may open your eyes to new horizons and new career directions.

 Curve ahead. Get your personal life in order. Anticipate changes in your schedule. Be adaptable, because the transition process is not predictable.

 Yield. You do not always have to be right. Consider alternatives and make compromises within your value system.

 Resume speed. Maintain a positive attitude. As you gain experience, you will become better organized and begin to really enjoy nursing. Be aware; sometimes as you resume speed, you may be experiencing another role transition as your career moves in a different direction.

Exit. Pay attention to your road signs; do not take an exit you do not really want. Before you exit your job, critically evaluate the job situation. "Look before you leap" by making sure the change will improve your work situation.

Slow traffic, keep right. You may be more comfortable in the slower traffic lane with respect to your career direction. Take all the time you need; it is okay for each person to travel at a different speed. Do not get run over in the fast lane.

School zone. Plan for continuing education, whether it is an advanced degree program or one to maintain your clinical skills or license. Allow yourself sufficient time in your new job before you jump back into the role of full-time student.

 Slow speed zone. Take time to get organized before you resume full speed! Have a daily organizational sheet that fits your needs and works for you both in your job and your personal life.

 Caution. Do not commit to anything with which you are not professionally or personally comfortable. Think before you act. Do not react. Do not panic. If in doubt, check with another nurse.

Roadside park ahead. Take a break, whether it is 15 minutes or 30 minutes a day to indulge yourself, or a week to do something you really want to do.

⊕ RELEVANT WEBSITES AND ONLINE RESOURCES

Commission on Collegiate Nursing Education (CCNE)
Accredited Nurse Residency Programs. http://www.aacnnursing.org/Portals/42/CCNE/PDF/CCNE-Accredited-Nurse-Residency-Programs.pdf

NCSBN
Transition to Practice. https://www.ncsbn.org/transition-to-practice.htm

NCSBN Learning Extension
Transition to Practice Online Program. https://ww2.learningext.com/newnurses.htm

BIBLIOGRAPHY

Beecroft, P. C., Dorey, F., & Wenten, M. (2008). Turnover intention in new graduate nurses: A multivariate analysis. *Journal of Advanced Nursing, 62*, 41–52. https://doi.org/10.1111/j.1365-2648.2007.04570.x.

Benner, P. (2001; 1984). *From novice to expert.* Menlo Park, CA: Addison-Wesley; Commemorative edition, Upper Saddle River, NJ: Prentice-Hall.

Berkow, S., Virkstis, K., Stewart, J., & Conway, L. (2008). Assessing new graduate nurse performance. *Journal of Nursing Administration, 38*(11), 468–474. https://doi.org/10.1097/01.NNA.0000339477.50219.06.

Candela, L., & Bowles, C. (2008). Recent RN graduate perceptions of educational preparation. *Nursing Education Perspectives, 29*, 266–271.

Casey, K., et al. (2004). The graduate nurse experience. *Journal of Nursing Administration, 34*(6), 303–311.

Duchscher, J. B. (2008). A process of becoming: The stages of new nursing graduate professional role transition. *Journal of Continuing Education in Nursing, 39*(10), 441–450.

Duchscher, J. B. (2009). Transition shock: The initial stage of role adaptation for newly graduated Registered Nurses. *Journal of Advanced Nursing, 65*(5), 1103–1113.

Duchscher, J. B., & Windey, M. (2018). Stages of transition and transition shock. *Journal of Nurses Professional Development, 34*(4), 228–232. https://doi.org/10.1097/NND.0000000000000461.

Institute of Medicine of the National Academies. (2011). *The future of nursing: Leading change, advancing health.* Retrieved from http://www.nap.edu/catalog/12956/the-future-of-nursing-leading-change-advancing-health.

Kramer, M. (1974). *Reality shock.* St. Louis, MO: Mosby.

Kramer, M., & Schmalenberg, C. (1977). *Path to biculturalism.* Rockville, MD: Aspen.

Lavoie-Tremblay, M., et al. (2002). How to facilitate the orientation of new nurses into the workplace. *Journal for Nurses in Staff Development, 18*(2), 80–85.

National Council of State Boards of Nursing (NCSBN). (2008). *NCSBN transition to practice report.* Retrieved from https://www.ncsbn.org/3924.htm.

NCSBN. (2013). *Outline of NCSBN's transition to practice modules.* Retrieved from https://www.ncsbn.org/2013_TransitiontoPractice_Modules.pdf.

NCSBN Learning Extension. (2017). *Transition to practice program.* Retrieved from https://learningext.com/new-nurses/.

Newton, J. M., & McKenna, L. (2007). The transitional journey through the graduate year: A focus group study. *International Journal of Nursing Studies, 44*(7), 1231–1237. https://doi.org/10.1016/j.ijnurstu.2006.05.017.

Oermann, M. H., Alvarez, M., O'Sullivan, R., & Foster, B. (2010). Performance, satisfaction, and transition into practice of graduates of accelerated nursing programs. *Journal for Nurses in Staff Development, 26*(5), 192–199. https://doi.org/10.1097/NND.0b013e31819b5c3a.

Robert Wood Johnson Foundation. (2011). *Value of nursing education and nurse residency programs.* Retrieved from http://campaignforaction.org/resource/value-nurse-education-and-residency-programs.

Roche, J., Lamoureux, E., & Teehan, T. (2004). A partnership between nursing education and practice. *Journal of Nursing Administration, 34*(1), 26–32.

Schumacher, K. L., & Meleis, A. I. (1994). Transitions: A central concept in nursing. *Image*, *26*, 119–127.

Spector, N., Blegen, M. A., Silvestre, J., Barnsteiner, J., Lynn, M. R., Ulrich, B., et al. (2015a). Transition to practice study in hospital settings. *Journal of Nursing Regulation*, *5*(4), 24–38. Retrieved from https://www.ncsbn.org/Spector_Transition_to_Practice_Study_in_Hospital_Settings.pdf.

Spector, N., Blegen, M. A., Silvestre, J., Barnsteiner, J., Lynn, M. R., & Ulrich, B. (2015b). Transition to practice study in nonhospital settings. *Journal of Nursing Regulation*, *6*(1), 4–13. https://doi.org/10.1016/S2155-8256(15)30003-X. Retrieved from https://www.ncsbn.org/Spector_2015.pdf.

Spector, N. (2015c). The National Council of State Boards of Nursing's transition to practice study: Implications for educators. *Journal of Nursing Education*, *54*(3), 119–120. https://doi.org/10.3928/01484834-20150217-13.

Steinmiller, E., Levonian, C., & Lengetti, E. (2003). Rx for success. *American Journal of Nursing*, *103*(11), 64A–66A.

Theisen, J., & Sandau, K. (2013). Competency of new graduate nurses: A review of their weaknesses and strategies for success. *Journal of Continuing Education in Nursing*, *44*(9), 406–414. https://doi.org/10.3928/00220124-20130617-38.

Varner, K. D., & Leeds, R. A. (2012). Transition within a graduate nurse residency program. *Journal of Continuing Education in Nursing*, *43*(11), 491–499.

2

Personal Management
Time and Self-Care Strategies

JoAnn Zerwekh, EdD, RN

ⓔ http://evolve.elsevier.com/Zerwekh/nsgtoday/.

Gain control of your time, and you will gain control of your life
Anonymous

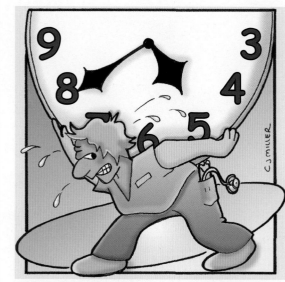

Is time managing you, or are you managing time?

After completing this chapter, you should be able to:
- Identify your individual time style and personal time-management strategies.
- Discuss strategies that increase organizational skills and personal priority setting.
- Describe early signs of compassion fatigue and burnout.
- Describe how compassion fatigue and burnout affect nurses.
- Discuss the importance of caring for yourself.
- Identify strategies for self-care.

There are so many activities that individuals need to accomplish at any one time that deciding "how to get it all done" and "what to do when" is a daily challenge—one that can sometimes be overwhelming. Nursing school complicates the daily routine. This relentless competition for our attention is described by the term *timelock* (Keyes, 1991).

MANAGING YOUR TIME

Regrettably, there is no way to alter the minutes in an hour or the hours in a day. Although we cannot create more actual time, we can alter how we use the time we have available. Employers of new graduates have identified lack of organizational and time-management skills as areas in which new nurses frequently need the most improvement and assistance. The methods and strategies identified by time-management experts can help you cope with timelock.

This section introduces you to the principles of effective time management. You will learn how to gain control of your time, increase your organizational skills, and reduce wasted time to your advantage. You will learn strategies for using those newly acquired hours to achieve your personal and professional goals.

Balance Is the Key

Making time to meet your individual, family, and professional needs and goals is vital to your overall success. If you neglect your health maintenance needs, completing school may be jeopardized. Integrating the principles of time management into your daily life can help you achieve both your personal and professional goals.

What Are Your Biological Rhythms, and How Do You Use Them?

Individuals have different biorhythms that affect their energy levels during the day and can even vary from season to season. Rest and sleep are essential for optimal health and emotional and physical responsiveness.

> Whenever possible, schedule difficult activities when you are most productive.

When possible, get 8 solid hours of sleep. Maintaining a regular sleep-wake rhythm (circadian rhythm) with adequate hours of sleep has both physiological and psychological restorative effects. Disruption of this rhythm causes chronic fatigue and decreases one's coping abilities and performance. Factors affecting rest and sleep include anxiety, work schedules, diet, and the use of caffeine, alcohol, and nicotine.

Fatigue, which can lead to impaired decision making, can occur with changes in the circadian rhythm and sleep deprivation. Physiological, psychological, and emotional problems have also been correlated to sleep deprivation; these include ischemic disease, increased peptic ulcers, indigestion, increased susceptibility to viral and bacterial infections, weight gain, sleep disturbances, and mood disorders. Therefore, if situations occur that interfere with your normal circadian rhythm, it is important to take measures to prevent these possible complications. Self-care tips to prevent complications caused by interferences in the normal circadian rhythm are presented in Box 2.1. Try these strategies, tossing out those that do not work for you.

> Engage in a relaxing activity 1 h before going to bed; for example, take a warm bath, read an interesting novel, or learn to initiate progressive relaxation techniques.

BOX 2.1   SELF-CARE TIPS WHEN CIRCADIAN RHYTHMS ARE DISRUPTED

- Reserve the bedroom for sleeping.
- Avoid watching television or using the computer while in bed.
- Leave your stressors at the door and pamper yourself just before sleeping by reading; stretching; meditating; or taking a warm, scented bath.
- Establish and maintain a consistent bedtime routine.
- Decrease noise or create "white noise" in the bedroom (e.g., use a bedroom fan).
- Charge or place your smartphone or mobile device in another room.
- Sleep with earplugs.
- Darken and cool down your sleeping environment.
- Use eye shields.
- Maintain a diet high in protein and low in carbohydrates to support your immune system.

What Is Meant by Right- and Left-Brain Dominance, and Where Is My Brain?

People think about and manage time differently, depending on their characteristic brain dominance—left, right, or both (Fig. 2.1).

Left-brain–dominant people process information and approach time in a linear, sequential manner. Their thinking structures time by minutes and hours. They tend to schedule activities in time segments and perform them in an ordered sequence. Left-brain–dominant people like to know the rules and play by them. They are usually able to meet their goals, but if this behavior is carried to an extreme, the individual is in danger of overwork at the expense of creative, artistic, and relaxing activities.

Right-brain–dominant people resist rules and schedules. They prefer to look at a project as a whole and to complete it in their own way and time. These are creative, flexible thinkers. However, if their behaviors are taken to an extreme, they can fail to meet needed completion times, which can induce guilt.

Some people are neither left-brain–dominant nor right-brain–dominant; hence they are more mixed in their behaviors. In fact, everyone uses both sides of the brain to some extent, thus tapping into the benefits of the brain's full capacities. The use of lists and calendars engages the left brain, whereas techniques such as the use of colored folders and whimsical office supplies helps individuals to use right-brain holistic thinking to solve problems.

Which Are You?

(Check out the Hemispheric Dominance Inventory at http://capone.mtsu.edu/studskl/hd/learn.html.)
1. I am left-brain–dominant.
2. I am right-brain–dominant.
3. I am left-brain–dominant and right-brain–dominant.

In addition to assessing your own dominant time style, it is helpful to be aware of the time styles of the people with whom you live and work. Rigid rules on a right-brain–dominant person will lead to increased resistance and frustration for everyone. Better to assign tasks such as cleanup of the kitchen or utility room to be completed by a specific time and inform them of the consequences of its not being done. It would be appropriate to have some right-brain–dominant persons on the recruitment and retention committee and some left-brain–dominant persons on the policy and procedures committee.

Knowing your time style can help you maximize your strengths and modify your weaknesses. Individual time styles can be modified, but it is wasted energy to fight or work against natural inclination.

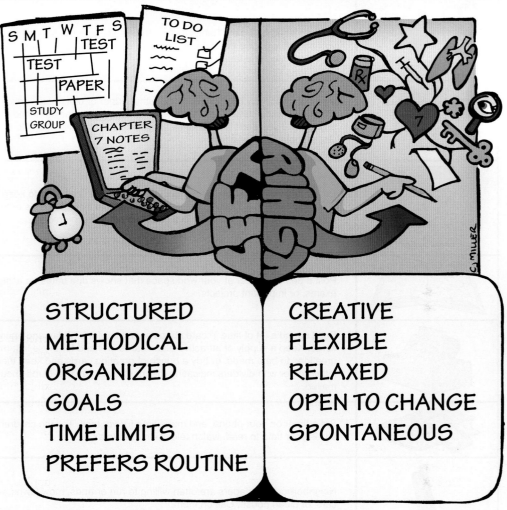

FIG. 2.1 Are you right- or left-brain–dominant?

After you are aware of your time style, you can begin to create more time for what you want to do and need to do by increasing your organizational skills.

How Can I Manage My Physical Environment?

A place for everything, and everything in its place.

Organizing and maintaining your physical environment at home, school, and work can dramatically reduce hours of time and the emotional frustration associated with "looking for stuff" (Fig. 2.2).

At home, set up a specific work area for such things as school supplies, papers, and books. A separate area or corner should be established where you can pay bills, send letters, order

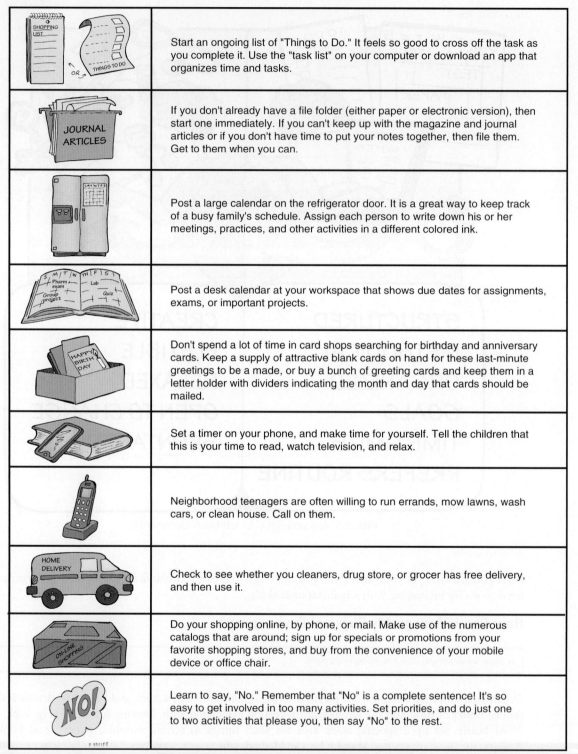

	Start an ongoing list of "Things to Do." It feels so good to cross off the task as you complete it. Use the "task list" on your computer or download an app that organizes time and tasks.
	If you don't already have a file folder (either paper or electronic version), then start one immediately. If you can't keep up with the magazine and journal articles or if you don't have time to put your notes together, then file them. Get to them when you can.
	Post a large calendar on the refrigerator door. It is a great way to keep track of a busy family's schedule. Assign each person to write down his or her meetings, practices, and other activities in a different colored ink.
	Post a desk calendar at your workspace that shows due dates for assignments, exams, or important projects.
	Don't spend a lot of time in card shops searching for birthday and anniversary cards. Keep a supply of attractive blank cards on hand for these last-minute greetings to be a made, or buy a bunch of greeting cards and keep them in a letter holder with dividers indicating the month and day that cards should be mailed.
	Set a timer on your phone, and make time for yourself. Tell the children that this is your time to read, watch television, and relax.
	Neighborhood teenagers are often willing to run errands, mow lawns, wash cars, or clean house. Call on them.
	Check to see whether you cleaners, drug store, or grocer has free delivery, and then use it.
	Do your shopping online, by phone, or mail. Make use of the numerous catalogs that are around; sign up for specials or promotions from your favorite shopping stores, and buy from the convenience of your mobile device or office chair.
	Learn to say, "No." Remember that "No" is a complete sentence! It's so easy to get involved in too many activities. Set priorities, and do just one to two activities that please you, then say "No" to the rest.

FIG. 2.2 Ten suggestions for organizing yourself.

take-out food, and take care of other household chores. When studying or working on major projects, find a space that provides a comfortable, but not too cozy, area. This space should have adequate lighting and be as free from distractions as possible. If you are studying, break your time into 50-minute segments followed by 10-minute breaks. Before beginning each study session, gather the appropriate tools—textbooks, paper, pens, highlighters, laptop, smartphone or handheld device, and reference material—to avoid wasting time searching for these items after you begin your work.

Compartmentalize
Place pens, notebooks, your smartphone or handheld device, or other reference materials in a designated holder or in a specific area of your workstation for quick access.

Color-Code
Do this for your files, keys, and whatever you can. Office supply stores are good sources of color-coded items. For example, color-coding keys with a plastic cover enables you immediately to pick out your car key or house key.

Convenience
Move and keep frequently used items nearest to where they are used.

Declutter the Clutter
At work, as well as at home, regularly clear your study and work areas.

What About All the Paperwork and/or Electronic Requests—How Can I Manage It?
Handling each piece of paper or electronic request only one time is a great time saver. Whenever possible, spend 30 seconds filing important information in the appropriate folder. This technique can save you time when you need the information again. Five ways to handle paper and electronic requests are as follows. Read each item, and then:
1. File it.
2. Forward it.
3. Respond to it—on the same sheet if possible.
4. Delegate it.
5. Discard it.

> One time-management principle is, "Don't agonize. Organize!"

What About Managing the Telephone?
Polite comments at the beginning and end of a telephone conversation are necessary to maintain positive interpersonal communications. However, when time limits are necessary, focus the conversation on the business at hand. Some possible phrases to move things along include "How can I help you?" or "I called to ...". To end the conversation, summarize the actions to be followed through: "I understand. I am to find out about ... and get back to you by the end of the week. Thanks for calling." Professional courtesy demands that you turn off your cellular phone while at work, in the classroom, during clinical rotation, and while attending a workshop.

Allocate a specific time during the day for business- or school-related telephone calls. Plan these calls by identifying key points that need to be discussed during the conversation. If you need to leave a message, provide enough detail, with the time and date, and a time when the individual can contact you. When making a call, (1) introduce yourself and your business or relationship to the individual; (2) relax—speak as if the individual is sitting in the room beside you; (3) smile—smiling will modify the tone of your voice; (4) keep the conversation short and to the point; and (5) summarize the conversation, review any action items, and thank the individual for his or her time.

Having conversations to maintain friendships, to touch base with a relative, to relax yourself, to vent your emotions, or to serve similar social purposes can be combined with routine housekeeping duties. Who has not swept the floor, put away dishes, sorted mail, or cleaned out a drawer while chatting with a friend?

What About All That E-Mail, Texting, or Social Media?

Restrict work- or school-related communications to one account, with another account designated for personal use. Turn off the notification chime and set aside a specific time during the day to read and answer your e-mail or texts instead of answering each one as it arrives. This could be the first task in the morning while you are enjoying your coffee. Do not let e-mail pile up in your inbox. Read it, answer it, and, if important, transfer it to a designated folder. Activate the junk e-mail function on your computer or read the subject line, determine whether a message is "junk," and delete it without even taking the time to read it. Your e-mail program may have parameters that allow you to designate specific messages to be sent directly into a special file. This helps move information out of the inbox and keeps you organized. Spend some time investigating the various features of your e-mail. Use your e-mail to your best advantage, because e-mail can become your best friend in terms of helping you organize your messages in folders. Specific tips for effective use of e-mail are provided in Box 2.2.

When communicating with your instructor by e-mail, be sure that you include your class number or title in the subject line. Many instructors manage their e-mail by sorting messages according to class, so a standardized subject line saves your instructor time. Identify yourself in the e-mail, and be sure to include a signature line with your contact information.

> Use your delete key aggressively and eliminate junk e-mail without reading it.

BOX 2.2   TIPS FOR EFFECTIVE ELECTRONIC COMMUNICATION

- Turn off those constant alerts and reminders.
- Check e-mail and texts at a specific time rather than constant monitoring.
- Take control—access an app that pushes messages at a designated time or explore features available through your current system that allow you to manage your inbox.
- Before sending, texting, or posting (committing)—THINK—could what you say be misinterpreted? Could it result in a misunderstanding?
- If it is in writing, you are accountable.
- Communication through electronic media (e-mail, texting) is not necessarily confidential.
- Use the "SUBJECT" line when appropriate.
- Proofread before you send or post.
- Follow the same principles of courtesy as you expect in face-to-face communication.
- Respect others' time and bandwidth.
- Keep flaming responses under control.
- Send responses to appropriate individuals only.
- Be brief, and always close with a farewell.
- Social media can drain your time—be aware of "friends" who are negative.

TABLE 2.1 **WEEKLY PERSONAL CALENDAR**				
MONDAY	**TUESDAY**	**WEDNESDAY**	**THURSDAY**	**FRIDAY**
Cleaners 9 a.m. workout	Pick up health insurance forms 3:30 p.m. carpool	4 p.m. workout 5:30 p.m. T-ball practice	4–7 p.m. Professional organization meeting	9 a.m. workout

How Can I Manage My Time?

Time management is a skill and involves planning and practice. Multiple time-management worksheets are available to assist in completing a personal analysis of your time. For example, the website *Mind Tools: Essential Skills for an Excellent Career* at http://www.mindtools.com/index.html provides multiple tools, worksheets, and strategies to assist in developing and refining time-management skills.

Calendars are available to schedule to-do activities by the month, week, and day. You gain control of your life by completing a schedule (Table 2.1). Scheduling provides you with a method to allocate time for specific tasks and is a constant reminder of your tasks, due dates, and deadlines. Schedule only what can realistically be accomplished and leave extra time before and after every major activity. Tasks, meetings, and travel can take longer than anticipated, so give yourself some time to transition from one project to another. Schedule personal time in your calendar. If someone wants to meet with you during this time, just say, "Thank you for the invite; however, I've got an important appointment. When would be another convenient time?" Or ask, "Could we meet tomorrow afternoon?" Color-code your appointments according to priorities or specific roles to stimulate the right side of your brain.

> Leave white space (nothing) in your schedule so you will have time for yourself and family, or schedule uninterruptible time for both.

At the beginning of each week, review the week's activities to avoid unexpected "surprises." Over-scheduling of more tasks than any human being can do in a single day inevitably leads to frustration. Build in some flexibility. It will not always be possible to follow your schedule exactly. However, when you do get "derailed," having a plan will help you get back on track with minimal time and effort (Critical Thinking Box 2.1).

? CRITICAL THINKING BOX 2.1

> Develop your time calendar—will it be a week-at-a-glance or a month-at-a-glance? Think about what works the best for you.

> Strategy: Leave some extra time before and after every major event to allow for transition.

MANAGING TASKS

How Do I Deal With Procrastination?

Everyone procrastinates, especially when a task is unpleasant, overwhelming, or cannot be done perfectly. Procrastination can lead to last-minute rushes that cause unnecessary stress. The time spent stressing about doing something takes more time than actually doing it! The anticipation itself can also be worse than the actuality, draining your energy and accomplishment. Alternatively, procrastination can lead to multitasking, which can impact your ability to give 100% of your attention to a task or project. Mokhtari, Delello, and Reichard (2015) surveyed college students by asking them if multitasking interfered with their ability to focus on their academic studies and guess what—multitasking was reported as a distractor to their learning. Considering this, here are some tips for preventing procrastination.

Consider the Consequences

Ask yourself what will happen if you do something and what will happen if you do not. If there are no negative outcomes of not doing something, there is no point in spending time doing it. You can eliminate that activity!

> If something will happen because you don't do it, then, of course, you need to get started.

The Earlier, the Better

Most projects take longer than planned, and glitches happen—for example, coffee spills all over your study notes the night before the test, your computer crashes, or your dog eats your notebook. To compensate for the inevitable delays and to avoid crises, start in advance and plan for your project to take three times longer than you think. Be realistic and use your common sense in scheduling this time frame.

> Schedule times to work on your project and track your progress on a calendar.

"By the Inch, It's a Cinch"

Break projects into small, manageable pieces; gather all the resources required to finish the project; and plan to do only the first step initially. For example, to study for a test, first collect all the related notes and books in one place. Next, review the subjects likely to be tested. If you are having difficulty getting started, plan to work on these steps for only 5 to 10 minutes. (Anybody can do just about anything for 5 to 10 minutes, eh?) Frequently, this will create enough momentum to get you going. When you have to stop, leave yourself a note regarding what the next steps should be. Here are some hints for effective studying.

1. Study difficult subjects or concepts first.
2. Study in short "chunks" of 50 minutes each.
3. Take a brief 10-minute break after every 50 minutes of studying.
4. Schedule study time when you are at your best (be aware of your internal clock).
5. Use waiting times. (Compile and carry 3 × 5 note cards or use Notes on your cell phone to organize critical information that you can review wherever you go—even when you are standing in that long line at the checkout counter.)
6. Keep a calendar for the semester that includes all of your assignments, tests, and papers. Use a different color for entering deadlines for each course.
7. Make a weekly to-do list. Prioritize this list and cross off each task as you complete it.
8. Before beginning a project, know what you are doing. Determine the goals, benefits, costs, and timetable for the endeavor. If you are working in a group, at the beginning of the project, make sure everyone understands his or her responsibilities. You should also designate someone to be in charge

of organizing group meetings. Leave time during the project for unexpected delays and to revisit and modify your goals. Be flexible.

If you are taking an online or web-enhanced course, remember these courses take as much, if not more time, than traditional face-to-face classes.

Here are some hints to assist with your time management related to online courses:

1. Print the syllabus, and place deadlines on your calendar before the first course meeting.
2. Identify how to contact your instructor, and schedule online office hours in your calendar.
3. Schedule daily times for logging into the class website.
4. Schedule a time for class work and select a specific site.
5. Cultivate collegial support groups with individuals who provide support and are good listeners.
6. Form an online or face-to-face study group with one or two peers. In your study group, make sure that all members are involved and your expectations for the study group align with your peers. One way to maximize a study group session is to come prepared to "teach" a section of the class material to your study group. Do not waste time reviewing your notes in the study group—you can do this by yourself.
7. Be active in the course by participating appropriately in discussion groups.
8. Establish an evidence-based file to download important articles (pdf format).
9. Bookmark websites (but before bookmarking these, review the information—don't assume all sites are up-to-date and evidence-based).
10. There are online sites that offer online storage and retrieval of documents and files. Check out the following links for more information on storing files via the Internet: www.justcloud.com, www.icloud.com, www.google.com/drive, and www.dropbox.com.

Reward Yourself

Bribing yourself with a reward can help you get started and keep going: "If I concentrate well for 1 hour on reading the assigned chapter, then I can watch my favorite television show guilt-free." Often, the stress reduction that comes from working on the project that has been put off is a reward in itself (Critical Thinking Box 2.2).

? CRITICAL THINKING BOX 2.2

What do you do to reward yourself for a job done well?

Schedule a time for celebration and self-reward with all of your projects.

Avoid the Myth of Perfection

Many of us were brought up with the well-intentioned philosophy that "Anything worth doing is worth doing well." Unfortunately, this is often interpreted as "Anything worth doing is worth doing *perfectly*." The fear of not doing something well enough or perfectly also feeds the tendency to procrastinate.

Certainly, everyone needs to make the best effort possible, but not everything needs to be done perfectly. Consider what the expected standard is—not the standard of perfection possible—and how you can meet it with a minimum amount of time and effort. Effective procrastination (i.e., pro-crastination that is used appropriately) is recognizing when a task should be purposefully postponed. This technique is a conscious decision and is used when time is needed to accomplish a task with a higher priority. Priority setting, delegating tasks when possible, eliminating wasted time by avoiding excessive social telephone calls, breaking tasks into separate small steps, and establishing realistic short-term goals are some additional strategies for managing procrastination.

MANAGING OTHERS

Communicating and getting along with other people can be challenging. Most people are supportive and easy to be with. They add to your energy and ability to function effectively, and they contribute to your goal attainment. However, some individuals drain energy from you and jeopardize organizational accomplishment through their whining, criticizing, negative thinking, chronic lateness, poor crisis management, overdependency, aggression, and similar unproductive behaviors. Avoid those individuals both online (through social media, texting, and e-mail) and in person. Occasional exhibitions of such behavior in relation to a personal crisis can be understood. Even in the best of human relationships, conflict and extreme emotions are inevitable. However, when people use these behaviors as their everyday *modus operandi* (method of operating), they interfere with attainment of individual and organizational goals. To protect your time and achieve your goals, it may be necessary to limit your time with such individuals. Learning to say "no" and practicing assertive communication can help as well. Chapters 12 and 13 provide assistance in learning these communication skills. Box 2.3 provides some hints for managing others.

What About Delegation and Time Management?

You do not have to handle everything personally. Use your delegation skills at home to identify tasks and activities that can be completed by others, leaving you more time to study and concentrate on important projects. The website *Mind Tools: Essential Skills for an Excellent Career*, at http://www.mindtools.com/index.html, provides multiple strategies related to delegation and a delegation worksheet to assist in determining whether a task can be delegated and to whom (see Chapter 14).

BOX 2.3   TIPS FOR MANAGING TIME AND MANAGING OTHERS

- Analyze how you spend your time.
- Maintain a "to-do" list.
- Organize material into files.
- Use an activity planner or calendar (paper copy or on your smartphone)—review it daily.
- Prioritize your activities.
- Make use of "mini" or waiting-time periods.
- AVOID PERFECTIONISM.
- Take "mini" vacations such as walk or do a load of laundry throughout the day to refresh your brain.
- Be aware of your internal clock—do critical tasks when you are most alert.
- Minimize the time spent with individuals who constantly complain and criticize.
- Use assertive communication with individuals with whom you are having a problem.
- Develop rituals (such as changing clothes) when you get home that say "I'm off duty."
- Avoid always saying yes. Before agreeing, take a deep breath—think about the real expectation of the project.
- Delegate when appropriate.
- Use technology.
- Don't let your e-mail, social media, and cell phone manage you and your time.
- Recognize "multitasking" as an excuse for "poor planning"—no one can do multiple tasks successfully and exceptionally.

MANAGING YOUR GOALS

Goals are the incremental steps required to achieve long-term success. Personal and professional goals are critical to lifestyle management. Keeping your goals in mind enables you to plan and perform activities that contribute to your goals and eliminate or reduce those that do not. Be realistic when setting your goals: allow enough time to complete them appropriately. Activities that contribute to goals are your high-payoff, high-priority activities; those that do not are low-payoff, low-priority activities. Your goals should be demanding enough that completion provides a feeling of satisfaction.

Many goal-directed activities need to be scheduled with completion times. This is sometimes called *deadlining* the to-do list. All kinds of calendars are available to schedule to-do activities by the month, week, and day. There are organizer apps available for your smartphone (check out www.rememberthemilk.com). It is also easy to make your own forms. Knowing your goals and priorities promotes flexible rescheduling, resulting in more effective time management and successful accomplishment.

Begin by Listing

It will be helpful to list all your goal-related activities on a master to-do list. Using all of the features of Microsoft Outlook by identifying tasks in the e-mail and/or calendar program and setting up reminders will be helpful for both tasks that are listed and tasks based on e-mails received or sent (e.g., assignments). Cross out items on your to-do list, your cards, and your schedule as you do them. This will give you immediate, positive feedback—an instant reward for your efforts and progress. When the inevitable interruptions occur, scan the to-do list and reevaluate your priorities in relation to your remaining time.

> Reward yourself as you cross out items on your to-do list.

Prioritize With the ABCD System

Other people are constantly demanding your time and energy; therefore you need to establish priorities but also be flexible. Being flexible will allow you to change your priorities throughout the day as situations change. In addition, as you work, always try to combine activities (multitask) or delegate tasks in an effort to manage your time appropriately.

Scan your to-do list and decide which are A, B, C, or D items (Box 2.4). The activities that are most closely related to your goals are the high-payoff ones; these are A priorities. Effective use of your time-management skills demands that you focus most of your energy on A-priority items. List these according to the urgency

---

BOX 2.4 PRIORITIZATION USING THE ABCD SYSTEM

A Absolute (immediate priority)—do it now or as soon as possible
B Better (as soon as possible)—necessary, but it can be done later
C Can wait until later—or when you get around to it
D Don't worry about it—let someone else take care of it
    OR ... the 4 **D**s
    Do it.
    Delay it (to a specific time).
    Dump it (unimportant; doing it just wastes your time).
    Delegate it.

BOX 2.5 TIME WASTERS

- Engaging in idle gossip.
- Constantly checking and responding to text and instant messages.
- Checking and responding to personal communication and social media sites (Facebook, Twitter, G-chatting) religiously.
- Multitasking.
- Watching TV, gaming, or online browsing/shopping instead of completing your "to-do" list.

of the time limits. Train yourself to do the hardest task first. Attending to the most difficult activity first reduces the nagging, anxiety-provoking thought that you "should be doing ___ instead" and helps you make early progress in identifying, gaining control of, and possibly preventing additional problems. This is an example of the classic time-management principle known as Pareto's 80/20 rule.

According to Pareto, an early 1900s economist, 20% of the effort produces 80% of the results. For example, spending 20% of your time studying the most difficult course can produce 80% success. In your home, 80% of what needs to be cleaned is in the kitchen and bathroom; spend 20% of your cleaning time on these two rooms and 80% of the cleaning will be done. Likewise, 80% of your nursing care will be with 20% of your patients. This illustrates that there are proportionally greater results in concentrating at least 20% of your efforts on higher payoff priorities. You will need to balance your priorities, because it is impossible to achieve our best at all times.

The B items on your list also contribute to goal achievement; thus they are high-payoff items but are generally less urgent than A items and can be delayed for a while. Eventually, many B items become A items, especially as completion times approach. It is also possible to "squeeze in" some B items in short periods of time—for instance, reading an article as you wait in a long line or as you "waste" time waiting for someone.

Items that do not substantially contribute to goals or do not have to be accomplished within a specific time frame are C items. These activities really can wait until you get around to them; they are things to be done when, or if, time permits. Of course, some C items become B or A priorities. However, many C items will fit the "nothing will happen if you do not do something" category and become D items. D items are those "nice to do" but not necessary. Some of these items could be classified as time wasters and can be ignored when you have only a limited amount of time (Box 2.5).

Keep It Going

Continuously review your lists, schedules, and outcomes, and reward yourself for achieving your goals. No one is perfect. Omissions and errors will occur, and these are good learning experiences. Do not waste time regretting failure or feeling guilty about what you did not do; consider these as learning experiences of "what not to do" and opportunities for learning "what to do." Remind yourself that there is always time for important things and that, if it is important enough, you will find the time to do it.

SELF-CARE STRATEGIES

The most beautiful people we have known are those who have known defeat, known suffering, known struggle, known loss, and have found their way out of the depths. These persons have an appreciation, a sensitivity and an understanding of life that fills them with compassion, gentleness, and a deep loving concern. Beautiful people do not just happen.

Elizabeth Kübler-Ross

As a professional nurse, you will be involved with providing care to individuals at their most vulnerable times. You will experience stressful and emotionally charged situations with your patients and their families that may leave you feeling emotionally and physically exhausted, resulting in compassion fatigue. Compassion fatigue has been extensively reported in nursing practice as the distress experienced by nurses who assume caregiving roles of patients experiencing pain and suffering from debilitating medical conditions (Berger et al., 2015; Figley, 2002; Yoder, 2010). Compassion fatigue can lead to burnout, dissatisfaction with work, and high nurse turnover. Therefore, it is important that you practice self-care measures to maintain your overall well-being, so that you are able to provide quality care to your patients (Fig. 2.3).

Self-care, the practice of engaging in activities that promote a healthy lifestyle, is the foundation that will assist you in thriving in nursing instead of just surviving. Engaging in the practice of self-care requires knowledge, motivation, time, and effort, but it is mandatory in your ability to manage stress. Self-care practices that decrease stress-related illness can be learned. Physical illnesses correlated to stress include cardiovascular problems, migraine headaches, irritable bowel syndrome, and muscle and joint pain. Mental health problems include unresolved anxiety, depression, and insomnia. Finally, stress and burnout among nursing personnel can contribute to organizational problems and attrition.

Is Burnout Inevitable for Nurses?

Much has been written about the concept of burnout in nurses. In early research, burnout was thought to be a problem within a nurse or a problem inherent in the nursing profession. However, the stressors

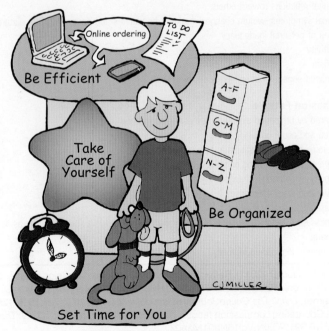

FIG. 2.3 Self-care strategies.

in the current workplace caused by staffing shortages, along with an increase in patient acuity and the accelerated rate of change in the health care environment, have increased the potential for burnout among nurses. What nurses are currently struggling with is that they may be working in environments that are not congruent with their personal philosophies of nursing care.

Burnout is generally associated with work overload and job stress that can leave nurses vulnerable to depression, physical illness, and withdrawal. Symptoms include a loss of energy, weariness, gloominess, dissatisfaction, increased illness, decreased efficiency, absenteeism, and self-doubt. Burnout typically starts gradually and worsens over time progressing through five stages that are particularly notable within the work setting: an initial feeling of enthusiasm for the job, followed by a loss of enthusiasm, continuous deterioration, crisis, and finally devastation and the inability to work effectively. Box 2.6 lists signs of burnout and compassion fatigue.

Compassion fatigue is a related to burnout and is caused by empathy; often referred to as the "cost of caring." Considered the natural consequence of stress resulting from caring for and helping traumatized or suffering people, symptoms of compassion fatigue occur suddenly with little warning and are more pervasive than burnout. In addition to regular burnout symptoms, a person experiencing compassion fatigue can feel a loss of meaning and hope and can have reactions associated with post-

---

BOX 2.6   SIGNS OF BURNOUT AND COMPASSION FATIGUE

Burnout
- Triggered by work-related issues and dissatisfaction
- Occurs gradually
- Irritability, anger, frustration
- Negative reactions toward others
- Physical symptoms: weight changes, frequent headaches and gastrointestinal disturbances, chronic fatigue
- Feeling of personal inadequacy
- Negativity
- Cynicism
- Decreased engagement and productivity at work

Compassion Fatigue
- Triggered by prolonged exposure to the trauma material of patients
- Sudden and acute onset
- Symptoms mirror post-traumatic stress disorder
- Insomnia, difficulty falling or staying asleep, nightmares
- Irritability or outbursts of anger
- Exaggerated startle responses
- Depression, sadness, grief
- "Witness guilt"—taking personal blame for inability to resolve a situation, such as easing the pain and suffering of a patient
- Addiction
- Detachment, diminished intimacy

Adapted from Sabo, B. (2011). Reflecting on the concept of compassion fatigue. *OJIN: The Online Journal of Issues in Nursing, 16*(1). doi: 10.3912/OJIN.Vol16No01Man01; Lombardo, B., & Eyre, C., (2011). Compassion fatigue: A nurse's primer. *OJIN: The Online Journal of Issues in Nursing, 16*(1). doi:10.3912/OJIN.Vol16No01Man03; and Boyle, D. (2011). Countering compassion fatigue: A requisite nursing agenda. *OJIN: The Online Journal of Issues in Nursing, 16*(1). doi: 10.3912/OJIN.Vol16No01Man02

traumatic stress disorder (PTSD), such as strong feelings of anxiety, difficulty concentrating, being jumpy or easily startled, irritability, difficulty sleeping, excessive emotional numbing, and intrusive images of another's traumatic material (Portnoy, 2011).

The increase in patient acuity, coupled with shortened hospital stays, is not compatible with the emphasis on high-quality, safe patient care and consumer satisfaction. These opposing philosophies create conflict for nurses and lead to burnout that is not as easily remedied as burnout caused by internal factors. Therefore, it is important to recognize clearly the mission of the hospital or corporation when you apply for your first job. Is their mission similar to yours? Will you be able to give the quality care that you want to deliver, or will you be required to compromise your values to fit into the system?

There are many strategies designed to combat burnout, and many of them are detailed in this chapter. However, nurses need to determine whether their burnout is caused by internal or external factors. A nurse who neglects his or her own needs can develop feelings of low self-esteem and resentment. These feelings could affect the care you provide to others. Therefore, by taking care of yourself, you are ultimately able to provide better care for others. In some cases, it may be necessary for the nurse to relocate to a place of employment that is more in line with her or his personal belief system.

Cultivating Mindfulness

Exactly what is mindfulness? Jon Kabat-Zinn (1990), who is considered a pioneer in bringing awareness to mindfulness, describes mindfulness as moment-to-moment awareness, cultivated by purposely and nonjudgmentally paying attention to the present moment. It is characterized by having an attitude of openness and curiosity, engaging the five senses, noticing your surroundings without holding on to or pushing away what you are experiencing. Essentially, it is responding thoughtfully versus reacting mindlessly to situations, thoughts, and emotions.

Are You Living on "Automatic Pilot?"

More than likely, you have had the experience of driving to work with your mind on something else—usually anticipating a future event or thinking and rehashing a past experience. The mind is busy scattering our thoughts and emotions as it constantly processes memories, plans, and past events, as well as processes information from our senses and keeps our bodily physiological functions moving seamlessly. No wonder we are mentally distracted and feel stress!

Mindfulness-based programs have proven to be a promising intervention in reducing stress experienced by nurses (Shapiro et al., 2005). Mindfulness has emerged in recent years as a self-care method that may confer protective effects against stressors at home and at work (Westphal et al., 2015). In addition to stress reduction, mindfulness-based interventions can also enhance the nurses' capacity for focused attention and concentration by increasing present moment awareness. When the nurse is fully present with coworkers by paying attention to one another, then the health care team is strengthened and is at the best able to deliver great service and nursing care (Battié, 2016). This can result in fewer errors, omissions, and other situations that lead to harm. Mindfulness techniques can be applied at work and at home with stressful situations. By acquiring the skills to be more mindful and present, nurses may be increasingly conscious of and attentive to their own self-care needs, thus being more present in both their personal and professional lives (Research for Best Practice Box 2.1).

RESEARCH FOR BEST PRACTICE BOX 2.1
Mindfulness to Promote Self-Care

Practice Issue

Nurses are often presented with hectic patient schedules, interruptions throughout the work day, and competing priorities of what needs to be done in the management of patient care. With the numerous demands and responsibilities placed on them, nurses must make timely, accurate decisions regarding patient care. It is no surprise that nursing is regarded as a stress-filled profession. This prolonged exposure to work-related stress and interpersonal and emotional stress can lead to burnout and compassion fatigue (often referred to as the "cost of caring"). It is important that nurses must first take care of themselves. The cultivation of daily mindfulness practice is one way that nurses may promote self-care and well-being.

Implications for Nursing Practice

- Awareness and acknowledgment regarding the intense and chronic nature of stress in the healthcare setting and its impact on nurses.
- Mindfulness can help relieve symptoms of burnout, depression, compassion fatigue, and anxiety among nurses and may improve patient care by providing an increased calmness and focused attention in the nurse.
- Short workplace courses on mindfulness strategies can be an effective approach to create organizational environments supporting healthy stress management and improved attentiveness and assist the nurse to be fully present to the task at hand.

Considering This Information

What aspects of mindfulness do you find appealing or not so appealing? Would you consider incorporating mindfulness activities into your daily routine?

References

Battié, R. N. (2016). Thriving with mindfulness. *AORN Journal, 103*(1), 1–2. https://doi.org/10.1016/j.aorn.2015.11.017.

Botha, E., Gwin, G., & Purpora, C. (2015). The effectiveness of mindfulness based programs in reducing stress experienced by nurses in adult hospital settings: A systematic review of quantitative evidence protocol. *JBI Database of Systematic Reviews and Implementation Report, 13*(10), 21–29. https://doi.org/10.11124/jbisrir-2015-2380.

Mahon, M. A., Mee, L., Brett, D., & Dowling, M. (2017). Nurses' perceived stress and compassion following a mindfulness meditation and self-compassion training. *Journal of Nursing Research, 22*(8), 572–583. https://doi.org/10.1177/1744987117721596.

Myers, R. E. (2017). Cultivating mindfulness to promote self-care and well-being in perioperative nurses. *AORN, 105*(3), 259–266. https://doi.org/10.1016/j.aorn.2017.01.005.

Pipe, T. B., Bortz, J. J., Dueck, A., Pendergast, D., Buchda, V., & Summers, J. (2009). Nurse leader mindfulness meditation program for stress management: A randomized controlled trial. *The Journal of Nursing Administration, 39*(3), 130–137. https://doi.org/10.1097/NNA.0b013e31819894a0.

What Are Mindfulness Exercises?

You have probably already experienced two types of mindful safety checkpoints:

- Hand-offs or hand-overs during **patient transitions** from different units or to other oncoming shift nurses.
- **Procedural time-outs** before any medical procedure to allow the staff to perform checks related to correct patient and correct procedure.

There are several easy methods you can use to bring your mind to the present moment, which leads us to the first one, which is called a **purposeful pause**. The purposeful pause takes only 10 to 60 seconds and may just be one deep breathing cycle (inhalation-exhalation). This type of deep breathing activity can help calm you and provide focus in the clinical setting. An Internet or literature search will locate many resources for you to promote mindfulness. Why, there are even apps for you to download to help you with your mindfulness practice—try Calm, Smiling Mind, Headspace, or Mindful.

Empowerment and Self-Care

Learning about self-care is really about empowerment. To empower means to enable—enable self and others to reach their greatest potential for health and well-being. However, the concept of "enabling" is seen in a negative light because it refers to doing things for others that they can do for themselves. Actually, preventing friends and loved ones from dealing with the consequences of their behavior is very disempowering.

With empowerment comes a feeling of well-being and effectiveness. There are times and situations in our lives when we feel more or less powerful. Examples of occasions when one feels powerful or powerless are listed in Box 2.7. You may find as you read through these lists that there are some situations in your life in which you do feel powerful and some in which you do not. Self-assessment of our sense of well-being and self-esteem helps us know where to begin. Because change is a constant, and all of us are in varying states of emotional, physical, and mental change at any given time, it is important to assess ourselves on a regular basis. As a matter of fact, knowing one's self is the very first step in learning to care for one's self. Empowerment in all spheres of our being is very important. Examine the Holistic Self-Assessment Tool (Critical Thinking Box 2.3), which includes measures of our emotional, mental, physical, social, spiritual, and choice potentials.

BOX 2.7 EXAMPLES OF TIMES WHEN ONE FEELS POWERLESS OR POWERFUL

I Feel Powerless When
- I'm ignored.
- I get assigned to a new hospital unit.
- I can't make a decision.
- I'm exhausted.
- I'm being evaluated by my instructor.
- I have no choices.
- I'm being controlled or manipulated.
- I have pent-up anger.
- I don't think or react quickly.
- I don't speak loudly enough.
- I don't have control over my time.

I Feel Powerful When
- I'm energetic.
- I receive positive feedback.
- I know I look good.
- I tell people I'm a nurse.
- I have clear goals for my career.
- I stick to decisions.
- I speak out against injustice.
- I allow myself to be selfish without feeling guilty.
- I tell a good joke.
- I work with supportive people.
- I'm told by a patient or family that I did a good job.

Adapted from Josefowitz, N. (1980). *Paths to power* (p. 7). Menlo Park, CA: Addison-Wesley. Reprinted with permission.

? CRITICAL THINKING BOX 2.3

Holistic Self-Assessment Tool

Directions: Place a check mark in the space before the statement that applies to you.

Emotional Potential

_____ I push my thoughts and feelings out of conscious awareness (denial).
_____ I feel I have to be in control.
_____ I am unable to express basic feelings of sadness, joy, anger, and fear.
_____ I see myself as a victim.
_____ I feel guilty and ashamed a lot of the time.
_____ I frequently take things personally.

Social Potential

_____ I am overcommitted to the point of having no time for recreation.
_____ I am unable to be honest and open with others.
_____ I am unable to admit vulnerability to others.
_____ I am attracted to needy people.
_____ I feel overwhelmingly responsible for others' happiness.
_____ My only friends are nurses.

Physical Potential

_____ I neglect myself physically—overweight/underweight, lack of adequate rest and exercise.
_____ I feel tired and lack energy.
_____ I am not interested in sex.
_____ I do not engage in regular physical and dental check-ups.
_____ I have seen a doctor in the past 6 months for any of the following conditions: migraine headaches, backaches, gastrointestinal problems, hypertension, or cancer.
_____ I am a workaholic—work is all-important to me.

Spiritual Potential

_____ I see that events that occur in my life are controlled by external choices.
_____ I find the world a basically hostile place.
_____ I lack a spiritual base for working through daily problems.
_____ I live in the past or the future.
_____ I have no sense of power greater than myself.

Mental Potential

_____ I read mostly professional literature.
_____ I spend most waking hours obsessing over people, places, or things.
_____ I am no longer able to dream or fantasize about my future.
_____ I can't remember much of my childhood.
_____ I can't see much change happening for myself, either personally or professionally.

Choice Potential

_____ I have difficulty making decisions, I am prone to procrastination, and I am frequently late for personal and professional appointments.
_____ I find it difficult to say no.
_____ I find myself unwilling to take reasonable risks.
_____ I find it difficult to take responsibility for myself.

From Zerwekh, J., & Michaels, B. (1989). Co-dependency: Assessment and recovery. *The Nursing Clinics of North America, 24*(1), 109–120.

Emotional wholeness is about our ability to feel. The ability to express a wide range of emotions is indicative of good mental health. Nurses are often very good at helping their patients "feel" their feelings but often have a difficult time feeling and expressing their own. Nurses frequently neglect their physical health. We make certain that our patients receive excellent health education and discharge instructions and worry when they are noncompliant. As nurses, however, we do not always follow through when it comes to such things as physical examinations, mammograms, and dental health for ourselves. We work long hours and do not plan adequate time for physical recuperation.

Because our profession is such a demanding one, we often do not take the time to cultivate our social potential. When we do spend time with friends, it is because they "need" us. When we get together with friends who are also nurses, we spend the time together talking about work. Spiritual potential simply means that we have a daily awareness that there is something more to living than mere human existence. With spiritual potential, nurses' lives have meaning and direction.

The ability to know that we have choices in life is the final area of the assessment tool. Nurses without "choice power" see life as black-and-white, with little gray in the middle. Awareness of our choices eliminates the black-and-white extremes and enables us to act rather than react in situations. Nurses with choice power are able to make decisions, take risks, and feel good about it.

Remember to use this tool not only to assess the negatives in your life but also to assess areas in which you are experiencing growth. You cannot survive nursing school, for example, without experiencing growth in all areas.

Suggested Strategies for Self-Care That Are Based on the Holistic Self-Assessment Tool

Not having life in a state of balance and not having a vision for the future often reflect a state of poor self-esteem. Nathaniel Branden (1992), who is often referred to as the father of the self-esteem movement, has identified several factors found in individuals with healthy self-esteem. These include the following:
1. Face, manner, and way of talking and moving that project the pleasure one takes in being alive
2. Ease in talking of accomplishments or shortcomings with directness and honesty
3. An attitude of openness to and curiosity about new ideas, new experiences, and new possibilities of life
4. Openness to criticism and being comfortable about acknowledging mistakes, because one's self-esteem is not tied to an image of perfection
5. An ability to enjoy the humorous aspects of life in one's self and others (Branden, 1992, p. 43).

The key to developing a healthy self-esteem is to become aware of the areas that need the most repair and to work on them. However, it is essential to maintain a sense of balance; going overboard in one or two areas is counterproductive. For example, a nurse who exercises five times a week, follows a healthy diet, and sleeps well but is emotionally numb and does not have a clear vision for her future is out of balance.

Am I Emotionally Healthy/Emotionally Intelligent?

Being emotionally healthy means that you are aware of your feelings and are able to acknowledge them in a healthy way. In the best-selling book *Emotional Intelligence*, Goleman (1995) states that emotional intelligence consists of the following five domains: knowing one's emotions, managing emotions, motivating one's self, recognizing emotions in others, and handling relationships.

Nurses who have good emotional health know when they are feeling fearful, angry, sad, ashamed, happy, guilty, or lonely, and they are able to distinguish these feelings. They have found appropriate ways to express their feelings without offending others. When feelings are not expressed or at least acknowledged, they frequently build up, which results in emotional binging. Sometimes our bodies take the brunt of unacknowledged feelings in the form of headaches, gastrointestinal problems, anxiety attacks, and so on.

Feelings or emotions are neither good nor bad. They are indications of some of our self-truths, our desires, and our needs. Critical Thinking Box 2.4 is an exercise to help access and acknowledge feelings.

? CRITICAL THINKING BOX 2.4

Exercises to Help Access and Acknowledge Feelings

1. Turn your attention to how you are feeling. What part of your body feels what?
2. Acknowledge that this is how you are feeling, and give it a name. If you hear an inner criticism for feeling this way, just set it aside. Any feeling is acceptable.
3. Allow yourself to experience the sensations you are having. Separate acknowledging these feelings from having to do anything about them.
4. Ask yourself whether you want to express your feelings now or some other time. Do you want to take some other action now or later? Remind yourself that you have choices.

What About Friends and Fun? How Do I Find the Time?

An occupational hazard of nursing is overcommitting, both personally and professionally. Nurses who do this frequently have difficulty in meeting their social potential.

Student nurses often say they do not engage in recreational activities because of the cost and that all their money goes toward living expenses. First, it is important to include some money in your monthly budget for fun. Depriving yourself of time for recreation on a regular basis may lead to impulsive recreational spending, such as a shopping binge with credit cards or with money allotted for something else. Second, there are many pleasurable things to do and fun places to go that do not cost a lot of money. Several examples are found in Box 2.8.

Another social area in which many nurses have difficulty is in forming relationships outside of nursing. If you spend all your free time with nurses, chances are that you will "talk shop." Nursing curricula are very science-intensive, because there is so much to learn in such a short time. Cultivate some friends who have a liberal arts or fine arts background. Choose friends who have different political opinions or come from a different part of town, a different culture, or a different socioeconomic class.

BOX 2.8 SOME PLEASURABLE ACTIVITIES

- Go on a picnic with friends.
- Invite friends over for a potluck dinner.
- Go to a movie.
- Plan celebrations after exams or completion of a project.
- Introduce yourself to three new people.
- Visit a new city.
- Call an old friend.
- Play with your children.
- "Borrow" someone else's children for play.
- Volunteer for a worthwhile project.
- Get involved in religious or spiritual activities.
- Spend some time people-watching.
- Take up a new hobby.
- Invite humor into your life.

How Do I Take Care of My Physical Self?

Nurses are great when it comes to patient education; it is one of the strengths of the nursing profession. Sometimes, though, we have difficulty applying this information to ourselves. Taking care of ourselves physically is extremely important. Our profession is both mentally and physically challenging. This physical self-care entails getting the proper nutrition, maintaining a healthy weight, obtaining adequate sleep, quitting smoking, limiting alcohol consumption to one drink daily, and exercising on a regular basis (Critical Thinking Box 2.5). Engaging in some form of relaxation will trigger the relaxation response, which prevents chronic stress from harming your health (Stark et al., 2005). According to Kernan and Wheat (2008), health and learning are linked; optimal learning cannot be achieved unless the environment is supportive and promotes the development of effective learning skills. They identified mental health concerns (stress, anxiety), respiratory tract infections, interpersonal concerns, and sleep difficulties as the greatest threats to academic success.

? CRITICAL THINKING BOX 2.5

What am I doing that interferes with my health and well-being?

Self-Care Activities

Physical exercise. Incorporate 30 minutes or more of moderate-intensity physical activity, such as walking, into your schedule (preferably daily). A good exercise program is one that includes activities that foster aerobic activity, flexibility, and strength. A very important part of an exercise program is that it be a regular habit. To be effective, the program should take 3 to 6 hours a week. And it does not have to cost money. You do not need to belong to a gym or invest in exercise equipment. Aerobic activities include walking, jogging, swimming, bicycling, and dancing. Minimal fitness consists of raising your heart rate to 100 beats/min and keeping it there for 30 minutes. Other strategies to increase your physical activity could include the following:

1. Park your car farther away from the entrance door.
2. Use the stairs instead of the elevator whenever possible.
3. Stretch during your breaks from homework or housework.
4. Take your dog for a walk (or volunteer to walk someone else's pet).

Laughter. Seek 20 minutes of laughter every day. Laughing promotes deep breathing and releases neuropeptides that decrease stress and lower blood pressure. (Check out www.laughteryoga.org for inspiring thoughts and affirmations.)

Mental exercise. Engage in some activity daily for at least 30 minutes that challenges your way of thinking. This activity will increase the number of connections between your brain cells (rewiring your brain). Activities that could promote brain function include:

1. Take a walk in the park to stimulate all your senses.
2. Try out a new restaurant.
3. Listen to new music.
4. Try brain games (see www.lumosity.com).

Motivate yourself. In the morning, read an inspiring quote, listen to upbeat music, or do stretching exercises. Take time for a balanced breakfast, and visualize your day. Take periodic breaks or switch activities throughout your day to maintain a high energy level. Tension can be released by simple stretching exercises and laughter.

Schedule idle time. We live in a time in which any moment can be interrupted by individuals, e-mail, texting, or phone calls. We need to give ourselves permission to relax—to unwind. Take care of your physical and mental health by scheduling idle time. Idle time is time you schedule away from interruptions—no phone calls, no e-mail, no texting. This is time in which you disconnect from technology to think and reflect. Take a walk in the park, just sit in your backyard and listen to the birds, or get a massage, but turn all your electronic devices off.

> Alternate mental and physical tasks. This strategy includes taking periodic breaks from studying to engage in a short game of basketball or a short run with the vacuum cleaner.

Strategies to Foster My Spiritual Self: Does My Life Have Meaning?

People who have a sense of spiritual well-being find their lives to be positive experiences, have relationships with a power greater than themselves, feel good about the future, and believe there is some real purpose in life. If we find that our lives lack meaning and our spiritual health is lacking, how do we go about finding spiritual well-being?

Daily prayer and meditation are very important in maintaining a spiritual self. Reading religious or philosophical material and studying the great religions are two examples of ways to foster spiritual growth.

In addition to reading what others have written about the subject, many people access their spiritual selves with the practice of meditation. Meditating allows us time to become quiet, heal our thoughts and bodies, and be grateful. The engagement of daily prayer or meditation allows for a time of self-reflection.

How Do I Increase My Mental Potential? Is It Okay to Daydream?

Nursing students are afforded considerable opportunity to exercise their mental potential while they are in nursing school. This activity, however, is primarily in the form of formal education. There are many other ways to exercise this potential. One of the first ways is to concentrate on removing negative thoughts or self-defeating beliefs from our minds. Here are some examples of statements that nursing students frequently make:

1. "I must make *A*'s in nursing school."
2. "I must have approval from everyone, and if I don't, I feel horrible and depressed."
3. "If I fail at something, the results will be catastrophic."
4. "Others must always treat me fairly."
5. "If I'm not liked by everyone, I am a failure."
6. "Because all my miseries are caused by others, I will have no control over my life until they change."

If you relate to any of these statements, you have some work to do on your belief system. You are setting yourself up for failure by having extremely high expectations of yourself. You are also giving other people power over your destiny. Remember, you cannot change others. The only person you can change is yourself. Wolf, Stidham, and Ross (2015) contend that using coping strategies such as positive thinking may be beneficial for reducing stress (specifically, for nursing students—that's you!).

One way that we can change these internal beliefs of negativity into positive thinking is to learn how to give ourselves daily affirmations—or daydream a little (Fig. 2.4). Simply put, affirmations are powerful, positive statements concerning the ways we would like to think, feel, and behave. Some examples are "I am a worthwhile person"; "I am human and capable of making mistakes"; and "I am able to freely express my emotions." Always begin affirmative statements with "I" rather than "you." This practice keeps the focus on self rather than others and encourages the development of inner self-worth.

The power of affirmation exercises lies in consistency—repetition encourages ultimate belief in what is being said. Begin each day with some affirmations. Try some of the examples in Box 2.9.

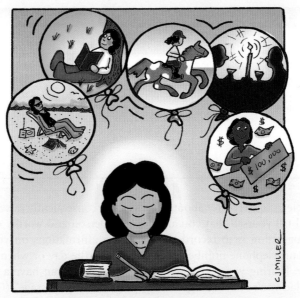

FIG. 2.4 Daydream: Send up your brain balloons!

BOX 2.9 AFFIRMATIONS

- I am a worthwhile person.
- I am a child of God.
- I am willing to accept love.
- I am willing to give love.
- I can openly express my feelings.
- I deserve love, peace, and serenity.
- I am capable of changing.
- I can take care of myself without feeling guilty.
- I can say no and not feel guilty.
- I am beautiful inside and out.
- I can be spontaneous and whimsical.
- I am human and capable of making mistakes.
- I can recognize shame and work through it.
- I forgive myself for hurting myself and others.
- I freely accept nurturing from others.
- I can be vulnerable with trusted others.
- I am peaceful with life.
- I am free to be the best me I can.
- I love and comfort myself in ways that are pleasing to me.
- I am automatically and joyfully focusing on the positive.
- I am giving myself permission to live, love, and laugh.
- I am creating and singing affirmations to create a joyful, abundant, fulfilling life.

BOX 2.10   EXAMPLES OF REACTIVE AND PROACTIVE LANGUAGE

Reactive	Proactive
There's nothing I can about do about it.	Let's look at our alternatives.
That's just the way I am.	I can choose a different approach.
He makes me so mad.	I control my own feelings.
They won't allow that.	I can create an effective presentation.
I have to do that.	I will choose an appropriate response.
I can't.	I choose.
I must.	I prefer.
If only.	I will.

These enable us to feel better about ourselves and consequently raise our self-esteem. Stand in front of a mirror and tell yourself that you are a special person and worthy of self-love and the love of others. Another suggestion is to record some positive affirmations on your telephone answering machine and call your telephone number in the middle of the day or when you are having a slump or attack of self-pity; hearing you own voice say you are okay can have a very positive effect. For example, "Hello—Glad you're having a great day, please leave a message" (Critical Thinking Box 2.6).

❓ CRITICAL THINKING BOX 2.6

What are some positive affirmations that work for you? How can you increase the effectiveness of these affirmations?

What Are My Choices, and How Do I Exercise Them?

Many of us negotiate our way through life never realizing that we have many choices. In his best-selling book *Seven Habits of Highly Effective People*, Stephen Covey (2004) states that the very first habit we must develop is to be proactive. We stop thinking in black-and-white and come to realize that in every arena of our lives, we have choices about how to respond and react. Covey differentiates between people who are proactive and people who are reactive. Examples of proactive versus reactive language are included in Box 2.10. Pay attention to your own language patterns for the next few weeks. Are there times when you could say "I choose"? You can choose to respond to people and situations rather than react. Exercising our choice potential also entails that we act responsibly toward others. We recognize that other people have the right to choose for themselves and to be accountable for their own behavior.

CONCLUSION

Before we can act responsibly toward others, we must first act responsibly toward ourselves. This involves self-acceptance and self-love. In his book *Born for Love: Reflections on Loving*, Leo Buscaglia (1994) states this very eloquently:

> *Being who we are, people who feel good about themselves are not easily threatened by the future. They enthusiastically maintain a secure image whether everything is falling apart or going their way. They hold a firm base of personal assuredness and self-respect that remains constant. Though they are concerned about what others think of them, it is a healthy concern. They find external forces more challenging than threatening. Perhaps the greatest sign of maturity is to reach the point in life when we embrace ourselves strengths and weaknesses alike and acknowledge that*

we are all that we have; that we have a right to a happy and productive life and the power to change ourselves and our environment within realistic limitations. In short, we are, each of us, entitled to be who we are and become what we choose. (p. 177)

When you get your personal life organized, you will become effective in getting priorities accomplished at home. When you get your school activities organized, you will study more effectively, be less stressed, and be able to prioritize more effectively. With these two areas organized, there will be more time for you to spend on yourself! You will find that after you get organized with your clinical schedule, you will become a more effective nurse and begin to have the time to perform the type of nursing care that you were taught. Often you will hear nurses complain about not having enough time in clinicals to provide the type of bath or teaching they would like to do because of the lack of time. Check them out; often they are the most guilty of wasting time (e.g., taking time to gossip after report, wasting time complaining that they do not have enough time, not delegating effectively, allowing unnecessary interruptions, not organizing their patient care, or not delegating when appropriate). Wow—all the things that this chapter is about!

🌐 RELEVANT WEBSITES AND ONLINE RESOURCES

Dartmouth College
Managing your time: Take the quiz. https://students.dartmouth.edu/academic-skills/learning-resources/time-management-tips.

MindTools.com
https://www.mindtools.com/pages/main/newMN_HTE.htm.

QS Top Universities
Best time management apps for students. https://www.topuniversities.com/blog/best-time-management-apps-students.

BIBLIOGRAPHY

Battié, R. N. (2016). Thriving with mindfulness. *AORN Journal, 103*(1), 1–2. https://doi.org/10.1016/j.aorn.2015.11.017.

Berger, J., Polivka, B., Smoot, E. A., & Owens, H. (2015). Compassion fatigue in pediatric nurses. *Journal of Pediatric Nursing, 30*(6), e11–e17.

Branden, N. (1992). *The power of self-esteem.* Deerfield, FL: Health Communications.

Buscaglia, L. (1994). *Born for love: Reflections on loving.* Thorofare, NJ: Random House.

Covey, S. (2004). *Seven habits of highly effective people.* New York: Simon & Schuster.

Figley, C. (2002). Compassion fatigue: Psychotherapists' chronic lack of self-care. *Psychotherapy in Practice, 58*(11), 1433–1441.

Goleman, D. (1995). *Emotional intelligence.* New York: Bantam Books.

Hopper, C. (2007). Hemispheric dominance inventory. *Practicing college study skills: Strategies for success* (3rd ed.). Boston, MA: Houghton Mifflin Company. Retrieved from http://capone.mtsu.edu/studskl/hd/learn.html.

Kabat-Zinn, J. (1990). *Full catastrophe living: Using the wisdom of your body and mind to face stress, pain and illness.* New York: Dell Publishing.

Kernan, W. D., & Wheat, M. E. (2008). Nursing students' perceptions of the academic impact of various health issues. *Nurse Educator, 33*(5), 215–219.

Keyes, R. (1991). *Timelock: How life got so hectic and what you can do about it.* New York: HarperCollins.

Knox, K. C. (2013). Getting a handle on email. *Information Today, 30*(1), 21.

Lerner, R. (1985). *Daily affirmations.* Pompano Beach, FL: Health Communications.

Lumosity. (2015). *Brain training games.* Retrieved from https://www.lumosity.com/en/brain-games/.

Mokhtari, K., Delello, J., & Reichard, C. (2015). Connected yet distracted: Multitasking among college students. *Journal of College Reading and Learning, 45*(2), 164–180.

Peck, M. S. (1978). *The road less traveled.* New York: Simon & Schuster.

Portnoy, D. (2011, July-August). *Burnout and compassion fatigue: Watch for the signs. Health Progress.* Retrieved from http://www.compassionfatigue.org/pages/healthprogress.pdf.

Remember the Milk. (2015). *Tour.* Retrieved from http://www.rememberthemilk.com/.

Shapiro, S. I., Astin, J. A., Bishop, S. R., & Cordova, M. (2005). Mindfulness-based stress reduction for health care professionals: Results from a randomized trial. *International Journal Stress Management, 12*(2), 164–176.

Stark, M. A., Maning-Walsh, J., & Vliem, S. (2005). Caring for self while learning to care for others: A challenge for nursing students. *Journal of Nursing Education, 44*(6), 260–270.

Westphal, M., Bingisser, M. B., Feng, T., et al. (2015). Protective benefits of mindfulness in emergency room personnel. *Journal of Affective Disorders, 175,* 79–85. https://doi.org/10.1016/j.jad.2014.12.038.

White, L. (2014). Mindfulness in nursing: An evolutionary concept analysis. *Journal of Advanced Nursing, 70*(2), 282–294. https://doi.org/10.1111/jan.12182.

Wolf, L., Stidham, A., & Ross, R. (2015). Predictors of stress and coping strategies of us accelerated vs. generic baccalaureate nursing students: An embedded mixed methods study. *Nurse Education Today, 35*(1), 201–205.

Yoder, E. A. (2010). Compassion fatigue in nurses. *Applied Nursing Research, 23*(4), 191–197.

3

Mentorship, Preceptorship, and Nurse Residency Programs

Ashley Zerwekh Garneau, PhD, RN

ⓔhttp://evolve.elsevier.com/Zerwekh/nsgtoday/.

Mentoring is a brain to pick, an ear to listen, and a push in the right direction
John Crosby

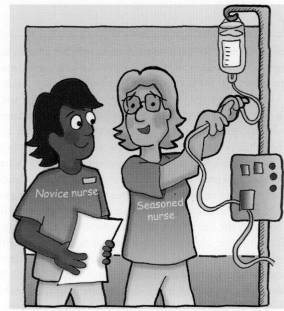

Mentoring is one of the broadest methods of encouraging human growth and potential.

After completing this chapter, you should be able to:
- Describe the difference between mentoring, coaching, and precepting.
- Identify characteristics of effective mentors, mentees, and preceptors.
- Implement strategies for finding a mentor.
- Discuss the types of mentoring relationships.
- Examine components of preceptorship programs and nurse residency programs.
- Evaluate the benefits of transitioning from mentee to mentor.

■ *Ashley*

It was my first day as a nurse extern in a busy medical intensive care unit. As I walked into my new place of work, I observed nurses on the phones, talking with doctors, and running in and out of patients' rooms with stern looks on their faces. So many questions were going through my mind. Which one of these nurses was my preceptor? What would my preceptor expect from me? Would he or she be receptive to helping me develop into my role as a professional registered nurse? I entered the room where the nurses receive hand-off report from the night staff. It was there that I had my first encounter with Julie, who would become my preceptor, nursing role model, and mentor in the months ahead.

HISTORICAL BACKGROUND

Did you ever wonder where the word *mentor* originated? It originated from Greek mythology. Mentor was the name of a wise and faithful advisor to Odysseus. When Odysseus (or Ulysses, as the Romans called him) left for his long voyage during the Trojan War, he entrusted the direction and teaching of his son, Telemachus, to Mentor. According to mythology, through Mentor's guidance, Telemachus became an effective and beloved ruler (Shea, 1999). Mentor's job was not merely to raise Telemachus but to develop him for the responsibilities he was to assume in his lifetime. Mentoring is one of the broadest methods for encouraging human growth and potential.

WHAT MENTORING IS AND IS NOT

A definition of mentoring in nursing is captured by Meier (2013) as "a nurturing process in which a more skilled or more experienced person, serving as a role model, teaches, sponsors, encourages, counsels and befriends a less-skilled or less-experienced person for the purpose of promoting the latter's professional and/or personal development" (p. 343). Oftentimes, the term *mentoring* is confused with *coaching* or *precepting*. Coaching is an approach to assisting an individual's growth through partnership with a colleague or other individual who is an equal. In coaching, one person focuses on the unique and internal qualities observed within the other person that may not be recognized or appreciated (MindTools, 2018). In the business world, executives often refer to themselves as coaches rather than managers, thus fostering a collaborative team-oriented approach. The International Coach Federation (2018) defines coaching as a partnership that enables and motivates the individual receiving coaching to attain his or her highest achievement in all areas of life. From a nursing perspective, the term *health coaching* describes the partnership between the nurse and patient, where the nurse assists the patient in identifying and engaging in healthy lifestyle choices. The National Society of Health Coaches (2015) offers an operational definition of health coaching in the organization's position statement as "the use of evidence-based skillful conversation, clinical strategies, and interventions to actively and safely engage clients in health behavior change to better self-manage their health, health risk, and acute or chronic health conditions resulting in optimal wellness, improved health outcomes, lowered health risk, and decreased healthcare costs" (p. 1). From these definitions, it is clear that coaches help individuals to find new ways to solve problems, reach goals, and design plans of action to motivate people to participate in activities that will advance and fulfill all aspects of their lives. According to Guest, "The strength of mentoring lies in the mentor's specific knowledge and wisdom, in coaching it lies in the facilitation and development of personal qualities. The coach brings different skills and experience and offers a fresh perspective, a different viewpoint. In both cases one-to-one attention is the key" (1999, p. 7). An effective coach does not need to have experience in the activities or context of what he or she is teaching. Rather, an effective coach has a unique set of qualities for coaching individuals in achieving knowledge and skills in a particular area.

Based on these definitions, coaches possess characteristics of mentors, and mentors share attributes of coaching. Considering this, mentoring and coaching complement one another and are often used concurrently in assisting individuals to grow both professionally and personally.

What about preceptors? The term *preceptor* simply means "tutor" and generally refers to a more formal arrangement that pairs a novice with an experienced person for a set time period, with a focus on policies, procedures, and skill development. Preceptors serve as role models and precept during their regularly scheduled work hours, which is part of their work assignment, in contrast with mentors, who are chosen, not assigned, and focus on fostering the mentee's individual growth and development during an extended period. Mentors develop a professionally based, nurturing relationship, which generally occurs outside of the work environment (Fig. 3.1).

What Is Preceptorship?

A preceptorship is a clinical teaching model in which a student is partnered with a preceptor and a faculty member, usually during the student's last semester of nursing school (Billings & Halstead, 2016; Bott, Mohide, & Lawlor, 2011). Nursing schools sometimes use the term *capstone course* synonymously with the term *preceptorship*. In a capstone course, the senior-level student works one-on-one with a preceptor who is a competent and experienced registered nurse (Fig. 3.2). The preceptor guides, observes, and assesses the student's ability to use the nursing process to make a clinical judgment about patient care. In addition, the preceptor may supervise the student performing clinical nursing skills to ensure safety and competency. Another component of the preceptorship is to provide the student with clinical experience in applying critical thinking and organization skills in managing a

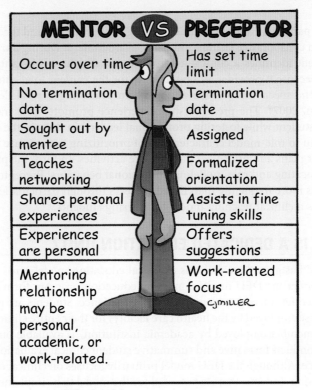

MENTOR VS PRECEPTOR	
Occurs over time	Has set time limit
No termination date	Termination date
Sought out by mentee	Assigned
Teaches networking	Formalized orientation
Shares personal experiences	Assists in fine tuning skills
Experiences are personal	Offers suggestions
Mentoring relationship may be personal, academic, or work-related.	Work-related focus

FIG. 3.1 Mentor versus preceptor.

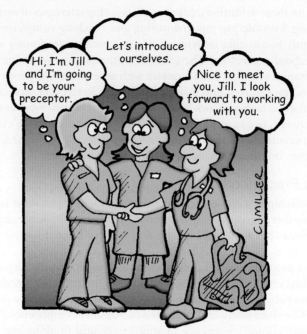

FIG. 3.2 Capstone course.

group of patients in a specific clinical setting. The preceptor and the nursing student identify goals and work in a collaborative fashion toward goal attainment. During a traditional preceptorship, the nursing student identifies a clinical area of interest that he or she anticipates working in after nursing school, because it provides an opportunity for the student to acquire and master nursing skills common to the specialization area and to begin practicing clinical decision making and prioritization (Emerson, 2007). The preceptorship experience promotes role transition and socialization for the nursing student while fostering professional leadership skills in the preceptor. For example, a student may begin to role-model characteristics of prioritizing patient care based on observations of how the preceptor plans and prioritizes patient-care activities. In turn, the preceptor gains leadership traits by communicating and role-modeling professional behaviors. Preceptors are currently acquiring leadership skills more frequently than in recent years through participation in the dedicated education unit (DEU) as a clinical teaching model for nursing students.

WHAT IS A DEDICATED EDUCATION UNIT?

The DEU has gained attention as a clinical education model across nursing programs in the United States. Under the DEU model, a nursing education program forms a partnership with a health care facility to offer nursing students a clinical experience. Students are paired up with a clinical preceptor (staff nurse employed by the health care facility) for their entire clinical rotation. The clinical instructor (faculty member employed by academic institution) is available on site for the student and the preceptor, conducts formative and summative student clinical evaluations, and oversees the entire clinical experience. Although the DEU model primarily focuses on clinical experiences for junior- and senior-level nursing students, there is potential for the model to be implemented throughout the nursing program beginning with first semester nursing students.

What is unique about the DEU model is that it offers health care facilities an opportunity to recruit new graduate nurses. Nursing students' perspectives about future employment can be positively influenced by gaining awareness of the nurse's responsibilities and the workflow of the unit through face-to-face interaction with staff nurses (Ahonen & Quinlan, 2013; Hunt, Milani, & Wilson, 2015). Although preceptorships and clinical teaching models like the DEU may offer you an opportunity to learn and practice real-world nursing alongside an experienced nurse, there may be certain times when your ideas or suggestions about nursing care may differ from your preceptor's viewpoint. In these situations, what can you do?

What Happens If I Experience a Challenge During My Preceptorship or Clinical Rotation?

When the time arrives for you to complete your preceptorship at the end of your nursing program or a clinical experience at any point in your nursing program, rest assured that those feelings of uncertainty and anxiety that you experienced on your first day of nursing school are normal and will subside with time. As you establish a professional relationship with your preceptor, it is important to understand your role and responsibilities as preceptee, as well as the preceptor's role and responsibilities. But what happens when you are placed with a preceptor who does not share the same excitement and interest as you do in participating in the preceptorship? Or what happens when your personalities do not blend well? What do you do?

First, it is important to identify the issues you are having with your preceptor. It may be helpful to write down what is concerning you and share this information with your clinical site supervisor before communicating your concerns to the preceptor.

> A word of advice: Never approach an issue with anyone (this includes your preceptor) when your emotions are running high. Give yourself a little time to cool down. It may help to write down your concerns and revisit your noted concerns the following day. Oftentimes, the issue that was a big deal to us the day prior is no longer a big deal after we have had time to calm down through reflection and a good night's rest!

After you have discussed your concerns with the clinical supervisor, arrange a time to meet with your preceptor to communicate your concerns in a professional manner, while also providing suggestions for a possible solution to the issue(s) you are having with your preceptor. Oftentimes, expressing your concerns to your preceptor will help the preceptor recognize and see your perspective on an issue. Equally important is for you to provide an opportunity for the preceptor to provide you feedback and offer suggestions on any concerns or issues related to the preceptorship experience. If neither you nor the preceptor is able to resolve the issue(s), then reach out to your clinical faculty for guidance and support. For additional conflict resolution strategies, refer to Chapter 13, Conflict Management.

A preceptorship has also been identified as a nurse residency program (NRP), where a new graduate nurse completes a formalized residency at his or her first place of employment as a professional nurse. NRPs are currently being implemented across many practice settings to ensure that new graduates deliver safe patient care.

WHAT IS A NURSE RESIDENCY PROGRAM?

The moment has finally arrived; you have passed the NCLEX-RN® and obtained your RN license. Now the next step in your professional career path as a nurse begins as you land your first position as a professional nurse. Making this step (what might feel like a big leap!) in your nursing career is like a moment of passage. You are no longer a student but a professional nurse. To that end, it is no surprise that you might be feeling a little bit scared or anxious as you start your first day working on the unit at your new place of employment. Remember your first day of nursing school? Similar feelings are sure to surface again as you begin working as a new graduate nurse.

In an effort to ease the transition into the clinical practice setting and reduce job turnover rates of new graduate nurses, NRPs are being employed by many health care organizations as a requirement for all newly hired graduate nurses. You might be asking yourself, what exactly is an NRP? An NRP is a formalized orientation that varies in length (anywhere between 6 and 18 months, but usually for approximately 1 year), where a new graduate nurse works full time on the unit where he or she will be working following completion of the residency program. NRPs vary at each institution but essentially serve the same purposes, which are to assist the new graduate nurse with transitioning into the nursing role through a formalized orientation experience. The new graduate nurse is provided an orientation to the unit to which he or she is hired and is usually assigned to work with a dedicated and experienced nurse, who serves as both a mentor and a coach, throughout the residency. In addition, residency programs provide additional specialty training, certification, and courses that may be a unit-specific requirement for the newly hired graduate nurse. Twibell and Pierre (2012) added that NRPs include a focus on curriculum and specific clinical experiences grounded in evidence-based practice, as well as offer new graduate nurses an opportunity for professional growth and socialization as members of the health care team (see the end of the chapter for a list of relevant websites and online resources). Following completion of an NRP, the nurses will work on the unit where they completed the residency. The American Nurses Credentialing Center (ANCC) offers a listing of nationally accredited NRPs.

Further support for requiring all new graduate nurses to complete an NRP following completion from a prelicensure degree program has been proposed by the Institute of Medicine (IOM). The IOM in collaboration with the Robert Wood Johnson Foundation conducted a 2-year initiative examining how nursing practice and education will transform the delivery of health care. In the 2010 IOM report, *The Future of Nursing: Leading Change, Advancing Health,* the IOM recommended that the following actions should be taken to implement and support NRPs:

- State boards of nursing, in collaboration with accrediting bodies such as The Joint Commission and the Community Health Accreditation Program, should support nurses' completion of a residency program after they have completed a prelicensure or advanced practice degree program or when they are transitioning into new clinical practice areas.
- The Secretary of Health and Human Services should redirect all graduate medical education funding from diploma nursing programs to support the implementation of NRPs in rural and critical access areas.
- Health care organizations, the Health Resources and Services Administration and Centers for Medicare and Medicaid Services, and philanthropic organizations should fund the development and implementation of NRPs across all practice settings.
- Health care organizations that offer NRPs and foundations should evaluate the effectiveness of the residency programs in improving the retention of nurses, expanding competencies, and improving patient outcomes (IOM, 2010, p. 12).

The American Association of Colleges of Nursing (AACN), in collaboration with Vizient, developed an NRP for graduate nurses following completion of their educational programs.

The Vizient/AACN NRP is 1 year long and uses an evidence-based curricular framework for preparing new graduate nurses to transition from their role of novice to competent practitioner. At the time of this publication, more than 400 hospitals and health care organizations currently offer the NRP (Vizient/AACN, 2018) (Research for Best Practice Box 3.1). The benefits of an NRP have also been extensively studied by the National Council of State Boards of Nursing (NCSBN).

🔍 RESEARCH FOR BEST PRACTICE BOX 3.1

Nurse Residency Program

Practice Issue

The clinical environment presents an engaging and rewarding experience for nursing students to begin applying nursing concepts and skills learned in the classroom setting to the practice setting. However, changes impacting health care, decreased clinical site availability, increased student enrollment, and faculty shortages have required key stakeholders in both academia and practice to develop alternative models of clinical education that will prepare future professional nurses to practice competently and safely. Nurse residency programs are a move in that direction, where a graduate nurse participates in a 1-year program that fosters role transition and clinical decision-making skills grounded in evidence-based practice. Providing a smooth transition into practice has also contributed to increased retention of new graduate nurses and decreased job burnout following completion of the nurse residency program (Crimlisk et al., 2017; Vizient/AACN, 2018).

Implications for Nursing Practice

* Health care organizations consider adopting a nurse residency program new graduate nurses are required to complete at the beginning of their employment.
* Implement an evidence-based curriculum under the nurse residency program that includes an emphasis on leadership, patient outcomes, and professional development and that aligns to established core competencies implemented by the health care institution.
* Collaborate with academic institutions to align nurse residency program objectives with nursing educational program outcomes.
* Vizient/AACN Nurse Residency Program had a first-year retention rate of 92.7% for nurses who graduated from the program as compared with the national average of 82.5% (Vizient/AACN, 2018a).
* Nurse residency programs promote socialization and facilitate understanding of the workplace setting (e.g., policies and procedural guidelines) for new graduate nurses (Crimlisk et al., 2017).
* Nurse residency programs provide a collaborative network for nurses to further develop after their internship.

Considering This Information

What are your thoughts on completing a nurse residency program as a requirement of your employer following graduation from nursing school? What area(s) of your professional nursing practice do you feel would stand to benefit from participating in a nurse residency program?

References

Crimlisk, J. T., Grande, M. M., Krisciunas, G. P., Costello, K. V., Fernandes, E. G., & Griffin, M. (2017). Nurse residency program designed for a large cohort of new graduate nurses: Implementation and outcomes. *MEDSURG Nursing, 26*(2), 83–104.

Vizient, American Association of Colleges of Nursing (AACN) (2018). *Vizient/AACN Nurse Residency Program*. Retrieved from: Vizient/AACN. http://www.aacnnursing.org/Nurse-Residency-Program.

Vizient, American Association of Colleges of Nursing (AACN) (2018a). *Vizient/AACN Nurse Residency Program—About the program*. Retrieved from: Vizient/AACN. http://www.aacnnursing.org/Portals/42/AcademicNursing/NRP/Nurse-Residency-Program.pdf.

The NCSBN implemented a transition to practice study for new graduate nurses employed in their first nursing position (NCSBN, 2016). The aim of the study was to examine the effectiveness of a transition to practice program on new graduate outcomes with regard to safety, competence, stress, job satisfaction, and retention as compared with current onboarding programs used by hospitals participating in the study (Spector et al., 2015, p. 26). The NCSBN Transition to Practice (TTP) model employed in the study consisted of an extensive institution-based orientation program, trained preceptors who assisted the new graduate with onboarding processes specific to the unit he or she was working in, and Quality and Safety Education for Nurses (QSEN) online educational models that

BOX 3.1 ESSENTIAL ELEMENTS OF TRANSITION PROGRAMS

- Be formalized in the institution, and have support and involvement of key stakeholders (chief nursing officer and administration)
- Be at a minimum 6 months in duration
- Include a preceptorship program into the transition program
- Include Quality and Safety Education for Nurses competencies of patient safety, teamwork, evidence-based practice, communication, informatics, quality improvement, clinical reasoning, and patient-centered care
- Be customized to the learning needs of the new graduate working on the unit
- Allow ample time for new graduates to learn and apply content, obtain feedback, and share their reflections.

Adapted from Spector, N., Blegan, M. A., Sivestre, J., Barnseiner, J., Lynn, M. R., Ulrich, B., et al. (2015). Transition to practice study in hospital settings. *Journal of Nursing Regulation, 5*(4), 24–38.

the new graduate nurses completed during the study. Findings from this study support the utilization of TTP programs to improve new graduate readiness for practice and increase retention. Based on findings from the study, researchers (Spector et al., 2015) suggest that nurse transition programs have essential elements that are evidence based (Box 3.1). As you begin your career as a professional nurse, here are additional questions you may want to ask your employing institution or agency:

1. Is a formalized orientation program, preceptorship, internship, and/or NRP available to graduate nurses? If so, what is the duration of the NRP?
2. Will I be paired with one or several preceptors?
3. What is the structure of the NRP? Face-to-face? Online? Hybrid? Simulation?
4. Is the NRP nationally accredited?
5. Does the NRP offer continuing education or professional development opportunities?

■ *Ashley*

When I was in nursing school, I thought that a preceptor was fancy terminology for mentor. However, I found out that these two terms are very different from each other.

In nursing, the word *mentor* has become synonymous with trusted advisor, friend, teacher, guide, and wise person. There have been many attempts at deriving a single definition of mentoring. Gibbons (2004) provides a detailed listing of 16 (yes, 16!) different definitions for *mentor*. What makes mentoring so different, so "special," and more encompassing than precepting and coaching?

- Mentoring requires a primary focus on the needs of the mentee and an effort to fulfill the most critical of these needs.
- Mentoring requires going the extra mile for someone else. The rewards of mentoring are enormous: a sense of personal achievement, mentee appreciation, and a sense of building a better organization.
- Mentoring is a partnership created between two people; the mentor possesses the educational degree to which the mentee aspires (Shea, 1999).

As you read through this chapter, begin to develop your own definition of a mentor.

Since the beginning of time, storytelling has been an important way to teach one another. A story about a starfish follows:

A beachcomber is walking along the beach one morning when he sees a young man running up and down by the water's edge throwing something into the water. Curious, he walks toward the runner and watches him picking up the starfish stranded by the tide and tossing them back into the ocean. "Young man," he says, "there are so many starfish on the beach. What difference does it make to save a few?" Without pausing, the young man picks up another starfish and, flinging it into the sea, replies, "It made a difference for this one."

> That is what mentors do. They make a difference for one person at a time.

According to Peddy, the process of mentoring can be described in eight words, "Lead, follow, and get out of the way" (2001, p. 16). What does this mean?

Lead

Mentors are leaders. They encourage another's growth and development, professionally and personally. Mentors help and inspire mentees by acting as role models. The focus is on wisdom and judgment. The mentor plays a very active role: teaching, coaching, and explaining while supporting and shaping critical thinking skills, providing invaluable advice when asked, and introducing the mentee to committees, advancements, and honors.

Follow

This is where mentees need to "get their feet wet." At this stage, the mentor and mentee walk the path together, but the advisor (mentor) assumes a more passive role. It is now up to the learner (mentee) to seek actively the advice or listening ear of the mentor.

Get Out of the Way

This means knowing when it is time to let go. If you have ever taught a child to swim or ride a bike, you know how hard it is to "let go" and let the child soar on his or her own. A helping relationship is a freeing relationship. This does not mean the relationship has to end; you share common values and beliefs in lifelong learning.

This process of mentoring is dynamic, not static. A mentor's task of self-development, learning, and mastery is never done. Each person in the mentoring process has a role. Mentors generally have more experience and are dedicated to helping mentees advance in their careers, especially in work and/or life skill issues. Mentoring is a two-way street, a partnership, with both parties freely contributing to the relationship as equals—working together in mutual respect.

■ *JoAnn*

On a personal note, when I think about mentors that I have had, one person comes to mind: Satora. She was my first mentor when I started working in the ICU after graduating with my diploma in nursing. She personified all that a new graduate would want in a mentor. She was understanding, patient, and compassionate, and she possessed extensive experience. She had an important, long-lasting impact on my nursing career. She nurtured me and encouraged me to reach within myself to become the nurse that I am today. I will never forget her.

Approximately 25 years after I left the ICU, I had the opportunity to talk with Satora by phone. It was one of those coincidences or synchronistic moments in which I was able, via a mutual friend, to find out where she was working. I had lost contact with her over the years in the several moves that I had made to different places. She was so surprised that I had called, and I shared with her how important our mentoring relationship had been to me. It made me feel good to pass along my gratitude for her willingness to mentor me.

How to Find a Mentor

The key to finding a mentor is having an open mind, being flexible, and remaining optimistic. As you finish nursing school and while you are in school, write down the goals you feel a mentor might help you achieve. Keep this list of goals with you while you are working, and try to get a feel for the different personality types that you will see as a nurse among your coworkers.

■ *Ashley*

During my orientation program as a newly licensed professional registered nurse, my mentor Julie shared with me a saying that I will share with you: "Always remember, the patient comes first." This stuck with me because it helped me gain greater awareness of the profound impact that we, as nurses, have in our patients' lives and in assisting them to an optimal level of wellness.

As you progress through your nursing program, consider establishing a mentoring relationship. Having the feeling of comfort and building trust with this person is crucial to the process of mentoring. Here are some ideas and strategies to think about:

- Look for common background in either nursing education or an area of expertise/practice or interest.
- Tell the person about yourself. When you disclose something about yourself, it is especially helpful if you can laugh about yourself in a given situation. This sets the tone of the interaction. It is helpful to keep it light, friendly, and positive.
- Find out the best mode for communicating (e.g., in person, by e-mail, phone) with your mentor.
- Ask broad, open-ended questions such as "How are things going?" that stimulate open discussion rather than direct questions such as "Do you like working here?" or "What kinds of problems are you having?" that may make the other person feel vulnerable.
- By starting out with these basic questions, you can begin to determine a level of comfort about the person. Next, let us examine the characteristics of a successful mentor.

What Are the Characteristics of a Successful Mentor?

When I think about the desired characteristics or competencies of a successful mentor, the following qualities come to mind:

- A mentor communicates **high expectations**. Mentors push mentees and provide avenues and opportunities for them to grow. They allow the mentees to learn through many of their own failures. The mentee grows and develops through active listening, role modeling, and open communication with the mentor. When mentors act as sources of intellectual stimulation and encouragement, they encourage their mentees to trust their own abilities and skills. Mentors open doors and encourage their mentees to search out and seek professional avenues that mentees might not have known about or would have taken longer to discover on their own. Rather than being the "sage on the stage," the mentor is the "guide on the side."
- A mentor is also a **good listener**. Mentors provide a nonjudgmental, listening ear (without taking on the mentee's problems, giving advice, or joining the mentee in a game of "Ain't it awful?"). This can serve as a powerful aid to a mentee. Many mentors believe that respectful listening is the premier mentoring act. When two people really listen to each other, a wonderful sense of synergy is created.
- A mentor has **empathy**. A mentor possesses a degree of sensitivity and perception about the needs of the mentee and has an ability to teach others in an unselfish, respectful way that does not blame but stays neutral. Mentors know what it is like to be the "new kid on the block."
- A mentor offers **encouragement**. By providing subtle guidance and reassurance regarding decisions made by the mentee, the mentor values the mentee's experience, ideas, knowledge of how things work, and special insights into problems. Mentors strive to promote independence in their mentees by offering suggestions but not pushing—mentors know that growth depends on the mentee solving his or her own problems.
- A mentor is **generous**. Mentors are willing to share their time and knowledge with others. Much of what the mentor offers is personal learning or insight (Shea, 1999) (Critical Thinking Box 3.1; Fig. 3.3).

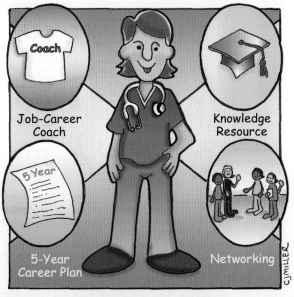

FIG. 3.3 Expectations of a mentor.

CRITICAL THINKING BOX 3.1

- Which of these traits appeals to you the most?
- Which ones would be the most important for your mentor to have?

What Is a Mentoring Moment?

Have you ever experienced a flash of insight or revelation? Peddy (2001) calls this a "mentoring moment." How do you know when that moment arrives? Someone once said, "When the student is ready, the teacher appears" (Peddy, 2001, p. 52). According to Peddy, mentoring is often built on a just-in-time principle, whereby the mentor offers the right help at the right time. A potential mentor must recognize when the mentee feels free to expose a deep-felt need, thereby enabling the mentor to provide the right help at the right time to the best of the mentor's ability.

When Do We Need Mentors?

A mentor is an established professional (selected by you) who takes a long-term personal interest in your nursing career. The mentor not only serves as a role model or counselor for you but also actively advises, guides, and promotes you in your career. A mentor can be any successful, experienced nurse who is committed to a professional career and to being a key figure in your life for a number of years while you are going through school, as well as when you graduate. Mentors should have your best interest at heart and should bolster your self-confidence. Mentors should be able to give feedback in a highly constructive, supportive atmosphere. As a result, trust and caring are hallmarks of the bonding that occurs between mentor and mentee. In short, a mentor is "a wise and trusted adviser" who can serve you well as you experience both professional and personal growth (Fig. 3.4).

A mentoring relationship is an evolving, personal experience for both mentor and mentee. It involves a personal investment of the mentor in the direction of the mentee's professional

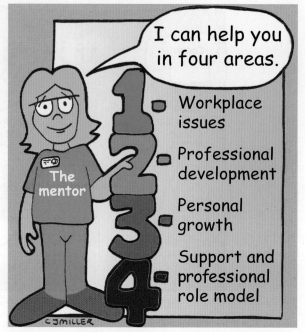

FIG. 3.4 The mentor role.

development. The mentor also benefits from the association by gaining an awareness and perspective of the recent mentee's role in nursing. Take note of the characteristics of successful mentors listed in Box 3.2.

What Is the Role of the Mentee?

As a mentee, you will be learning and absorbing the useful information that the mentor provides. Before seeking a mentor, there are a few questions you may want to ask yourself that may help you to get exactly what you need from the mentoring relationship (Critical Thinking Box 3.2) (Shea, 1999).

BOX 3.2 CHARACTERISTICS OF SUCCESSFUL MENTORS

- Make a personal commitment to be involved with mentee for an extended period of time
- Be trustworthy and sincere
- Show mutual respect
- Do not be in a position of authority over the mentee
- Promote an easy give-and-take relationship, and be flexible and open
- Listen and accept different points of view
- Be experienced
- Have values and goals compatible with those of the mentee
- Be able to empathize with mentee's struggles
- Be nurturing
- Have a good sense of humor, and enjoy nursing

What Are the Characteristics of the Mentee?

Just exactly what are important characteristics that you, as a mentee, should project in your interpersonal communications with your mentor? Use the checklist in Table 3.1 to answer the questions in the table.

How did you score? Are there areas in which you need to improve your interpersonal skills as a mentee?

What Are the Types of Mentoring Relationships?

There are several types of mentoring relationships that you may experience when you develop an active relationship with your mentor (Table 3.2). Formal, informal, and situational mentoring relationships are three types that are commonly encountered (Shea, 1999).

Mentoring Through Reality Shock

The hospital setting is the largest setting where nurses work. In this setting, formal orientation programs are usually established for new graduate nurses, and a mentoring environment is fostered so the new graduate can address the issues of reality shock. This type of mentoring setting appeals to many new graduates because it provides support from other health care team members. Remember Kramer's

TABLE 3.1 MENTEE CHECKLIST

WHEN MEETING WITH YOUR MENTOR, DO YOU …	ALWAYS	FREQUENTLY	USUALLY	SELDOM	NEVER	SCORE
Communicate clearly						
Welcome your mentor's input (express appreciation or tell him or her how it will benefit you)						
Accept constructive feedback						
Practice openness and sincerity						
Take initiative to maintain the relationship with your mentor						
Actively explore options with your mentor						
Share results with your mentor						
Listen for the whole message, including mentor's feelings						
Be alert for mentor's nonverbal communication, and use it as data						

Score yourself as follows: *Always*, 10; *frequently*, 8; *usually*, 6; *seldom*, 4; *never*, 2. According to Shea, a score of 80 or better means you are among the limited group of individuals who have good mentee interaction skills (Shea, 1999, p. 46).
Adapted from Shea, G. F. (1999). *Making the most of being mentored: How to grow from a mentoring relationship.* Lanham, MD: Crisp Publications.

TABLE 3.2 **TYPES OF MENTORING RELATIONSHIPS**			
	FORMAL	**INFORMAL**	**SITUATIONAL**
Structure	Traditional/structured	Voluntary/very flexible	Brief contact/often casual
Characteristic	Driven by organizational needs	Mutual acceptance of roles	A one-time event
Effectiveness	Results measured by organization frequently	Periodic check-ups by supervisors	Results assessed later

Adapted from Shea, G. F. (1999). *Making the most of being mentored: How to grow from a mentoring partnership* (pp. 73–75). Lanham, MD: Crisp Publications.

phases of reality shock in Chapter 1? Let us see how an effective mentorship relationship could address each of the phases.

Honeymoon Phase

The mentor can be supportive by listening and understanding when the mentee shares the excitement of starting the new position and passing the NCLEX exam. The mentor can act as an intermediary with other staff members and as a professional role model.

Shock or Rejection Phase

Mentors can encourage mentees to discuss their feelings of disillusionment and frustration, as well as share their own personal transition processes through this phase. Asking mentees to write down their feelings (keep a reflection journal) or sharing ideas for a possible resolution to a situation can be helpful in mitigating the feelings associated with this phase.

Recovery Phase

The mentor's role during this phase, as mentees begin to accept the reality of the situation and put issues in perspective, is to maintain an open channel of communication and encourage mentees to "step outside their comfort zone" and try new things without stifling the mentee's transition as a new graduate nurse.

Resolution Phase

Mentors are instrumental during this phase to reinforce positive qualities that the mentee possesses and to encourage the mentee in solving problems related to any issues involving the desire either to change nursing positions or to stay put. In addition, this phase can also bring the mentee opportunities to develop leadership skills that may be implemented when the mentee becomes the mentor.

Transitioning from Mentee to Mentor

The moment has arrived, and you are officially flying solo as a professional registered nurse. Your preceptor or mentor is no longer by your side and readily available to answer your questions, validate your concerns, and reassure you that those feelings of inadequacy and wanting to give up were completely normal during this first year of transitioning from nursing student to graduate nurse. As you become more confident and acquire knowledge and skills in your role as a professional nurse, take note that your employer may approach you and ask you to serve as a mentor or preceptor for a newly hired graduate nurse. Making this transition from mentee to mentor can feel scary, but central to mentoring is the idea of passing on your knowledge and clinical expertise to advance the future generation of professional nurses. In addition, mentoring can advance the nursing profession by promoting civility and professionalism among nurses (Research for Best Practice Box 3.2).

🔍 RESEARCH FOR BEST PRACTICE BOX 3.2

Promoting Civility Through Mentoring

Practice Issue

Workplace incivility exists in the nursing profession. Of particular concern, new graduate nurses are often the victims of workplace incivility. The impact of this type of bullying on retaining new graduate nurse in the workplace setting is a chief concern for nurses, health care administrators, and employers. Weaver (2013) contends that workplace incivility is a contributing factor as to why new graduates leave their job and even the profession of nursing. Mentoring can be an effective strategy for abolishing incivility in the workplace by promoting a culture of compassion and kindness shared between mentor and mentee through effective communication (Frederick, 2014).

Implications for Nursing Practice

- Frederick (2014) suggests that effective communication between mentor and mentee can contribute to a positive mentoring relationship. Mentors can use the following techniques when communicating with their mentee to foster receptivity of the mentee's message: questioning, thinking aloud, and debriefing.
- Questioning allows the mentor to assess the mentee's understanding of the issue under discussion. Questioning also allows the mentee to process through information and come up with a solution on his/her own.
- Thinking aloud is another communication technique that a mentor can use to get the mentee to problem-solve and arrive at a clinical decision through debate and "what if" scenarios.

  The debriefing component is vital to the mentoring relationship. During debriefing, the mentee and mentor engage in dialogue through reflection. It is during the debrief, where learning occurs as the mentor assists the mentee in processing through an issue or event by discussing what worked, what went wrong, what could have been done differently, and a plan for what could be done going forward in a similar situation.

- When unsure about something or trying something new, mentees should feel welcomed by their mentor and not scared when asking for help. Mentors should be receptive to answering the mentee's questions and helping out the mentee when the time arises (Frederick, 2014).

Considering This Information

What additional communication guidelines would you carry out with your mentor to foster civility in your workplace?

References

Frederick, D. (2014). Bullying, mentoring, and patient care. *AORN Journal, 99*(5), 587–593. https://doi.org/10.1016/j.aorn.2013.10.023.

Weaver, K. B. (2013). The effects of horizontal violence and bullying on new nurse retention. *Journal for Nurses in Professional Development, 29*(3), 138–142. https://doi.org/10.1097/NND.0b013e318291c453.

So, when will you know that you are ready to mentor or precept a graduate nurse or assist with orienting a seasoned nurse recently hired on the unit where you work? Although there is no minimum amount of time that you must go through to feel ready to mentor or precept another nurse, gaining confidence in clinical knowledge and decision making usually occurs 1 to 2 years after entering into practice (Nickitas, 2014). However, the mentee or preceptee oftentimes finds you and wants you to serve as their mentor or preceptor. Look at the following characteristics demonstrated by both mentors and preceptors in Box 3.3.

What Does the Future Hold?

The future of mentoring programs is changing. Because of technological advancements that have made it possible to offer nursing programs online, an innovative mentoring model has evolved, known

BOX 3.3 ATTRIBUTES OF MENTORS AND PRECEPTORS

- They have acquired a wealth of experience—they are the nurse you would go to on your unit for pretty much anything (e.g., unsure about a policy or procedure, unable to contact a prescriber, trouble logging in to the computer to document patient care).
- They serve as role models.
- They exhibit excellent communication skills.
- They consistently provide constructive feedback (both good and bad) to the mentee.
- They demonstrate professionalism both professionally and personally.
- They empower the mentee by believing them and highlighting their successes.

as e-mentoring. The term *e-mentoring* simply means any type of mentoring partnership that takes place in an online modality. The National Research Mentoring Network (NRMN) offers college students and graduate students continuing their education and research in a biomedical, behavioral, clinical, or social science–related field an opportunity to participate in an online mentorship program for networking and professional development (NRMN, 2018). An advantage of e-mentoring is that mentoring can occur at any time; there are no time or physical constraints that may occur in a face-to-face mentoring partnership. Moreover, the internet has made it possible for NRPs to be offered online (Research for Best Practice Box 3.3).

Q RESEARCH FOR BEST PRACTICE BOX 3.3

Transition to Practice via E-Learning

Practice Issue

Formalized orientation programs traditionally are offered onsite at the new graduate nurses' employing institution following their hire. Throughout the orientation, the new nurse is paired with a preceptor and begins to acquire increased confidence and problem-solving abilities by working with the preceptor in delivering patient care, performing nursing skills, delegating, and communicating with other members of the health care team for a set period. A shortage of nursing staff, coupled with an increase in the number of nurses retiring from the workforce and limited institutional resources, pose as a myriad of factors affecting the new graduate nurse's transition into practice.

Implications for Nursing Practice

- Develop or adopt an e-learning transition to practice model where a portion of the new graduate nurse's orientation program occurs in a blended learning environment consisting of both an online component and onsite at the nurse's employing institution.
- The Future of Nursing Iowa Action Coalition in collaboration with the University of Iowa has implemented a 12-month online nurse residency program for new graduate nurses. The competency-based online residency program's curriculum includes essential competencies that new graduate nurses often struggle with early in their nursing practice. The online program consists of the following interactive modules: transitioning from student to nurse, communication, professional nursing responsibilities, and clinical decision making at the point of care. Another feature of the online residency program is that it offers the nurse resident peer support via online discussion groups. In additional, the new graduate nurse acquires confidence by working with a clinical mentor onsite at the employing health care institution throughout their residency (The University of Iowa College of Nursing, 2018).
- The National Council of State Boards of Nursing (NCSBN) has an online e-learning transition to practice program for newly licensed professional nurses. The online program consists of five online courses that focus on communication and teamwork, patient- and family-centered care, evidence-based practice, quality improvement, and informatics. The program also offers an online program for nurse preceptors (NCSBN, 2017).

Considering This Information

What are your thoughts about online residency programs for onboarding newly licensed nurses? What do you feel will benefit your practice the most as a new graduate nurse participating in an online residency program?

🔍 RESEARCH FOR BEST PRACTICE BOX 3.3—cont'd

References

National Council of State Boards of Nursing (NCSBN) (2017). *NCSBN launches transition to practice online e-learning program.* Retrieved from https://www.ncsbn.org/10224.htm.

The University of Iowa College of Nursing (2018). *Online nurse residency program.* Retrieved from https://uiowa.edu/ionrp/.

Peer mentoring programs continue to be used on campuses throughout the United States. These programs allow senior-level nursing students to mentor entering freshman nursing students. Peer mentoring can be an effective collaborative clinical teaching model for use as a capstone course or an interprofessional clinical simulation experience for nursing students (Research for Best Practice Box 3.4).

🔍 RESEARCH FOR BEST PRACTICE BOX 3.4
Peer Mentoring

Practice Issue

Peer mentoring involves a shared learning experience where a senior nursing student mentors a beginning or freshmen nursing student in fine-tuning nursing skills, assisting with test-taking strategies and study tips, and in sharing strategies for success in nursing school. According to Sweeney (2018), peer mentoring has the potential to provide academic and psychosocial support to community college nursing students transferring into a baccalaureate program. In the clinical lab setting, senior nursing students' serve as lab mentors for junior nursing students in learning how to perform physical assessments, operate medical equipment, and perform essential nursing skills.

Peer mentoring can also take place as an interprofessional experience among allied health, medical, and nursing students in a simulated setting to foster interprofessional teamwork and role development (MacDonald et al., 2018). In addition, an interprofessional learning experience benefits a variety of health-related disciplines in recognizing the unique responsibilities and roles of each team member in providing safe, patient care (Disch, 2017).

Implications for Nursing Practice

* Peer mentoring can alleviate the mentee's perceived stress and loneliness and increase self-efficacy by receiving pertinent information on effective study habits and time-management skills from the peer mentor; these essential skills and peer support may also increase student retention (Raymond & Sheppard, 2018).
* The mentor maintains competency with nursing skills as he or she is continually teaching the skills to mentees in the nursing laboratory.
* The mentees gain experience in learning nursing skills and may be less anxious performing these skills during their clinical experience (Walker & Verklan, 2016).
* Working with students from other disciplines and professions can support nursing students in understanding their roles and responsibilities as a member of the health care team, as well as provide innovative learning opportunities (Disch, 2017).

Considering This Information

What learning opportunities could an interprofessional experience in working with students from the following disciplines offer you?

* Physical Therapy
* Occupational Therapy
* Respiratory Therapy
* Nutrition
* Dental Hygiene
* Forensic Psychology
* Social Work

Continued

RESEARCH FOR BEST PRACTICE BOX 3.4—cont'd

Since beginning your nursing program, reflect on a time when you experienced stress. What was the source of your stress? How might a peer mentor assist you in coping with stress? What attributes would you look for in a peer mentor to assist you in performing various nursing functions in the skills lab? Do you feel that a peer mentor would lessen your anxiety with performing a skill? What do you feel might be a potential challenge(s) in working with a peer mentor? How will you plan to overcome these challenges?

References

Disch, J. (2017). Combining skills and knowledge from different disciplines enhances patient care. *American Nurse Today, 12*(7), 26–30.

MacDonald, S., Manuel, A., Dubrowski, A., Bandrauk, N., Law, R., Curran, V., et al. (2018). Emergency management of anaphylaxis: A high fidelity interprofessional simulation scenario to foster teamwork among senior nursing, medicine, and pharmacy undergraduate students. *Cureus. 10*(7). e2915. https://doi.org/10.7759/cureus.2915.

Raymond, J. M., & Sheppard, K. (2018). Effects of peer mentoring on nursing students' perceived stress, sense of belonging, self-efficacy and loneliness. *Journal of Nursing Education and Practice, 8*(1), 16–23. https://doi.org/10.5430/jnep.v8n1p16.

Sweeney, A. B. (2018). Lab mentors in a two-plus-two nursing program: A retrospective evaluation. *Teaching and Learning in Nursing, 13*(3), 157–160. https://doi.org/10.1016/j.teln.2018.03.006.

Walker, D., & Verklan, T. (2016). Peer mentoring during practicum to reduce anxiety in first-semester nursing students. *Journal of Nursing Education, 55*(11), 651–654. https://doi.org/10.3928/01484834-20161011-08.

CONCLUSION

Here is one final note about mentorship: There is a short anecdotal story about "Everybody, Somebody, Anybody, and Nobody" that has become part of internet lore. I think you will understand that Everybody has to realize the importance of advancing the field of nursing through mentorship; your task will be to find that Somebody who is willing to extend a hand to guide you through the process.

There was an important job to be done, and Everybody was sure that Somebody would do it. Anybody could have done it, but Nobody did it. Somebody got angry about that because it was Everybody's job. Everybody thought Anybody could do it, but Nobody realized that Everybody wouldn't do it. It ended up that Everybody blamed Somebody, when Nobody did what Anybody could have.

Mentoring is a complex, interpersonal, emotional relationship. All parties involved in a mentoring relationship benefit from a mutual exchange of information, life experiences, and diversity. *Mentoring* is defined as a developmental, empowering, and nurturing relationship that extends over time (Vance & Olson, 1998). It involves mutual sharing, learning, and growth that occur in an atmosphere of respect and affirmation (Bower, 2000). A mentor has been described as a role model and guide who encourages and inspires. We leave you with this thought:

"There are two ways of spreading light: to be the candle or the mirror that receives it."
Edith Wharton

🌐 RELEVANT WEBSITES AND ONLINE RESOURCES

American Association of Colleges of Nursing (AACN) and Vizient
Vizient/AACN Nurse Residency Program. http://www.aacnnursing.org/Nurse-Residency-Program

American Association of Colleges of Nursing (AACN)
Academic Practice Partnerships. http://www.aacnnursing.org/Academic-Practice-Partnerships/The-Guiding-Principles

American Nurses Credentialing Center (ANCC)
List of Practice Transition Accreditation Programs (PTAP). https://www.nursingworld.org/organizational-programs/accreditation/find-an-accredited-organization/

Institute of Medicine of the National Academies (IOM)
The Future of Nursing: Leading Change, Advancing Health (Consensus report). http://www.nationalacademies.org/hmd/Reports/2010/The-Future-of-Nursing-Leading-Change-Advancing-Health.aspx

NRMN (National Research Mentoring Network)
About the National Research Mentoring Network. https://nrmnet.net/about-nrmn-2/

Twibell, R. St. Pierre, J., Johnson, D., Barton, D., Davis, C., Kidd, M., & Rook, G.
Tripping over the welcome mat: Why new nurses don't stay and what the evidence says we can do about it. https://www.americannursetoday.com/tripping-over-the-welcome-mat-why-new-nurses-dont-stay-and-what-the-evidence-says-we-can-do-about-it/

U.S. Department of Health & Human Services
HHS Mentoring Program. https://mentoring.hhs.gov/index.aspx

BIBLIOGRAPHY

Ahonen, K. A., & Quinlan, C. M. (2013). Role of the staff nurse in undergraduate nursing education. *American Nurse Today, 8*(5), 52–53.

Billings, D., & Halstead, J. (2016). *Teaching in nursing: A guide for faculty* (5th ed.). St. Louis, MO: Elsevier.

Bott, G., Mohide, A., & Lawlor, Y. (2011). A clinical teaching technique for nurse preceptors: The five minute preceptor. *Journal of Professional Nursing, 27*(1), 35–42. https://doi.org/10.1016/j.profnurs.2010.09.009.

Bower, E. (2000). Mentoring others. In E. L. Bower (Ed.), *Nurses taking the lead* (pp. 11–14). Philadelphia: Saunders.

Emerson, R. J. (2007). *Nursing education in the clinical setting.* St. Louis, MO: Elsevier.

Gibbons, A. (2004). *Mentoring definitions.* Retrieved from http://www.coachingnetwork.org.uk/information-portal/Articles/ViewArticle.asp?artId=54.

Guest, A. B. (1999). A coach, a mentor...a what? *Success Now, 13.* Retrieved from http://www.coachingnetwork.org.uk/information-portal/Articles/ViewArticle.asp?artId=72.

Hunt, D. A., Milani, M. F., & Wilson, S. (2015). Dedicated education units: An innovative model for clinical education. *American Nurse Today, 10*(5), 46–49.

Institute of Medicine of the National Academies (IOM). (2010). *The Future of Nursing: Leading Change, Advancing Health (Report recommendations).* Retrieved from http://www.nationalacademies.org/hmd/Reports/2010/The-Future-of-Nursing-Leading-Change-Advancing-Health/Recommendations.aspx.

International Coach Federation. (2018). *Core competencies.* Retrieved from https://coachfederation.org/core-competencies.

Meier, S. R. (2013). Concept analysis of mentoring. *Advances in Neonatal Care, 13*(5), 341–345. https://doi.org/10.1097/ANC.0b013e3182a14ca4.

MindTools. (2018). *What is coaching?* Retrieved from https://www.mindtools.com/pages/article/newTMM_15.htm.

National Council of State Boards of Nursing (NCSBN). (2016). *Transition to Practice. Why Transition to Practice (TTP)?* Retrieved from https://www.ncsbn.org/transition-to-practice.htm.

National Research Mentoring Network (NRMN). (2018). *About NRMN.* Retrieved from https://nrmnnet.net/about-nrmn-2/.

National Society of Health Coaches (NSHC). (2015). *Position Statement. Health Coaches & Health Coaching: Definition, Qualifications, Risk and Responsibility, and Differentiation from Wellness Coaching.* Retrieved from https://www.nshcoa.com.

Nickitas, D. M. (2014). Mentorship in nursing: An interview with Connie Vance. *Nursing Economics, 32*(2), 65–69.

Peddy, S. (2001). *The art of mentoring.* Houston, TX: Bullion Books.

Shea, G. (1999). *Making the most of being mentored: How to grow from a mentoring relationship.* Lanham, MD: Crisp Publications.

Spector, N., Blegan, M. A., Sivestre, J., Barnseiner, J., Lynn, M. R., Ulrich, B., et al. (2015). Transition to practice study in hospital settings. *Journal of Nursing Regulation, 5*(4), 24–38.

Twibell, R., & St. Pierre, J. (2012, June). Tripping over the welcome mat: Why new nurses don't stay and what the evidence says we can do about it. *American Nurse Today, 7*(6). Retrieved from https://www.americannursetoday.com/tripping-over-the-welcome-mat-why-new-nurses-dont-stay-and-what-the-evidence-says-we-can-do-about-it/.

Vance, C., & Olson, R. K. (1998). Discovering the riches in mentor connections. *Reflections on Nursing Leadership: Sigma Theta Tau International Honor Society of Nursing, 26*(3), 24–25.

4

Employment Considerations: Opportunities, Resumes, and Interviewing

JoAnn Zerwekh, EdD, RN

ⓔ evolve.elsevier.com/Zerwekh/nsgtoday/.

School is almost over and the dream of being paid as an RN (Real Nurse) will soon come true!

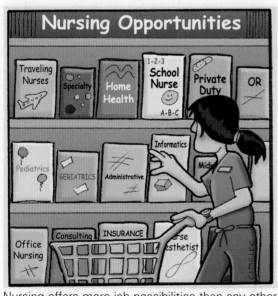

Nursing Opportunities

Traveling Nurses • Specialty • Home Health • 1-2-3 School Nurse A-B-C • Private Duty • OR

Pediatrics • GERIATRICS • Administrative • Informatics • Midw...

Office Nursing • Consulting • INSURANCE • ...rse ...esthetist

Nursing offers more job possibilities than any other aspect of health care. So if your first choice doesn't work out, select another specialty!

After completing this chapter, you should be able to
- Assess trends in the job market
- Identify the primary aspects of obtaining employment
- Describe the key aspects of an e-portfolio and a resume
- Describe the essential steps involved in the interviewing process
- Discuss the typical questions asked by interviewers
- Analyze your own priorities and needs in a job
- Develop short-term career goals

With graduation in sight, you are excited but probably also a little anxious about moving into the workplace, looking for the perfect match to your hard-earned degree. As you consider possible employment opportunities, prepare for the upcoming job search as you would for any graded class assignment: Do your homework! Careful preparation is the key to finding a job you really want. Very few worthwhile job offers come to someone who just happens to walk into the human resources department. The continued expansion of the health care field and the growing nursing shortage have created tremendous opportunities for recent graduates. You have developed marketable skills that are in demand, but to sell yourself successfully to prospective employers and get the job you really want, you must do some homework.

> Take some time to brainstorm about a career—if you could go anywhere you wanted to in nursing, where would it be?

In addition to evaluating the possibilities and limitations of the job market under consideration, give yourself plenty of time to consider what type of position you want and need. You can compare the process with the selection of a marriage partner, car, home, or any other major life choice. It is important for nurses to take the time to create their career plans. Your first professional position is a stepping stone in a long nursing career; it will help define who you are and influence your career path. Only *you* can determine the path you want to travel, so it is important that you become informed and selective in the process. Too often, new graduates accept their first job without sufficient awareness of their own needs or knowledge about the employer they select. Your work is a major factor in your life. If you simply go to work every day, put in your time, and go home, then your job will manage you. If your work enriches your life, is exciting, and you have a feeling of fulfillment, then you are in charge. As a graduate nurse, you have a choice—to do nothing or to take charge of the direction in which you want to go. However, as the Cheshire Cat was well aware, only Alice could make the choice as to the direction in which she should go (Fig. 4.1). Although there is no guarantee that a job will be a perfect fit, career dissatisfaction and turnover can be decreased if careful consideration is given to possible job selection *before* you send out your resume and schedule an interview.

This chapter provides some guidelines to a thorough background preparation for your job search. Critical Thinking Box 4.1 will help you identify your clinical interests and the possible reasons for these preferences. Hint: This will also help you answer interview questions about your professional interests.

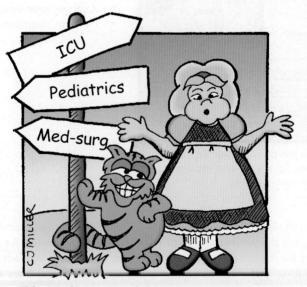

FIG. 4.1 Choose carefully where you want to go.

? CRITICAL THINKING BOX 4.1

Assess Your Wants and Desires, Likes and Dislikes

Identify your interests and the possible reasons for them.

INTERESTS	REASONS
1. I prefer to work with patients whose age is _____.	
2. I prefer to work in a small hospital versus a large medical center _____.	
3. I prefer rotating shifts versus straight shifts _____.	
4. I prefer an internship versus general orientation _____.	
5. I prefer to have a set routine or a constantly changing environment _____.	
6. I prefer these areas (e.g., geriatrics, pediatrics, community, health, medical) _____.	
7. Which of my religious or cultural beliefs or values might have an impact on where I work? _____.	

WHAT IS HAPPENING IN THE JOB MARKET?

There is a cyclic flow of nursing shortages and nursing surpluses. Since 1998 it has been impossible to read an article about the health field that does not mention the nursing shortage, the "looming nursing shortage," or the "worst nursing shortage in U.S. history." Many research studies have shown that the United States would be facing an unprecedented shortage of up to 1 million registered nurses (RNs) by 2020, primarily because of the aging RN workforce, the growing elderly population, and the downswing in the number of younger nurses (Zhang, Tai, Pforsich, & Lin, 2017). The U.S. nursing shortage is projected to grow to 130,000 RNs by 2025, but not the overwhelming shortage that researchers had earlier predicted (Auerbach, Buerhaus, & Staiger, 2015). Let's look at a chronological order of current and projected shortage indicators that have been published since the statement by Buerhaus, Auerbach, and Staiger (2009) about the current easing of the nursing shortage due to the recession in 2008.

■ 2010—The Institute of Medicine (IOM) *Future of Nursing* report called for increasing the number of baccalaureate-prepared nurses in the workforce to 80% and doubling the population of nurses with doctoral degrees. Only 55% of RNs are prepared at the baccalaureate or graduate level.

■ 2017—In a recent issue of the *American Journal of Medical Quality* a group of researchers reevaluated the RN supply-and-demand numbers from 2016 to 2030 using a previously published forecast model with more recent workforce data. There will be a shortage of 154,018 RNs by 2020 and 510,394 RNs by 2030. The South and West regions will have higher shortage ratios than the Northeast and Midwest regions. This reflects a nearly 50% overall improvement when compared with the authors' prior study (United States Registered Nurse Workforce Report Card and Shortage Forecast) reported by Juraschek and colleagues in 2012 (Zhang et al., 2017).

■ In the Bureau of Labor Statistics' *Employment Projections* 2014 to 2024, registered nursing is listed among the top occupations in terms of job growth through 2024. From 2.71 million expected nurse positions in 2014 to 3.2 million needed in 2024, the predicted increase is 16%, or an increase of 439,300 RNs. Due to growth and replacements, approximately 1.09 million nurses will be needed in 2024 to cover the number of job openings for RNs (American Association of Colleges of Nursing [AACN], 2017).

Over the last three decades, the Health Resources and Services Administration (HRSA) has reported every 4 years on the supply of RNs through the National Sample Survey of Registered Nurses (NSSRN). Data collection from the most recent, and final, NSSRN was completed in 2008. The 2008 survey noted that the average age of all licensed RNs increased to 47 years in 2008, from 46.8 in 2004, which represents a stabilization after many years of continuing large increases in average age. Nearly 45% of RNs were 50 years of age or older in 2008, a dramatic increase from 33% in 2000 and 25% in 1980 (HRSA, 2010). Sponsored by the U.S. Department of Health and Human Services' HRSA, the National Sample Survey of RNs examines the characteristics of RNs and their experiences in the nursing field. The U.S. Census Bureau is responsible for the NSSRN data collection, and the survey is now in its 10th cycle. The 2018 NSSRN is the first administration of the survey by the Census Bureau (https://www.census.gov/programs-surveys/nssrn/about.html).

In 2017, the National Council of State Boards of Nursing (NCSBN) and the National Forum of State Nursing Workforce Centers worked together to conduct a survey to provide data on the national nursing workforce. The publication is titled *The National Council of State Boards of Nursing and the Forum of State Nursing Workforce Centers 2017 National Nursing Workforce Survey* (NCSBN, 2019; Smiley et al., 2018). Their findings include the following:

- Male RNs continue to be a growing minority in the workplace.
- The average age of those working in nursing is 51; these findings are consistent with the 2015 study findings.
- Approximately 19.3% of responding RNs were minorities, which includes other and two or more races: Asian (7.7%), Black/African American (6.2%), other (2.8%), and two or more races (1.8%).
- The hospital setting was reported by over half of the RN workforce as their primary place of employment.
- Over half (54.1%) of RNs reported providing nursing services using telehealth technologies.
- 41.7% of RNs had a bachelor of science in nursing (BSN) or higher degree as their initial credential (NCSBN, 2019; Smiley et al., 2018).

The graying of the American population will have a large impact on the health care industry. There will continue to be a substantial increase in the number of older patients, and their levels of care will vary widely from assisted living settings to high-tech environments. This affects the growing need for nurses in the geriatric setting. As the general population ages, so do nurses.

What will happen with nursing employment, the job market, and health care when a large percentage of nurses become part of the older generation? What effort will hospitals make to retain older nurses as the economic recession recovers? Who will mentor the new nurses and help them develop critical decision-making skills at the bedside? How will the role of simulation help bridge the gap between textbook learning and clinical decision making? According to the Bureau of Labor Statistics' *Occupational Outlook Handbook* (2018), "Employment of registered nurses is projected to grow 15 percent from 2016 to 2026, faster than the average for all occupations. Growth will occur for a number of reasons, including an increased emphasis on preventative care; growing rates of chronic conditions, such as diabetes and obesity; and demand for healthcare services from the baby boomer population, as they live longer and more active lives." The current and continuing shortage of nursing personnel in some areas of the country will dramatically heighten the need for increased efficiencies in clinical education for new graduates. How will the job market continue to evolve for the graduate nurse during the next 5 years? Only one thing is certain—everything will continue to change at an increased pace (Critical Thinking Box 4.2).

? CRITICAL THINKING BOX 4.2

What changes have you observed as a result of the nursing shortage? What impact has the shortage had on salaries and staffing in your community? If the signs of a nursing shortage were beginning to surface as far back as the late 1990s, why haven't we (education, health care employers, government) yet created effective solutions for this growing problem?

SELF-ASSESSMENT

What Are My Clinical Interests?

Begin by jotting down possible settings where you could pursue your areas of clinical interest. Depending on your interests, there will be a number of possible paths to pursue. As you identify clinical areas that interest you, try to prioritize them. This step may seem like a nonissue if you tend to "eat, sleep, and drink" one nursing specialty; however, many people have two or more strong interests, and this step helps to outline more possibilities. Believe it or not, some graduating students confess to liking *every* clinical rotation and feel pulled in multiple directions when they consider where to begin a job search. If that description fits you, hang in there—you are not alone! Keep in mind that all nursing experiences, both negative and positive, can contribute to your career in a productive way. The more areas you sample, the broader your knowledge base will be as you gradually build a career.

Recruiters like to see flexibility in new graduates, but let us try to narrow your professional interests just a bit before your actual job search. Perhaps you can identify what you liked about each clinical rotation through reflective journaling and then prioritize possible interests or identify common experiences.

What Are My Likes and Dislikes?

Another way to approach self-assessment involves identification of your likes and dislikes in the work setting. This is related to interests but on a more personal level. The job you eventually select may have some drawbacks, but it should meet many more of your likes than dislikes in order to be a good "fit" (Fig. 4.2).

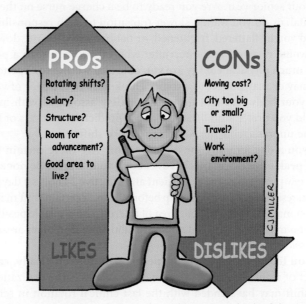

PROs
Rotating shifts?
Salary?
Structure?
Room for advancement?
Good area to live?

CONs
Moving cost?
City too big or small?
Travel?
Work environment?

LIKES   DISLIKES

FIG. 4.2 Assess your personal needs and interests. Is the job a good fit?

Write out your responses to the following questions:

1. Do you enjoy an environment that provides a great deal of patient interaction, or do you thrive in a technically oriented routine? Think back to your clinical rotations and see if you can find a pattern to what was most enjoyable or disagreeable.
   - I liked opportunities for using many technical skills.
   - I was bored with slower-paced routines (e.g., mother–infant care).
   - I liked to see the results of care as soon as possible (e.g., perioperative anesthetic care unit [PACU]).
   - I disliked the constant turnover of patients every day (e.g., emergency department).

2. **Do you enjoy caring intensively for one or two patients at a time with a high acuity level and a potential rapid change in patient status, or do you prefer a less acute patient assignment with opportunities for family education and observing increased patient independence? Why did you like or dislike one type or the other?** Discuss your responses with some friends who may have had other experiences and get their opinions. Consider how you will explain your preferences to a nurse recruiter on the phone, in an online cover letter, or in person.

3. **Do you learn best in a highly structured environment or in more informal on-the-job training situations?** Knowing your learning style can guide your interest and narrow your selection of an internship or orientation program. For example, internships range from formal classes with lengthy preceptorships to more informal orientations of fairly short duration. Remember, a program that meets *your* needs may not be the answer for your best friend. Write down what you would like from an orientation or internship program. Look over your list and prioritize what you need and want most.

4. **Do you feel comfortable functioning with a significant degree of autonomy, or do you want and need more direction and supervision at this point in your professional development?** Soon you will have completed nursing school, backed up by employment on a telemetry unit throughout your senior year. Are you ready to be a charge nurse on the 3- to 11-p.m. shift in a small rural hospital, or do you want a slower transition to such responsibility? If this situation were offered, would you be flattered, frightened, or flabbergasted? Write down your reaction and consider how you would respond to the recruiter who offered you such a position.

5. **How much physical energy are you able and willing to expend at work?** Running 8 to 12 hours a day may or may not act as a tonic. Think back to the pace of your clinical rotations and consider how your body reacted (minus the anxiety associated with instructor supervision, if you can!). Would you prefer a unit that has some predictable periods of frenzy and pause, or do you thrive on the unpredictable for your entire work shift?

6. **Are you a day, evening, or night person? Are there certain times of the day when you are at your peak of performance? How about your worst?** Be honest and realistic with your answers. Very few people are equally efficient and effective 24 hours a day. If your body shuts down at 10 p.m. or you resist all efforts to wake up before 9 a.m., a certain shift may have to be eliminated. However, if the job market is tight in your area of interest, the available positions may be on a less desirable shift and you may have to make temporary adjustments in other areas of your life to acclimate better to a professional position.

7. **Do you like rotating shifts or, perhaps more realistically, can you work rotating shifts?** One aspect of reality shock for many new graduates is the realization that jobs involving working the day shift may have ended with the last clinical rotation in school. Hospital and long-term-care staffing is 24 hours a day, 7 days a week. It is a "24/7 profession"—a possibly unpleasant aspect of nursing but a real one nonetheless. Assess your ability to work certain shifts and try to strike a

flexible approach before you speak with nurse recruitment. Working 12-hour shifts (7 a.m. to 7 p.m. or 7 p.m. to 7 a.m.) can be very demanding on the days assigned, but this option is very popular with many nurses because of the increased days off.

8. **Consider the impact of these choices on your family, your social life, and other needs.** If there are certain shifts you must rule out, recognize that this may limit your job choices and plan accordingly. Giving some thought to your flexibility ahead of time will help you avoid committing to any and all shifts during an interview and will facilitate your job hunt. On the other hand, it is probably not realistic to request a Monday-through-Friday schedule in an acute care setting unless the organization has a separate weekend staff or a high level of personnel who ask to work only weekends. Shift patterns may vary significantly within a city—and in different areas of the country as well— so do your homework online or through job fairs about available shifts before you go in for an actual interview.

9. **Can you work long hours (e.g., 12-hour shifts) without too much tension and fatigue?** The 12-hour staffing option offers flexibility (e.g., six 12-hour days of work in an 80-hour pay period) but leaves some people exhausted and irritable. Consider your personal needs outside of work when you respond to this item. Can you climb into bed or put your feet up after a nonstop 12-hour shift, or do you need to pick up family responsibilities as soon as you walk in the door? The 4 days off may well compensate for 3 days of fatigue, but map out your needs before you begin your job search.

10. **Do you like making decisions quickly or generally favor a more relaxed approach to clinical problems?** In general, intensive care units (ICUs) and step-down units require more immediate reactions than an adolescent psych unit or orthopedics. Does the ICU environment excite or overwhelm you? Would you prefer a slower pace? Do not criticize yourself for your likes or dislikes. Slower-paced units require different strengths, not less knowledge. You have nothing to gain by working in an ICU if you dislike the setting. Meet your own needs, not someone else's. You will spend a great deal of your time at work. Make the choice for *you*, not according to someone else's idea of the perfect job.

11. **What do you need in a job to be happy?** This question does not mean money or benefits but rather the sense that the job is worth getting excited about. Think about past employment you have had, whether in health care or not. What did you like or dislike about the job? What made you stay? Possible answers include opportunities for growth, advancement, working with people you respect, or collegiality. Remember, your answers should include things that are important to you. These are the kinds of issues that make you eager to go to work or to help you work through difficult clinical days. You may want to compare your answers with those of others whose opinions you value to gain a broader perspective.

After thoroughly reflecting on the questions listed, you will have to reflect on yourself as a person and explore what interests you have in the many facets of nursing.

What Are My Personal Needs and Interests?

A third aspect of self-assessment focuses on personal needs and interests. How much time and effort are you willing and able to give to your career at this point in time? Will work be a number-one priority in your life, or does family or continued education take precedence?

Is relocation a possibility? If you are considering relocation, decide how you will gather information on possible job opportunities in the area or areas under consideration. Include Internet websites, professional journals, and professional and family contacts as possible sources of information. In addition to reviewing online job possibilities, research the hospital's website for details about the organization's overall philosophy, its department of nursing, and a sense of "fit." Prospective employers want to know that applicants have taken the time to become knowledgeable about them and appreciate it when applicants ask more informed questions about employment.

If this is a voluntary move, develop a list of pros and cons for each location under consideration. Include your personal interests in the decision (e.g., cost of living, commuting time, possible relocation allowance, access to recreational activities, opportunities for advanced education, and clinical opportunities).

What salary range are you willing to consider? Although starting salaries for new graduates are generally nonnegotiable, differentials for evenings, nights, and weekends create a range of salary possibilities. If you want an extended internship, a lower starting salary may be offered. Are you willing and able to trade this for the benefits of an extended internship? The quality of the internship may be worth a lower salary temporarily because of later advancement opportunities. Some areas of the country offer considerably higher salaries than others, but factor in the cost of living before you move out of town. You may be unpleasantly surprised by a monthly rent that swallows up a significant percentage of your salary.

What Are My Career Goals?

The final step of your self-assessment is the development of career goals. Yes, you really do need to have some goals! You are the architect of your professional future, so take pen to paper or fingers to the keyboard and start designing. Consider your answers to the following questions:

What do you want from your first nursing position? Possible answers might include developing confidence in decision making, more proficiency with technical skills, increased organizational abilities, and gathering skills to move into a more favorable position.

What are your professional goals for the first year? Third year? Fifth year? If you cannot imagine your life let alone your career beyond 1 to 2 years, relax. Many people feel uneasy planning beyond their initial position and first paid vacation.

Develop a comfortable response to a question regarding your goals for the first year, and consider what you might want to be doing after that time. Remember, it is far easier to gauge how your career is progressing if you have established some benchmark goals to which you can refer. This is also a favorite question posed during interviews, so spend some time thinking about it! Recruiters are interested in nurses with a plan.

RESEARCHING PROSPECTIVE EMPLOYERS

What Employment Opportunities Are Available?

You have a world of nursing to choose from; there are opportunities available to begin your practice as a graduate nurse. The largest employers are hospitals or acute care facilities. In hospitals, a wide variety of positions are available, although new graduates are almost always placed in staff nurse positions. If it is a general hospital, you must choose what areas interest you most. Your first position may not be exactly what you want, but remember, it is the first step toward your career goal. As you build your competence and self-esteem, you may find just the position you want. In many hospitals, staff positions represent different levels of proficiency, especially if the hospital participates in clinical or career ladders (Fig. 4.3).

> The staff nurse position can be one of the most challenging. It can also be like an "incubator" from which to develop your nursing career.

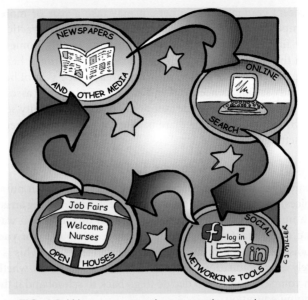

FIG. 4.3 Ways to research prospective employers.

Charge nurse positions may involve responsibility for a particular staff or a particular day, or they may involve managing staff for an entire unit. New graduates should not be placed in charge positions until they have mastered a staff nurse role, but the marketplace may result in new graduates being offered the charge position, especially in more rural settings. If this is a situation that you face soon after graduation, make sure that you identify your resources and consider whom you can contact for professional support and backup. Do not allow your ego to let you accept an unsafe position that could endanger patients and your hard-earned nursing license.

Entry-level positions in the hospital are usually staff nurse positions. Staff nurse positions in medical-surgical nursing are among the most demanding—and rewarding—positions. Frequently nurses begin their careers here with the intention of moving on to greener pastures; however, the rewards and challenges may more than fulfill their needs. It is important that your first position offers you an opportunity to further develop your nursing skills. Surely you have heard at least one person in nursing school say to you, "You should get a year's experience in Med-Surg first." Is this a true statement? Yes and no. Yes, if you want to work in a medical-surgical field, and no, if you do not. Yes, the experience will help sharpen your assessment skills and some technical skills, but every area of work has advantages and potential drawbacks. If you know in your heart that med-surg makes you miserable, turn around and go in a different direction. Life is too short to be miserable for 8 to 12 hours a day. Furthermore, chances are that you will not give your best to the patients if you are unhappy.

Whether it is working in the emergency department, day surgery, specialty units, or medical-surgical units, staff nurse positions give you a very valuable opportunity to polish your time management, patient care organization, and nursing skills. Once you are confident with skills, procedures, and the overall practice of nursing, you may be ready to move on to new challenges. This may take 6 months for some recent graduates. For others, it may take a year or more. Take the time to reinforce your nursing competencies; it will prepare you for your future practice in nursing. Other areas in which nurses may find employment include community health, home health care, and nursing agencies. Working in the community in such positions as occupational health, school health, and the military may require a bachelor's degree in nursing and at least 1 year of hospital nursing. If you want to work in a community setting, concentrate initially on refining your assessment and critical thinking skills in the acute care setting, because the autonomy of the community setting means more decision making on your own without the immediate backup of experienced peers, who are usually available in the acute care setting.

What About Advanced Degrees in Nursing?

There are many advantages to earning an advanced degree in nursing (review Chapter 7 for the different choices). One of the most important aspects of obtaining an advanced degree is using your experience as a nurse to help you determine in what direction you want to go. If you have an associate degree, you might want to consider the basic requirements for your baccalaureate degree, including what schools are available and what their requirements are. This is an area you can begin to work on immediately after graduation. As you interview for jobs, ask whether the prospective employer will work with your schedule if you decide to go back to school and if they provide tuition reimbursement for continuing education.

HOW DO I GO ABOUT RESEARCHING PROSPECTIVE EMPLOYERS?

Employment Considerations: How Do You Decide on an Employer?

In your search for a job, it is important to look for organizations and hospitals that create a work environment supporting professional nursing practice. In 1980, the American Academy of Nursing identified criteria for the designation of "magnet hospital." This designation recognized certain hospitals for their lower turnover rates, their visionary leaders, the value they placed on education, and the ability to keep lines of communication open. To identify magnet hospitals in your area, check the website http://www.nursecredentialing.org/Magnet/FindaMagnetFacility (ANCC, 2015). Inquire about the last accrediting agency survey results. This may be a state survey in long-term and subacute care or The Joint Commission in acute care. The survey results will give you information about the quality of care delivered at that employment agency. Showing an interest in being a part of a quality organization will put you in a positive light as a candidate for hire. In your search for a job, it is important to look for organizations and hospitals that create a work environment supporting professional nursing practice. In the current job market, finding magnet hospitals in your community will help you in your job search.

Media Information

Newspapers. Although many people no longer look at the newspaper for information, preferring the internet for data, the newspaper is still a good place in which to look for information about jobs as well as articles about hospitals or other health care employment opportunities. This will vary considerably depending on the area of the country where you are hoping to work. Scan the advertisements to see whether any are targeted specifically to graduating seniors. Focus on these initially because they will include information on possible job fairs, internships, or specialized orientations in addition to specific openings for graduate nurses.

Online searches. Electronic job searches have replaced newspaper searches for many people as the best places in which to start looking for employment. This is an efficient way to search because you can access information for both local and distant nursing opportunities with the ease of a few clicks—assuming that the sites are kept current. As a new graduate, consider the value of looking at employer websites rather than generic nursing employment sites because employer sites are better focused for new graduates. Additionally, many employer websites offer services for building a profile that allows you to customize based on the department or unit you are interested in working for. It is also a terrific way to review the positions available within the entire organization. If you intend to use this method to follow up on a job posting, be prepared to submit your flawless resume electronically—and be sure to spell-check all of your correspondence before you click the "Send" button! Many organizations now require electronic applications, occasionally raising issues of software compatibility for applicants. Know and be prepared to comply with human resources requirements for submitting your resume and cover letter. Patience in the application process is essential for your professional success. With the availability of computer spell-checking and editing support, there is no excuse for a poorly written resume or cover letter. Take the time to review your documents for errors. Recruiters pay attention to these details.

Social networking. Social networking is the way in which people of the 21st century seem to communicate with one another through online websites that comprise a community of individuals with like-minded interests. According to the 2018 Pew Research Center report, the majority of Americans now use Facebook (68%) and YouTube (73%)—two platforms out of the eight surveyed—as well as Instagram (35%), Pinterest (29%), Snapchat (27%), LinkedIn (25%), Twitter (24%), and WhatsApp (22%). "As was true in previous Pew Research Center surveys of social media use, there are substantial differences in social media use by age. Some 88% of 18- to 29-year-olds indicate that they use any form of social media. That share falls to 78% among those ages 30 to 49, to 64% among those ages 50 to 64 and to 37% among Americans 65 and older" (Smith & Anderson, 2018). Other interesting findings from the Pew social media use report are these:

- Pinterest is more popular with women users (41% of whom say they use the site) than with men users (16%).
- LinkedIn is very popular among college graduates and those in high-income households.
- The messaging service WhatsApp is popular in Latin America, and this popularity also extends to Latinos in the United States.
- The typical (median) American uses three of the eight sites. Younger adults tend to use a greater variety of social media platforms. The median 18- to 29-year-old uses four of these platforms, but that figure drops to three among 30- to 49-year-olds, to two among 50- to 64-year-olds, and to one among those 65 years old and older.
- Most social media users say that it *would not* be hard to give up social media (59%) with 40% saying it would be hard to give it up (Smith & Anderson, 2018).

Thus, if you are trying to make a good impression, your appearance on the social networking website will be what an employer first sees. Begin by doing an internet search on yourself and fix anything that may have a negative connotation. Be sure to use a professional photo, perhaps just a headshot, and—if you want to use the Facebook account for family and friends—make your Facebook account private to prevent employers from searching for you there. Potential employers may dismiss you as a candidate after viewing inappropriate photographs or information. A study by Careerbuilder (2016) noted that approximately 60% of employers are using networking sites to obtain additional information about a potential applicant, which is up 11% from a decade ago, when the first survey was conducted. Approximately 49% of employers who research job applicants on social media said that they had found content that caused them to eliminate a candidate. This screening process is not only for potential employees; 41% of employers say they use social networking sites to research current employees, with 26% having found content that led to employee reprimand or termination.

As the amount of personal information available online grows via sources such as Facebook, Twitter, and the like, first impressions are being formed long before the interview process begins, warns David Opton, ExecuNet's chief executive officer (CEO) and founder. "Given the implications and the shelf-life of Internet content, managing your online image is something everyone should address—regardless of whether or not you're in a job search," he says (Lorenz, 2009).

LinkedIn (2018) operates the world's largest professional network on the internet with over 562 million users in over 200 countries and territories. LinkedIn has become the place for reconnecting with colleagues and classmates as well as powering your career with a vast network of contacts and employers looking for the right employee. Recruiters often search this site. If you do not have a profile on LinkedIn, you may be left out of finding the right type of position. LinkedIn allows you to link to your professional Twitter, Facebook, or blog pages and upload your resume to your profile, which definitely comes in handy for interested employers.

Job fairs/open houses. You may have the opportunity to attend a nursing job fair or hospital open house as a soon-to-be graduate nurse. Take advantage of these opportunities to collect information about specific employers and possibly make initial contacts for later interviews. Leave your jeans and tennis shoes at home on these occasions and put on your professional best. Take some time with your appearance, because first impressions are important (Fig. 4.4)!

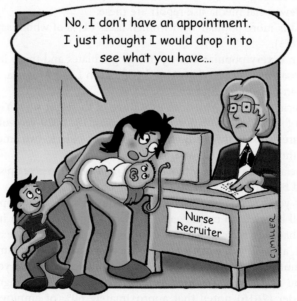

FIG. 4.4 The first impression is a lasting one, so make it count *for* you, not against you.

Employee contacts. If you have a friend or family member—or simply know someone—who works at an organization you are considering for employment, make an effort to speak with him or her about the job environment. As an insider, this person may be able to provide you with a perspective about the employer that the advertisement, recruiter, or interview cannot. Possible questions you may want to ask such an insider may include these: "Why do you enjoy working there? What was orientation like? How is employee morale? What is the turnover rate for nursing or for other employees? Does management show appreciation for employee effort and welcome employee input?"

Recruitment Contacts

Letter-writing campaign. Plan to send your resume with a cover letter and triple-check both documents for grammatical errors. Your resume and cover letter are the first impression you will make with a prospective employer. Make it a positive one!

Telephone contact. Before you pick up the telephone, get out your calendar and start planning likely dates for possible interviews, as well as the approximate date you want to begin working. Armed with this information, you can comfortably answer questions beyond the fact that you would like the employer to send you a brochure and an application. Depending on the organization you contact, the human resources or nurse recruitment department may want you to first submit a resume online or may ask you to set up an appointment for an interview. Do not commit to an interview if you are not ready.

Personal contact. If you plan to just stop by human resources or nurse recruitment for a brochure and an application, make sure you give some thought to your appearance. Tee shirts, shorts, and jeans are not appropriate and have caused otherwise well-qualified applicants to be passed over for further consideration. Again, remember that first impression!

WHAT DO I NEED TO KNOW TO ASSESS THE ORGANIZATION?

Now that you have described yourself and have thought about the kind of setting in which you work best, continue these exercises on a consistent basis. This ongoing analysis will help you to make decisions about the kind of organization that is best for you and put you in a position to determine what kind of organization fits you.

How Do You Go About Assessing an Organization to Find What You Want?
Talk to People in the Organization

One obvious answer is to ask the people who work in that organization. When you interview for a position, you can meet people who work in the specific setting in which you are interested. Ask questions that will help you learn about certain situations. Take some time to think about questions and situations you would like to present when you talk to people in various facilities. Keep in mind that the values of the organization will affect your work on a daily basis. If both patients and employees are valued, you will see this reflected in the quality of patient care and in the retention of nurses.

Read and Analyze the Recruitment Materials

Organizations also present themselves to you through their documents. Carefully analyze the materials presented to you—this is another way of determining the values the organization lives by and deems important. All of these materials are intended to make a statement to you about who they are.

Review the Mission or Philosophy Statement

There are other written documents to examine. For example, a specific nursing unit may have a mission statement that tells you who they are and what they are about. The department of nursing will have a philosophy statement or possibly a nursing theory that should be the organizing framework around which the members structure themselves in delivering nursing care. In some organizations, the staff knows what this mission statement says and how it provides direction to them. In other organizations, the staff will be unfamiliar with the statement of philosophy and may react with confusion when you ask them. All of these written materials should send a message to you about the organization. Do your observations during the interview process support the organization mission/philosophy statements (Critical Thinking Box 4.3)?

? CRITICAL THINKING BOX 4.3

What are some observations that you could have during your interview process that would cause you to have second thoughts about accepting a position at the organization?

Evaluate the Reputation of the Leadership

Organizations are guided by people at the top and take on the characteristics these people support. What do you know about the CEO? This person sets the stage and the direction for the organization. You can gather information about the CEO by checking the organization's website and asking people during the interview what this person is like. People in the community will also be familiar with this person and can give you insight into the values and characteristics that this person represents.

    The same can be said for the chief nursing officer (CNO). This person sets the direction for the nursing organization, either by active design or benign neglect, and sets into motion an organization that structures the beliefs about patients, staff, and nursing. It is important to talk with nurses who are working with the CNO to determine how they feel about the leadership in the organization. Has he or she had a successful track record? Is this person well respected? Can people point to a strategic direction and philosophy this person has given to the organization?

PORTFOLIOS

Portfolios have been used in nursing education to document a student's knowledge, skills, abilities; to track the student's progress within a curriculum; and to monitor and evaluate his or her performance at strategic checkpoints. A professional portfolio is like a scrapbook that is a collection of past events, documents, certificates, and other artifacts (*artifacts* meaning all information, documents, and so on placed in the portfolio). Portfolios take time to develop and maintain; however, the payoff is that the collection of information is available for job seeking, promotion, and evaluation. Don't confuse a portfolio with a resume or curriculum vitae (CV). The resume or CV is a component of the professional portfolio. If you haven't already started a portfolio during your nursing program, you can start by compiling the supporting documents to include in the portfolio. Box 4.1 provides a list of supporting documents to include in the portfolio as a new graduate seeking employment. Your portfolio will be a work in progress and must be updated throughout your academic and professional journey. As you collect your documents, you'll be wise to scan them into an electronic format and keep a backup on either a removable disk drive or in the "cloud." By having your portfolio documents in electronic format, you can create an e-Portfolio.

BOX 4.1 PORTFOLIO SUPPORTING DOCUMENTATION

- Degree from nursing school attended
- Clinical evaluation document for all clinical rotations, including a narrative notation from the clinical instructors about your progress in the clinical and simulation setting
- Documentation of nursing skills list
- Group projects or assignments demonstrating your involvement in working with a team
- Certificates of attendance for any nursing student or professional development conferences attended
- Supporting documentation for any service learning projects that you planned or participated in (i.e., health fair, flu vaccination clinics)
- Resume or curriculum vitae (CV)

What Is an E-Portfolio?

The electronic portfolio, or e-portfolio, is a relatively new tool being used by students to secure their first position after graduation by showcasing their talents and skills and focusing attention on the unique attributes they have for the prospective employer and desired position. The e-portfolio is pre-ferred by employers. In addition, the e-portfolio clearly demonstrates the new graduate's web writing skills and ability to create and update their e-Portfolio website. Many health care employers use the e-portfolio as an additional tool to review the prospective employee in the prehire period beyond the resume, employment application, and interview (McMillan, Parker, & Sport, 2014) (Critical Thinking Box 4.4). Hannans (2017) states that an estimated 60% to 80% of employers do online searches of potential hires and warns that your digital identity should not be taken lightly.

? CRITICAL THINKING BOX 4.4

Are you wondering where to find a website or hosting for your e-Portfolio? Type the following in your web browser, "free e-Portfolio website providers," to locate some suggestions. What obstacles do you feel you will encounter in creating your e-Portfolio?

Make sure your online identity reveals information about you personally and professionally, as it often mediates the first impression you will make with recruiters and nurse managers.

As you acquire e-portfolio documents, now is a good time (if you have not already started) to develop your resume and to showcase your academic, professional, and past employment experience. So let's focus on resumes.

TRADITIONAL AND EMPLOYER-FOCUSED RESUMES

A trend in writing a resume is the employer-focused resume, which basically has the same elements as the traditional resume but requires a change in focus. The traditional resume provides an inventory of your professional work background and skills and highlights the background first, followed by matching it to attributes noted for a desired job position. The employer-focused resume approach requires the prospective job applicant to know the audience (employing agency) and what they want, so that the resume can be written to demonstrate that the applicant has the required competencies for employment (i.e., the applicant is a "good fit" for the agency). Let's look at some techniques used in writing an effective resume.

How Do I Write an Effective Resume?

> Design your resume by using the KISS principle: Keep It Simple, Sincerely! (That is, use concise wording and make it easy to read, informative, and simple.)

Your resume conveys the first impression a prospective employer will have of you. It will give the employer a basic idea of who you are professionally and what your objectives are for your nursing career. While you define your strengths, it is also important not to overstate your skills. Everything that you include on your resume should be true. Expect the employer to check all facts. Do not jeopardize a job possibility by intentional misstatements or careless attention to dates of prior employment or education.

Most employers are willing to train you on all or some of the components of the position you are applying for. A resume is a concise, factual presentation of your educational and professional history (Box 4.2). Do not be surprised if a recruiter suggests other areas to you in addition to what you have initially indicated on your resume or in your interview. Be open to suggestions; they may have some ideas or considerations you have not even thought about.

What Information Is Necessary for a Resume?

Here are the components of a resume. Be sure to proofread what you write for correct spelling and grammar. Do not forget that this is the first impression someone may get of you.

Demographic Data: Who Are You?

Your name, address, telephone number, and e-mail address should be at the top of the page. Be sure to give correct, current information so that the employer can easily contact you. If you need to give an alternative telephone number or e-mail address, provide the prospective employer with the contact person's name and advise the person that a potential employer may be calling for you. Keep in mind that you never put personal information such as your social security number, marital status, number of

---

BOX 4.2   RESUME GUIDELINES

- Catch all typos and grammatical errors. Have someone proofread your resume.
- Present a clear summary of qualifications that emphasize your skills and strengths.
- A good first impression is critical, so if written, your resume should be neat and printed on white or off-white paper.
- Avoid using "I" or "me" in your resume.
- Keep the information concise, preferably limited to one or two pages.
- The rule of thumb on work experience is to show your most current work experience. This generally means the last 10–15 years unless there is something in your more distant background that is critical to note.
- Do not try to impress anyone with big words. Jargon specific to the profession is okay if everyone knows what it is.
- Do not inquire about salary or benefits in your resume. That is not the right place for that.
- Do not exaggerate about what you can and cannot do, because the potential employer will check it out.
- Present yourself in a positive light.
- Your resume should be neat and visually appealing. If sending by email, save to a PDF file to preserve formatting.
- Do not list all of your references. Be prepared to provide them on a separate list when asked. You may want to have different references for different types of positions.

children, or picture on a resume. Your e-mail address conveys a message, so don't include anything that sends a "cutesy" or possibly offensive message to a prospective employer. Consider the image you want to convey.

Summary of Qualifications (Professional Objective): What Position Are You Applying For?

There are many ways in which to address this element. With the traditional resume, it is important that you describe the position you are applying for and specify what department or area of nursing you are interested in. The professional objective statement focuses on the job applicant's wishes and needs and not on the prospective employer's needs. With the widespread use of the internet, it is easy to view job openings and be more educated and decisive about what you are looking for. This is the first step in developing your employer-focused resume by determining what the employer wants in a job applicant. The **summary of qualifications** has become more common today than the professional objective. The qualification summary notes the specific skills and competencies you have that fit the job position. Typically, the qualification summary is 5 to 10 lines or bullet points providing a brief overview of your critical skills and competencies. The qualification summary functions like an abstract for a journal article (Welton, 2013). See Fig. 4.5 for an example of the summary of qualifications.

Education: Where Did You Receive Your Education?

List your education in chronological order, beginning with the most recent. List the month and year of graduation and what degree you received, if any. If you have degrees other than nursing, include these

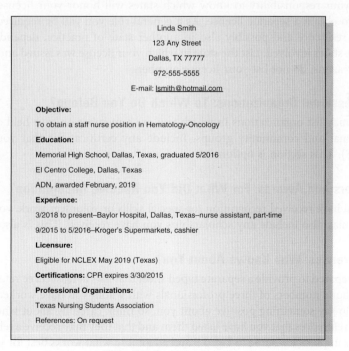

Linda Smith

123 Any Street

Dallas, TX 77777

972-555-5555

E-mail: lsmith@hotmail.com

Objective:

To obtain a staff nurse position in Hematology-Oncology

Education:

Memorial High School, Dallas, Texas, graduated 5/2016

El Centro College, Dallas, Texas

ADN, awarded February, 2019

Experience:

3/2018 to present–Baylor Hospital, Dallas, Texas–nurse assistant, part-time

9/2015 to 5/2016–Kroger's Supermarkets, cashier

Licensure:

Eligible for NCLEX May 2019 (Texas)

Certifications: CPR expires 3/30/2015

Professional Organizations:

Texas Nursing Students Association

References: On request

FIG. 4.5 Sample resume.

in the chronological order in which you received them. This section will contain any certifications (BLS, ACLS, PALS) and special training you have received, where you received them, and the date you completed them. If you are currently enrolled in school, be sure to include that as well.

Professional Experience: What Do You Know How to Do?

"Easy to read" is the goal. It is very important to put this section in chronological order beginning with the present. You want the prospective employer to see what you have been doing most recently. List your current or previous employer, position held, dates from and to, and a brief description of your responsibilities. This is a good place to reinforce special skills that you highlighted in your summary of qualifications that you feel may be important to your prospective employer. This section will differ for an experienced nurse versus a recent graduate nurse. However, it is important to list your employment history through the past 7 years, including those areas of employment that may not be associated with nursing or the health care field. All the experiences you have had as an employee help to demonstrate your ability to work with people, handle stress, be flexible, and so forth. It is not necessary to list clinical rotations you have completed during nursing school, as these are generally standardized. If you have not had any work experience and this will be your first job, state that also. It is important for managers and staff educators to be aware of the levels of experience of recent graduates they consider. If you had an opportunity to take a clinical elective in a specialty area, include that information because it may enhance your application, especially if you apply for a position in that specialty.

Licensure: What Can You Do and Where Can You Do It?

This is a very important area of information for nurses. With the implementation of the multistate Nurse Licensure Compact (see Chapters 5 and 17), you may need to be licensed in only one state. It is your responsibility to know which states will honor your license and which ones will require you to obtain a separate license. As a general rule you will be required to be licensed in the state of your residence and possibly also in another state of practice, depending on the licensure compact of the states involved. List the state in which your license was issued and the expiration date. For security reasons, do not list your license number.

Professional Organizations: To Which Do You Belong?

You may list organizations in which you are a member or have held an office. You should list professional and community groups. Include any certifications that you have obtained (BLS, ACLS, PALS). This section is optional.

Honors and Awards: For What Did You Receive Recognition?

If you have received recognition for special skills or volunteer work, you may want to include it here. You may also include any scholarships you have received. This is also an optional section.

References: Who Knows About You?

Be prepared to provide a separate typed sheet that lists at least three references. Provide the names and telephone numbers of three professionals with whom you have worked. These professionals must be able to say something positive about you, so think carefully about whom you choose. Always notify your references that you have listed them and that they may receive a telephone call about you. Look at the example of a resume in Fig. 4.5 and adapt it to what works best for you. Make every effort as a new graduate to keep your resume on one page because recruiters generally scan the resume in less than

2 minutes. As you gain professional experience, a longer resume may become necessary. If you need further examples of resumes or formats, check the Internet for samples (www.resume.monster.com). Many word processing programs also have resume formats that you can access.

What Else Should I Submit With My Resume?

Along with your resume, you should enclose a cover letter that serves as a brief introduction (Box 4.3). Summarize your important strengths or give information regarding change of specialty, but remember that this letter should be brief—about three to five well-written paragraphs on one or two pages (www.csuchico.edu/plc/cover-letters.html). If you have spoken with a recruiter and have a specific name, address the letter to him or her. However, you do not have to address it to a specific person; it will be distributed to the recruiter who handles the units in which you have indicated an interest. Simply addressing it to "Nurse Recruitment" will usually ensure that it gets to the right person. Large organizations may have several recruiters, so a general address to recruitment will often suffice. However, if you have spoken with a recruiter and have a specific name, address your letter to that person.

BOX 4.3 REMINDERS FOR COVER LETTERS

Content and Format
- Business letter format
  Date
  Employer's Name and Title
  Company Name
  Address
- Salutation: Use person's name and title (e.g., Mr. John Smith, Outpatient Supervisor)
- Opening Paragraph: Should state what position you are interested in and how you heard about it.
- Middle Paragraph: Should detail how you are qualified for the position based on experience, skills, and abilities. Discuss your interest in working for this agency. Carefully check for grammar, as the cover letter provides a short glimpse of your writing skills.
- Closing Paragraph: Refer the person to your resume and focus on the steps or actions that need to be taken to initiate an interview.

If Mailed
- 8½- by 11-inch paper—white, off-white, or light blue
- Typed, with no mistakes (your first opportunity to wow them with professional style)
- No smudges
- 1½- to 2-inch margins on all sides
- Signed, usually in black ink
- No abbreviations
- Business letter format

If E-Mailed
- Follow good writing skills.
- Create resume in a Word document using standard fonts (Times New Roman, Arial, Helvetica), and save to PDF to preserve formatting.
- Attach the cover letter and resume or complete forms on an agency human resources website.
- Save files using your name and date (e.g., John-Adams_resume_5-2019; John-Adams_coverletter_5-2019).

What Are the Methods for Submitting Resumes?

There are a variety of ways to submit a resume: hand-carry it, submit it electronically by means of e-mail or the hospital website, or mail it through the post office. Your prospective employers will likely have a preferred method for submission. If their website states that electronic submission is required, do not place a printed version in the mail. It is likely to be ignored. One of the most popular methods for nurses to send resumes is through the website of the medical organization where they are interested in obtaining an interview. This is an excellent way to submit your resume, but remember to follow up with a telephone call if you have not heard from a recruiter within 1 week. You can also directly e-mail your resume to a recruiter. E-mail addresses are readily available through business cards, websites, and word of mouth. If you e-mail your resume, be sure to convert it to a PDF file so as to preserve the formatting and make it easy to read. But beware: Your e-mail first page will serve as the cover letter when you submit your resume by using an e-mail attachment of the PDF file. The same resume-writing principles apply to all electronically submitted resumes because your resume will be printed out for review.

There are also many large job-search websites available on the internet. You can post your resume on any of these by using their specific formats, but remember that businesses must pay a fee to search for applicants. It is important to remember that not all organizations belong to every job-search website. Use discretion regarding where you want to post your resume; if you are interested in a specific organization, it is best to review its website directly for positions available and guidelines for submitting resumes.

Now that you have your resume ready to submit, you will need to identify prospective employers. Remember, one of the first things you can do is network. Networking is contacting everyone you know and even some people you do not know to get information about specific organizations or institutions. Places where you can network are at your facility, during your clinical rotation, at nursing student organization programs, at career days at colleges, and at career opportunity fairs. Attend local chapter meetings of nursing organizations. Read nursing journal employment sections. When you have identified the organizations where you would like to discuss possible employment, send them your resume. If you have not heard from them within 7 to 10 days, give them a call to make sure your resume was received and to schedule an interview. Keep a record of contacts and resumes sent so that you will have easy access to all this information (Fig. 4.6). It will be important to document your follow-up actions and results—do not forget to keep copies of correspondence and notes about any conversations with

Employer Address and Phone Number	Interviewer and Title	Date Resume Sent	Date and Time of Interview	Inquiry of Application Letter	Application Submitted	"Thank You" Letter Sent After Interview	Job Offer Received	Confirmation of "No Thank You" Letter Sent	Comments or Notes

FIG. 4.6 Record of employer contacts and resumes sent.

BOX 4.4 YOUR CHECKLIST FOR FINDING A JOB

- Define your goals.
- Develop your resume.
- Identify potential employers.
- Send your resume and cover letter.
- Make a follow-up phone call.
- Schedule an interview.
- Send a follow-up letter.
- Keep a record of employer contacts (see Fig. 4.6).
- Make an informed decision as to where to work.

---

potential employers. Date all entries, briefly note any information received, and indicate all interviews requested and granted, resumes sent, and job offers received. Box 4.4 presents a summary of the steps to finding the job you want.

THE INTERVIEW PROCESS

How Do I Plan My Interview Campaign?

Set Up Your Schedule

Keep the following points in mind:

- Agencies usually have specific dates for orientations, internships, and preceptorships.
- Identify when you want to begin employment and mark your calendar.
- Work backward from this date to plan dates and times for interviews.
- Plan no more than two interviews a day. If you do, beware of information overload and the risk of being late for at least one interview. Have two or three possible dates available on your calendar before calling the human resources or nurse recruitment office. Advance planning will keep you from fumbling on the telephone when they tell you that your first choice is unavailable! It is also a good idea to get a contact name and phone number in the event that you need to reschedule the interview.

While you are on the telephone, ask questions about the interview process. How much time should you plan for the interview? It may range from under an hour to a half day. If you have not already read the job description in the newspaper or online, ask where you can access it when you call. Becoming familiar with both the job description and the prospective employer is critical to interview success.

What does the interview process involve? It may involve tours and multiple interviews including human resources, nurse recruitment, one or more clinical managers, and, possibly, staff nurses. If you are applying for an internship, it is not unusual to be interviewed by a panel of three or four people. Knowing this ahead of time may increase your anxiety, but it is less stressful than being surprised by this fact at the door.

Will more than one interview be required? Some organizations will use the first interview as a screening mechanism. You may be asked to come back for a follow-up interview.

How do you get to the human resources or nurse recruitment office? Ask for directions ahead of time if you are unfamiliar with the area. Have a good idea of the time involved for travel. Arriving late for an interview may create a very poor initial impression.

Will you be able to meet with clinical managers from different areas on the same day? Are there new graduates in the area with whom you can talk? This is important if you are interested in more than one clinical area. Will a tour of the unit be included? If this is not a standard part of the interview process, express interest in having one so that you can get a more realistic idea of the setting and possibly meet some of the staff.

Prepare to Show Your Best Side

Develop your responses to probable interview questions. If you do not plan possible responses, you run the risk of looking wide-eyed as you fumble for an answer or ramble on around the subject. Despite the reality of a nursing shortage in most areas of the country, organizations still give considerable weight to the interview, and an employment offer is far from automatic to anyone who walks in the door with a diploma or license in hand.

Critical Thinking Box 4.5 includes examples of interview questions with which you should be familiar. How would you answer these questions?

? CRITICAL THINKING BOX 4.5

Sample of Interview Questions

The following is a sample list of interview questions you should be familiar with. Prepare your responses.

Traditional interview
1. What area or areas of nursing are you interested in and why?
2. Tell me about your clinical experiences. Which rotations did you enjoy the most? Why?
3. Tell me about yourself. What do you see as your strengths? Why?
4. Tell me about your weaknesses. What do you see as your weaknesses? Why?
5. Tell me about a staff nurse who most impressed you and why.
6. How would your most recent nursing instructor describe your performance in the clinical setting?
7. What skills do you feel you have gained from your past work experiences that may help you in this position?
8. Tell me a little about yourself. How would others describe you?
9. What are your future career plans? Where do you expect to be in 2 or 3 years? In 5 years?
10. We do not have any openings at the present time in the areas in which you have indicated an interest. Would you be willing to accept a position in another area? If so, what other areas interest you?

Behavioral interview
1. Tell me about your most challenging clinical assignment and what you learned from it.
2. Tell me about a time when you had to establish priorities during one of your clinical work.
3. Tell me about a time when you went out of your way to assist a family or patient even though you really did not have the time.
4. Tell me how you have worked under pressure.
5. What do you do when faced with a challenging patient situation? Staff conflict situation?
6. What is the biggest mistake you ever made, and how was the problem resolved?
7. Provide an example of how you set a goal and how you achieved it.
8. Tell me how you work with a team.
9. How do you respond when you have a disagreement with a staff member? Patient? Family member?
10. Tell me of an example where you motivated a coworker? A patient?
(Spend some time looking over your answers. Do they describe you accurately? Rework your answers until you feel comfortable with them, but do not try to memorize the words. They should serve as a guide for the upcoming interview.)

Rehearse the Interview

If you role-play a possible interview, it will probably increase your comfort level for the real thing. Following are some suggestions for a rehearsal:
- Dress for the part. It will add some authenticity to the situation.
- Choose a supportive friend, recently employed new graduate, or family member to role-play the interview while video recording, which will allow you to view your nonverbal communication. Sometimes we make facial expressions and display body language that may be unfavorable.
- Practice your verbal responses to sample questions in front of the mirror.

- Ask for constructive feedback regarding your appearance, body language, and responses.

Many applicants say they have no questions at the end of the interview. This may be true, or it may reflect the urge to end the interview and relax! Some words of advice: Prepare a few questions! This will be your opportunity to gather important details and possibly impress the interviewer with your interest. The following is a sampling of possible questions:

- What are your expectations for recent graduates?
- What is your evaluation process like?
- Who will evaluate me, and how will I get feedback about my performance?
- I would like some more information about your preceptorship program. How long will I have a preceptor, and what can I expect from the preceptor?
- What is the nurse-to-patient ratio on each of the shifts I may be working?
- What is your policy regarding weekend coverage?
- What opportunities are there for professional and leadership development?
- When do you plan to fill the position?
- How will I be notified if I am offered the position?

Strategies for Interview Success

One of the most important strategies for successful interviewing is to dress for success (Box 4.5). Pay attention to your interviewing etiquette; your nursing instructors have taught you professional standards, and this is an opportunity to put that education to good use. Also, make sure you know the name and title of the individual who is scheduled to meet with you.

BOX 4.5 THE *DOS* AND *DON'TS* OF DRESSING FOR INTERVIEWS

Do

- Look over your wardrobe and select a conservative outfit. The tried-and-true rule for job interview attire is this: Dress conservatively and professionally. Although a nursing shortage may loosen the rules a bit, the impression you convey by your appearance is likely to be remembered. Also, remember that you may be touring the facility, so wear comfortable shoes.
- Cover any body art and remove any visible jewelry piercings.
- Women: If you own a suit, consider wearing it, but do not blow your budget buying something you will never wear again. Other acceptable outfits include a business-type dress or skirt with coordinated top. Dress pants and a conservative blouse are also acceptable.
- Be conservative with your perfume, makeup, and hairstyle.
- Wear minimal jewelry; you do not want to jingle and rattle with every move.
- Wear hose with a skirt or a dress; bare legs may be fashionable, but they are not appropriate for a professional interview.
- Men: Consider wearing a suit or jacket with coordinated slacks and shirt, but do not blow your budget buying something you will never wear again. A tie is optional. A dress shirt and slacks are also acceptable. Be conservative with your cologne, aftershave, and hairstyle.
- Take a few minutes to look yourself over in the mirror.

Don't

- Wear casual clothes such as tee shirts, jeans, tennis shoes, or sandals. They may reflect the "real" you, but this is not the place to show that aspect of your personality.
- Be guilty of poor grooming or hygiene.
- Chew gum during the interview.
- Wear brand-new shoes, which may turn your day into a painful experience.
- Bring your children with you. Do not expect the staff to act as babysitters.
- Wear wrinkled or revealing clothing.

CRITICAL FIRST 5 MINUTES!

> The decision to hire or not is usually made within the first 60 seconds. You will need to put your best foot forward from the start. Show up at least 10 to 15 minutes early. Smile at everyone you meet, and shake hands firmly (Restifo, 2002).

Arriving early may give you a chance to look over additional information about the organization or possibly give you more time for your interview. If you are delayed or cannot keep the appointment, call the interviewer as soon as possible to reschedule. Under no circumstances should you present yourself for an interview with your children or spouse in tow. They do not belong at a job interview and will create a negative impression with the interviewer. Human resources cannot provide babysitting services, and the presence of children in the waiting area is a safety concern without adult supervision. If you experience a childcare emergency, call and reschedule the interview.

Be aware of your body language; establish eye contact with the interviewer and maintain reasonable eye contact during the interview. Try to avoid or minimize distracting nervous mannerisms. Keep your hands poised in your lap or in some other comfortable position. If you tend to "talk with your hands," try not to do this continually. If you cross your legs, do not shake your foot. If offered coffee or another drink, decide whether this will relax you or complicate your body language. Show enthusiasm in your voice and body language. Do not chew gum or have anything in your mouth. Give a winning smile when you are introduced and offer to shake hands.

Demonstrate interest in what the interviewer has to say. Do not argue with or contradict the interviewer! Wait to ask about salary and benefits until all other aspects of the interview have been completed, including your other questions! Salary and benefits are important aspects, but they should not dominate your conversation. If the salary offer is lower than you expected, do not argue with the interviewer. You may point out that another organization is offering a higher starting salary, but do not try to use this information as a form of harassment or coercion. If you want to take some notes during the interview, ask the interviewer if he or she minds. This is generally quite acceptable. Bring along your list of questions, and if you cannot recall them when given the chance, ask to take out your list. Do not check off information during the interview as if you were grocery shopping!

PHASES OF THE INTERVIEW

The interview is generally divided into three areas, each of which serves a particular purpose. The first few minutes constitute the introduction. This is a "lightweight" section that is designed to help put you somewhat at ease. Some effort to "break the ice" will be made, and the communication may focus on the traffic, the weather, or the excitement you probably feel about your upcoming graduation. Take some slow deep breaths and make a conscious effort to relax.

The second phase involves fact finding. Depending on the skill and style of the interviewer, you may be unaware of the subtle change in conversation, but questions about you will most likely now be asked. Often the employer will use *behavioral interview questions*, which are different from *traditional interview questions* where you describe your various employment roles and/or share qualifications. Behavioral interview questions focus on obtaining information on how your skills and experiences relate to the position and how you handled various work situations in the past. Successful handling of previous work situations typically conveys to the interviewer your ability to handle those situations in the future.

Your resume may be used as a source of questions, so make sure you can speak about its contents and that every item on the resume can be verified. Be prepared to offer your references and possibly explain why you have selected these particular individuals. If you have a tendency to give short responses or avoid answering questions, a skilled interviewer will reword the question or possibly note that you do not answer questions well. Interviewers strive to have the applicant talk about 90% of the time, so consider this your audition. Be prepared to explain how you fit into carrying out the mission and values of the agency. They are really interested in getting to know you as a prospective "fit" with their organization, so you should be both enthusiastic and honest. Although many organizations offer a prolonged internship or preceptorship to increase both your confidence level and practical skill set, the interviewer is looking for prospective employees who are capable of being assertive team players— people who can be flexible but persistent. Critical Thinking Box 4.5 offers sample questions that you can practice with. Consider how you can best portray your background and experiences for the recruiter. Explaining how you have gone the extra mile for patients in a challenging situation is what a recruiter and nurse manager want to hear.

Some organizations are asking students or recent graduates to bring in a portfolio reflecting their school experiences. Included in this portfolio might be your skills check-off sheet, exemplar nursing care plans/concept maps, and any educational materials that showcase your best work. This is particularly beneficial if it is signed by the faculty with occasional positive comments.

The closing is the last phase of the interview process. The interviewer may summarize what has been discussed and give you some ideas about the next step in the process (e.g., a tour, a meeting with clinical managers, or a follow-up interview). This is your time to ask questions. However, if you feel full of facts and unable to ask any questions at this time, leave the door open to future contacts by saying, "I believe you answered all my questions at this time, but may I contact you if I have some questions later on?"

After the initial interview, you may have the opportunity to tour the area in which you will work. Show interest when this tour is offered and use it as a chance to observe the surroundings for such things as professional behaviors as well as organizational and environmental factors. If you have the chance, interact with the staff, especially with recent graduates. Ask what they enjoy about their unit and job position. Before leaving, make sure you thank the interviewer for his or her time and interest.

HOW DO I HANDLE UNEXPECTED QUESTIONS OR SITUATIONS?

So you did your homework and you are prepared for anything, but out of the blue you are asked a question you never expected. What should you do? Saying "No fair" is not a good answer! Take a deep breath, pause, and consider saying something like this: "That's an interesting question. I'd like to think about my answer for a minute if you don't mind. Can we come back to that subject later in the interview?" Given a temporary break, you will have time to develop your thoughts on the subject. Do not ignore the question, however, because a good interviewer will most likely bring it up again. Suppose you answer the question but feel that your response was incomplete or off the mark. Look for an opportunity at the end of the interview to bring up the subject again, saying something like, "I've had some time to think about an earlier question and want to add some additional information if you don't mind" (Box 4.6).

Now Can We Talk About Benefits?

At some point during the interview process, the interviewer might open the discussion on the salary and benefits the hospital has to offer. Salary, job responsibilities, and facility location are not the only major

---

BOX 4.6   KEY POINTS TO REMEMBER ABOUT YOUR RESPONSES DURING AN INTERVIEW

- Answer honestly.
- Do not brag or gloat about your achievements but do show yourself in a positive light. It might be helpful to have your portfolio available from your prelicensure nursing program to showcase your clinical experiences, exposure to nursing skills, and other academic accomplishments.
- Remember that you are your best salesperson!
- Do not criticize past employers or instructors. It is more likely to reflect unfavorably on you than on them.
- Do not dwell on your shortcomings. Turn them into areas for future development: "I want to improve my organizational skills. Managing a group of patients will be a challenge, but I am looking forward to it."
- Demonstrate flexibility and a willingness to begin work in an area of second or third choice if the job market is limited in the area in which you are applying.

BOX 4.7   BENEFIT PACKAGE OPTIONS

Check with human resources regarding which benefits you are eligible to receive and when they are effective.
- Health and life insurance
- Accidental death and dismemberment coverage
- Sick or short-term disability pay
- Vacation pay
- Retirement plan
- Long-term disability leave
- Dental and/or vision care
- Parking
- Tuition reimbursement
- Loan programs
- Dependent care programs
- Health and wellness programs

---

considerations in choosing an employer; do not forget to consider the total compensation package (that is, your benefits). Often, benefits are overlooked by new graduates because their value is less visible than an exciting new salary. Some organizations spend as much as 40% of their total employee payroll to provide this extra compensation. You should consider benefits as your "hidden paycheck" (Box 4.7).

Sign-on Bonuses

This has become a marketing tool for some organizations. Be cautious: carefully read and evaluate what is connected with the sign-on bonus. How long will you have to work for the employer to receive any or all of the bonus, and when will it be paid? Is the sign-on bonus in any way tied to the area in which you will be working? If you originally wanted to work in an ICU but decided after 6 months that that was not the area for you, can you transfer to another unit without losing your sign-on bonus?

When doing your job search, reviewing benefits is a major part of your decision. Therefore, as a new graduate, be sure to familiarize yourself with all the options that are available to you. The human resources department of the hospital or organization will be able to answer your questions. The decisions you make soon after graduation and in the early months of employment will have a far-reaching effect on your future.

JOB OFFERS AND POSSIBLE REJECTION

Let us consider a positive outcome first. If you are offered a position during or at the end of the interview, you are likely to have one of three possible reactions:

1. You are not ready to say yes or no. This is your first interview, and you have two more interviews scheduled.
2. You would like very much to work here. The job offer is just what you are looking for.
3. You do not want the position. It is not what you thought it would be, or something about the organization has created a negative impression.

Whichever decision you make about the job offer, the following are helpful tips for forming a response:

- Be honest. If you have other interviews to complete, say so. Be prepared to tell the interviewer when you will make your decision about the job offer.
- Avoid being pressured to say yes if you are not ready to commit to the job or feel that the position does not meet your needs.
- Be polite. Ask for some time to consider the offer if you are unsure of what you want to do at present.
- If you know the offer does not interest you, decline the offer graciously and express appreciation for the company's interest in you.
- Accept the offer and smile!

Suppose you receive a rejection or no job offer for the position despite your interest and preparation. Before you leave in a state of dejection, find the courage to ask for a possible explanation if it has not been made clear at this point. If you do not find out about the rejection until later, consider calling the interviewer for this information. Check the following list for common reasons an organization may not offer you a job. Consider whether any of these factors might apply to you:

- *Lack of opening for your interests and skills.* They liked you but could not find a spot right now, or a more qualified candidate was selected for the position.
- *Poor personal appearance, including inappropriate clothes.* You stopped by for the interview on your way to the gym.
- *Lack of preparation for the interview.* You were unable to answer questions intelligently or showed a lack of knowledge of, or interest in, the employer. Your answers were superficial or filled with "I don't know."
- *Poor attitude.* You conveyed an attitude of "What's in this for me?" instead of "How can I contribute to the organization?" Your first question focused on salary and perks.
- *Your answers and behavior reflected conceit, arrogance, poor self-confidence, or lack of manners or poise.* They should hire you just because you showed up! Or you submitted a resume and responses that did not reflect initiative, achievements, or reliable work history.
- *You have no goals or future orientation.* After all, you just want a job, and they should hire you because there is a nursing shortage.
- *Perceived lack of leadership potential.* You like being a follower in all situations and do not want to make decisions. If this scenario sounds like you, rethink your approach. All nurses are expected to be leaders, whether in a formal or informal role. In your next interview, ask the interviewer how the organization supports the development of leadership in new graduates.
- *Poor academic record without a reasonable explanation.* You worked as hard as you could in school, but the teachers did not like you; you lacked appropriate references; or your references were not available or did not reflect favorably on you. All experiences provide us with an opportunity for growth, especially the negative ones. Avoid blaming others for your shortcomings and look for ways to grow from the experience.

- *Lack of flexibility.* You were unwilling to begin work in an area that is not your first or second choice. Consider how rigid you can afford to be at this particular point in time or in this organization.

> If at first you don't succeed, try, try again.

Postinterview Process

Now that the interview is over, you may want to relax, celebrate, or jump in your car to get to your next interview appointment. However, stop for a few minutes and jot down some notes about the interview. This is particularly important if you have another interview on the same day. Critique the interview you just had. Consider the following questions:

- What do you think were your strengths and weaknesses?
- Is there anything you wish you had or had not said? Why?
- Were there any surprises?
- How do you feel you handled the situation?
- What could you do differently the next time?

Write down details about the job that will help you decide on its relative merits and drawbacks. If you do not do this, you may not be able to distinguish job A from job B by the time the interviews are finished. You may experience information overload after a number of interviews, but if you have taken notes about each, the sorting-out process will be easier.

After the interviews are over, rank your job offers against your personal list of priorities to make an informed choice. This may be an unnecessary step for you if you were sold on a particular interview. However, it is a good idea to consider interviewing with at least two organizations, if only to strengthen your decision about the first interview. It will help to eliminate possible doubts about your choice later on. If there is a job you think you are really interested in, do a couple of other interviews first. This will give you some experience in interviewing. You may then be able to conduct a more positive interview for the position in which you are most interested. More interviews may also open your eyes to other possibilities.

Follow-up Communication

Remember how nice it is to get a thank-you note in the mail or a telephone call of appreciation? Well, the same idea carries over to the work world: Write those letters!

Follow-up Letter

Take a few minutes to write a note of thanks to the interviewer for the time and interest spent on your behalf. You may want to include additional information in the note: your continuing interest in the position if you hope an offer will be made, the date you will be making your job decision, additional thanks for any special efforts extended to you (lunch, individualized tour), and any change in telephone numbers and appropriate times when you can be reached. Use plain thank-you note cards, not frilly or cute ones. This is a situation where a handwritten note is certainly acceptable; just make sure it is legible and neat. Recruiters frequently comment on the positive aspect of a follow-up letter, and this attention to interpersonal communication may serve to keep your name at the top of the list. This step also helps to separate you from the pack of applicants.

An electronic note of thanks is acceptable. However, in the blur of daily e-mail, a personal handwritten note will particularly stand out.

Letters of Rejection

As soon as you make up your mind regarding job offers, notify other prospective employers of your decision. Decline their job offer graciously and include an expression of appreciation for their interest in you. The format for this letter should follow the standard rules of business letters. Remember, you have accepted a position elsewhere, but your career might take a turn in the future that could bring you back to the organization you are now declining. Leave a positive impression with human resources and recruitment.

Telephone Follow-up

On the basis of the interview, you should have a pretty clear idea of the "how" and "when" of further contact. A telephone call may be appropriate when you have not heard from a recruiter by an agreed-upon date. You can contact a recruiter or interviewer by telephone to decline a job offer, but a personal letter is preferable to leaving a telephone message. Remember to be unfailingly polite to everyone you speak with on the telephone. Administrative assistants and other support personnel will remember and pass on unfavorable impressions to their superiors. Recruiters do not want to hire staff members who are rude or impatient. They know that this behavior is likely to be shown toward patients and families as well. Administrative assistants often act as gatekeepers for their bosses and can be counted on to report both positive and negative perceptions of the job applicants with whom they have contact.

What If I Do Not Like My First Position?

It is not uncommon to experience frustrations during your first work experience. Return to Chapter 1 on transitions and reality shock and review it for some suggestions on how to handle your situation. You also need to keep in touch with the nurse recruiter who hired you. Nurse recruiters can offer further support and assistance. Recruiters know where other recent graduates are working in the organization and may provide you with a network of individuals who can offer suggestions and support to improve your situation. In addition, recruiters know the staffing needs of other areas in the hospital and may suggest transferring. A good way to get an idea of other areas where you may be interested in working is to "shadow" a staff nurse in that area. This means you would spend a day observing this staff nurse performing his or her job. This provides you with a good insight as to what the job requires and the working conditions of that area. When you take your first position, plan on staying there for at least a year. You want to avoid "job hopping," or changing jobs whenever you do not like what is going on with your current position. Remember, other positions also have their benefits and problems; the grass may not be greener on the other side of the fence.

> Don't trade one set of problems for another set that may be even more difficult.

What If It Is Time to Change Positions?

If you think it is time to change positions or explore other options, it is important to submit a letter of resignation (Fig. 4.7). Give at least 2 weeks' notice. Check your contract to see whether you agreed to give more than that; if so, give 4 weeks' notice if possible. If you are leaving on less than amicable terms, do not express this in your resignation letter. You can always report grievances to the personnel or human resources department. As a means of improving retention, many organizations conduct an exit interview or call former employees at some time after their departure to explore their reasons for leaving. If you are given this opportunity, make every effort to provide objective feedback and avoid character assassination. Do not "burn any bridges," since you may want to work at the organization

February 1, 2020

Linda Smith
101 Anywhere Street
Dallas, TX 77777
214-555-8888

Ms. Joan Winter
Assistant Vice President
Children's Medical Center of Dallas
1935 Hospital Street
Dallas, TX 75235

Dear Ms. Winter:

It is with regret that I must submit my resignation. I have been offered a position with Hancock Hospital. My period of employment at Children's has been very positive. I feel I have gained much experience that will be of great benefit to me in my career. My last day of employment will be November 20, 2019.

Thank you for the opportunity to work at your facility and your kind consideration.

Sincerely,

Linda Smith
Linda Smith

FIG. 4.7 Letter of resignation.

again later in your career. Maintain a professional attitude as you develop a network of contacts. Always "take the high road" and avoid petty comments.

CONCLUSION

Searching for and finding your niche in the workplace can sometimes be an overwhelming task. Take the plunge and start looking. Keep a positive outlook, because the job you are looking for is out there. This is one of those situations in which a little preparation and investigation go a long way toward finding what you want. Get your resume together and start investigating what is out there for you. A basic understanding of the process of job hunting can minimize the frustrations and promote a positive first-job experience. Take a look further on in this chapter for additional online resources for interviewing and securing a position. Good luck with your job search!

> Success lies not in achieving what you aim at but in aiming at what you want to achieve.

🌐 RELEVANT WEBSITES AND ONLINE RESOURCES

American Nurses Association
Nursing Career Center. Retrieved from https://jobs.ana.org/.

Nursing Job Interview
Retrieved from http://www.best-job-interview.com/nursing-job-interview.html.

Top15 Nursing Interview Questions (Sample Answers Included)
Retrieved from https://theinterviewguys.com/nursing-interview-questions/.

Worst Answers to Nursing Interview Questions
Retrieved from http://nursinglink.monster.com/benefits/articles/8211-10-worst-answers-to-nursing-interview-questions.

BIBLIOGRAPHY

American Association of Colleges of Nursing. (2017). *Fact sheet: Nursing shortage. In AACN.* Retrieved from http://www.aacnnursing.org/News-Information/Fact-Sheets/Nursing-Shortage.

American Nurses Credentialing Center. (2015). *Find a magnet organization.* Retrieved from http://www.nursecredentialing.org/Magnet/FindaMagnetFacility.

Andre, M., & Heartfield, K. (2011). *Nursing and midwifery portfolios: Evidence of continuing competence* (2nd ed.). Sydney: Elsevier Publishing. Retrieved from http://www.us.elsevierhealth.com/media/us/samplechapters/9780729540780/Andre_Nursing&MidwiferyPortfolios_Sample.pdf.

Auerbach, D. I., Buerhaus, P. I., & Staiger, D. O. (2015). Will the RN workforce weather the retirement of the baby boomers? *Medical Care, 53*(10), 850. https://doi.org/10.1097/MLR.0000000000000415.

Buerhaus, P. I., Auerbach, D. I., & Staiger, D. O. (2009). The recent surge in nurse employment: Causes and implications. *Health Affairs, 28*(4), 657–668.

Bureau of Labor Statistics. (2018, April). *U.S. Department of Labor. Occupational Outlook Handbook: Registered Nurses.* Retrieved from http://www.bls.gov/ooh/healthcare/registered-nurses.htm.

Careerbuilder. (2016). *Number of employers using social media to screen candidates has increases 500% over the last decade.* Retrieved from http://www.careerbuilder.com/share/aboutus/pressreleasesdetail.aspx?sd=4%2F28%2F2016&id=pr945&ed=12%2F31%2F2016.

Hannans, J. (2017). Craft a positive nursing digital identity with an ePortfolio. *American Nurse Today, 12*(11), 48–49.

Health Resources and Services Administration. (2010). *The registered nurse population: Initial findings from the 2008 national sample survey of registered nurses.* Retrieved from http://bhpr.hrsa.gov/healthworkforce/rnsurvey/initialfindings2008.pdf.

Juraschek, S. P., Zhang, X., Ranganathan, V., & Lin, V. W. (2012, November). United States registered nurse workforce report card and shortage forecast. *American Journal of Medical Quality, 27*(3), 241–249. https://doi.org/10.1177/1062860611416634.

Linked-In (2018). *About us.* Retrieved from https://press.linkedin.com/about-linkedin.

Lorenz, K. (2009). *Warning: Social networking can be hazardous to your job search.* Retrieved from http://www.careerbuilder.ca/blog/2006/07/12/cb-warning-social-networking-can-be-hazardous-to-your-job-search/.

McMillan, L., Parker, F., & Sport, A. (2014). Decisions, decisions! E-portfolio as an effective hiring assessment tool. *Nursing Management, 45*(4), 52–54. https://doi.org/10.1097/01.NUMA.0000444882.93063.a7.

National Council of State Boards of Nursing (NCSBN). (2019). *National nursing workforce study.* Retrieved from https://www.ncsbn.org/workforce.htm.

Restifo, V. (2002). *The successful interview how to market yourself for career advancement. NSNA Imprint,* 37–41. Retrieved from http://www.nsna.org/Portals/0/Skins/NSNA/pdf/Career_successint.pdf.

Smiley, R. A., Lauer, P., Bienemy, C., Berg, J. G., Shireman, E., Reneau, K. A., & Alexander, M. (2018, October). The 2017 national nursing workforce survey. *Journal of Nursing Regulation, 9*(3), 1–88. Retrieved from https://www.journalofnursingregulation.com/article/S2155-8256(18)30131-5/fulltext.

Smith, A., & Anderson, M. (2018). *Social media update in 2018.* Pew Research Center. March 1, 2018. Retrieved http://www.pewinternet.org/2018/03/01/social-media-use-in-2018/

Welton, R. H. (2013). Writing an employer-focused resume for advanced practice nurses. *AACN, 24*(2), 203–217.

Zhang, X., Tai, D., Pforsich, H., & Lin, V. W. (2017). United States registered nurse workforce report card and shortage forecast: A revisit. *American Journal of Medical Quality, 33*(3), 229–236. https://doi.org/10.1177/1062860617738328.

5

NCLEX-RN® Exam and the New Graduate

JoAnn Zerwekh, EdD, RN

ⓔhttp://evolve.elsevier.com/Zerwekh/nsgtoday/.

The way I see it, if you want the rainbow, you gotta put up with the rain.
Dolly Parton

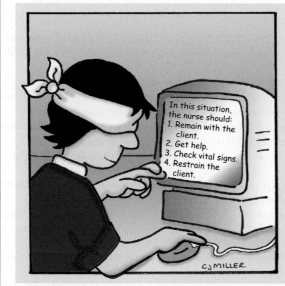

In this situation, the nurse should:
1. Remain with the client.
2. Get help.
3. Check vital signs.
4. Restrain the client.

CJ MILLER

Don't take any chances ... understand the NCLEX-RN® exam process.

After completing this chapter, you should be able to
- Discuss the role of the National Council of State Boards of Nursing (NCSBN)
- Discuss the implications of computer-adaptive testing
- Identify the process and steps for preparing to take the National Council Licensure Exam for Registered Nurses (NCLEX-RN®).
- Identify criteria for selecting a NCLEX-RN® exam review book and review course
- Identify the characteristics of the alternate item format questions on the NCLEX-RN® exam

The NCLEX-RN® exam is the really big test for which you have been preparing since you entered nursing school. Consider the opportunity to take the NCLEX-RN® exam a privilege; it took a lot of hard work to achieve this level, and you should have confidence you are prepared to pass the NCLEX-RN® exam and begin your professional practice as an RN. As with other aspects of transition, planning begins early, before you graduate. Planning ahead will help you develop a comprehensive plan for how to attack that mountain of material to review.

When you plan ahead and know what is expected, your anxiety about the exam will be decreased. Being prepared and knowing what to expect will help you maintain a positive attitude.

THE NCLEX-RN® EXAM

Who Prepares It and Why Do We Have to Have It?

The National Council of State Boards of Nursing (NCSBN) is the governing body for the committee that prepares the licensure exam. Each member board or state determines the application and registration process as well as deadlines within the state. The NCLEX-RN® exam is used to regulate entry into nursing practice in the United States. It is a national exam with standardized scoring; all candidates in every state are presented with questions based on the same test plan. Every state requires the same passing level or standard. There is no discrepancy in passing scores from one state to another. In other words, you cannot go to another state and expect the NCLEX-RN® exam to be any easier.

According to the NCSBN, the NCLEX-RN® exam is designed to test "knowledge, skills, and abilities essential to the safe and effective practice of nursing at the entry level" (NCSBN, 2018a). On successful completion of the exam, you will be granted a license to practice nursing in the state in which you applied for licensure. The status of state licensure continues to be in a transition process of its own. There are many nurses who maintain a current license in multiple states. The increase in nursing practice across state lines, the growth of managed care, distance education, and the advances in "telehealth" medicine prompted a research project conducted by the NCSBN in the late 1990s. Results of the research resulted in the development of the Mutual Recognition Model for Multistate Regulation. This was referred to as the *Nurse Licensure Compact* (NLC). In May 2015, the NCSBN overwhelmingly approved enhancement of the NLC, referred to as the enhanced Nurse Licensure Compact (eNLC). If you live in a state that has enacted the eNLC, you will have multistate privileges. As of September 2018, the eNLC has been enacted by the legislatures of 30 states (NCSBN, 2018h).

How Will the Nurse Licensure Compact Affect Your License?

The nursing license in the participating compact states will function much like a driver's license, where the individual holds one license issued in the state of residence but is also responsible for the laws of the state in which he or she is driving. The individual nurse will be licensed to practice in his or her state of residence but may also practice nursing in another state; however, the nurse must comply with the Nurse Practice Act of the state in which he or she practices. The transition process for the Nurse Licensure Compact began in 2000 and is continuing to progress. The eNLC must be passed by the state legislature in each participating state. Watch your state nursing organization and Board of Nursing newsletters or check the NCSBN website (www.ncsbn.org) to see where your state is in the process of implementing the eNLC (Critical Thinking Box 5.1).

> ### ❓ CRITICAL THINKING BOX 5.1
>
> What is the status of the Nurse Licensure Compact in your state?

> "If you need to work in a state that has not yet joined the eNLC, you will need a separate license to practice in that state. Understanding these changes is important, in order for nurses, faculty, and employers to know where they can legally practice in person, provide telehealth care or teach distance education." (NCSBN, 2017b)

Before the eNLC is implemented, the respective states will continue to require the nurse to be licensed in the individual state of practice. Transfer of nursing licenses between states is a process called "licensure by endorsement." If you wish to practice in a state in which you are not currently licensed, you must contact the State Board of Nursing in the state in which you wish to practice. The State Board of Nursing will advise you of the process for becoming licensed in that state (see Appendix A, State Boards of Nursing, on the Evolve website). Transferring your license to practice from one state to another does not negate your successful completion of the NCLEX-RN® exam, nor do you have to take the exam again. All states recognize the successful completion of the NCLEX-RN® exam regardless of the state in which you took the exam or where your initial license was issued. You can get the most recent list of state boards of nursing from the NCSBN website (https://www.ncsbn.org/contact-bon.htm).

What Is the NCLEX-RN® Exam Test Plan?

The content of the NCLEX-RN® exam is based on a test blueprint determined by the NCSBN. The blueprint reflects entry-level nursing practice as identified by research published in an RN practice analysis study of newly licensed registered nurses. The NCSBN conducts this research study every 3 years. The RN practice analysis research in 2017 indicated that the majority (82.2%) of new graduates were continuing to work in hospitals, with approximately 7.2% working in long-term care and 6.8% in community-based facilities. The overall practice settings were in medical-surgical (27.6%) and critical care settings (23.3%), which represent a slight increase in these settings from the previous practice analysis study in 2014. There was a significant decrease in nursing home, skilled, and intermediate care (11.2% to 5.2%) and an increase in step-down/progressive care (4.3% to 6.5%). Most entry-level nurses indicated that they cared for acutely ill clients (55%). The other percentages noted for entry-level nurses indicated that they cared for adult and geriatric clients with stable chronic conditions (38.2%), unstable chronic conditions (34%), and behavioral/emotional conditions (27.2%). The majority of the new graduates (96.6%) surveyed responded that they were receiving some form of formal orientation. Hospitals were the primary employers of new graduates. Respondents (32.9%, down from 43.4%) reported having a primary administrative position. Newly licensed RNs working in long-term care facilities were more likely to report having primary administrative responsibilities than those working in hospitals (56.6% in long-term care vs. 11.4% in hospitals). The test plan in this chapter was implemented in April 1, 2019, and will be used through March 31, 2022. A new test plan is implemented every 3 years. This represents the time required to conduct the research, analyze the data, and implement the new test plan for the NCLEX-RN® exam (NCSBN, 2018a).

The exam is constructed from questions designed to test the candidate's ability to apply the nursing process and to determine appropriate nursing responses and interventions to provide safe nursing care. The distribution of content is based on the areas of client needs. The nursing process is integrated throughout the exam. Four levels of client needs are identified in the *2019 NCLEX-RN® Detailed Test Plan* (NCSBN, 2018b). Each level of client need is assigned a percentage reflecting the weight of that category of client need on the NCLEX-RN® exam. The approximate percentages of each area are as follows:

Safe, Effective Care Environment	
Management of care	17%–23%
Safety and infection control	9%–15%
Health promotion and maintenance	6%–12%
Psychosocial integrity	6%–12%
Physiological integrity	
Basic care and comfort	6%–12%
Pharmacological and parenteral therapies	12%–18%
Reduction of risk potential	9%–15%
Physiological adaptation	11%–17% (NCSBN, 2018b)

In April 1994, the NCSBN implemented computer-adaptive testing (CAT) for the NCLEX-RN® exam for both practical/vocational nurses (NCLEX-PN/VN) and registered nurses (NCLEX-RN). The information presented here is a brief introduction to the NCLEX-RN® CAT. It is important that you download the Candidate Bulletin for your testing year from www.ncsbn.org and carefully follow the instructions; you will receive additional information from your state board of nursing.

Pearson VUE is the company contracted by the NCSBN to schedule candidates, administer, and score the NCLEX-RN® exam. The NCSBN is responsible for the content and development of the test questions, the test plan, policies, and requirements for eligibility for the NCLEX-RN® exam. Pearson VUE will assist you in scheduling your exam and will provide a location and equipment for the administration of the exam.

What Does Computer Adaptive Testing (CAT) Mean?

With CAT, each candidate receives a different set of questions via the computer. The computer develops an exam based on the test plan and selects questions to be presented on the basis of the candidates' responses to the previous question. In this way, every time a candidate answers a test question, the computer re-estimates the candidate's ability based on all the previous answers and the difficulty of those items. The number of questions each candidate receives and the testing time for each candidate will vary. As candidates answer questions correctly, the next question will be either at a degree of difficulty equal to the previous question or at a higher level of difficulty. All of the questions presented will reflect the categories of the NCLEX-RN® exam test plan (NCSBN, 2018b).

"Pretest" questions have been integrated into the exam in the past and will continue to be integrated into the current exam. The NCSBN Exam Committee evaluates the statistical information from each of these "pretest" questions to determine whether the question is valid and to identify the level of difficulty of the test item (NCSBN, 2018b). Do not be alarmed—these questions are not counted in the grading of your exam, and time has been allocated for you to answer these questions. It is impossible to determine which questions are "pretest" questions and which are "scored" test questions, so it is important that you answer every question to the best of your ability. These pretest items ensure that each question that counts toward your score has been thoroughly evaluated for content as well as statistically validated.

What Is the Application Process for the NCLEX-RN® Exam Computer-Adaptive Test?

In the beginning of your final semester, your school of nursing will have each student complete an application form and send it to the state board of nursing. When you complete the nursing program, the school will verify your graduate status with the state board of nursing. After the forms have been processed, you will receive an Acknowledgement of Receipt of Registration. You will then receive by email the Authorization to Test (ATT), with instructions regarding how to schedule your exam with Pearson VUE. You cannot schedule your exam until you have received your ATT. Read your instruction packet and your *Candidate Bulletin* carefully (the *Candidate Bulletin* may be found at www.ncsbn.org). All registrations must be processed via the Pearson VUE website or through the Pearson VUE call center. After you schedule your appointment, you will be emailed a Confirmation of Appointment from Pearson VUE. First, verify that all information is correct. Then, call or go online to check that your appointment has been scheduled/rescheduled. If you do not receive a confirmation every time that you schedule or reschedule an appointment, contact Pearson VUE NCLEX Candidate Services immediately to correct any errors to the appointment (NCSBN, 2018d). Your ATT will contain your authorization number, candidate ID number, and an expiration date. The expiration date cannot be extended for any reason; *you must test within the validity dates on the ATT*. It is to your advantage to schedule your exam date shortly after receiving your ATT even if you do not plan to take the test for several weeks. Testing centers tend to fill up early; if you wait too long, you may not be able to get your desired testing date. Pearson VUE will email a confirmation of your testing appointment. As a first-time test taker, you will be offered an appointment within 30 days of the request to schedule an appointment (NCSBN, 2018d).

When you provide an email address at the time you register for the NCLEX-RN® exam, all future correspondence from Pearson VUE will be via email, regardless of whether you registered by telephone or via the internet. To gain access to the NCLEX-RN® exam, you must present one form of identification that matches exactly the name you provided when registering. The first and last name on your identification must match exactly the name you provided when registering. You will be required to provide your digital signature and a palm vein scan and will have your photograph taken (NCSBN, 2018e; Pearson, 2013).

What About Testing Accommodations?

Students who qualify to take the NCLEX can receive testing accommodations through authorization from the state board of nursing; this should be done before the NCLEX registration is submitted to Pearson VUE. The following are some important aspects about the process:

- Send request early to the state board of nursing.
- Do not schedule an appointment to take NCLEX until you have received confirmation of your accommodations and your ATT email listing the granted accommodations.
- Candidates approved for testing with accommodations must schedule their testing appointment by calling Pearson VUE NCLEX Candidate Services at the telephone number listed on their ATT and asking for the NCLEX Accommodations Coordinator.
- Candidates who seek to test with accommodations cannot schedule their appointments through the NCLEX Candidate website (NCSBN, 2019, p. 4).

Where Do I Take the Test?

There are testing sites in every state. A candidate may take the test at any of the Pearson VUE testing sites listed in the *Candidate Bulletin*. However, the license to practice will be issued only in the state where the candidate's application was submitted. Information regarding the location of the centers can be found at the candidate area on the NCSBN website. There will be multiple testing stations at each center.

When Do I Take the Test?

After receiving the ATT, a candidate may contact the exam Candidate Services at the phone number provided in the *Candidate Bulletin* or go to the NCLEX exam area of the Pearson VUE website (www.pearsonvue.com/nclex) to schedule the exam. The location and telephone numbers of the testing centers will be included in the information from the NCSBN. Remember, you *must* test within the validity dates on your ATT. You may schedule your exam as soon as you receive the emailed ATT. This means that you could receive the ATT on Wednesday; call or go online to the location of your choice; and, if you wish, take the exam the next day if there is space available. Or you can call and/or go online and schedule your exam date within the next 2 to 3 weeks.

During the last 2 months of school, begin to make plans for when you would like to take the exam. The exam should be taken within approximately 4 to 6 weeks of graduation. Allow for some study time and consider whether you want to take a formal review course. It is important that you take the exam soon after graduation. If you wait too long, your level of comprehension of critical information will be decreased. Finish school, take a review course if you desire, obtain your ATT, and go take the exam. It is not a good time to plan a vacation, get married, or engage in other activities that could cause a crisis in your life (Critical Thinking Box 5.2).

? CRITICAL THINKING BOX 5.2

When do you want to take your NCLEX-RN® exam? Refer to this book's *Evolve* website for information on selecting an NCLEX-RN® exam review course to help you start thinking about this process and assist you in deciding how to select a review book.

How Much Time Do I Have and How Many Questions Are There?

Each candidate is scheduled for a 6-hour time slot. You should plan to be at the site for 6 hours. Each candidate must answer at least 75 questions. Within those first 75 questions there are 15 pretest items that are not scored. The number of questions you answer and the length of time that you test are not indications of whether you will receive a pass or fail score. The length of your exam depends on how you answered the questions. When the computer indicates that you are finished, regardless of how long you have been testing or how far past 75 questions you have gone, it just means you have "turned your test in," and your test is completed. The exam will end when the student:

- Measures at a level of competence above or below the established standard of competency and at least 75 questions have been answered
- Completes a maximum of 265 questions
- Has been testing for the maximum time of 6 hours (NCSBN, 2018e)

Do I Have to Be Computer-Literate?

It is not necessary to study from a computer, nor is it necessary that you be "computer-literate." Research has demonstrated that candidates who were not accustomed to working on a computer did as well as those who were very comfortable with a computer (NCSBN, 2018e). So previous computer experience is not a prerequisite to passing the NCLEX-RN® exam!

How Will I Keep the Computer Keys Straight and Deal With a Mouse?

At the testing site, each candidate is given a tutorial orientation to the computer. This tutorial will introduce you to the computer, demonstrate how to use the keyboard and the calculator, as well as how to use the mouse to record your answers (Fig. 5.1). It will also explain how to record the answers for the alternate-format items (more about this later). If you need assistance with the computer after the exam starts, a test administrator will be available. Every effort is made to ensure that you understand and are comfortable with the testing procedure and equipment.

Only one question will be on the screen at any time. You will read the question and select an answer. After you have chosen the answer, select "enter" from the lower right corner of the screen, and the computer will present another question. Previously answered questions will not be available for review. An onscreen optional calculator is built into the computer. The tutorial program will demonstrate the use of the calculator in calculating numerical answers.

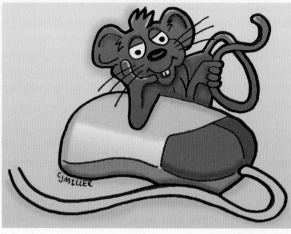

FIG. 5.1 The use of the computer mouse makes navigating the computer-adaptive test (CAT) easier. (From Zerwekh, J. [2019]. *Illustrated study guide for the NCLEX-RN® exam* [10th ed.]. St. Louis: Mosby.)

What Is the Passing Score?

Every state has the same passing criteria. Specific individual scores will not be available to you, your school, or your place of employment. You cannot obtain your results from the testing center. Your score will be reported directly to you as pass or fail. A composite of student results will be mailed to the respective schools of nursing. There is no specific published score or number that represents passing.

How Will I Know I Have Passed?

The exam scores are compiled at the Pearson VUE center and transmitted directly to state boards of nursing. Most boards of nursing can advise the candidates in writing of their results within 4 to 6 weeks of taking the exam. Some states allow you to access your "unofficial" results after 48 business hours through the quick results service of Pearson VUE. There is a small fee for this service. Check your *Candidate Bulletin* as well as online verification from your state board of nursing regarding the availability of results online or from an automated telephone verification system. *Do not call* the state board of nursing, NCLEX Exam Candidate Services, or the Pearson VUE Professional Centers to inquire about your pass or fail status; they cannot release information over the telephone.

What Types of Questions Will Be on the NCLEX-RN® Exam?

Most of the questions are in multiple-choice format, with four options. Each question will stand alone and will not require information from previous questions to determine the correct answer. All of the information for the question will be available on the computer screen. You will be provided with an erasable board for any notes or calculations you would like to make. You may not take calculators into the exam; the "drop-down" calculator will be available on the screen for math calculations. Everyone will be tested according to the same test plan, but candidates will receive different questions. There is only one correct answer to each question; you do not get any partial credit for another answer; it is either right or wrong. All questions must be answered, even if you have to make a wild guess. The computer selects the next question based on your response to the previous question. (You do not get another question until the one on the screen has been answered.) You will not be able to go back to a previous question after that question has been removed from the screen. (This means that you cannot go back and change your answer to the wrong one!) There will be an optional break after 2 hours of testing. If you need to take a break before the 2 hours are up, notify one of the testing center administrators. A second optional break is offered after 3.5 hours of testing. The tutorial and all breaks are considered part of the 6 hours allowed for testing (NCSBN, 2018e).

There is not much storage space at the testing sites, although there are some small lockers for your personal items. Therefore do not take your textbooks, your notes from school, your lucky stuffed bear, or any other materials you have been carrying around in that pack for the past 2 years! All electronic devices (cell/mobile/smartphones, tablets, pagers, or other electronic devices) are required to be sealed in a plastic bag provided by the Pearson VUE Testing Center. If you refuse to store your mobile device or devices in the plastic bag provided, you will not be allowed to take the exam and will have to repay a $200 exam fee and reschedule to take the exam another time (NCSBN, 2019).

What Are Some of the Other Things I Really Need to Know About the NCLEX-RN® Exam?

What If I Need to Change the Time or Date I Have Already Scheduled?

You can change your testing date and time if you advise NCLEX Exam Candidate Services 24 hours or 1 full business day before your scheduled exam appointment. You may go to the NCLEX candidate website (www.Pearsonvue.com/nclex) to reschedule or you may speak with an agent at Pearson VUE and receive confirmation of the unscheduled/rescheduled appointment letter. The phone number will be listed in your *Candidate Bulletin*. You can then reschedule the test at no additional cost. If a candidate does not reschedule within this time frame or does not come at the scheduled testing time, the ATT is invalidated and the candidate will be required to reregister and repay the $200 registration fee. There are *no exceptions* to this policy (NCSBN, 2019).

What About Identification at the Testing Site?

At the testing site, you will submit a digital signature and will be digitally fingerprinted and photographed. An additional security screening is the palm vein screening. It will be required for admission to the exam. You will also be required to provide one form of identification. All identification documents must be in the original form; no copies will be accepted. Be sure that the first and last name printed on your identification match exactly the first and last name printed on your ATT. The following are acceptable forms of identification (must be in English, valid and not expired, with a photograph and a signature):

- US driver's license
- US state-issued identification
- Passport
- Permanent residence card
- US military identification (NCSBN, 2019)

What Are the Advantages of the Computer Adaptive Test for the Candidate?

The environment is quiet and conducive to testing. The work surface is large enough to accommodate both right-handed and left-handed people, with enough room for the computer. Each candidate can work at his or her own pace and is allowed to test up to 6 hours. Each candidate has his or her own testing station or cubicle. There should be a minimal amount, if any, of distraction by the other candidates who are testing at the same time. If a candidate has to retake the exam, the parameters for retesting are established by the respective state board of nursing. The NCSBN requires the candidate to wait at least 45 days before rescheduling the exam. Some individual boards of nursing require a waiting period of 90 days after the first exam before rescheduling. Candidates who take the exam again will not receive the same questions (NCSBN, 2019).

PREPARING FOR THE NCLEX-RN® EXAM

Where and When Should I Start?

Six Months Before the NCLEX-RN® Exam

Make sure you know the dates and deadlines in the state in which you are applying for licensure. Your school will advise you of the specific dates on which the forms are due to the state board of nursing. If you are registering individually, contact the state board of nursing in your state of residence (or in the state where you wish to file for licensure) and find out the filing deadlines. Make sure you follow the directions exactly. State boards of nursing will not accept applications that are not submitted on time or are submitted in an incorrect format. A listing of the state boards of nursing can be found on the Evolve website. If you plan to apply for licensure in a state other than the one in which you are graduating, it is your responsibility to contact the board of nursing in that state to obtain your papers for application. Plan early (at least 6 months ahead) to investigate the feasibility of taking the exam in another state.

Investigate review courses, review books, and practice tests. Review courses, review books, and practice tests can be excellent resources in your preparation for the NCLEX-RN® exam. Review courses will help you to organize your study materials and identify the areas where you must focus your study time. These courses will help you to understand the NCLEX-RN® exam test plan. Understanding the test plan will help you to prioritize your studying. Review books are helpful throughout your nursing program to assist you when you study. Practice testing is an important component to sharpen your test-taking skills.

Plan an expense account for the end of school and for the NCLEX-RN® examination. Frequently students face unexpected expenses at the end of school; one of these expenses may be the fees for the NCLEX-RN® exam. Start a small savings plan—maybe $10 a week—to help defray these expenses. As for family and friends who want to give you something for graduation, you might tell them of your "wish list," including those expenses incurred at graduation (Box 5.1).

Two Months Before the NCLEX-RN® Exam: What Do I Need to Do Now?

If you have a job, discuss your anticipated NCLEX-RN® exam test date with your employer. You can estimate your test date by checking your graduation date, determining from previous students or nursing faculty the approximate time to receive the ATT in your state, and then considering review courses and study time and how these might affect when you want to schedule your exam. Remember, you can change your testing appointment without penalty as long as you do it within 24 hours (or one full business day) of your scheduled appointment and within the dates on the ATT. Submit your request for days off work in writing as soon as you have confirmed your exam date; you want to make sure that your manager understands. Plan to take off the day or two before the exam and, if possible, the day after as well. This will give you time to relax and, if necessary, travel to and from the testing site.

Decide how you are going to get to the test site and whether it will be necessary for you to stay overnight. If the closest testing site is not easily accessible, is more than an hour's drive away, or involves driving through heavily congested traffic, you may consider staying overnight in a hotel close

BOX 5.1 BUDGET FOR THE END OF SCHOOL AND THE NCLEX-RN® EXAM

How Much Is It Going to Cost Me to Complete School?

Required Expenses
Graduation fees from college or university _____
Application fees for NCLEX-RN® exam _____
Application fee to state board of nursing_____

Expenses to Take NCLEX-RN® Exam
Travel (e.g., car, bus, airfare) _____
Hotel accommodations at NCLEX exam testing site _____
Miscellaneous (e.g., food, cab fare, parking) _____

Optional Expenses
School pin _____
Uniform or cap and gown for graduation _____
Graduation expenses passed on to graduate _____
Graduation pictures (class or individual) _____
Graduation invitations _____
NCLEX-RN® exam review course (need to plan this before school is out) _____
NCLEX-RN® exam review books (get these early—they really help with the last year of nursing school!) _____
NCLEX-RN® Practice Exam _____

Expenses After Graduation (It's Not Over Yet!)
Professional organizations (most organizations will give a new membership discount to the graduate nurse) _____
Professional journals _____
Uniform, scrub suits, and shoes to begin new job _____
Professional liability insurance (check with the school regarding transfer from school policy to individual policy) _____

to the site. For some graduates, this will prevent unnecessary hassle and may alleviate anxiety on the day of the exam.

Are you going with a group or by yourself? How will you feel if the group is finished and you are still working on your exam? Will you feel rushed because everyone else is waiting for you? Do not create a situation that will increase your anxiety at one of the most important times of your nursing career. If you are okay with the group waiting for you and everyone understands the situation, then it may be a source of support for you. If a group of graduates is traveling together and everyone is able to schedule the exam on the same day, consider planning hotel accommodations if they are necessary. Do not have a crowd in your room. Five people in a room designed for two or four will not be conducive to sleep the night before the exam. If you are rooming with another person, select someone you like and can tolerate in close quarters for a short period of time. Surround yourself with people who have a positive attitude; you do not need complainers and negative thinkers.

Develop a plan for studying. Do you need to study alone, or do you benefit from group study time? Set yourself a study schedule that you can realistically achieve. About 2 to 3 hours a day for 2 or 3 days a week is realistic; 8 hours a day on your days off does not work. If you take a formal review course, plan your study time to gain the most from the course. A review course is not meant to be your only study time. When you finish a review course, you should have a much better idea of what is going to be tested, how it will be tested, and where you need to focus some extra study time. Priority areas to study are those in which you are the weakest; focus on those first.

The Day Before the BIG DAY

Make sure you have the identification required for admission. Read your *Candidate Bulletin* again. The information that you receive should have all of the necessary information and directions needed for the test site. Check whether there is anything else you will need to take with you to the site.

Make a "test run" the evening before the test. Go to the site and evaluate traffic patterns and driving time. Find the parking area. If your hotel is within four to six blocks of the test site, walk to the site; this is a terrific way to help reduce anxiety and get the blood to your brain! Whether you drive or walk to the site, go the day before to make sure you know where you are going.

Go to bed early; do not study, cram, or party! Plan to eat a light dinner, something that will not upset your stomach—you do not need to be up half of the night with heartburn and/or diarrhea!

The BIG DAY Is Here

Eat a well-balanced breakfast, not sweet rolls and coffee. Protein and complex carbohydrates will help sustain you during the exam. Eat light, something that is nourishing but not heavy. Do not drink a lot of coffee; you do not need to have the caffeine jitters or be distracted by frequent bathroom trips.

Dress comfortably, but look nice. Anticipate that the temperature at the testing sites will be a little cool rather than too warm. Do not wear tight clothes that restrict your breathing when you sit down! Dress casually and comfortably; you may not wear hats, scarves, or jackets in the testing room. The NCSBN requests that you arrive at the testing site about 30 minutes early. This will allow you time to get checked in and prevent anxiety about being late. If you arrive more than 30 minutes after your scheduled appointment, you may be required to forfeit your exam appointment as well as the exam fees (NCSBN, 2019).

How Do I Select an NCLEX-RN® Exam Review Course?

Many review courses are available to help the graduate nurse prepare for the NCLEX exam. Before you sign up, evaluate which course will be most beneficial to you. In considering a review course, remember that the objective is review, not primary learning. (See the Evolve website for selecting an NCLEX-RN® Exam Review Course.)

What Types of Review Courses Are Available?

Live (face-to-face) review courses. Evaluate your geographic location. Which review courses are easily accessible? Are you considering traveling to another city to attend a review course? If you have a prospective employer, check with the nurse recruiter to determine whether the facility provides a review course. Collect data on all of the courses; then compare them to see which one best meets your needs and budget. Also, check with the nurse recruiter or the nursing manager regarding time off and scheduling. Plan ahead and make an intelligent decision regarding review courses. Do not feel that you must sign up with the first review company that contacts you!

NCLEX-RN® exam online review courses. How well do you study at the computer? If you find that studying at the computer is very easy for you, you may want to consider an online review course. When you are investigating online review courses, determine whether the course provides an online book, study questions, and/or additional online study materials as well as the availability of a review faculty. Most students need a resource person or faculty to answer questions (either about nursing content or the NCLEX-RN® exam) and to assist in developing a study plan. Consider the length of time for which the online course is available—is it over several weeks or an indefinite time? With online courses, it is critical to set aside study time, plan how you are going to progress through the course, and evaluate how long you think you will need to complete the course. Online review courses can be beneficial if you plan your study time, take advantage of the course resources available, and follow the suggested activities within the online course.

Carefully evaluate your need for a review course. Are you the type of student who can plan study time, establish a study review schedule, and stick to it? Were you in the top 25% of your graduating class? Have you had experience working in a hospital with adult medical-surgical clients other than while you were in school? As a new graduate, do you feel prepared for this exam? If you can answer "yes" to all of these questions, you may not have to consider a review course in your preparation for the NCLEX-RN® exam. Most graduates can say yes to one or two of these questions but not to all of them.

What Are the Qualifications of the Review Course Instructors?

To teach a review course effectively, the instructor must be familiar with the NCLEX-RN® exam. That ability is most often found in instructors who have teaching experience in a school of nursing. Some hospitals provide in-house review courses taught by excellent educators and clinical specialists. Determine whether these instructors are familiar with the NCLEX-RN® exam test plan. Information that is not a focus of the NCLEX-RN® exam test plan does not have to be included in a review course. It is also important to find out whether the review course instructor is from a school of nursing in your immediate area. It is possible that you will be paying for a review course to be taught by someone from your nursing school faculty. A review course may be more effective if someone other than your school faculty teaches it. You need to hear information from a different perspective. This helps to anchor information and reinforce previous learning. Look for a course that brings faculty in from areas outside your school.

What Types of Instructional Materials Are Used in the Course?

Are the materials required for the course an additional expense or part of the registration fee? Do you get to keep the materials after the course is finished? Can you print copies of the materials if you are taking an online course? Are handouts, workbooks, CDs, flash drives, audiotapes, books, and other materials used to enhance learning? Be concerned if there are no course outlines, workbooks, handouts, or books; you might spend all of your time writing and miss listening to the necessary information. Do the course materials include practice test questions that are similar in format to the NCLEX-RN® exam? Ask about the format used to organize the material (e.g., integrated, blocked, systems). How does the format compare with the NCLEX-RN® exam plan of client needs and nursing process that is described in your *Candidate Bulletin* from the NCSBN?

Does the Course Include Instruction in Test-Taking Skills and Testing Practice?

Test-taking skills and testing practice are very important aspects of a review course. Graduates have to practice test-taking strategies and use them in answering questions written by someone other than their nursing school faculty. This is important to evaluate in the face-to-face review as well as in the online review.

How Much Does the Course Cost?

Most review courses cost between $300 and $500. Frequently, there is a discount for early registration, and there may also be a discount for group registration. Make sure you understand and review company policy regarding deposit, registration fees, and cancelation policy. Check out the possibility of organizing a group; some courses give a free review or a discount to the group organizer.

How Long Does It Last?

Is the face-to-face course 3, 4, or 5 consecutive days? Is it offered only in the evenings? Is it taught only on the weekend for 6 weeks? The answers to these questions are very important to determine early in your evaluation of review courses. Notify your employer as soon as possible if you must fit the review course into your work schedule. Most hospitals will arrange the new graduate's schedule to allow attendance at a review course. It is important to provide adequate advance notice to your employer so that staffing schedules may be planned.

If you are considering an online course, how long will it take you to work through the course? Is the course set up in "real time," similar to the face-to-face review, or is it self-paced? How long does the provider recommend that you spend in the course? Do you want to study for 2 to 3 hours every day for 4 weeks, or do you want to work faster and study 4 to 6 hours a day and complete it in 2 weeks? If you plan to study 4 to 6 hours in 1 day, you should not plan to work that day.

Some hospitals even provide a review course or reimburse the review course registration fee as a benefit to the graduate nurse employee! After you have determined which review course as well as what type of review course you wish to take, discuss it with your prospective employer or notify your current employer as soon as possible.

Where Is the Face-to-Face Course Held?

Are you going to have to drive for an hour every day? Will you have to arrange for a hotel room? Ask about parking. What is the availability of inexpensive restaurants in the area? These are additional expenses you must consider if you plan to take a live review course.

What Are the Statistics Regarding the Pass Rate for the Company?

It is appropriate to inquire how the review company determines the pass rate statistics. Check the NCSBN website (www.ncsbn.org/index.htm) to determine the most current statistics for passing the NCLEX-RN® exam. The review company must obtain NCLEX-RN® exam results directly from course participants. The NCSBN or a school of nursing will not provide this information to review companies. Find out whether the advertised pass rate is based on actual responses from participants or on projected figures from the company.

Does the Review Company Offer Any Type of Guarantee?

Some review companies will offer a guaranteed "refund," a free review course, or further assistance if you are not successful on the exam. Find out what the guarantee means and who is eligible for it. Sometimes the "guaranteed refund" is not easily obtainable and may require completing 100% of the course resources and additional materials. Make sure you obtain in writing what you must do to be eligible and to file for the benefit.

When Is the Course Offered?

Some graduates prefer to take a review course just before the exam so that the information will still be fresh in their minds. Most graduates prefer to take the review within 1 to 2 weeks before the exam. This time frame generally works very well; the review course may be scheduled during the time you are waiting for your Authorization to Test (ATT). When you receive your authorization, you will have completed your review course and be ready to schedule the exam. This schedule allows time to organize and study those areas that are your weakest. If you have only one review course available, how does it fit with your plans for scheduling the exam? Another aspect to consider is your employment schedule. Arrange your review course time so that you can truly focus on the material. If you have to work nights or evenings during the course, you will not benefit as much from the review.

Call the review company for answers to your questions. Does the representative spend time on the phone with you, or does he or she rush you off the phone? Or do you get an automated response instead of a live conversation? Is the company representative friendly and knowledgeable, and does that person demonstrate concern for answering all of your questions?

The online review course eliminates the problem of scheduling a specific time for you to take a review course. However, you must still plan the time to spend working through the online course in order for the review to be beneficial. Ultimately each graduate must decide whether to take a review course and what type of review course to take. The more informed you are regarding a review course, the more intelligent your decision will be.

NCLEX-RN® Exam Review Books: Which One Is Right for You?

It is important to select a review book that meets your study needs. The first step is to check out your choices. Nursing faculty, friends who have review books, the school library, and the local bookstores that stock nursing textbooks are all sources of information regarding review books. There are two types of nursing review books: those with content review and those that consist totally of review test questions. Evaluate how you are going to use the book. Is it for study during school or is it specifically for review for the NCLEX-RN® exam? For example, if you bought the review book to study pediatric nursing, you may be disappointed. The focus of the NCLEX-RN® exam is not on pediatrics; therefore pediatrics is not often a strong component in review books. If you wish to use a review book to identify priority aspects of care in the medical-surgical client, a review book can be of great benefit. The following discussion of review book selection is directed primarily toward review books that contain content review. Take notes as you read the different selections; it is hard to remember all the positive and negative points of each book (Box 5.2) (see "Selecting a Review Book: Where Do I Start?" in the Evolve resources). Frequently students find the review books to be of great benefit during school in assisting them to organize and consolidate a large amount of information. Plan to purchase a review book while you are still in nursing school.

Scan the Table of Contents

Is the information presented in a logical sequence? How is the information organized? It is important that the information be organized in a manner that you find logical. The NCLEX-RN® exam is based on an integrated format, with a focus on the nursing process and client needs. Read the introduction to see how these areas were considered in the organization of the text. Quickly scan the table of contents and check the number of pages in various areas of subject material. Where is the focus of the material?

Evaluate Chapter Layout

How well is the material organized within the chapter? Are there major headings and subheadings to assist you in finding information quickly? Some texts use boxes or color to highlight divisions of content or priority information. These characteristics help to decrease the monotony of constant reading and increase interest in the material presented.

Evaluate Content

Select a topic or topics you would like to read about in each of the review books you are considering. Select the priority nursing concepts and interventions you want to identify (e.g., nursing care of a client with diabetes). Evaluate the information regarding the adult, pediatric, and obstetric client. How does the information compare in the review books you are considering? Is the material logically organized? Does it contain the major concepts of care for that particular example? The focus of the review book

BOX 5.2 SELECTING AN NCLEX-RN® EXAM REVIEW COURSE

Here Are Some Questions to Consider:

Where Am I Going to Work?
Will the institution pay for the review? _____
Will the institution pay the initial fee or do I have to plan for reimbursement? _____

Does the Institution Provide an On-Site Review?
Who teaches it? _____
Is it organized and presented by an independent company or by hospital employees? _____

Review Course Instructors
Who will teach the class? Your faculty from school? Or review course faculty trained by the review company? _____

What Type of Instructional Material Is Used?
Does it cost extra beyond the registration fee? _____
If it is additional to the registration fee, where do I get it? _____
Can I keep all of the instructional materials (e.g., books, testing booklets, online modules, DVDs, CDs)? _____
Does the instructional material include practice test questions in the NCLEX-RN® exam format? _____

How Are the Classes Conducted?
How many days? _____
Are days consecutive or spread across several weeks? _____
What are the hours each day? _____
What is the teaching style (e.g., group work, lecture, home study, group participation, testing practice, online)? _____
What is the average size of the class for the area? _____

How Much Does It Cost?
What is the total price? _____
Does this include all of the class materials? _____
Are there group rates? If yes, what are they? _____
Does the group organizer receive a special rate? _____
Are there early registration discounts? _____
When does the money have to be in? _____
Are there any "extra incentives"? _____

How Do I Pay for it?
Is there a payment plan? _____
Can I make an early deposit to hold my space? _____
When is the deposit due? When is the final amount due? _____
If I change my mind after I make the deposit, can I get the deposit back? _____

Is There a Guarantee?
What is the guarantee? _____
Can I take the review again? _____
Does it have to be in the same location as the first time? _____
What do I have to do to qualify for the guarantee? _____

What Is the Pass Rate, and How Is It Determined?
How does the company determine the pass rate for the review course? (Remember—the review company does not have access to NCLEX-RN® exam results.) _____
Is the pass rate determined by a company survey of review participants after the NCLEX-RN® exam? _____
Is it based on all participants or only the first-time takers? _____
Is it based on the company's projected success rate? _____
Did the review company answer all of my questions in a courteous manner, and did they seem interested in my business? _____
Do you know anyone who has taken a review? What are their recommendations? _____

should be toward nursing concepts and delivery of safe nursing care. In evaluating the currency of content, keep in mind that you cannot expect information that came out last month to be reflected in any textbook. The purpose of the NCLEX-RN® exam is to determine whether a candidate can perform safely and effectively as an entry-level nurse. This is the content that should be included in the review book. Based on the detailed test plan and the areas where new graduates are employed, the NCLEX-RN® exam is more heavily weighted toward the medical-surgical adult client.

Evaluate the Index

Look up several common topics in the index. A good index is critical to finding information in a timely manner.

Test Questions

Are test questions included in the text? Questions may be found after each of the main chapters or grouped together at the end of the book. Check to see if a rationale for the correct answer is included for each question and the rationale for why the other options are incorrect. Does an online test bank come with the book? How many questions are available? Are alternate-item-format test questions included?

Test-Taking Strategies

Does the book include information on test-taking strategies for multiple-choice and alternate item format questions? Test-taking strategies help you to be more "test wise." These strategies can be of great benefit while you are still in school and also for practice as you prepare for the NCLEX-RN® exam.

NCLEX-RN® Practice Exam

The NCSBN offers a practice exam for $150; it is available on this website: https://www.nclex.com/. The practice exam provides the look and feel of the CAT NCLEX exam that you will take on your test day. It is composed of previously used NCLEX exam questions. Your score on the NCLEX practice exam is not a predictor of whether you will pass or fail your actual NCLEX exam. Each exam will be available for a one-time use. The following information is provided about the practice exam:

- Two separate exams with 125 questions on each.
- Six continuous hours to take each practice exam.
- A tutorial to demonstrate the different question types.
- Each exam is good for one-time use.
- Exams must be used within 45 days of purchase.
- A score report is provided giving the percentage of questions answered correctly (NCSBN, 2018f).

Test Anxiety: What Is the Disease? How Do You Get Rid of It?

Frequently students and graduates focus on their "test anxiety" as the reason for not doing well on exams. Test anxiety is something that only you can change. You are the one allowing the anxiety to affect you in a negative way. The only person responsible for your test anxiety is you, and the only one who can do anything about it is you. Address your test anxiety while you are still in school. Look at some simple steps to decrease your anxiety regarding testing.

- **Plan ahead.** Do not wait until the last minute to read 150 pages in your textbook, all your classroom notes, and the 10 articles assigned for the test. Plan study time and stick to it!

- **Set aside study time for when you are at your best.** Frequently study time is squeezed in only after everything else (laundry, meals, housecleaning, yard work, and so on) has been completed. You are defeating your purpose and increasing your anxiety when you try to study at a time when you are tired and not receptive to learning.
- **Study smart.** Plan for 45 minutes to an hour of review on the day after a 90-minute class lecture. This will greatly enhance your retention of the classroom information. Plan for an hour to review/scan assigned reading or information before class so that you will know where information is located and what you will need for note-taking in class.
- **Give yourself a break!** Plan your study time to include a break about every hour. Your retention of information begins to decrease after about 30 minutes and is significantly decreased after an hour.
- **Think positively!** If your friends are "negative thinkers," do not plan to study with them. Go to the movies or play sports with them, but do not study with them. Anxiety and negative thinking are contagious—do not expose yourself to the disease!
- **Do not cram.** Whether you are studying for a unit exam in school or for the NCLEX-RN® exam, cramming is not an effective study method, and it will increase your anxiety. The NCLEX-RN® exam is not written to evaluate memory-based information. Test questions focus on the higher levels of cognitive ability. Application of principles and the analysis of information will be required to determine an appropriate nursing response or action. Do not jeopardize your critical thinking skills by staying up late and cramming.

Just thinking about an exam can cause some students to become more anxious. It seems as though during the last year of school, particularly the last semester, tests become a major source of anxiety. Everyone knows fellow students who become obsessed with the idea that they are going to fail an important exam. View an exam as a positive step—an opportunity to demonstrate your knowledge.

> Put yourself in charge of your feelings.
> Get rid of those negative thought "tapes"!
> Replace negative thoughts and ideas with positive ones:
> I WILL pass this test!
> I will be SO glad to get this test behind me.

Write down positive affirmations and put them on your bathroom mirror, on your refrigerator, or any place where you will see them often. Potential employers, state boards of nursing, your spiritual advisers, and your neighbors are not going to think less of you if you are not at the top of the class. Keep in mind that your employers and the state boards do not care what your grades were in school or on the NCLEX-RN® exam—they just want to know that you can pass the NCLEX-RN® exam and practice nursing safely. Give yourself permission to be in the middle—an average student on grades but one who is concerned about professional safe nursing practice.

What Kinds of Questions Can I Expect on the NCLEX-RN® Exam?

It is anticipated that most of the questions on the NCLEX-RN® exam will be in a multiple-choice format; they have a stem in which the question is presented and four options from which to choose an answer. Of these four options, three are meant to distract you from the correct answer.

With the four-item multiple-choice questions, there is only one correct answer. The multiple-choice NCLEX-RN® exam questions provide a choice of four answers, not a combination of the four options (Fig. 5.2).

> The focus of the NCLEX-RN® exam is on nursing care. The questions ask you to use nursing concepts and judgment in the situation presented.

What Are Alternate Item Format Questions?

Alternate item format questions are different from the four-option multiple-choice questions. They are included in the test bank of questions that will be used to select the test items for a candidate's exam. There is no preset number of alternate item format questions that will be presented to a candidate; the question or items will be randomly selected as the adaptive testing process selects questions that meet the parameters of the test plan.

No special or additional nursing knowledge is needed to answer the alternate item format questions. There is no attempt to hide or camouflage the questions; they are randomly selected to be included in a candidate's exam. The same nursing concepts are being tested, and the questions are based on the same test plan. The question is simply asked in a different format. All test item types may include multimedia such as charts, tables, graphics, sound, and video. You do not have to do anything differently with regard to the alternate item format questions; just be aware of the types of alternate item format questions and implement good testing strategies to answer them (NCSBN, 2018e).

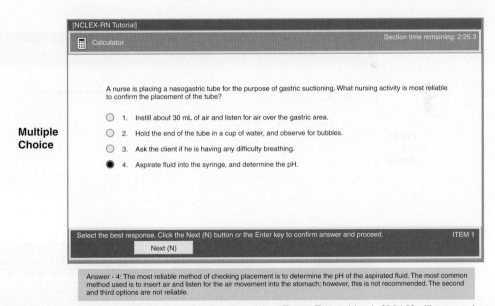

Multiple Choice

[NCLEX-RN Tutorial]

Calculator   Section time remaining: 2:25.3

A nurse is placing a nasogastric tube for the purpose of gastric suctioning. What nursing activity is most reliable to confirm the placement of the tube?

1. Instill about 30 mL of air and listen for air over the gastric area.
2. Hold the end of the tube in a cup of water, and observe for bubbles.
3. Ask the client if he is having any difficulty breathing.
4. Aspirate fluid into the syringe, and determine the pH.

Select the best response. Click the Next (N) button or the Enter key to confirm answer and proceed.   ITEM 1

Next (N)

Answer - 4: The most reliable method of checking placement is to determine the pH of the aspirated fluid. The most common method used is to insert air and listen for the air movement into the stomach; however, this is not recommended. The second and third options are not reliable.

FIG. 5.2 Sample of a multiple-choice test question. (From Zerwekh, J. [2019]. *Illustrated study guide for the NCLEX-RN® exam* [10th ed.]. St. Louis: Mosby.)

What Are the Different Types of Alternate Item Format Questions?

Fill-in-the-blank. A short answer is required for fill-in-the-blank questions. These may be questions that require a drug calculation, an intake and output calculation, or an assessment scoring. In these questions, only the numbers should be entered in the space provided. No units of measurement can be included with the answer because the unit of measurement is already on the screen (Fig. 5.3).

Multiple-response item. This is a different type of multiple-choice question. More than four options will be presented, and the question will very clearly ask you to select all of the options that correctly answer the question. With the mouse, you will select each option you want to include in the answer; then you'll click *enter* to confirm your answers and continue to the next question. There is only one correct combination of answers (Fig. 5.4).

Hot spot. These items present a diagram or a graphic and require you to select an area on the diagram to answer the question. For example, let's assume that the diagram is an illustration of the anterior thorax. The question for this diagram might ask you to click on the area where you would place the stethoscope to listen for the apical heart rate or where you would listen for the characteristic sounds of the mitral valve (Fig. 5.5).

Ordered response (drag and drop). For this type of question, you will be presented with a list of activities, clients, or steps in a procedure. The question will ask you to click on each item and "drag" it to another area of the screen, placing the items, for instance, in the order in which they would be performed or in order of priority of care. Pay close attention to how the question asks you to rank the options. After you have determined how your answer should be ranked, click on the option you want to place first, "drag" that option over, and place it in the box. You will then select the option you want to place second, "drag" that option over, and place it in the box. You will continue this process until you have used all of the options available. You can change your answer any time before you click the "next" button. This type of question is called an ordered response (Fig. 5.6).

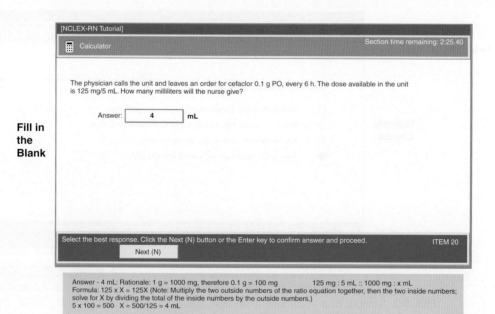

FIG. 5.3 Fill-in-the-blank question. (From Zerwekh, J. [2019]. *Illustrated study guide for the NCLEX-RN® exam* [10th ed.]. St. Louis: Mosby.)

[NCLEX-RN Tutorial]

📋 Calculator   Section time remaining: 3:15.20

The nurse is caring for an 85-year-old client who has a diagnosis of vancomycin-resistant enterococci (VRE) pneumonia. What precautions will the nurse implement in assisting the client with morning care?

Select all that apply:

Multiple Response

1. ☑ Wear clean gloves.

2. ☐ Remove all extra suctioning supplies from the room.

3. ☐ Dispose of the gown and mask in container outside client's door.

4. ☑ Wear face mask when working within 3 feet of the client.

5. ☑ Put on a gown prior to entering the room.

6. ☐ Remove the stethoscope from the room if it did not come in contact with the client.

Select the best response. Click the Next (N) button or the Enter key to confirm answer and proceed.   ITEM 21

Next (N)

Answer: The answer is based on standard precautions, plus respiratory precautions for the pneumonia. Nothing should be removed from the room and the gown should be removed prior to leaving the room, not outside the room.

FIG. 5.4 Multiple-response question. (From Zerwekh, J. [2019]. *Illustrated study guide for the NCLEX-RN® exam* [10th ed.]. St. Louis: Mosby.)

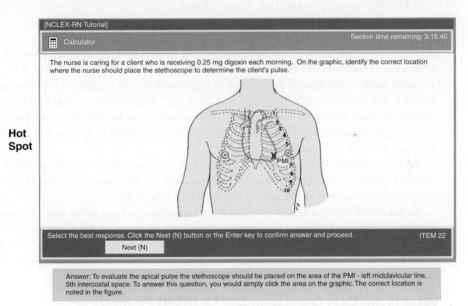

[NCLEX-RN Tutorial]

📋 Calculator   Section time remaining: 3:15.40

The nurse is caring for a client who is receiving 0.25 mg digoxin each morning. On the graphic, identify the correct location where the nurse should place the stethoscope to determine the client's pulse.

Hot Spot

Select the best response. Click the Next (N) button or the Enter key to confirm answer and proceed.   ITEM 22

Next (N)

Answer: To evaluate the apical pulse the stethoscope should be placed on the area of the PMI - left midclavicular line, 5th intercostal space. To answer this question, you would simply click the area on the graphic. The correct location is noted in the figure.

FIG. 5.5 Hot spot. *PMI*, Point of maximal impulse. (From Zerwekh, J. (2019). *Illustrated study guide for the NCLEX-RN® exam* [10th ed.]. St. Louis: Mosby.)

Chart/exhibit item. These questions will present a problem and then provide exhibit information stored in tabs. You will click on each tab to find information that will help you to solve the problem being presented. The tabs frequently contain information from a chart or data collection from a client. There will still be four options from which to select the correct answer, but you will have to evaluate the

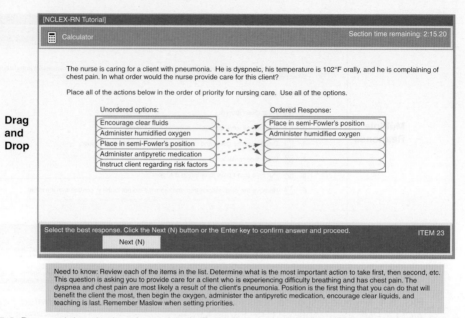

[NCLEX-RN Tutorial]

Calculator   Section time remaining: 2:15.20

The nurse is caring for a client with pneumonia. He is dyspneic, his temperature is 102°F orally, and he is complaining of chest pain. In what order would the nurse provide care for this client?

Place all of the actions below in the order of priority for nursing care. Use all of the options.

Drag and Drop

Unordered options:
- Encourage clear fluids
- Administer humidified oxygen
- Place in semi-Fowler's position
- Administer antipyretic medication
- Instruct client regarding risk factors

Ordered Response:
- Place in semi-Fowler's position
- Administer humidified oxygen
-
-
-

Select the best response. Click the Next (N) button or the Enter key to confirm answer and proceed.   ITEM 23

Next (N)

Need to know: Review each of the items in the list. Determine what is the most important action to take first, then second, etc. This question is asking you to provide care for a client who is experiencing difficulty breathing and has chest pain. The dyspnea and chest pain are most likely a result of the client's pneumonia. Position is the first thing that you can do that will benefit the client the most, then begin the oxygen, administer the antipyretic medication, encourage clear liquids, and teaching is last. Remember Maslow when setting priorities.

FIG. 5.6 Drag and drop (ordered response). (From Zerwekh, J. [2019]. *Illustrated study guide for the NCLEX-RN® exam* [10th ed.]. St. Louis: Mosby.)

data in each of the tabs to determine the correct answer. Do not attempt to select the correct answer without evaluating all of the information provided on each of the tabs (Fig. 5.7).

Audio item. In this type of item, you will be presented with a question that has an audio component. You will put on the headset provided and click the "play" button to listen to the audio for the information required to answer the question. The volume may be adjusted, and you can click the "play" button again to repeat the audio information. Listen carefully to the audio clip and select the option that best answers the question (Fig. 5.8).

Graphic options. The graphic option type of alternate item format question presents you with graphics instead of text for the answer options. You will be required to select the correct answer from the graphics presented at the end of the question (Fig. 5.9).

As the NCSBN continues to research the development of test items that evaluate the reasoning and nursing judgment of nursing graduates, other types of alternate item format questions will be developed. Don't be alarmed if you encounter one of these other types of alternate item format questions—focus on what the question is asking, follow the directions, and select the option that reflects the best client care.

What Is the Next Generation NCLEX (NGN) Project?

The NCSBN is conducting research on the reliability of using innovative types of test items to assess clinical judgment and decision making; this involves the Special Research Section as part of the NCLEX exam administration. Thus, once an exam candidate completes his or her NCLEX exam, an introductory screen will launch to begin the Special Research Section. The question numbering will continue with the last numbered question the candidate had when the exam was completed (e.g., if the exam ended on question 97, the Special Research Section would begin on question 98). *These new questions will have no impact on NCLEX scoring or results.* Not all candidates will be given the Special

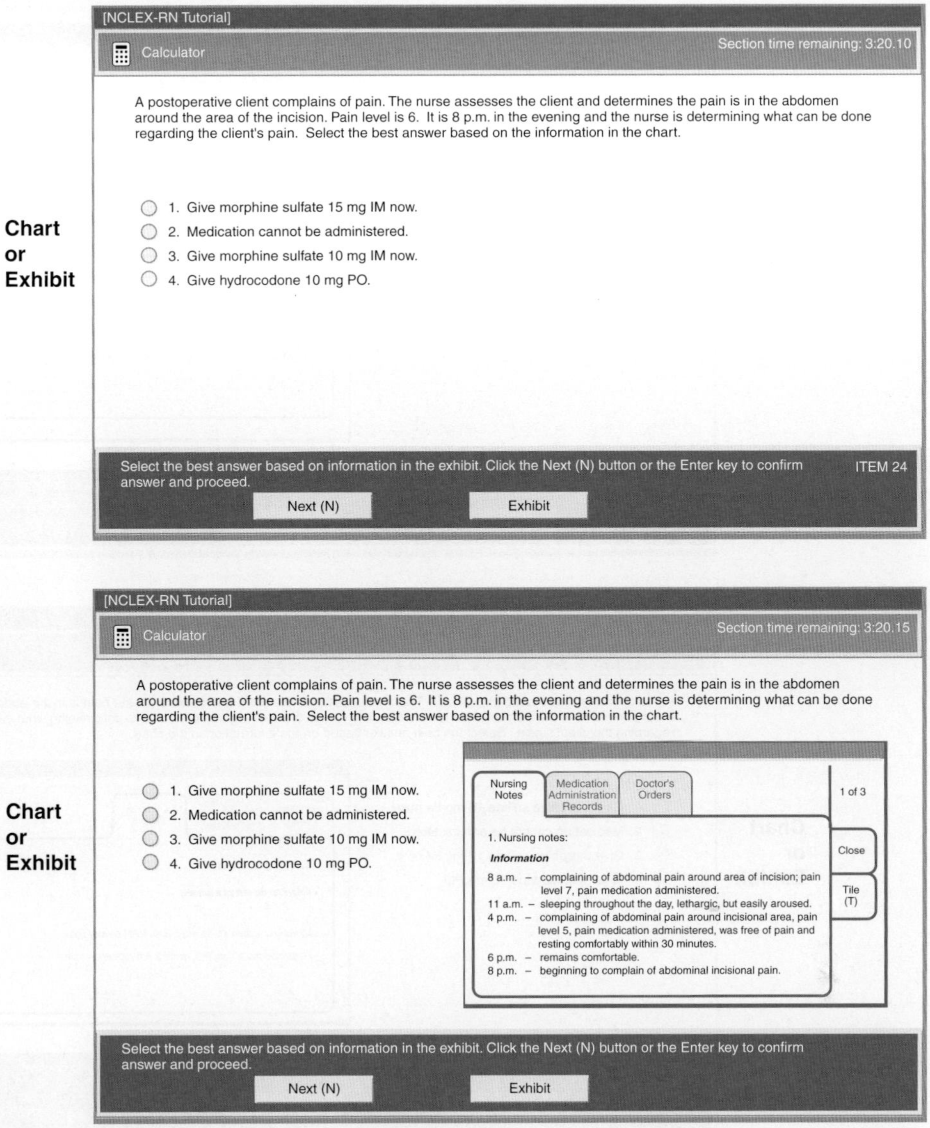

FIG. 5.7 Exhibit. (From Zerwekh, J. [2019]. *Illustrated study guide for the NCLEX-RN® exam* [10th ed.]. St. Louis: Mosby.)

Research Section questions because of various factors, such as the time remaining in the NCLEX appointment. Typically, it will take the candidate approximately 30 minutes to complete the section. It is important that candidates understand that whether they receive the Special Research Section has no relationship to how they performed on their NCLEX. In addition, there is no penalty if the candidate chooses not to participate, as the Special Research Section is optional. At any time during the Special Research Section, a candidate can choose to exit and not finish.

[NCLEX-RN Tutorial]

🖩 Calculator   Section time remaining: 3:20.15

A postoperative client complains of pain. The nurse assesses the client and determines the pain is in the abdomen around the area of the incision. Pain level is 6. It is 8 p.m. in the evening and the nurse is determining what can be done regarding the client's pain. Select the best answer based on the information in the chart.

**Chart
or
Exhibit**

○ 1. Give morphine sulfate 15 mg IM now.
○ 2. Medication cannot be administered.
○ 3. Give morphine sulfate 10 mg IM now.
○ 4. Give hydrocodone 10 mg PO.

| Nursing Notes | Medication Administration Records | Doctor's Orders | | 2 of 3 |

Close

Tile (T)

2. Medication administration record (MAR):

Morphine sulfate 10 mg IM administered at 8 a.m.

Hydrocodone 10 mg, PO administered at 4 p.m.

Select the best answer based on information in the exhibit. Click the Next (N) button or the Enter key to confirm answer and proceed.   ITEM 24

Next (N)   Exhibit

[NCLEX-RN Tutorial]

🖩 Calculator   Section time remaining: 3:20.30

A postoperative client complains of pain. The nurse assesses the client and determines the pain is in the abdomen around the area of the incision. Pain level is 6. It is 8 p.m. in the evening and the nurse is determining what can be done regarding the client's pain. Select the best answer based on the information in the chart.

**Chart
or
Exhibit**

○ 1. Give morphine sulfate 15 mg IM now.
○ 2. Medication cannot be administered.
○ 3. Give morphine sulfate 10 mg IM now.
○ 4. Give hydrocodone 10 mg PO.

| Nursing Notes | Medication Administration Records | Doctor's Orders | | 3 of 3 |

Close

Tile (T)

3. Doctor's orders:

Orders for the last 24 h include:

Morphine sulfate 10-15 mg q 3-4h PRN severe pain.

Hydrocodone 10 mg PO, every 3-4 h moderate pain.

Select the best answer based on information in the exhibit. Click the Next (N) button or the Enter key to confirm answer and proceed.   ITEM 24

Next (N)   Exhibit

FIG. 5.7, cont'd

What Difference Do Test-Taking Strategies Make?

Knowing how to take an exam is a skill that is developed through practice. Look back at the beginning of nursing school and your first nursing exam; you have come a long way from there! How many times during school have you reviewed a test and discovered you knew the right answer but marked the wrong one? Nursing faculty and those responsible for the NCLEX-RN® exam are not sympathetic to your claim that you "really meant this answer and not the one I marked." How many times did

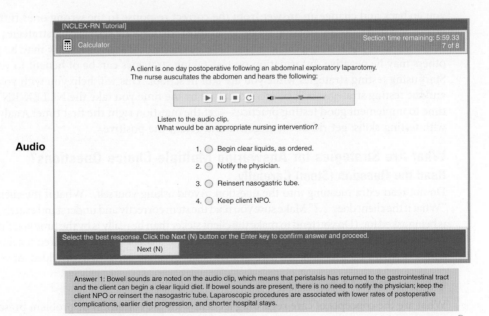

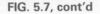

FIG. 5.7, cont'd

FIG. 5.8 Audio. (From Zerwekh, J. [2019]. *Illustrated study guide for the NCLEX-RN® exam* [10th ed.]. St. Louis: Mosby.)

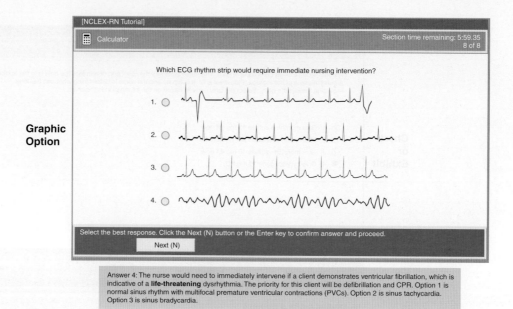

Graphic Option

[NCLEX-RN Tutorial]

Calculator   Section time remaining: 5:59.35
                                                                              8 of 8

Which ECG rhythm strip would require immediate nursing intervention?

1. ○
2. ○
3. ○
4. ○

Select the best response. Click the Next (N) button or the Enter key to confirm answer and proceed.

Next (N)

Answer 4: The nurse would need to immediately intervene if a client demonstrates ventricular fibrillation, which is indicative of a **life-threatening** dysrhythmia. The priority for this client will be defibrillation and CPR. Option 1 is normal sinus rhythm with multifocal premature ventricular contractions (PVCs). Option 2 is sinus tachycardia. Option 3 is sinus bradycardia.

FIG. 5.9 Graphic option. (From Zerwekh, J. [2019]. *Illustrated study guide for the NCLEX-RN® exam* [10th ed.]. St., Louis: Mosby; rhythm strips from Lewis, S. L., Bucher, L., Heitkemper, M. M., & Dirksen, S. R. [2014]. *Medical-surgical nursing* [9th ed., pp. 799, 793, and 800, respectively]. St. Louis: Elsevier.)

you go back and change an answer from the correct response to the wrong one? If these are common errors you make during nursing school, you must incorporate test-taking strategies into your testing skills. Some of the testing practices you have developed through the years may be positive, whereas others may be negative. Information on test-taking strategies can be of benefit to you now and later. Start using testing strategies while you are still in school. This will help you with your current exams, and the testing strategies will be second nature by the time you take the NCLEX-RN® exam. Take the time to implement good testing practices—get the question right the first time! Analyze where you are with testing skills; get rid of the negative and retain the positive.

What Are Strategies for Answering Multiple-Choice Questions?
Read the Question (Stem) Carefully
Do not read extra meaning into the question. Avoid asking yourself, "What if the client should …?" or, "What if the client does …?" Make sure you read the stem correctly and understand exactly what information is being asked for. (Do you tend to make the client sicker than he really is by the time you finish the question?) Do not add information to the question or think about a client whom you cared for during clinicals or at your job. All the information you need to answer the question correctly is provided for you in the question.

Create a Pool of Information
What are the concepts of care regarding a client with the condition or problem presented? Get a general idea of the condition and type of care required before you read the options. Do not try to predict a correct answer.

Look for Critical Words

Evaluate the question for critical words that make a difference in what the question is asking. Watch for *priority, initial, first action, side effect,* and/or *toxic effect.*

Evaluate All the Options in a Systematic Manner

Focus on what information is being requested and then carefully go through each option. Do not stop with the first correct answer; the last option may be more correct or more inclusive of information.

Eliminate Options You Know Are Not Correct

And leave them alone! After you have eliminated an option, do not go back to it unless you have gained more insight into the question. Frequently your initial response in evaluating an option will be correct. Go through all the options and eliminate the incorrect ones. What is left is frequently the correct answer even if it is not what you were looking for.

Identify Similarities in the Options

Look for an option that is unique from the rest. For example, in a question dealing with a low-residue diet, three of the options might contain a vegetable with a peel but one might not—that one is probably the correct answer. Evaluate options that contain several suggested client activities. Are three of the activities similar and is one different from the rest? The option that is different may be the correct answer.

Evaluate Priority Questions Very Carefully

Keep in mind the nursing process and Maslow's hierarchy of needs. You must have adequate assessment information before proceeding with the nursing process. If assessment information is presented in the stem of the question, the answer may require a nursing intervention. If a client in the question is presented as experiencing severe chest pain, it would not be appropriate to conduct a cardiac assessment before putting the client to bed and starting the oxygen! (*If in distress, don't assess!* If a client is presented in a distressed condition, then adequate assessment data have already been provided in the stem of the question, so you will have to look for an immediate nursing intervention to address the problem.) According to Maslow, physical needs must be met before psychosocial needs—the physical needs of your mental health client must be met before you can focus on the mental health needs. When you are considering the physical needs, respiratory needs come first. (You've got to breathe first!) But a word of caution—do not give a client a respiratory problem if he doesn't have one!

Select Answers That Focus on the Client

Choices that focus on hospital rules and policies are most often not correct. Consider that you have enough time and adequate staff to perform whatever action is necessary for safe client care.

Analyze your testing skills so that you will know where to start to improve them. After you have identified your testing weaknesses, organize a plan to correct the problem areas. One of the most difficult things to do is to change the way you are used to doing something, even when the change makes life easier. Get an early start on evaluating testing skills; it can make a significant difference in the remaining exams in nursing school.

NCLEX-RN® Exam Testing Tips
NCLEX Hospital

For the NCLEX-RN® exam to be appropriate to all candidates nationwide, it is important that there be a base for the vast knowledge that is to be tested. Therefore, when you are taking the NCLEX-RN®

exam, consider yourself as working in the "NCLEX Hospital." It is a great place to work; everything you need is provided—great equipment that works the way it's supposed to, plenty of staff, and enough time to provide the best and safest nursing care possible. The clients (*patients* are most frequently referred to as *clients* on the NCLEX-RN® exam) all have conditions that respond just as the book says they are supposed to respond. Study according to your textbooks. Your clinical experience is complementary to your academic study. Do not focus on the unusual, unexpected, or strange things that happened to you during clinical rotations. Avoid thinking, "this is the way we actually do it where I work."

NCLEX Clients

Focus on the client in the question you are working on. As far as the NCLEX Hospital is concerned, that is the only client you are to be concerned about. Do not worry about the five or six other clients you may have assigned to your care. In the NCLEX Hospital, you are taking care of one client at a time unless stated otherwise. Your priority concern is the client in the question you are currently trying to answer.

Medication Administration

Know the Six Rights and the common nursing implications of medications. The generic name will be in the question because it is more consistent, whereas a brand or trade name may vary (NCSBN, 2018e). A good strategy is to study the medications according to the classification. For example, study the nursing implications regarding administration of corticosteroid medications and be able to identify the generic name of common corticosteroids and their nursing implications.

Calling for Assistance

Be careful with questions for which the right answer appears to be to call someone else to take care of the problem. This is a nursing exam; therefore identify the best nursing management. This includes questions that include calling the doctor, respiratory therapist, housekeeping, chaplain, or social worker. Be sure there is not something you need to do for the client before notifying someone else regarding the problem. If the client is experiencing difficulty, their condition is changing, and there is nothing you can do, call the doctor. This is particularly true in situations where the client is experiencing a problem with circulatory compromise. However, if the client is having difficulty breathing, the priority focus may be to position the client to maintain an open airway and/or to begin oxygen as well as to assess the status of the client quickly before calling the doctor.

Positioning

Watch for questions that have particular positions in the stem of the question or those that include positions in the options. Is the client's position necessary to prevent complications or to treat a current problem or is it primarily for comfort? As you are reviewing, be aware of questions that include conditions that require a specific position in the care of a client.

Delegation and Supervision

The NCLEX-RN® exam includes questions in these areas. Some common considerations to make when evaluating these questions include the following:

- Delegate to someone else the care of the most stable client with the most predictable response to care.
- Delegate tasks to the most qualified person to perform the task.
- Delegate to nursing assistants those tasks that have the most specific guidelines (e.g., collecting a urine sample, feeding, providing hygiene, assisting ambulation).

Note: Chapter 14 provides more details about delegation and supervision.

Setting Priorities With a Group of Clients

A question may present a group of clients and ask you to determine which client you would take care of first, or it may ask you to rank the clients according to when you would take care of them. Determine the most unstable client who requires nursing care to prevent immediate problems and take care of this client first. Keep in mind Maslow's hierarchy of needs.

Prescriber's Orders

For most of the questions, you can consider that you have a prescriber's order to perform any of the options presented in the question. However, you should watch for questions that may specifically ask for a "dependent nursing action," where you will have to consider whether you need a prescriber's order to perform the nursing action. It would be difficult to present questions while continuing to repeat that a physician's or health care provider's order was present. Standing orders and state nurse practice acts all have implications for orders. This is a standardized test that is administered nationally; therefore there has to be consistency. Consequently unique aspects of nurse practice acts and standing orders are not tested.

> Be aware that the answer you are looking for may often not be included in the options! This is not uncommon on NCLEX-RN® exam questions. Consider the principles and concepts of care for a client with the problem presented. Eliminate the wrong answers and evaluate what is left.

CONCLUSION

Wow! NCLEX-RN® exam deadlines, review courses, testing skills, review books, money, license—and you thought all you needed to do was graduate from nursing school! A lot happens between graduating from nursing school and being successful on the NCLEX-RN® exam. The key to surviving it all with a smile is careful planning and implementing those plans during your role transition. (That sounds a lot like the nursing process, doesn't it?) The NCLEX-RN® exam is one of the most incredible opportunities of your life. This exam will open the doors for you as you begin one of the most fantastic experiences of a lifetime: a career in nursing. A listing of relevant websites and online resources follows.

> Just say to yourself, "I can do it. I WILL pass the NCLEX-RN® exam!"

🌐 RELEVANT WEBSITES AND ONLINE RESOURCES

National Council of State Boards of Nursing (NCSBN)
http://www.ncsbn.org
    Candidate Bulletin
    (Updates every year in January: https://www.ncsbn.org/1213.htm).
    Detailed Test Plan
    https://www.ncsbn.org/testplans.htm

Pearson VUE Testing
This is also the location for the Online Tutorial for the NCLEX Exam. http://www.pearsonvue.com/nclex/

BIBLIOGRAPHY

Livanos, N. (2017). *Reconstructing licensure mobility: eNLC.* National Council of State Boards of Nursing. Retrieved from https://www.ncsbn.org/10734.htm Video transcript: https://www.ncsbn.org/Transcript_2017DCM_NLivanos.pdf

National Council of State Boards of Nursing (2017a). *Transition to the eNLC – New compact states.* Retrieved from https://www.ncsbn.org/10799.htm Video transcript: https://www.ncsbn.org/Transcript_eNLC-New_States.pdf

National Council of State Boards of Nursing (2017b). *Transition to the eNLC – Original compact states.* Retrieved from https://www.ncsbn.org/10802.htm Video transcript: https://www.ncsbn.org/Transcript_eNLC-Original_States.pdf

National Council of State Boards of Nursing (2018a). 2017 *RN Practice analysis: Linking the NCLEX-RN® exam to practice.* Retrieved from https://www.ncsbn.org/17_RN_US_Canada_Practice_Analysis.pdf

National Council of State Boards of Nursing (2018b). *2019 NCLEX-RN® detailed test plan.* Retrieved from https://www.ncsbn.org/2019_RN_TestPlan-English.pdf.

National Council of State Boards of Nursing (2018c). *Application & registration.* Retrieved from https://www.ncsbn.org/nclex-application-and-registration.htm.

National Council of State Boards of Nursing (2018d). *Authorization to test.* Retrieved from https://www.ncsbn.org/1212.htm.

National Council of State Boards of Nursing (2018e). *NCLEX FAQs.* Retrieved from https://www.ncsbn.org/nclex-faqs.htm.

National Council of State Boards of Nursing (2018f). *NCLEX practice exam FAQs.* Retrieved from https://www.ncsbn.org/12749.htm.

National Council of State Boards of Nursing (2018g). *Next generation NCLEX (NGN) project.* Retrieved from https://www.ncsbn.org/next-generation-nclex.htm.

National Council of State Boards of Nursing (2018h). *Nurse licensure compact.* Retrieved from https://www.ncsbn.org/compacts.htm.

National Council of State Boards of Nursing (2019). *2019 NCLEX examination candidate bulletin.* Retrieved from https://www.ncsbn.org/2019_Bulletin_Final.pdf.

Pearson, V. U. E. (2013). *State of the art identification: Palm vein pattern recognition for the NCLEX examination.* Retrieved from https://www.ncsbn.org/NCLEX_Palm_Vein_Recognition_FAQ.pdf.

Pearson, V. U. E. (2018). *Pathway to practice NCLEX examinations.* Retrieved from https://portal.ncsbn.org/.

Nursing: A Developing Profession

6

Historical Perspectives
Influences on the Present

JoAnn Zerwekh, EdD, RN

🌐 http://evolve.elsevier.com/Zerwekh/nsgtoday/.

History repeats itself because each generation refuses to read the minutes of the last meeting.
Anonymous

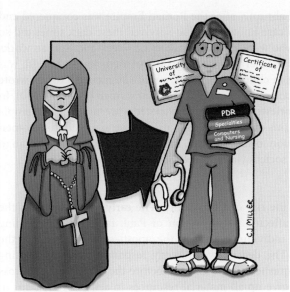

Nursing has come a long way; it is not what it used to be.

After completing this chapter, you should be able to:
- Discuss the importance of the nursing profession understanding its own history.
- Explain the early European contributions to nursing.
- Explain the events that have affected the roles of American nurses.
- Discuss the history of nursing education programs.
- Identify contributions of key historical nursing leaders.

S o, you have to study the history of nursing. In general, the topic is considered boring. Well, be prepared for a different approach to the topic. Knowing the history of our profession guides our understanding of why we do what we do today. This understanding can be useful to us as we set our professional goals. Threads of nursing history can be found throughout the book. Understanding the history can often help in deciding what changes are needed, what changes are helpful, and what changes may be unnecessary. Let us begin with a look at where nursing began.

NURSING HISTORY: PEOPLE AND PLACES

Where Did It All Begin?

Most nursing historians agree that nursing, or the care of the ill and injured, has been done since the beginning of human life and has generally been a woman's role. A mother caring for a child in a cave and someone caring for another ill adult by boiling willow bark to relieve fever are both examples of nursing. The word *nurse* is derived from the Latin word *nutricius*, meaning "nourishing."

Roman mythological figures associated with nursing include the goddess Fortuna, who was usually recognized as being responsible for one's fate and who also served as Jupiter's nurse (Dolan, 1969). Even before Greek and Roman times, ancient Egyptian physicians and nurses assembled voluminous pharmacopoeia with more than 700 remedies for numerous health problems. Great emphasis was placed on the use of animal parts in concoctions that were generally drunk or applied to the body. The physician prescribed and provided the treatments and usually had an assistant who provided the nursing care (Kalisch & Kalisch, 1986). Some ancient medicine was based on driving out the evil spirit rather than curing or treating the malady (i.e., condition or illness). The treatments were often very foul and frequently included fecal material. By now you may be thinking of the saying: "The treatment was successful, but the patient died."

Advancement of medical knowledge halted abruptly after the Roman Empire was conquered and the Dark Ages began. Any medical and health care knowledge that survived these dark times did so only through the efforts of Jewish physicians who were able to translate the Greek and Roman works (Kalisch & Kalisch, 1986). One bright spot was in Salerno, where a school of medicine and health was established for physicians and women to assist in childbirth. In fact, a midwife named Trotula wrote what may be considered the first nursing textbook on the cure of diseases of women (Dalton, 1900). In general, nursing was performed by designated priestesses and was associated with some type of temple worship. Little information has survived about this early period. Historians have assumed that women assisted Hippocrates, but there is little information to support that. From these roots, nursing began to develop as a recognized and valued service to society (Jamieson & Sewall, 1949).

Why Deacons, Widows, and Virgins?

Paralleling the fall of the Roman Empire was the rise of Christianity. The early organization of the young Christian church, which was directly affected by the vision of Paul, included a governing bishop and seven appointed deacons. These individuals assisted the apostles in the work of the Church (the word *deacon* means "servant"). The deacon was directly responsible for distributing all the goods and property that apostles relinquished to the Church before they "took up the cross and followed." The apostles were required to give up all material resources to achieve full status in the Church.

Women sympathetic to the Christian cause of aiding the poor were encouraged in this work by bishops and deacons. Eventually, deacons relinquished this work to women and established the position of deaconess for that purpose. To maintain a pure heart, these women were required by the Church either to be virgins or widows. The stipulation for widows, however, was that they had to have been married only once (Jamieson & Sewall, 1949). The deaconesses carried nursing forward as they ministered to the sick and injured in their homes. Phoebe, a friend of Paul's and the very first deaconess in the young Christian church, has been called the first visiting nurse (Dana, 1936).

Treatments continued to be a mixture of scientific fact, home remedies, and magic. Eventually, an order of widows evolved that was composed of women who were free from home responsibilities and thus able to commit fully to working among the poor. The widows, although not ordained, continued to do the same work as the deaconesses. This was soon followed by the creation of the Order of Virgins as the Church began placing greater value on purity of body. Although deaconess orders were abolished in the Mediterranean countries, they thrived in other European countries. The traditional commitment to care for the poor and sick became invaluable in a society that generally had neither the time nor the inclination to aid them. Eventually, these women became known as *nuns* (from *non nuptae*, meaning "not married").

This was a time of tremendous upheaval in the world. Wars, invasions, and battles were constant, and as a result of these encounters, the number of widows was significant. Society during this time did not have the sophistication or the means to handle the dependents of the soldiers killed in battle. As a means of survival, women joined the nuns as a form of protection from starvation and poverty. This was a dark and dreary time in which superstition, witchcraft, and folklore were predominant influences. Because of the need for physical protection, convents were built to shelter these women (Jamieson & Sewall, 1949). The convents became havens into which women could withdraw from ignorance and evil and be nurtured in traditional Christian beliefs (Donahue, 1985). The deaconesses, widows, and virgins continued to minister to and nurse the ill within the safety of the convent.

How Did Knighthood Contribute to Nursing?

The Holy Wars furthered the development of nursing in an interesting way. Because many Christian crusaders became ill while in Jerusalem, a hospital known as the Hospital of St. John was built to accommodate them. Those who fought in these Holy Wars had taken oaths of chivalry, justice, and piety, and were known as knights. Often men trained in the healing arts accompanied the knights into battle. These male nurses cared for wounded or otherwise stricken knights. They usually wore a red cross emblazoned on their tunics so that in the heat of battle they could be easily identified and thus avoid injury or death (Bullough & Bullough, 1978).

The Hospital of St. John provided excellent nursing care. Many of the nurses who survived stayed to work with the hospital organizers. As the battles in the Holy Land continued, the nurses and knights organized a fighting force with a code of rules and a uniform consisting of a black robe with a white Maltese cross, the symbol of poverty, humility, and chastity. They ventured out to rescue the sick and wounded and transport them to the hospital for care; thus, they became known as the Hospitalers (Kalisch & Kalisch, 1986). Male nurses dominated these orders. Other orders that emulated the Hospitalers developed in Europe, and more hospitals were opened based on the Hospital of St. John model (Donahue, 1985).

The altruistic spirit of nursing was also seen in the craftsmen's guilds. Although their primary purpose was to provide training and jobs through the practice of apprenticeship, the guilds provided care and aid for their members when they became old and could no longer work at their trade. The guilds also assisted members and their families in times of illness and injury. The apprenticeship system—in which experience is gained on the job but no formal education is provided—once served as a model for the training of nurses (Donahue, 1985). This system is no longer used and is now considered to have been detrimental to the evolution of nursing.

What nursing gained during this period of history was status. The altruistic ideal of providing care as a service performed out of humility and love became the foundation for nursing. The recognition of the value of hospitals grew; all across Europe, cities were building their own hospitals. A general resurgence in the demand for trained doctors and nurses contributed to the building of medical schools and the development of university programs in the art and science of healing.

What About Revolts and Nursing?

Revolts—not the kind that led to battles, but revolts of a social nature—were common. There were battles, too; however, the social revolts had a more direct impact on nursing. The revolution of the spirit, more commonly known as the Renaissance, ushered in new concepts of the world: the discovery of the laws of nature by Newton, the exploration of unknown lands, and the growth of secular interests (humanism) over spiritual ones. In this era emerged several outstanding humanists who were to become saints (Donahue, 1985). Interestingly, these saints are shown in depictions as needing nursing care or as giving care to a wounded or injured person.

In Europe, the Protestant Reformation began primarily as a religious reform movement but ended with revolt within the Church. Many hospitals in Protestant countries were forced to close, and those loyal to the Church that operated them were driven out of the country, resulting in a significant short-age of nurses (mostly nuns) to care for the ill and injured. The poor and ill were considered a burden to society, and those hospitals that remained operational in the Protestant countries became known as "pest houses." To fill the need for nurses, women (many of whom were alcoholics and former pros-titutes) were recruited. In general, during this period, a nurse was a woman serving time in a hospital rather than a prison (Donahue, 1985; Jamieson & Sewall, 1949).

The industrial and intellectual revolutions that followed the Reformation all had significant impacts on nursing. During the Industrial Revolution, as production of much-needed goods was streamlined through industrial innovation, craftsmen left the rural life to work in factories. The intellectual contributions of scientists, many of whom were physicians, combined with the inventions of the microscope, thermometer, and pendulum clock, advanced our knowledge and understanding of the world. The invention of the printing press allowed for easier sharing of infor-mation, which further contributed to experimentation. Finally, a disease that was feared worldwide was conquered when Edward Jenner (1749–1823) proved the effectiveness of the smallpox vaccination.

Throughout these revolutions, however, the maternal and infant death rates continued to be high. In fact, before his pioneering work in antisepsis in obstetrics, Ignaz Phillipp Semmelweis (1818–1865) observed that patients giving birth in hospitals under the care of educated physicians had significantly higher death rates than women giving birth at home or in clinics with the assistance of midwives.

Despite all the knowledge gained during this time of revolution, society was generally callous toward the plight of children. Children were abandoned without apparent remorse, and poor families who were desperate to reduce the number of mouths to feed practiced infanticide. These families had no reliable form of birth control except abstinence. Because it was common practice for the woman hired as a wet nurse to sleep with the infant, many infants were inadvertently suffocated. Donahue (1985) reported that, during this period, 75% of all children baptized were dead before they reached the age of 5 years. Because of the persistence of these sad conditions, children's and foundlings' hospitals were established. Eventually, laws were enacted to aid these unfortunate victims (Donahue, 1985).

Existing health care conditions for the ill and injured continued to contribute to high mortality rates. Some sources reported hospital mortality rates as high as 90%. Conditions in the armies were no better. In any military action, mortality rates were high. Reports from the battlefront during the Crimean War suggested that battles were postponed because there were too few able-bodied soldiers to fight. Dysentery and typhoid were the military's nemeses. If a soldier was wounded, infection invari-ably resulted. Hospitals generally offered no guarantee of survival. In any event, these occurrences had a serious effect on military strategies. If men are ill or injured, battles cannot be won.

Upon this scene entered Florence Nightingale.

Florence Nightingale: The Legend and the Lady

First, let us discuss the legend. Published works about Florence Nightingale before the 1960s generally presented the legend. Most authors agreed that she was beautiful, intelligent, wealthy, socially successful, and educated. She certainly had an ability to influence people and used every Victorian secret to accomplish her desires. Although Nightingale believed it improper to accept payment for her services, she did demand financial support for materials, goods, and staff to accomplish her programs and goals. Some historians believe that it was through Nightingale's influence that Jean Henri Dunant, a Swiss gentleman, provided the aid to the wounded that laid the foundation for the organization of the International Red Cross (Bullough et al., 1990; Dodge, 1989; Dossey, 2000).

Regardless of what actually happened between Dunant and Nightingale, her interest and ambition lay in becoming a nurse. Her family was upset because of this decision. As described by Dossey (2000), Florence (or "Flo" as her family and friends called her) began her journey as a mystic when she was 16 years old. Her experience of a sudden, inner "knowing" took place under two majestic cedars of Lebanon in Embley (England), one of her sacred spots for contemplation. She claimed to receive the following in her awakening moment: "That a quest there is, and an end, is the single secret spoken." Energized by her contact with the Divine Reality or Consciousness, Florence "worked very hard among the poor people" with "a strong feeling of religion" for the next 3 months (Dossey, 2000, p. 33; Critical Thinking Box 6.1, Fig. 6.1, and Box 6.1).

? CRITICAL THINKING BOX 6.1

Consider all that you have heard about Florence Nightingale. Now, think about the idea that she was a mystic. What does that mean?

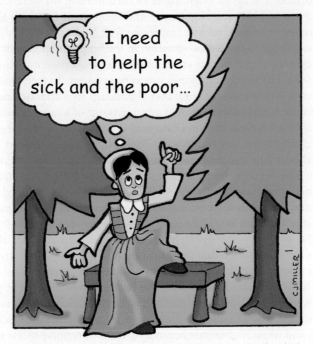

FIG. 6.1 Florence Nightingale: the legend (mystic, visionary, healer) and the lady.

BOX 6.1 NIGHTINGALE AND MYSTICISM

What is mysticism? It is considered to be a universal experience of enlightenment obtained via meditation or prayer that focuses on the direct experience of union with divinity, God, or Ultimate Reality, and the belief that such experience is a genuine and important source of knowledge. It is characterized by a call to personal action, because the person is uncomfortable with the world as it is. Underhill (1961) describes five (nonlinear or nonsequential) phases in the spiritual development of a mystic: awakening, purgation, illumination, surrender, and union.

Awakening: At age 16, Nightingale experienced her first call from God and on three other occasions later in life when she heard the voice of God again.

Purgation: Nightingale spent her later teen years and young adulthood (approximately 17 years) separating herself from the affluent lifestyle and worldly possessions that characterized her early life.

Illumination: For Nightingale, this period began when she accepted her first superintendent position at Harley Hospital in London, which propelled her to battle for better conditions during the Crimean War invasion and later, when she returned to England, to fight for reform of the army medical department.

Surrender: This "dark night of the soul" period for Nightingale is thought to have begun approximately 6 years after the Crimean War when she was in her late 30s and continued to her late 60s, a time characterized by her chronic ill health and episodes of stress, overexertion, and depression.

Union: The last 20 years of Nightingale's life (ages 70–90) were engendered with an appreciation of the blessings in her life and feelings of peace, joy, and power. Social action and issues no longer spurred the driving force in her life.

Data from Dossey, B. (2005). *Nursing as a spiritual practice: The mystical legacy of Florence Nightingale*; Underhill, E. (1961). *Mysticism.* New York: Dutton.

Nightingale's parents felt that hospitals were terrible places to go and that nurses were, in most cases, the dregs of society. Hospitals were certainly not places for women of proper social upbringing. Although she was forbidden to do so, Nightingale studied nursing (in secret). After a fortuitous meeting, a relationship developed between Nightingale and Sidney and Elizabeth Herbert, an influential couple who were interested in hospital reform. Impressed with Nightingale's analytical mind and her ability to apply nursing knowledge to the critical situation in the hospitals (Bullough & Bullough, 1978; Bullough et al., 1990), they encouraged her to study nursing at Kaiserswerth School, run by Lutheran deaconesses (Dolan, 1969). Her family, of course, was very unhappy. In fact, Dodge (1989) reported that the event precipitated a family crisis, because they threatened to withdraw financial support.

Nightingale accepted a position as administrator of a nursing home for women, the Institution for the Care of Sick Gentlewomen in Distressed Circumstances. She hired her own chaperone and went to work at reforming the way things were done. Nightingale's interest in hospital reform was insatiable. She visited hospitals and took copious notes on nursing care, treatments, and procedures. She sent reports on hospital conditions to Sidney Herbert, the British Secretary of War. Secretary Herbert then assigned her other hospitals to review. The reviews always included recommendations for improving nursing care. From this early background of experiences, Nightingale was now ready for her greatest mission—the Crimean War. The legend was on her way (Bullough et al., 1990).

In 1854, soldiers were dying, more from common diseases than from bullets. Bullough and colleagues (1990) reported that the Crimean War was a series of mistakes. No plan was made for supplying the troops, no plan was in place to maintain the environment in camps, and no provisions were available to care for the injured after the battle. When Herbert appointed Nightingale as head of a group of nurses to go to Crimea, she had already developed a plan of action. In fact, some historians believe that she was already planning to go in an unofficial capacity. The announcement caused a sensation, and when Nightingale began a rigorous selection process for accepting nurses, many volunteered, but few were chosen. She cleaned up the kitchens, the wards, the patients, and improved the general hygiene. From there, the legend grew.

She was clever; after demonstrating the effectiveness of her methods, she withdrew her services. Naturally, all that she had accomplished was done under the scrutiny, skepticism, suspicion, and anger of the physicians. Without the services of the nurses, the abominable conditions quickly returned, and finally the physicians begged her to do whatever she wished—just help! Nightingale responded to the pleading. The actual number of soldiers who benefited from the care of her nurses was immeasurable.

> The nurses made rounds day and night, and the legend of the lady with the lamp was born.

Nightingale's great success prompted her to begin developing schools of nursing based on her knowledge of what was effective nursing. Eventually, many schools in Europe and America used the Nightingale model for nursing education. The program was generally 1 year in length, and classes were small. Many women wanted to become nurses; however, only 15 to 20 applicants were accepted for each class. The goals of her programs included training hospital nurses, training nurses to train others, and training nurses to work in the district with the sick poor (Dolan, 1969). Nightingale had changed society's view of the nurse to one of dignity and value and worthy of respect. As a tribute to Nightingale, Lystra Gretter, an instructor of nursing at the old Harper Hospital in Detroit, Michigan, composed "The Nightingale Pledge," which was first used by its graduating class in the spring of 1893. It is an adaptation of the Hippocratic Oath taken by physicians (Box 6.2).

In any legend, the truth is often mixed with myth. The stories surrounding Florence Nightingale are many. What is interesting is that, before the 1970s, authors tended to deify Nightingale or establish her as a saintly person. These myths make for interesting reading. Early nurse historians also contributed to these myths by their interpretations of Nightingale's work. But myths have a purpose. They can be used to explain worldviews of groups of people or professions at a given time, and they provide explanations for practice beliefs or natural phenomena. Myths tend to maintain a degree of accuracy when the truth is lost. The trick is to separate myth from fact and story from legend and to draw conclusions regarding the occurrences. This is no easy task when one studies Florence Nightingale. Therefore, it is important to read a variety of studies across several time periods before drawing conclusions about the legend and the lady.

In summary, Florence Nightingale had certain characteristics that enabled her to achieve success during the strict Victorian times in which she lived. She was extremely well educated for her time. She had traveled throughout the world and had the advantage of personal wealth and a gift for establishing relationships with persons of influence and philanthropic spirit. Most portraits depict her as an attractive woman with pleasant features. Contemporary historians agree she had tremendous compassion for all who suffered. She was very strong-willed, a characteristic that carried her through the period of the Crimean War. She had the ability to analyze data and draw relevant conclusions, on which she based her recommendations. Her students of nursing received better preparation than most physicians. She was 36 at the end of the war, and when she returned home, she became a virtual recluse until she died at age 90. She did have some physical ailments: Crimean fever, sciatica, rheumatism,

---

BOX 6.2 NIGHTINGALE PLEDGE

I solemnly pledge myself before God and in the presence of this assembly, to pass my life in purity and to practice my profession faithfully. I will abstain from whatever is deleterious and mischievous, and will not take or knowingly administer any harmful drug. I will do all in my power to maintain and elevate the standard of my profession and will hold in confidence all personal matters committed to my keeping and all family affairs coming to my knowledge in the practice of my calling. With loyalty will I endeavor to aid the physician, in his work, and devote myself to the welfare of those committed to my care.

and dilation of the heart, each of which could have crippling side effects and contributed to her becoming bedridden (Bullough et al., 1990). According to Dossey (2000), "In 1995, D.A.B. Young, a former scientist at the Wellcome Foundation in London, proposed that the Crimean fever was actually Mediterranean fever, otherwise known as Malta fever; this disease is included under the generic name brucellosis" (p. 426). Because of the widespread Crimean fever that the soldiers encountered, it is thought that Nightingale was most likely exposed to this disease through ingesting contaminated food, such as meat or raw milk, cheese, or butter. It seems a logical assumption that Nightingale's 32-year history of debilitating, chronic symptoms is compatible with a diagnosis of chronic brucellosis. In any event, the legend and the lady had a significant effect on American nursing as we know it today (Bullough & Bullough, 1978; Bullough et al., 1990; Dodge, 1989; Dolan, 1969; Dossey, 2000).

AMERICAN NURSING: CRITICAL FACTORS

What Was It Like in Colonial Times?

In colonial times, all able-bodied persons shared nursing responsibilities; however, when there was a choice, women were preferred as nurses. Early colonial historians described care for the ill and house chores as the responsibilities of nurses. Although most women of this era were considered dainty (Bradford, 1898), nurses were usually depicted as willing to do hard work. Some colonies organized nursing services that sought out the sick and provided comfort to those who were ill with smallpox and other diseases (Bullough & Bullough, 1978). There were few trained nurses, however, and most of the individuals who delivered nursing care in the five largest hospitals were men (Dolan, 1969). Eventually, women were hired at the command of George Washington to serve meals and care for the wounded and ill. The era ended with the enactment of the first legislation to improve health and medical treatment and to provide for formal education for society as a whole (Dolan, 1969).

What Happened to Nursing During the U.S. Civil War?

The period of the U.S. Civil War witnessed an improvement in patient care through control of the environment in which the patient recovered. The greatest problems for the army stemmed from the poor sanitary conditions in the camps, which bred diseases such as smallpox and dysentery. The results were many deaths from inadequate nutrition, impure water, and a general lack of cleanliness.

Nurses who had some formal training were recognized as being major contributors to the relative success of hospital treatments. It was in this era that the value of primary prevention, or the prevention of the occurrence of disease by measures such as immunization and the provision of a pure water supply, became understood. Volunteer nurses, mostly women, served in hospitals caring for those wounded soldiers fortunate enough to have survived the trip from the battlefield. Their patients were nursed in a clean environment and were provided with adequate nutrition. The likelihood of their recovering was significantly improved. Astute physicians observed that patients cared for by nurses generally recovered well enough to return to the battlefield. Families, too, saw that when nurses had control over the environment, their ill or injured loved one was more likely to recover—and return home.

As the United States moved into the industrial age of the early 1900s, Victorian values began to permeate the middle and upper middle classes. Social concerns focused on protecting families from the diseases of the crowded urban areas, and the demand for improved health care increased.

How Did the Roles of Nurses and Wives Compare During the Victorian Era?

The Victorian era had a significant effect on nurses, primarily because they were women. The parallelism between the idealized view of the Victorian woman and the traditional nurse is stunning. The effect of many of the values and beliefs of this era, some historians report, is still felt by women today.

The typical upper-class Victorian household consisted of a husband, who earned a living outside of the home and maintained total control of the family finances, and his wife, who maintained harmony within the home and raised their children. Women's work was generally restricted to philanthropic and voluntary work; women attended teas and other social functions to raise money for organizations and people in need.

Most women were considered fragile and dainty. They were often ill. It has been suggested that some women used illnesses and frailty as a form of birth control to prevent the numerous pregnancies that most women experienced. Some historians concluded that it was through their weaknesses that women gained control and attention. If the wife was ill or frail, maids or servants were hired, but if the wife was healthy, the husband would expect more from her. The Victorian wife was expected to "be good." She was esteemed by her husband but had limited power within the confines of the home and society. She was expected to be hardworking and able to maintain harmony, while at the same time being submissive to the demands of her husband. In general, this fostered dependence on the dominant male figure—the Victorian husband (Rybczynski, 1986).

Let us examine nursing during this same time, especially within the hospital organization. Nurses generally were women who wanted to avoid the drudgery of a Victorian marriage. They were required to be single to make a complete commitment to their vocation. Schooled in submission, women were expected to be equally accommodating within the hospital organization. A good nurse worked for harmony within the hospital. She was expected to be hardworking and submissive. The doctor and the hospital administrator were frequently the same person, usually a man who expected position and power to go hand in hand. Patients were admitted only if they had income and could afford to pay for the services. It was the physician who generated income, and good nurses were expected to help him continue to maintain power. Because the system rewarded people for being ill, there was little incentive to be healthy. Social values contributed to dependence on the health care system. From this milieu came the reformers (Bullough & Bullough, 1978; Davis, 1961; Kalisch & Kalisch, 1986; Stewart, 1950).

Who Were the Reformers of the Victorian Era?

The Victorian era, although a time of repression for women, was also a time of reform. A list of important names in nursing reform includes M. Adelaide Nutting, Minnie Goodnow, Lavinia L. Dock, Annie W. Goodrich, Isabel Hampton Robb, Lilian D. Wald, Isabel M. Stewart, and Sophia Palmer, among others (Jamieson & Sewall, 1949; Kalisch & Kalisch, 1986). These women, who had in common a comfortable upper middle-class background, intelligence, and education, also had in common a desire to reach beyond the constraints that society imposed on them. As society began to realize the important role that nurses played in treating the ill and injured, it also began to understand the need for training programs that would better educate nurses. Reformers focused on establishing standards for nursing education and practice. Among their accomplishments were the organization of the American Nurses Association (ANA) and the creation of its journal (until 2006, when *American Nurse Today* became the official journal of the ANA), the *American Journal of Nursing*, and the enactment of legislation to require the licensure of prepared nurses. This protected the public from inadequate care provided by people who were not trained as a nurse (Christy, 1971; Dock, 1900; Maness, 2006).

What Were the Key Challenges and Opportunities in 20th- and 21st-Century Nursing?

Wars, influenza, the Great Depression, HIV/AIDS, and rapid technological advancements during the twentieth century affected the nursing profession. Table 6.1 summarizes some key historical and nursing events along a timeline. Box 6.3 lists key influential American nurses.

TABLE 6.1 TIMELINE OF EVENTS IN THE 20TH AND 21ST CENTURIES

1900–1910	1910–1920	1920–1930	1930–1940	1940–1950
1820–1910 Influence of Florence Nightingale 1900 First publication of the *American Journal of Nursing* 1901 U.S. Army Nurse Corps established 1908 U.S. Navy Nurse Corps established 1909 American Red Cross Nursing Service formed 1909 University of Minnesota establishes the first baccalaureate nursing program 1910 Florence Nightingale dies	1914–1918 World War I 1918–1919 21.5 million people died as a result of the 1918–1919 pandemic. More recent estimates have placed global mortality from the 1918–1919 pandemic at anywhere between 30 and 50 million	1923 Goldmark Report—study focused on nursing student preparation in hospital programs and faculty preparation 1924 Yale School of Nursing becomes the first autonomous school of nursing in the United States with its established nursing department meeting the standards of the university 1925 Establishment of the Frontier Nursing Service—first organized midwifery program 1925 Establishment of the Frontier Nursing Service—first organized midwifery program 1929 Stock market crashes, leading to the Great Depression	1932 Teachers College establishes the first EdD in nursing 1934 First PhD program in nursing started at New York University 1935 Social Security Act enhances and promotes public health nursing	1939–1945 World War II 1943 Nurse Training Act provided federal funding for nursing education 1943 U.S. Cadet Nurse Corps established During this decade the rise of "team nursing" occurs because of a shortage of nurses

RESOURCES

American Association for the History of Nursing: *Nursing history calendar,* 2016. Retrieved from http://www.aahn.org/nursinghistorycalendar.html.

American Journal of Nursing: *The state board test pool exam, 52*(5):616, 1952. Retrieved from http://www.jstor.org/discover/10.2307/3468023?uid=3739552&uid=2129&uid=2&uid=70&uid=4&uid=3739256&sid=21101634154573.

American Nurses Association: Historical Review, 2016. Retrieved from http://www.nursingworld.org/FunctionalMenuCategories/AboutANA/History/BasicHistoricalReview.pdf.

Haase PT: *The origins and rise of associate degree nursing education,* Durham and London, 1990, Duke University Press.

National Council of State Boards of Nursing. (2016): *NCSBN Historical Timeline.* Retrieved from https://www.ncsbn.org/70.htm.

Texas Organization for Associate Degree Nursing: *History,* n.d. Retrieved from http://www.toadn.org/history/index.php?PHPSESSID=53455f97767bc71c0a89009780fb7676.

1950–1960	1960–1970	1970–1980	1980–1990	1990–2000	2000 to current
1950 Associate degree education for nursing began as part of an experimental project at Teachers College, Columbia University, New York 1950–1953 Korean War 1953 Establishment of the National Student Nurses' Association 1950 Nursing became first profession to use the same licensing exam in all states, called the State Board Test Pool Exam 1952 Publication of first issue of *Nursing Research* 1959 Beginning of the Vietnam War that would last until 1975	1964 Nursing Training Act—first federal law to give comprehensive assistance for nursing education 1965 Medicare and Medicaid Acts 1965 American Nurses Associations (ANA's) "Position Paper on Educational Preparation for Nurse Practitioners and Assistants to Nurses" 1965 Establishment of the first nurse practitioner (NP) role, developed jointly by Loretta Ford, a nurse educator, and Henry Silver, a physician at the University of Colorado 1968 Adoption by ANA of a new Code for Nurses	1973 Establishment of the American Academy of Nursing 1978 First test-tube baby born 1978 Establishment of the National Council of State Boards of Nursing (NCSBN) to lead nursing regulation 1985 Establishment of the American Association of Nurse Practitioners (AANP)	1981 Release of the first IBM personal computer 1982 Centers for Disease Control and Prevention (CDC) begins formal tracking of all AIDS cases 1984 Formation of Texas Organization of Associate Degree Nursing (TOADN) 1985 Establishment of the National Institute of Nursing Research (NINR) at the National Institutes of Health (NIH) 1986 National Organization for the Advancement for Associate Degree Nursing (NOAADN) is established	1991 American Nurses Credentialing Center operational 1990 Explosion of medical technologies and the access to information via the Internet 1994 NCSBN Implements computer adaptive test (CAT) for nurse licensure 1996 Publication of a free online electronic journal, *Online Journal of Nursing Issues (OJIN)*	2000 NCSBN initiates the Nurse License Compact (NLC) 2001 9/11 Terrorist attack 2004 American Association of Colleges of Nursing (AACN) recommends all advanced practice nurses earn a Doctor of Nursing Practice (DNP) 2010 Affordable Care Act signed into law 2012 Canada chooses to use the NCLEX exam for licensing

Kansas University Medical Center: *100-year timelines of world history, nursing, medicine, science & industry advances, U.S. economic & healthcare market, U.S. social policy, and U.S. presidents*, n.d. Retrieved from http://www2.kumc.edu/instruction/nursing/pqe/timelinehistory.htm.

National Institute of Nursing Research: *Important events in the National Institute of Nursing Research History*, n.d. Retrieved from https://www.ninr.nih.gov/aboutninr/history.

U.S. Department of Health & Human Services: *The great pandemic: The United States in 1918-1919*, n.d. Retrieved from http://www.flu.gov/pandemic/history/1918/.

University of Minnesota School of Nursing: *School of nursing: about*, 2013. Retrieved from http://www.nursing.umn.edu/about/index.htm.

BOX 6.3   KEY INFLUENTIAL AMERICAN NURSES

- Dorothea Dix (1802–1887) was an advocate and reformer for the mentally ill and Civil War nurse. With no formal medical or nursing education or experience she was appointed Superintendent of the United States Army Nurses in 1861.
- Clara Barton (1821–1912) was the founder of the American Red Cross and was nicknamed "The Angel of the Battlefield" during the Civil War.
- Linda Richards (1841–1930) is considered America's first trained nurse with her diploma archived in the Smithsonian Institute in Washington, DC, and she was instrumental in developing an organized system of notetaking and medical record keeping.
- Mary Eliza Mahoney (1845–1926) became the first African-American woman to complete nurse's training in 1879 and is noted for becoming the first African-American licensed nurse. She was one of the first black women to join the American Nurses Association.
- Lillian Wald (1867–1940) helped to develop the community health care system and pioneered public health and school nursing, was instrumental in the development of the National Association for the Advancement of Colored People (NAACP), and persuaded Columbia University to appoint the first professor of nursing.
- Mary Adelaide Nutting (1858–1948) became the first professor of nursing at Teachers College of Columbia University.
- Mary Breckenridge (1881–1965) was a nurse midwife, who founded the Frontier Nursing Service in the Appalachian Mountains of eastern Kentucky.
- Mildred Montag (1908–2004) developed the concept of associate degree nursing, as the topic of her doctoral dissertation in 1951.
- Florence Wald (1917–2008) is credited with being the "mother of the American hospice movement."
- Loretta Ford (born 1920) partnered with pediatrician Henry Silver in Colorado and started the first pediatric nurse practitioner program in 1965.
- Eddie Bernice Johnson (born 1935) was elected to a Texas congressional seat in 1972 and in 1992 was the first registered nurse elected to the US Congress, as a democrat from Texas.

References

American history: Influential female nurses. (n.d.). Regis College. Retrieved from https://onlinenursing.regiscollege.edu/family-nurse-practitioner/american-history-influential-female-nurses/.

Daniels, J. Z. (2015). *From the bedside to the halls of Congress: Our national nurses. Minority Nurse.* Retrieved from https://minoritynurse.com/from-the-bedside-to-the-halls-of-congress-our-national-nurses/.

Kennedy, M. S. (2015). Securing our place in history: Why it matters. *AJN, 115*(3), 7. https://doi.org/10.1097/01.NAJ.0000461788.76291.a2.

How Did the Symbols (Lamp, Cap, and Pin) of the Profession Evolve?

As mentioned previously, Florence Nightingale acquired the nickname "Lady with the Lamp" while caring for soldiers during the Crimean War. Throughout the night, she would carry her lamp while checking on each soldier. For many historical scholars, this image of Nightingale more accurately represents Longfellow's poetic imagination in his 1857 Santa Filomena than the historical record (Grypma, 2010). Here is a link to this famous poem: www.theatlantic.com/past/docs/unbound/poetry/nov1857/filomena.htm.

The nurse's cap design evolved from the traditional garb of the early deaconesses or nuns, who were some of the earliest nurses to care for the sick. More recently, the cap's use was to keep a female nurse's hair neatly in place and present a professional appearance. There were two types of cap styles: one was a long nurse's cap, which covered most of the nurse's head; the other was a short nurse's cap, which sat on top of the head. The design of the cap identified the nurse's alma mater, which differentiated graduates from their respective nursing programs. Typically, a black band sewn on the cap signified a senior-level student or graduate status and sometimes identified the head nurse on a clinical unit. The origin of the black or navy band is unknown; some historical scholars believed the black band was a sign of mourning for Florence Nightingale. By the late 1970s, the hat had disappeared almost completely, as have "capping" ceremonies when the new students passed a probationary period of the program to receive their nursing cap. Also, the rapid growth of the number of men in nursing necessitated a unisex uniform.

The nursing pin is a 1000-year-old symbol of service to others (Rode, 1989). The Maltese cross worn by the knights and nurses during the Crusades is considered the origin of the nursing pin. The most recent ancestor of the pin is the hospital badge that has been worn to identify the nurse since its inception more than 100 years ago. The nursing pin was given by the hospital school of nursing to the graduating students to identify them as nurses who were educated to serve the health needs of society. As schools of nursing flourished, each designed their own unique pin to represent their unique philosophy and beliefs. The pin is still worn as part of nurses' uniforms today.

What Are the Key Events and Influences of the 21st Century?

The beginning of the current millennium was marked with the Year 2000 problem, or Y2K, signifying problems that originated from mainframe computers that were keeping computer documentation data in an abbreviated two-digit format (98, 99, 00) rather than a four-digit year (1998, 1999, 2000). The computer would interpret 00 as 1900 rather than 2000. In newspapers and magazines, there were reports of widespread fear and concern that a massive computer calamity would lead to a global financial crisis, hospital support system shutdown, nuclear meltdowns, collapse of air-traffic control systems, loss of power, and so on. Throughout the world, organizations had to fix and upgrade their computer systems.

Dramatic events following the World Trade Center attacks in New York City on September 11, 2001, affected all aspects of life, including more focus on nursing disaster management and emergency preparedness. Natural disasters, such as Hurricane Katrina in 2005 (Gulf Coast) and Superstorm Sandy in 2012 (East Coast), called on nurses to respond to events that they had not previously experienced. The Ebola outbreak that began in West Africa and spread to the United States in the fall of 2014 pushed nursing to focus on early identification, isolation, monitoring, and quarantine (Centers for Disease Control and Prevention [CDC], 2014).

In early 2010, the passage of the Affordable Care Act (ACA), also referred to as "health care reform" or "Obamacare," was signed into law. Although it will take 10 years to fully implement the reform, it provides for a comprehensive national health insurance program requiring everyone to have health insurance. There continues to be controversy since the passage of the act, with some states suing the federal government, stating that it is unconstitutional to mandate that individuals buy health insurance. The Supreme Court ruled that the health care law was constitutional in 2012; however, politicians and the public still have dividing opinions on the implementation of the reform. In early 2018, the ACA Individual Mandate was repealed (which takes full effect in 2019), which was the requirement that individuals must sign up for health insurance or face a tax penalty. Whether the ACA will remain in effect is a question that only history will reveal.

HISTORY OF NURSING EDUCATION

What Is the History of Diploma Nursing?

The oldest form of educational preparation leading to licensure as an RN in the United States is the diploma program. Education in diploma schools emphasized the skills needed to care for the acutely ill patient. Graduates received a diploma in nursing, not an academic degree. From 1872 until the mid-1960s, the hospital diploma program was the dominant nursing program. Currently, there are approximately 42 diploma programs accredited by the Accreditation Commission for Education in Nursing (ACEN); this represents the smallest percentage (4%) of all basic RN programs (ACEN, 2016; National

League for Nursing [NLN], 2014b). Perhaps one of the reasons for this decline was that the courses offered by hospitals frequently did not provide college credit. Although most diploma programs are associated with institutions of higher learning, where the graduates receive some college credit, graduates still may not receive college credit for the nursing courses.

What Is the History of Associate Degree Nursing?

The associate degree nursing program has the distinction of being the first and, to date, only educational program for nursing that was developed from planned research and controlled experimentation. Since its beginning in 1951, the associate degree nursing program has grown to more than 1092 programs, producing more graduates annually than either diploma or baccalaureate programs (NLN, 2014a). Approximately 58% of all graduates are from associate degree programs, which has been a steady percentage since 1994 (NLN, 2014b).

In 1951, Mildred Montag published her doctoral dissertation, *The Education of Nursing Technicians*, which proposed education for the RN in the community college. Dr. Montag suggested that the associate degree program be a terminal degree to prepare nurses for immediate employment. According to Dr. Montag, there was a need for a new type of nurse, the "nurse technician," whose role would be broader than that of a practical nurse but narrower than that of the professional nurse. The technical nurse was to function at the "bedside." The duties of the technical nurse, according to Dr. Montag, would include (1) giving general nursing care with supervision, (2) assisting in the planning of nursing care for patients, and (3) assisting in the evaluation of the nursing care given (Montag, 1951).

In 1952, the American Association of Junior Colleges established an advisory committee. Along with the NLN, this committee was to conduct cooperative research on nursing education in the community college. The goals of this Cooperative Research Project were threefold: (1) to describe the development of the associate degree nursing program, (2) to evaluate the associate degree graduates, and (3) to determine the future implications of the associate degree on nursing. The original project was directed by Dr. Montag at Teachers College of Columbia University and included seven junior colleges and one hospital from each of the six regions of the United States.

In the proposed technical nursing curriculum, there was to be a balance between general education and nursing courses. Unlike the diploma programs, the emphasis was to be on education, not service. At the end of 2 years, the student was to be awarded an associate's degree in nursing and would be eligible to take the state board examinations for RN licensure (now called the NCLEX-RN® Exam).

What Is the History of Baccalaureate Nursing?

The early baccalaureate nursing programs were usually 5 years in length and consisted of the basic 3-year diploma program with an additional 2 years of liberal arts. In 1909, the University of Minnesota offered the first university-based nursing program. It offered the first Bachelor of Science in Nursing degree and graduated the first bachelor's degree–educated nurse. By 1916, there were 13 universities and 3 colleges with baccalaureate nursing programs. A 2017 survey conducted by the American Association of Colleges of Nursing (AACN) found that total enrollment in entry-level nursing programs leading to the baccalaureate degree was 338,802 with graduation numbers at 128,852 (AACN, 2017a). Approximately 38% of all graduates are from baccalaureate degree programs, which has been a steady percentage since 2006 (NLN, 2014b). According to NLN's (2014a) biennial survey of schools of nursing, there are 710 baccalaureate nursing programs.

What Is the History of Graduate Nursing Education?

Graduate nursing programs in the United States originated during the late 1800s. As more nursing schools sought to strengthen their own programs, there was increased pressure on nursing instructors to obtain advanced preparation in education and clinical nursing specialties.

The Catholic University of America, in Washington, DC, offered one of the early graduate programs for nurses. It began offering courses in nursing education in 1932 and conferring a master's degree in nursing education in 1935.

The NLN's Subcommittee on Graduate Education first published guidelines for organization, administration, curriculum, and testing in 1957. These guidelines have been revised throughout the years and reflect the focus in master's education on research and clinical specialization.

Until the 1960s, the master's degree in nursing was viewed as a terminal degree. The goal of graduate education was to prepare nurses for teaching, administration, and supervisory positions. In the early 1970s, the emphasis shifted to developing clinical skills, and the roles of clinical specialists and nurse practitioners emerged. By the late 1970s, the focus again shifted back to teaching, administration, and supervisory positions (McCloskey & Grace, 2001).

In response to health care reform, the number of master's programs has increased. In 2014, NLN reported that 113,788 students were enrolled in master's programs with current enrollment at 158,941 (AACN, 2017a). Considering the 158,941 enrollment number, 95,232 are advanced practice students, with nurse practitioner enrollments having the highest enrollment of 87,750, CRNA at 4333, CNM at 1768, and CNS at 1381 (AACN, 2017a).

With a historic decision made in 2004, nursing leaders called for moving the current level of preparation necessary for advanced nursing practice from the master's degree to the doctorate-level by the year 2015. Essentially, the Doctor of Nursing Practice (DNP) is a terminal degree in nursing practice and offers an alternative to research-focused doctoral programs (see Chapter 7 on nursing education). The DNP degree mirrors other professions who have moved to a doctorate practice degree: Pharmacy (PharmD), Psychology (PsyD), Physical Therapy (DPT), and Audiology (AudD). The Commission on Collegiate Nursing Education (CCNE) began accrediting DNP programs in Fall 2008. To date, 259 DNP programs have been accredited by CCNE. From 2015 to 2016, the number of students enrolled in DNP programs increased from 21,995 to 25,289. During that same period, the number of DNP graduates increased from 4100 to 4855, while the number and growth of research-focused doctoral programs have remained steady with around 100 programs (AACN, 2017b).

THE NURSE'S ROLE: THE STRUGGLE FOR DEFINITIONS

What Do Nurses Do?

As a student, you study nursing texts that explain theories, skills, principles, and the care of patients. Every text has at least one introductory chapter that describes nursing and its significance. By examining many of these introductory chapters of nursing texts, you can generate a rather extensive list of roles (Anglin, 1991). From this list of roles, six major categories can be determined (Table 6.2). The most traditional role for nurses is that of caregiver. The nurse as teacher or educator is often referred to when discussing patient care or nursing education. The role of advocate had been very controversial in the early 1900s; however, patient advocacy has become the essential nursing role since the 1980s and has become more of a priority of the profession (Hanks, 2008). Nurses were also expected to be managers ever since the first formal education or training program was instituted. Another interesting role for the nurse is that of colleague. The final role is that of expert.

What Is the Traditional Role of a Nurse?

The role of the nurse as caregiver has engendered the least amount of controversy. This role has been thoroughly documented, not only in writing but also through art, since early times. Nurses and nursing leaders agree that this is their primary role. As students, your caregiving skills will be measured constantly through skill laboratories, clinical evaluation proficiency, and, eventually, through licensure testing and staff evaluations. All of these mechanisms are used to evaluate your ability to be a caregiver.

TABLE 6.2 WHAT NURSES DO

CAREGIVER	EDUCATOR	ADVOCATE	MANAGER	COLLEAGUE	EXPERT
Care provider	Patient educator	Interpreter	Administrator	Collaborator	Academician
Comforter	Family educator	Learner	Coordinator	Communicator	Historian
Healer	Counselor	Protector	Decision maker	Facilitator	Nursing instructor
Helper	Community teacher	Risk-taker	Evaluator	Peer reviewer	Professional educator
Nurturer		Change agent	Initiator	Professional	Researcher
Practitioner			Leader	Specialist	Research consumer
Rehabilitator			Planner		Teacher
Support agent					Theorist
					Practitioner
					Leader

Caregiving is probably the only role about which there is agreement as to what it means and how we do it.

Imagine a nurse providing care. In general, the picture that most often comes to mind is someone, usually female, in a white uniform caring for a patient who is ill. This picture is the romanticized version of caregiving continually portrayed in movies, television, and novels. We know that caregiving takes place in many settings: clinics, homes, hospitals, offices, businesses, and schools, among others. We can probably agree that caregiving is an important role for nurses and that it is why most of us chose nursing. Studies examining the role of caregiver continue to be undertaken, and our understanding of the role is expanding (Benner, 1984; Leininger, 1984; Watson, 1985). Without a doubt, caregiving is an important role, one that is essential to nursing.

Did You Know You Would Be a Teacher or Educator?

Teaching patients about their therapy, condition, or choices is critical to the successful outcome of some prescribed treatments. For example, nurses have learned through research that knowledge can reduce anxiety before and after surgery. Teaching becomes especially important when patients have to make treatment choices and decisions about their care. With the volumes of information available regarding health care, it is even more important that nurses help patients understand what they need to know to make wise decisions regarding their health. Discharge plans also provide an opportunity for patient education. Home care includes teaching as a reimbursable activity. Agency charting procedures all require documentation of patient education. All nursing textbooks include sections on what the nurse needs to emphasize regarding patient education. With all this evidence, there is little doubt that the educator role is an important one for the nurse (Fig. 6.2).

Teaching is planned to strengthen a patient's knowledge regarding making decisions about treatment options, and it is an essential nursing intervention (Alfaro-LeFevre, 1998). In many ways, the nurse as an educator is also an interpreter of information, and this leads us to the next role for discussion.

When Did the Nurse Become an Advocate? Nurse in the Role of Advocate

A useful definition of the term *advocate* is "one who pleads a cause before another." The first advocacy issue, arising early in the 1900s, concerned nursing practice. Public health and visiting nurses were the majority (approximately 70%), and hospital nurses were the minority (approximately 30%) of working nurses. Working as a private duty nurse or visiting nurse was a source of income for women who had

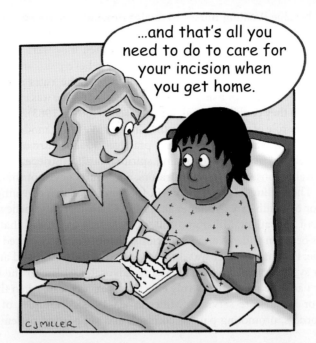

FIG. 6.2 Did you know you would be a teacher?

no other means of support. Because there was no way to determine the credentials of the visiting nurse, many impostors worked in that capacity. Lavinia L. Dock, Sophia Palmer, and Annie W. Goodrich, three nursing leaders, deplored this situation and endeavored to protect the public from unscrupulous "nurses" (Dolan, 1969; Goodnow, 1936). Dock was an excellent nurse who believed in fairness to qualified nurses and to the public. She advocated that all practicing nurses be measured by a "fair-general-average standard," as determined by written examination, and be rewarded with licensure on attainment of the standard (Christy, 1971).

Palmer's proposed solutions were similar. Many hospitals were sending out inexperienced undergraduates to do private duty nursing while not reporting the income. She advocated a training school in which students of nursing would learn to provide care under a qualified nurse, and she supported the implementation of a registration process for all qualified nurses to protect the public from incompetent, unqualified nurses.

Goodrich advocated compulsory legislation that would ensure that graduates or trained nurses would be the only ones who could work as nurses. She pleaded for the registration of qualified nurses, not only for the protection of the nurse but also for the protection of the community. Goodrich also fought against correspondence or home-study programs for nurses, which were a greater menace to the public's safety than people realized. Such legislation, she believed, would encourage talented young women who were intellectually prepared for scientific education to select nursing as a career. The role of the advocate, as understood by these three early nursing leaders, was to protect the public from unqualified nurses (Christy, 1969; Dock, 1900; Palmer, 1900).

From this beginning, the role of advocate grew. Public health nurses served as advocates in factories and communities during the Industrial Revolution. Many municipal boards of health hired visiting nurses to work as inspectors in the factories to protect the workers from health hazards and to help prevent accidents. Communities were finding that the nurse as advocate for the factory worker had inestimable value. Visiting nurses were also proving very effective in preventing the spread of communicable diseases. Hospital nurses also worked as advocates for the patients while giving care. Nurses were crucial in protecting patients from harm when they were too ill to protect themselves. Nurses were also responsible for providing measures to relieve pain, and they strove to make their patients happy and comfortable, even if it meant breaking the rules sometimes (Hill, 1900). During the 1970s and 1980s, the responsibility of the nurse as advocate was expanded to include speaking for their patients when they could not speak for themselves (Sovie, 1983). Nurses returned to work in churches in the primary role of advocate under the Granger Westberg model for parish nursing. The members of the congregation where a parish nurse practiced found affirmation and support as they reached to improve their physical, emotional, and spiritual health (Striepe, 1987).

Historically, consumers, administrators, and courts have not shared the perception of the nurse as advocate. The findings of a study done in 1983 indicated that consumers did not recognize the nurse as an initiator of health care (Miller et al., 1983). Consumers also believed that physicians would protect the rights of the patient. Miller and colleagues (1983) concluded that although nurses were serving as mediators between patients and institutions, changes rarely occurred within the institutions as a result of this role. Patient advocacy was directly related to the power and authority allowed the nurse by the particular system. Nurses generally became advocates whenever the issue involved patient care; however, they had little power to be truly effective as an advocate when the concerns involved the medical regimen or health care services (Miller et al., 1983). Examples of advocacy included questioning doctors' orders, promoting patient comfort, and supporting patient decisions regarding health care choices.

> Advocacy is a critical role for nurses today. Nurses are in a vital position to be effective in this role.

With the need for informed consent, advance directives, and treatment choices, patients more than ever need an advocate to interpret information, identify the risks and benefits of the various treatment options, and support the decision they make. However, nurses are extending their roles as advocates in providing patient care to initiatives that improve patient safety and recognize the nursing profession as a key player in providing all individuals access to quality health care.

For example, the ANA has endorsed the *Registered Nurse Safe Staffing Act of 2015*. If passed, this law would require Medicare-funded hospitals to develop and implement safe staffing plans for nurses. Nurses providing direct patient care along with nurse managers would comprise a nurse staffing committee that would evaluate staffing needs of the health care institution with an overall goal of ensuring nurse-to-patient acuity ratios are optimal to deliver safe patient care, reduce patient readmissions, and improve nursing staff retention (ANA, 2015). With the inception of the ACA, ensuring access to health care for the public remains an ongoing concern.

Considering this, the Coalition for Patients' Rights (CPR) consists of more than 35 organizations with dedicated members who are on the front line in ensuring that all health care professionals be able to practice fully to the extent of their education, scope, and practice in providing quality health care (CPR, 2016). With registered nurses comprising the largest group of health care professionals, CPR in collaboration with several professional nursing organizations recognize that nurses are and will continue to play an integral role in providing quality health care to the public. For a complete listing of current CPR coalition members, check out https://www.patientsrightscoalition.org/resources.html.

What Is the Role of Manager of Care?

Even Florence Nightingale recognized the need for nurses to be managers. She insisted that nurses needed to organize the care of the patient so that other nurses could carry on when they were not present. There were four major eras in the development of the nurse as manager. During the first period, lasting until about 1920, a nurse manager was known as the *charge nurse*. Charge nurses were responsible for teaching the nursing students what they needed to know and for directing the care that the students provided. The charge nurse was autocratic. This nurse had absolute authority over the student.

During the second era, lasting until 1949, the term *supervisor* was used to describe the role of nurse manager. The supervisor continued to be responsible for the students; however, the role had expanded to include enforcing agency policies, developing improvements in the care of the ill, and being responsible for the effective use of the ward's resources. Nurses were more involved in the patient care process. Hospital administrators were relying on nursing expertise to establish policies for patient care and hospital administration. This era ended with the publication of Esther Lucille Brown's report (1948) recommending that nursing education be separated from hospital administration.

During the third period, lasting until 1970, the nurse was referred to as a *coordinator*. The nurse coordinator no longer had responsibility for the nursing education of the students but was expected to motivate staff, be innovative, and solve problems. Coordinators were active in improving patient care and were expected to maintain harmony within the institution. Many nurse coordinators had few skills in and little knowledge of middle management. They basically learned by trial and error how to be effective.

The last period, from 1970 to the present, is a series of waves. Nurses gained recognition as managers and were able to function in that role. Hospital nurses gained middle-management positions and proved their abilities. The period before diagnostic-related groups (DRGs) saw escalating hospital costs and growth in the numbers of employees and services. From this growth came significant efforts to control the costs of health care. The term *manager* is used most often now in the nursing literature, but you may find it used to describe any of the four periods.

> No matter what era in history you study, the expectation is that the nurse-manager will coordinate patient care and supervise nurses in the delivery of quality care.

Can Nurses Be Colleagues?

The role of colleague is a vital one in any profession. The status of colleague within health care generates pictures of nurses, doctors, and pharmacists discussing, on an equal basis, problems and concerns related to health care. In nursing, we have made great progress in achieving the status of colleague. Interprofessional collegial relationships are strengthening, due in part to the increasing utilization of health care–related services taking place in community and homecare settings (Naylor, 2011). Interprofessional collaboration is essential to the changes taking place with health care delivery models.

Between 1960 and the present, the term *collaborator* has been adopted for this role. The definition of this word means "a person who works jointly on an activity or project; an associate." A secondary definition means "a person who cooperates traitorously with an enemy; a defector."

The primary definition may be the most fitting description of the role. Nurses are interested in developing collaborative relationships with doctors, pharmacists, and other health professionals. The literature is abundant with discussions of these relationships and consistently describes these relationships as collaborative (Hahm & Miller, 1961; Kelly, 1975; Quint, 1967; Seward, 1969; Tourtillott, 1986; Wisener, 1978).

Where Does This Leave the Role of Colleague?

Nursing education has promoted the term *collaborator* over *colleague*. Students in their educational experiences are seldom offered the opportunity to practice the role of colleague and therefore have only a vague understanding of the role. However, public health nurses throughout American history have not only understood the role but probably have attained a greater degree of collegiality than any other practice area of nursing. Public health nurses are not the majority within the profession. Nevertheless, they continue to enjoy and maintain the essence of the role (Anglin, 1991). As a colleague, one recognizes nurses with expertise and relies on those nurses for their expertise in the interest of improving patient care and advancing the profession. The essence of the role is mutual respect and equality among professionals, both intradisciplinary and interdisciplinary (Anglin, 1991). The Interdisciplinary Nursing Quality Research Initiative (INQRI) recognizes the valuable role nurses play in advancing and improving patient care and continues to validate the nurse as a deliverer of quality patient care through conducting extensive interdisciplinary research (INQRI, n.d.).

What About Experts?

There is one other role in which nurses are often found. This role is called *expert*. It is a conglomerate of advanced formal or informal education, certification, and acquired or recognized expertise. The role includes academicians, historians, nursing educators, clinicians, professional educators, researchers, research consumers, theorists, nurse technologists, and the leaders within the profession. The American Academy of Nursing recognizes some of these individuals and votes to bestow on them the honor of Fellow. There are many nurses who are experts in an area of practice, whether it be in clinics, at the bedside, in nursing homes, or in other settings. As nurses with special expertise, they are called on to provide testimony in courts and at government hearings or to share information and knowledge with other nurses, which is their obligation to the profession. This sharing can be done through mentoring, guest speaking, performing in-services, offering continuing-education programs, contributing to publications, and writing technical articles. These experts are usually the nurses who create the momentum that moves the profession forward. This is a role that should be recognized, encouraged, and rewarded.

CONCLUSION

The history of nursing provides a wealth of knowledge about where we have been and illustrates for us the lessons that have been learned. Few of us know the specifics of how nursing evolved into the discipline that it is today; however, the study and review of our rich history provides the context for where we will be tomorrow. At the end of this chapter is a listing of relevant websites and online resources on the history of nursing.

So, history naturally informs nursing knowledge, both imaginatively and practically. As historian Joan Lynaugh observed, nursing history is "our source of identity, our cultural DNA." Nurses love nursing history when it illuminates their imaginations and they can feel its meaning in their bones. Indeed, nursing history offers all nurses an exciting future in ideas (Meehan, 2013, p. 13).

What do nurses do? There is no simple answer. We agree that nurses care for patients—hence nurses are caregivers. We agree that nurses teach patients what they need to know to make informed choices—and therefore nurses are educators. We also agree that the role of manager exists in some form, and so we manage our practice and patients' care. We can even define the role of advocate. The role of colleague is gaining clarity with an increased focus on nurses' role in interprofessional collaboration. We are consistent in using the term *collaborator*; however, the term *colleague* is frequently referenced in nursing education and research, as compared with clinical practice, but progress is being made in recognizing the nurse as a colleague in all settings where nurses practice.

Finally, we have experts whom we may or may not recognize—and on whom the profession depends to provide the leadership for the whole. These roles merely provide a beginning for you to understand the profession you have chosen—nursing. May you become proficient in these roles and develop into an expert who will then provide the leadership for nursing in the future.

The future is not the result of choices among
Alternative paths offered;
It is a place that is created,
Created first in the mind and will,
Created next in activity.
The future is not some place we are going to,
But one we are creating.
The paths to it are not found, but made.
And the activity of making them
Changes both the maker and the destiny.
Anonymous, 1987

🌐 RELEVANT WEBSITES AND ONLINE RESOURCES

American Association for the History of Nursing
http://www.aahn.org/

Barbara Bates Center for the Study of the History of Nursing
www.nursing.upenn.edu/history/

Black Nurses in History
http://libguides.rowan.edu/blacknurses

Canadian Association for the History of Nursing
http://cahn-achn.ca/

Clendening History of Medicine Library — Florence Nightingale Resources
http://clendening.kumc.edu/dc/fn

Florence Nightingale Museum
http://www.florence-nightingale.co.uk/

Frontier Nursing Service
http://www.frontiernursing.org

History of Nursing Education: In Our Past Lies Our Future
http://www.nursingeducationhistory.org

Images from the History of Medicine
http://www.ihm.nlm.nih.gov/

Margaret M. Allemang Society for the History of Nursing (Canadian)
http://allemang.on.ca/

Museum of Nursing History
http://www.nursinghistory.org/

Nursing History and Health Care
www.nursing.upenn.edu/nhhc

Regis College American History: Influential Female Nurses
https://onlinenursing.regiscollege.edu/family-nurse-practitioner/american-history-influential-female-nurses/

BIBLIOGRAPHY

Accreditation Commission for Education in Nursing (ACEN). (2016). *Online directory of accredited programs.* Retrieved from http://www.acenursing.us/accreditedprograms/programSearch.htm.

Alfaro-LeFevre, R. (1998). *Applying nursing process: A step-by-step guide.* New York: Lippincott Williams & Wilkins.

American Association of Colleges of Nursing (AACN). (2017a). *2016-2017 Enrollment and graduations in baccalaureate and graduate programs in nursing.* Washington, DC: Author.

American Association of Colleges of Nursing (AACN). (2017b). *Fact sheet: The doctor of nursing practice (DNP).* Washington, DC: Author. Retrieved from http://www.aacnnursing.org/Portals/42/News/Factsheets/DNP-Factsheet-2017.pdf.

American Association of Colleges of Nursing (AACN). (2017c). *The changing landscape: Nursing student diversity on the rise.* Washington, DC: Author. Retrieved from http://www.aacnnursing.org/Portals/42/Policy/PDF/Student-Diversity-FS.pdf.

American Nurses Association. (2019). The history of the American Nurses Association. Retrieved from https://www.nursingworld.org/ana/about-ana/history/.

American Nurses Association. (2015). *Safe staffing.* Retrieved from http://www.rnaction.org/site/PageNavigator/nstat_take_action_safe_staffing.html.

Anglin, L. T. (1991). *The roles of nurses: A history, 1900 to 1988.* Ann Arbor, MI: University of Michigan.

Benner, P. (1984). *From novice to expert: Excellence and power in clinical nursing practice.* Menlo Park, CA: Addison-Wesley.

Bradford, W. (1898). *History of Plymouth plantation: Book II (1620).* Plymouth: MA: Wright & Potter.

Brown, E. L. (1948). *Nursing for the future.* New York: Russell Sage Foundation.

Bullough, V., & Bullough, B. (1978). *The care of the sick: The emergence of modern nursing.* New York: Prodist.

Bullough, V., Bullough, B., & Stanton, M. P. (1990). *Florence Nightingale and her era: A collection of new scholarship.* New York: Garland.

CDC. (2014). *Cases of Ebola diagnosed in the United States.* Retrieved from http://www.cdc.gov/vhf/ebola/outbreaks/2014-west-africa/united-states-imported-case.html.

Christy, T. E. (1969). Portrait of a leader: Isabel Hampton Robb. *Nursing Outlook, 17*(3), 26–29.

Christy, T. E. (1971). First fifty years. *American Journal of Nursing, 71*(9), 1778–1784.

CPR. (2016). *Coalition for Patients' Rights.* Retrieved from http://www.patientsrightscoalition.org/.

Dalton, R. (1900). Hospitals: Their origins and history. *Dublin Journal of Medical Science, 109*(3), 17–19.

Dana, C. L. (1936). *The peaks of medical history.* New York: Paul B. Hoeber.

Davis, M. D. (1961). I was a student over 50 years ago. *Nursing Outlook, 61,* 62.

Dock, L. (1900). What may we expect from the law? *American Journal of Nursing, 1*(9).

Dodge, B. S. (1989). *The story of nursing* (2nd ed.). Boston: Little, Brown and Company.

Dolan, J. A. (1969). *History of nursing.* Philadelphia: Saunders.

Donahue, M. P. (1985). *Nursing: The finest art.* St. Louis: Mosby.

Dossey, B. (2000). *Florence Nightingale: Mystic, visionary, healer.* Springhouse, PA: Springhouse.

Goldmark, J. (1923). *Nursing and nursing education in the United States: Report of the Committee for the Study of Nursing Education.* New York: Macmillan.

Goodnow, M. (1936). *Outlines in the history of nursing.* Philadelphia: Saunders.

Grypma, S. (2010). Revis(it)ing nursing history. *Journal of Christian Nursing, 27*(2), 67.

Hahm, H., & Miller, D. (1961). Relationships between medical and nursing education. *Journal of Nursing Education, 39,* 849–851.

Hanks, R. G. (2008). The lived experience of nursing advocacy. *Nursing Ethics, 15*(4), 468–477. https://doi.org/10.1177/0969733008090518.

Hill, J. (1900). Private duty nursing from a nurse's point of view. *American Journal of Nursing, 1*(2), 129.

INQRI. (n.d.). *Program overview. The Interdisciplinary Nursing Quality Research Initiative.* Retrieved from http://www.inqri.org/about-inqri/program-overview.

Jamieson, E. M., & Sewall, M. F. (1949). *Trends in nursing history.* Saunders: Saunders.

Kalisch, P. A., & Kalisch, B. J. (1986). *The advance of American nursing.* Boston: Little, Brown and Company.

Kelly, L. Y. (1975). *Dimensions of professional nursing* (3rd ed.). New York: Macmillan.

Leininger, M. (1984). *Care: The essence of nursing and health.* Thorofare, NJ: Charles B. Slack.

Maness, P. F. (2006). Introducing the new voice of nurses. *American Nurse Today, 1*(1). Retrieved from https://americannursetoday.com/introducing-the-new-voice-of-nurses/.

Meehan, T. C. (2013). History and nursing knowledge. *Nursing History Review, 21,* 10–13.

McCloskey, J., & Grace, H. K. (2001). *Current issues in nursing* (6th ed.). St. Louis, MO: Mosby.

Miller, B. K., Mansen, T. J., & Lee, H. (1983). Patient advocacy: Do nurses have the power and authority to act as patient advocate? *Nursing Leadership, 6*(2), 56–60.

Montag, M. L. (1951). *The education of nursing technicians.* New York: GP Putnam's Sons.

National League for Nursing (NLN). (2019). *NLN biennial survey of schools of nursing academic year 2017–2018: Executive summary.* Retrieved from http://www.nln.org/newsroom/nursing-education-statistics/biennial-survey-of-schools-of-nursing-academic-year-2017-2018.

National League for Nursing (NLN). (2014a). *Number of basic RN programs, Total and by program type: 2005 to 2014.* Retrieved from http://www.nln.org/docs/default-source/newsroom/nursing-education-statistics/number-of-basic-rn-programs-total-and-by-program-type-2005-to-2014.pdf?sfvrsn=0.

National League for Nursing (NLN). (2014b). *Percentage of basic RN programs by program type: 1994 to 1995 and 2003 to 2012 and 2014.* Retrieved from http://www.nln.org/docs/default-source/newsroom/nursing-education-statistics/distribution-of-nursing-programs-by-region-and-program-type-2014-%28pdf%29.pdf?sfvrsn=0.

Naylor, M. D. (2011). *Viewpoint: Interprofessional collaboration and the future of healthcare.* Retrieved from http://www.americannursetoday.com/viewpoint-interprofessional-collaboration-and-the-future-of-health-care/.

Orsolini-Hain, L., & Waters, V. (2009). Education evolution: A historical perspective of associate degree nursing. *Journal of Nursing Education, 48*(5), 266–271.

Palmer, S. (1900). The editor. *American Journal of Nursing, 1*(4), 166–169.

Quint, G. C. (1967). Role models and the professional nurse identity. *Journal of Nursing Education, 6*(1).

Rode, M. W. (1989). The nursing pin: Symbol of 1000 years of service. *Nursing Forum, 24*(1), 15–17.

Rybczynski, W. (1986). *Home: A short history of an idea.* Middlesex, England: Penguin.

Seward, J. M. (1969). Role of the nurse: Perceptions of nursing students and auxiliary nursing personnel. *Nursing Research, 18*(2), 164–169.

Sovie, L. (1983). Nursing. In N. Chaska (Ed.), *The nursing profession.* New York: GP Putnam's Sons.

Stewart, I. M. (1950). A half-century of nursing education. *American Journal of Nursing,* 617.

Striepe, J. (1987). *Nurses in churches: A manual for developing parish nurse services and networks.* Spencer: Iowa Lake Area Agency on Aging.

Tourtillott, E. A. (1986). *Commitment—a lost characteristic.* New York: JB Lippincott.

Watson, J. (1985). *Nursing: Human science and human care—a theory of nursing.* East Norwalk, CT: Appleton-Century-Crofts.

Wisener, S. (1978). *The reality of primary nursing care: Risks, roles and research. Role changes in primary nursing.* New York: National League of Nursing.

7

Nursing Education

Ashley Zerwekh Garneau, PhD, RN*

(e)http://evolve.elsevier.com/Zerwekh/nsgtoday/.

Unless we are making progress in our nursing every year, every month, every week, take my word for it we are going back.
Florence Nightingale

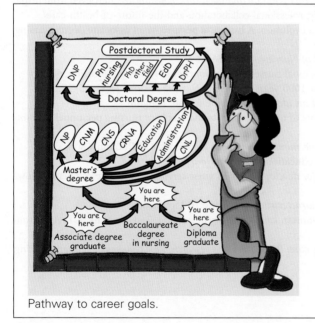

Pathway to career goals.

After completing this chapter, you should be able to:

- Compare the various types of educational preparation for nursing.
- Describe the educational preparation for a graduate degree.
- Compare nontraditional pathways of nursing education.
- Describe the purpose of nursing program accreditation and regional accreditation.
- Set personal educational goals for yourself.

What an exciting time to be a nurse. Never before have the doors been so open for nurses to further their education. The Institute of Medicine (IOM) report, *The Future of Nursing: Leading Change, Advancing Health* (2010), set forth recommendations that would change the future of nursing and nursing education in ways never dreamed possible. Recommendation 4 discussed increasing the number of nurses with baccalaureate degrees

*We would like to thank **Gayle P. Varnell, PhD, MSN, RN, CPNP-PC** for her previous contributions on this chapter.

to 80% by the year 2020, whereas Recommendation 5 proposed doubling the number of nurses with doctorate degrees by 2020. Recommendation 6 explained the need for nurses to engage in lifelong learning. Based on these three recommendations alone, educational systems across the country began diligently brainstorming and working collaboratively to address these goals.

A Joint Statement on Academic Progression for Nursing Students and Graduates was made by the Tri-Council for Nursing and endorsed by both community college–registered and university-registered nursing programs with the understanding that both student nurses and practicing nurses need to be encouraged and supported to achieve higher levels of education (Tri-Council for Nursing, 2010). Additionally, national nursing accrediting organizations including the Accreditation Commission for Education in Nursing (ACEN), the Commission on Collegiate Nursing Education (CCNE), and the National League for Nursing Commission on Nursing Education Accreditation (NLN CNEA) further support nurses advancing their education by encouraging community colleges and universities to offer seamless educational pathway nursing programs to further meet the demands of the nursing workforce and patient needs of the future (Accreditation Agencies Joint Statement on Academic Progression, 2015, para 1). What does all this mean to you as a nurse? It means that educational programs and employers throughout the country are striving to find ways to make it easier for nurses to further their education. More community colleges and universities are expanding their nursing programs to increase diversity in the nursing workforce and meet the needs for health care reform. Add to this the advancing computer technology that makes it easier to provide comparable education via distance learning and simulation, and you have an environment that beckons nurses to further their education. Whatever your basic nursing education program, you will now find it easier to advance in your profession. Instead of seeing roadblocks, you will see more doors and windows opened to allow you to advance your education. Are you ready for the challenge?

After completing your initial educational preparation for nursing, you are probably looking forward to that first paycheck as a registered nurse (RN). The last thing on your mind is returning to school for more education! The purpose of this chapter is not to discuss the issue of entry into practice or to debate which educational program is best. Instead, the goal of this chapter is to help you look at where you are educationally and to offer guidance regarding educational opportunities to enhance your career goals and to continue on the path of lifelong learning. Before looking down the path at the variety of educational offerings available to help you meet those goals, let us look at the various pathways that lead to the initial educational preparation for an RN.

Which path did you travel? There are three primary paths (diploma, associate's degree, and bachelor's degree) that lead to one licensing examination: the National Council Licensure Examination for Registered Nurses (NCLEX-RN® Examination). These programs usually require a high school diploma or the equivalent for admission. Some of the other paths include master's and doctoral nursing degree programs, both of which accept college graduates with liberal arts majors. Other paths include career ladder programs (from practical nurse to associate degree or baccalaureate degree nurse), accelerated baccalaureate programs for non-nursing college graduates, entry-level master's and doctorate programs, and community college–based bachelor of science in nursing (BSN) programs. Another source for nursing education is the online option. Online programs are particularly popular for people who are place-bound and unable to travel to distant sites to obtain or continue their education. Some of these programs require brief visits to a campus, whereas others are exclusively online.

The distribution of the RN population according to basic nursing education is illustrated in Fig. 7.1. The *2017 National Workforce Survey of Registered Nurses* indicates that initial preparation in a diploma program accounted for 12%, the associate's degree accounted for 36.3%, and the baccalaureate degree program accounted for 41.7% of the RNs. Furthermore, 3.8% of RNs received their initial nursing education at either a master's or doctoral level (Smiley et al., 2018, p. 15).

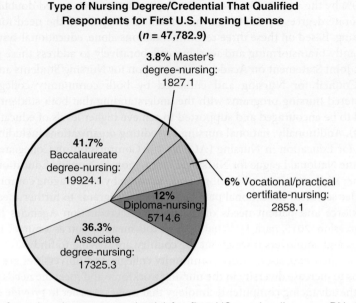

Type of Nursing Degree/Credential That Qualified Respondents for First U.S. Nursing License

(*n* = 47,782.9)

3.8% Master's degree-nursing: 1827.1

41.7% Baccalaureate degree-nursing: 19924.1

6% Vocational/practical certifiate-nursing: 2858.1

12% Diploma-nursing: 5714.6

36.3% Associate degree-nursing: 17325.3

FIG. 7.1 Type of nursing degree or credential for first US nursing license—RN. (Smiley, R. A., Lauer, P., Bienemy, C., Berg, J. G., Shireman, E., Reneau, K. A., et al. (2018). The National Council of State Boards of Nursing (NCSBN) 2017 national nursing workforce survey [supplement]. *Journal of Nursing Regulation, 9*(3), 4–88.)

PATH OF DIPLOMA EDUCATION

What Is the Educational Preparation of the Diploma Graduate?

The current preparation of a diploma nurse varies in length from 2 to 3 years. This type of program may be under the direction of a hospital or incorporated independently. The diploma program may include general education subjects, such as biology and physical and social sciences, in addition to nursing theory and practice. Because there is a close relationship between a nursing school and a hospital, many diploma graduates are employed by that same hospital and therefore may experience an easier role transition. Graduates of diploma programs are awarded a certificate or diploma and are eligible to take the NCLEX-RN examination for licensure.

PATH OF ASSOCIATE DEGREE EDUCATION

What Is the Educational Preparation of the Associate Degree Graduate?

The current preparation of an associate degree nurse usually begins in a community college, although some programs are based in senior colleges or universities. The associate degree program lasts 18 to 21 school calendar months. In some programs, the student must complete the general education and science course requirements before beginning the nursing courses. At the end of the program, the student receives an associate's degree in nursing (ADN), associate of applied science in nursing (AAS), or an associate of science in nursing (ASN).

The student population of associate degree programs is increasing in diversity. Many of these individuals have baccalaureate and higher degrees in other fields of study and are seeking a second career.

Students 25 years of age and older comprised over 50% of the student population among associate degree nursing programs nationwide (NLN, 2016). Along with their maturity, these students bring life experiences that are applicable to nursing. The community college curriculum is conducive to students who want to attend school on a part-time basis. Graduates of associate degree programs are eligible to take the NCLEX-RN examination for licensure.

The associate degree program has provided students with the motivation to further their education and the opportunity for career mobility. Although many nursing students end their education with an associate's degree, many others enter the associate degree program with every intention of continuing their nursing education to the baccalaureate level or even further.

PATH OF BACCALAUREATE EDUCATION

In this discussion, only the "generic" baccalaureate programs are addressed. A generic student is one who enters a baccalaureate nursing program with no training or education in nursing. A traditional generic baccalaurcate program includes lower-division (freshman and sophomore) liberal arts and science courses with upper-division (junior and senior) nursing courses. RNs entering baccalaureate programs are discussed later in this chapter.

What Is the Educational Preparation of the Baccalaureate Graduate?

The current preparation of a baccalaureate nurse is 4 to 5 years in length (120 to 140 credits) and emphasizes courses in the liberal arts, sciences, and humanities. To qualify for a baccalaureate program, the student must first meet all of the college or university entrance requirements.

During the first 2 years of a traditional baccalaureate nursing program, the student is usually enrolled in liberal arts and science courses with other non-nursing students. It is usually not until late in a student's sophomore or early junior year that nursing courses are introduced. However, some baccalaureate programs incorporate nursing courses throughout the 4-year nursing curriculum. The emphasis in the baccalaureate nursing program focuses on preparing students to work in a variety of practice settings (i.e., community and public health).

The graduate of a baccalaureate program must fulfill both the degree requirements of the nursing program and those of the college. On completion of the program, the degree awarded is a BSN. Graduates of baccalaureate nursing programs are eligible to take the NCLEX-RN® examination for licensure.

OTHER TYPES OF NURSING EDUCATION

What Are the Other Available Educational Options?

Following the IOM report, nursing organizations, regulatory bodies, nursing accreditation agencies, and nursing education programs have developed innovative pathways for advancing nursing education. Besides the traditional pathways for entering the nursing profession, such as diploma, associate degree, and baccalaureate programs, new pathways are growing. Entry-level master's programs, accelerated programs for non-nursing graduates, community college–based baccalaureate programs, and RN degree completion programs for licensed practical nurses and other health care providers are a few of the many options, and it is anticipated that there may be others in the near future.

Just as there are new pathways to enter the nursing profession, there are also new pathways for those nurses who are interested in advancing their nursing education including baccalaureate to doctoral programs, master's degrees for advanced generalist roles such as the clinical nurse leader (CNL), and the doctor of nursing practice (DNP).

It truly is an exciting time to be in nursing, and there is no one right career pathway for everyone. Each person needs to consider what his or her professional end goal is and what works best for him or her (Critical Thinking Box 7.1). It is important to ask yourself what you are willing to invest in your education besides the time and monetary expenses.

? CRITICAL THINKING BOX 7.1

Is an online program that provides more flexibility in scheduling for family and work obligations the best choice or perhaps a blended or hybrid program?

Is the program respected in the nursing community and known for producing great nurse educators, researchers, or advanced practice nurses?

Is it an accredited program?

Will course work/credits transfer?

In assessing the available educational options, one source of information is the American Association of Colleges of Nursing (AACN) website (https://www.aacnnursing.org/Students). There is a section for students that includes information on nursing careers, financial aid, scholarships, and nursing programs. Potential students should also contact individual schools for information regarding their particular programs. After you are ready to begin the application process, you will also find that the Nursing Centralized Application Service (Nursing CAS) has simplified the process by providing a service that enables students to apply to participating nursing programs offered at all levels nationwide (https://www.aacnnursing.org/Students/Apply-to-Nursing-School). The end of this chapter provides a complete list of additional relevant websites and online resources for advancing your nursing education—be sure to check it out!

The career ladder or bridge concept focuses on the articulation of educational programs to permit advanced placement without loss of credit or repetition. There are many variations on this type of program. Multiple-exit programs provide opportunities for students to exit and reenter the educational system at various designated times, having gained specific education and skills. An example is a program that ranges from practical nurse to RN at the associate's, baccalaureate, master's, and doctoral levels. A student in such a program may decide to leave the educational system at the completion of a specific level and be eligible to take the licensure examination applicable to that educational level. On termination, the student may choose to work for a while and later return for more education at the next level without having to repeat courses on previously acquired knowledge or skills. Information on the three types of articulation agreements—individual, mandated, and statewide—can be found on the AACN website.

What Is a Concurrent Enrollment BSN Completion Program?

Growing numbers of nursing education programs within the community college setting are now offering students innovative pathways for advancing their education (Fig. 7.2). These dynamic programs are known by several names, including concurrent enrollment, dual-enrollment, and A-to-B (associate-to-baccalaureate) programs. Whatever the terminology, these programs are successfully empowering students to attain BSN degrees at a much faster pace. In the white paper, *"Meeting current and future nursing needs through progression and innovation—the concurrent enrollment program at MaricopaNursing"* (Schultz, 2016), Dr. Margi Schultz adds the following:

Concurrent or dual-enrollment programs layer nursing coursework, blending both the associate and RN to BSN curricula. Students meet all criteria for the community college associate program and then have the opportunity, based on a number of factors, to explore and select a university partner

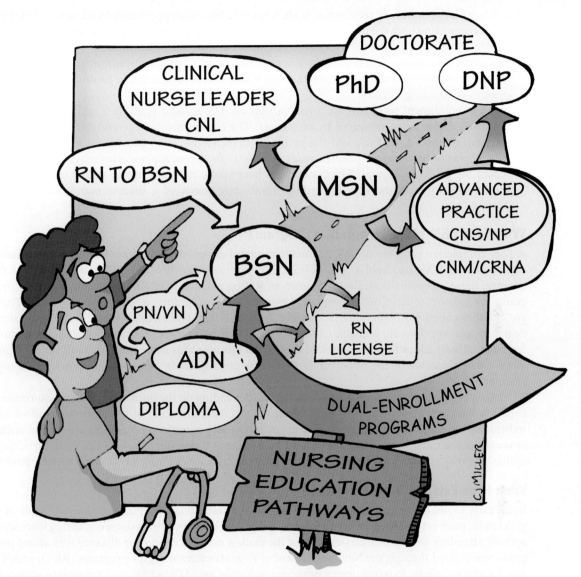

FIG. 7.2 What are other available education programs?

school. The student will complete all prerequisites for both the community college and the university and will make application to both colleges.

The concurrent or dual pathway program will often begin with the student taking a university course the semester before beginning the community college nursing program. This is generally an introductory course that reviews nursing theory, the history of nursing, or an introduction to professional nursing practice. Following the initial course, the student will enter the nursing program at the community college, and the RN to BSN courses, which are most often offered online or in a hybrid format, will either be layered with the associate degree courses during traditional semesters or spaced during breaks, summers, and/or intercessions.

Depending on the university requirements, students may have the opportunity to accelerate their program, completing both the associate and the baccalaureate degrees at approximately the same time. Students may elect to take the baccalaureate courses at a slower pace, finishing the BSN in one or two terms following completion of the associate degree. In most concurrent programs the student will complete the associate degree and take the National Council Licensing Examination (NCLEX) prior to completing the BSN.

Concurrent enrollment programs are a win/win for all. The student saves time and money, earning a nursing degree often preferred by employers. The community college and the university have engaged, motivated students and the ability to share resources to provide an affordable career ladder, placing competent, practice-ready graduates in the workplace who may then return to school for graduate degrees. The community benefits by having a highly skilled nursing workforce ready to meet the ever-expanding health care needs of a diverse population (Schultz, 2016, p. 1).

What Is a BSN/MSN Completion Program?

A BSN-completion program is a baccalaureate program designed for students who already possess a diploma or an ADN and hold a current license to practice as an RN. Depending on the part of the country, these programs may also be known as RN baccalaureate (RNB) programs, RN/BSN programs, baccalaureate RN (BRN) programs, two-plus-two programs, or capstone programs. There are 747 BSN-completion programs. In addition to the BSN-completion programs, 230 RN-to-master's degree program options are available (AACN, 2017c). In most of these programs, nurses receive transfer credit in basic education courses taken at other institutions plus some transfer credit for their previous nursing courses or the opportunity to receive nursing credit by passing a nursing challenge examination.

The usual length of such programs is 1 to 2 years, depending on the number of course requirements completed at the time of admission to the program. To meet the needs of the returning student and individuals residing in outlying geographic areas, many BSN-completion programs are offered online or on-site at the nurses employing institution. More than 600 programs have part of their curriculum online, whereas an increasing number of programs are available completely online (AACN, 2017c).

What Is an External Degree Program?

In the early 1970s, the external degree program was a nontraditional program that allowed a student to gain credit, meet external degree requirements, and obtain a degree from a degree-granting institution without attending face-to-face classes. One of the earliest external degree (or distance education) programs was offered through the New York Board of Regents external degree programs (REX), which is now Excelsior College. External degree programs may offer an ADN, a BSN, and a master of science in nursing (MSN). These programs are designed to allow individuals to obtain degrees in nursing without leaving their jobs or their communities.

Nursing education online is a rapidly expanding part of the Internet. In the past, these programs were called external degree or distance education; however, these programs are now more commonly considered online nursing education. Online nursing programs are accredited by the ACEN (formerly the National League for Nursing Accrediting Commission [NLNAC]), the NLN CNEA, or the CCNE, which is an autonomous accrediting agency associated with the AACN. In undergraduate nursing programs, all students are required to pass specific college-level tests and performance examinations in two components: general education and nursing. On completion of the undergraduate external degree programs, students are eligible in most states to take the RN licensure exam.

Online (Web-Based) Programs

More and more traditional colleges and universities are offering courses and even entire programs through the Internet. In fact, it is possible to earn ADN, BSN, master's, and doctoral degrees in web-based or web-enhanced formats. At times, it can be confusing and overwhelming to find the right programs. Several sites are available to help users locate specific web-based or web-enhanced courses (and course descriptions). See the Internet resources listed on this book's Evolve website. When considering which program is the best fit for your career goals, it is important to consider the cost of an online program but also if the program is in an enhanced nurse licensure compact (eNLC) state. See Chapter 20 for more information on the eNLC.

Proprietary Nursing Schools

In addition to the colleges and universities that are offering these types of courses, an influx of new proprietary nursing programs has occurred. A proprietary nursing school is a for-profit school with a nursing program. Many proprietary schools have nursing programs in more than one state. Because not all nursing boards have the same requirements for licensure, it is important to review the requirements in your state to make sure that you will be eligible for licensure once you complete the program. A prospective student should also make sure that the program is accredited and review the pass rates on the NCLEX examination for their graduates.

What Is an Accelerated Program?

Accelerated programs are offered at both the baccalaureate and master's degree levels; they are designed to build on previous learning to help a person with an undergraduate degree in another discipline make the transition into nursing. In 2016, there were 272 accelerated baccalaureate programs and 69 accelerated master's programs available at nursing schools nationwide. In addition, 24 new accelerated baccalaureate programs are in the planning stages, and 9 new accelerated master's programs are also taking shape (AACN, 2017a).

NONTRADITIONAL PATHS FOR NURSING EDUCATION

What About a Master's Degree as a Path to Becoming a RN?

MSN programs are particularly attractive to the growing number of college graduates who decide to enter nursing later in life. Generally, the program is 24 to 36 months long. Upon graduation, these students are expected to demonstrate the same entry-level competencies in nursing as baccalaureate graduates. MSN graduates from these programs are then eligible to take the NCLEX-RN examination. Currently, there are 69 entry-level master's programs in the United States (AACN, 2017a).

What About a Doctoral Path to Becoming a RN?

The last and least-common path leading to the RN licensure examination is the doctoral degree in nursing, where the graduate has a non-nursing baccalaureate degree. A doctoral nursing program provides basic nursing courses, along with advanced nursing courses. Upon completion, the graduate is eligible to take the NCLEX-RN examination. Currently, the University of Colorado and Case Western University are the only universities to offer a doctoral nursing program as an entry-level degree or prelicensure option (AACN, 2004).

GRADUATE EDUCATION

What About Graduate School?

Whatever path you chose to become an RN, one thing was certain: It was not easy! After putting life, liberty, and the pursuit of happiness on hold while you worked toward becoming an RN, it may seem like pure insanity to subject yourself to more education!

Graduate nursing education, like other graduate programs, is responding to changes in social values, priorities in the public sector, and student demographics, in addition to technological advances, knowledge development, and maturity of the profession. According to the 2017 *National Nursing Workforce Survey of Registered Nurses,* the percentage of nurses who indicate a BSN as their initial education to become an RN continues to grow, with 41.7% reporting this initial education path (Smiley et al., 2018, p. 15).

Graduate education programs are available on a part-time or a full-time basis. Graduate programs require a good grade point average (GPA) at the undergraduate level. Prerequisites for most graduate programs are satisfactory scores on the Graduate Record Examination (GRE) or the Miller Analogies Test (MAT). Although an increasing number of graduate programs are waiving the entrance examination requirements, it is strongly recommended that all students, whether they plan to pursue graduate studies or not, take the GRE after completing their undergraduate studies. Taking another test may be the last thing you want to do, but it is much easier to do it when the information is current in your mind, than later when you decide that you want to continue your education.

Why Would I Want a Master's Degree?

> You've got to be kidding! More school?

Sure, an advanced degree may not be in your career plans right now, but later, after you have been practicing nursing, you may change your mind. Policy statements from the nursing profession reflect the need for more education in preparation for the changing role of nursing, a result of health care reform. As care delivery moves increasingly from the acute care center to the community setting, there will be an increased need for advanced clinical practice nurses. Nursing programs are already responding to this changing need.

Master's nursing programs vary from institution to institution, as do the admission and course requirements and costs. The master of science (MS) and the MSN are the most common degrees. The usual requirements for admission include a baccalaureate degree from a program that is accredited in nursing by the ACEN, CCNE, or CNEA (the accrediting body of the NLN since 2013), licensure as an RN, completion of the GRE or MAT, and a minimum undergraduate GPA of 3.0.

The majority of programs are at least 18 to 24 months of full-time study. Unlike undergraduate students, master's students usually choose an area of role preparation, such as education or administration, and an area of clinical specialization, such as pediatrics or adult health. Some of the more common areas of role preparation include education, administration, case management, health policy/health care systems, informatics, and the increasingly popular advanced clinical practice roles. See Table 7.1 for typical educational preparation and responsibilities of various advanced nursing roles.

An evolving area of role preparation is that of the CNL. The CNL role is different from the role of manager or administrator. The CNL is prepared at the master's level as a generalist managing the health care delivery system across all settings. Any person interested in the CNL role is encouraged

TABLE 7.1 ADVANCED SPECIALTY NURSING ROLES

	EDUCATION	WHAT THEY DO
Certified nurse educator (CNE)	CNEs are registered nurses (RNs) who hold a master's or doctoral degree in nursing with an emphasis in nursing education.	The majority of CNEs are nurse educators who facilitate student learning by providing innovative teaching methods in a variety of academic and practice settings, which may include community colleges, universities, hospitals, and technical programs (NLN, 2018).
Certified academic clinical nurse educator (CNEcl)	The academic CNEcl is an RN who holds a BSN degree or higher and is employed by an educational institution to provide clinical instruction to nursing students (NLN, 2018).	The academic CNEcl supports the learning of nursing students throughout their clinical experiences in nursing school by serving as a clinical instructor or preceptor during the student's clinical rotation (NLN, 2018).
Advanced Practice Nursing Roles		
Nurse practitioner (NP)	Most of the approximately 330 NP education programs in the United States today confer a master's degree. The majority of states require NPs to be nationally certified by ANCC, AANP, or a specialty nursing organization. In 2018, more than 248,000 advanced practice nurses were NPs (AANP, 2018).	Working in clinics, nursing homes, hospitals, health maintenance organizations (HMOs), private industry or their own offices, NPs are qualified to handle a wide range of basic health problems. Most have a specialty—for example, an adult, family, or pediatric health care degree. At minimum, NPs conduct physical examinations, take medical histories, diagnose and treat common acute minor illnesses or injuries, order and interpret laboratory tests and radiographs, and counsel and educate patients. In all states they may prescribe medication according to state law. Some work as independent practitioners and can be reimbursed by Medicare or Medicaid for services rendered.
Certified nurse-midwife (CNM)	An average 1.5–2 years of specialized education beyond nursing school, either in an accredited certificate program or at the master's level. In 2017, there were an estimated 11,826 nurses prepared as CNMs in the United States (ACNM, 2018).	CNMs are well known for delivering babies in hospitals and homes, and providing well-woman gynecological and low-risk obstetrical care, including prenatal, labor and delivery, and postpartum care. The CNM manages women's health care throughout the lifespan, including primary care, gynecological exams, and family planning. CNMs have prescriptive authority in all 50 states.
Clinical nurse specialist (CNS)	CNSs are RNs with advanced nursing degrees—master's or doctoral—who are experts in a specialized area of clinical practice such as psychiatric/mental health, adult/gerontology, pediatric, women's health, and neonatal health. The majority of CNSs specialize in adult health or gerontology (NACNS, 2016).	Most CNSs work in the hospital setting, full time, and have responsibility for more than one department. CNSs can also work in clinics, nursing homes, their own offices, and other community-based settings, such as industry, home care, and HMOs. They conduct health assessments, make diagnoses, deliver treatment, lead evidence-based practice projects, and develop quality-control methods. In addition to delivering direct patient care, CNSs work in consultation, research, education, and administration. Some work independently or in private practice and receive reimbursement. Based on state laws where the CNS practices, CNSs are authorized to prescribe medications (NACNS, 2016).
Certified registered nurse anesthetist (CRNA)	CRNAs are RNs who complete a graduate program and meet national certification and recertification requirements. There are an estimated 42,260 CRNAs in the United States (Bureau of Labor Statistics, 2017).	In this oldest of the advanced nursing specialties, CRNAs safely administer approximately 43 million anesthetics to patients each year in the United States. In some states, CRNAs are the sole anesthesia providers in rural hospitals (AANA, 2016). This enables health care facilities to provide obstetrical, surgical, and trauma stabilization services. CRNAs provide anesthetics to patients in collaboration with surgeons, anesthesiologists, dentists, podiatrists, and other qualified health care professionals.

to read the *Competencies and Curricular Expectations for Clinical Nurse Leader Education and Practice* (AACN, 2013), which can be found on the AACN website. Upon completion of a formal CNL program, a graduate is eligible to take the CNL certification examination. At the time of this writing, 6856 nurses have attained CNL certification (Commission on Nurse Certification, 2018).

Areas of specialty within the master's nurse practitioner programs include family, emergency care, pediatric, psychiatric, and adult-gerontology nursing practice. Currently, the American Association of Nurse Practitioners (AANP) reports over 248,000 licensed nurse practitioners (NPs) in the United States (AANP, 2018). An excellent resource for nurses who are considering becoming an advanced practice registered nurse (APRN) can be found at the AANP website https://www.aanp.org/education/student-resource-center/planning-your-np-education.

The National Council of State Boards of Nursing APRN Advisory Committee and leading professional nursing organizations developed the *Consensus Model for APRN Regulation: Licensure, Accreditation, Certification, and Education* allowing APRNs to practice to the full extent of their education (NCSBN, 2010). In the APRN Consensus Model, APRNs are educated in one of four roles: certified registered nurse anesthetist (CRNA), certified nurse-midwife (CNM), clinical nurse specialist (CNS), or certified nurse practitioner (CNP) (NCSBN, 2010). All four of these roles are given the title of APRN. It is important for all potential APRNs to read this document, because it changes how APRNs are educated and obtain certification (https://www.nursingworld.org/certification/aprn-consensus-model/faq-consensus-model-for-aprn-regulation/). See Table 7.1 for typical educational preparation and responsibilities of various advanced nursing roles.

In the more traditional master's degree programs, the student takes the courses required for the degree and then, depending on institutional requirements, may also be required to take a comprehensive written or oral examination, or write a thesis, or both. There are also nontraditional models that include outreach programs, summers-only programs, and programs for RNs who have bachelor's degrees in other fields.

Advances in technology have also made it possible for graduate programs to become more creative in the way courses are offered. It is now possible for students to obtain all or part of their course offerings by means of the Internet, distance learning, computer-based programs, and teleconferencing. This flexibility makes it easier for students in rural communities and part-time students to obtain advanced degrees.

How Do I Know Which Master's Degree Program Is Right for Me?

Your career goals and interests will help you determine which choice is best for you. Do some reading on your area of special interest and find out how advanced education will help you attain your career goals. As an example, in most nursing programs, a nurse with a non-nursing master's degree would need to complete a master's in nursing to become an advanced practice nurse. If you think that you might want to become a nurse practitioner at some point in your life, be sure that you obtain your master's in nursing. You can always go back and obtain a post-master's certificate as a nurse practitioner. If your master's degree is in another field, this may not be possible, because most programs require a master's in nursing. Although the movement to change the entry level for an APRN to a DNP by the year 2015 did not materialize, it is important to note that this may be a reality in the future, and you might want to consider this as you set your educational goals.

After you have decided on a master's degree, there are several resources available online, such as *Peterson's Guide* (www.petersons.com), to help you find the right school. Consider all the options and do your homework. If you are considering an advanced practice degree, be sure to check with the Board of Nursing for the state in which you reside to see what the requirements are to be recognized as an APRN in your state. Believe it or not, the requirements are *not* the same for every state. After all, if you are going to expend the time, energy, and finances to obtain a graduate degree, you want to get the most from it.

Why Would I Want a Doctoral Degree?

Power, authority, and professional status are usually associated with a doctoral degree. Nurses with doctoral degrees provide leadership in the improvement of nursing practice and in the development of research and nursing education programs. It is no secret that the role of the nurse is changing and will continue to change as health care reform continues to be implemented. There is a growing need for administrators, policy analysts, clinical researchers, and clinical practitioners in the community and in governmental agencies. Nurses need to position themselves to take on these new leadership roles, and the way to do this is through advanced education, particularly at the doctoral level.

Until recently, there were two basic models of doctoral education in nursing: the academic degree, or doctor of philosophy (PhD); and the professional degree, or doctor of nursing science (DNS, DSN, or DNSc). For either of these degrees, you must first have a master's in nursing. Nurses have other doctoral degree options available to them, such as the doctor of education (EdD), the doctor of public health (DrPH), the PhD in a discipline other than nursing, the nontraditional external degree doctorate, and the practice-focused nurse doctorate (ND), which was initiated as an entry-level degree.

In October 2004, the AACN published a position statement on the doctor of nursing practice (DNP) degree. Since that time, the terms *research-focused* and *practice-focused doctorate* have been used to describe the different doctoral degrees offered in nursing. The DNP would become the educational preparation for all advanced practice nurses seeking a practice-focused degree. This move toward a DNP as the practice-focused degree in nursing is to take place throughout a 15-year period. There are currently 303 DNP programs with more than 124 additional nursing schools that are considering starting a DNP program (AACN, 2017b).

How Do I Know Which Doctoral Program Is Right for Me?

As with the master's degree, it is important to look at your career goals before deciding which doctoral program is best for you. To help you with that task, look at the NLN and AACN publications specific to doctoral education. Ask yourself how much time you can devote to obtaining a doctorate degree. Can you be a full-time student, or must you continue to work? What do you plan to do with the degree after you obtain it?

Is there an institution available to you that offers a doctorate in nursing, or would you have to consider moving? What are your career and professional goals? Do you want to teach? The PhD is considered the research-focused degree. It prepares an individual for a lifetime of intellectual inquiry and has an increased emphasis on postdoctoral study. In contrast, the DNP is viewed as the practice-focused degree. The goal of this program is to prepare an advanced practitioner for the application of knowledge with an emphasis on research.

At the end of this chapter are additional relevant websites and online resources for continuing your nursing education.

CREDENTIALING: LICENSURE AND CERTIFICATION

What Is Credentialing?

In the early days of nursing before the Nightingale era, anyone could claim to be a nurse and practice the "trade" as he or she wished. It was only during the past century that nursing became a credentialed profession. A credential can be as simple as a written document showing an individual's qualifications. A high school diploma is a credential that indicates a certain level of education has been attained.

A credential can also signify a person's performance. The attainment of a title—such as Fellow of the American Academy of Nursing (FAAN)—signifies excellence in performance; a postgraduate degree from an institution of higher learning (PhD or EdD) indicates success in terms of academic achievement and advanced nursing knowledge.

In nursing, the educational credentials that an individual holds indicate not only academic achievement but also the attainment of a minimum level of competency in nursing skills. An ADN, a diploma in nursing, or a baccalaureate degree in nursing (BSN or BS) represents academic achievement. After academic preparation and successful completion of the NCLEX, you will have a legal credential—your nursing license—that permits you to practice as an RN. Additional nursing credentials may reflect practice in special areas, such as critical care registered nurse (CCRN) and certified addictions registered nurse (CARN).

What Are Registration and Licensure?

Licensure affords protection for the public by requiring an individual to demonstrate minimum competency by examination before practicing certain trades. By 1923, 48 states (Alaska and Hawaii did not become states until much later) had some form of nursing licensure in place. Nursing licensure is a process by which a governmental agency grants "legal" permission to an individual to practice nursing. This accountability is maintained through state boards of nursing, which are responsible for the licensing and registration process. Boards of nursing vary in structure and are based on the design of the nurse practice act within each state. State boards of nursing also exercise legal control over schools of nursing within their respective states. In 1978, all boards of nursing formed a national council, the National Council of State Boards of Nursing (NCSBN), to present a more collective front on nursing education and licensure.

Foreign nurse graduates who want to practice nursing in the United States must contact the board of nursing in the state in which they want to practice to obtain licensure, because each state controls its own requirements for licensure. The state's board of nursing will review the candidate's nursing education and determine the requirements needed to obtain a license in that state. Most states require that foreign nurses take the Commission on Graduates of Foreign Nursing Schools (CGFNS) examination before the NCLEX-RN® examination. This examination determines proficiency in nursing and the English language, thus assisting in the prediction of success on the NCLEX-RN® examination. All foreign nurse graduates, regardless of licensure in their home countries, must successfully complete the NCLEX-RN® examination.

What Is Certification?

In the classic article on credentialing published by the ANA in the late 1970s, certification is defined as a "voluntary process by which a nongovernmental agency or association certifies that an individual licensed to practice a profession has certain predetermined standards specified by that profession for specialty practice" (ANA, 1979, p. 67). Certification is a different credential from licensure and has a variety of interpretations—both for the nursing profession and the public.

> The nursing license is recognized as indicating minimum competency, whereas the certification credential indicates preparation beyond the minimum level.

Since the establishment of the first certification program by the ANA in 1973, certification is the credential that provides recognition of professional achievement in a defined functional or clinical area of nursing practice. Credentials, such as professional certification, are the stamps of quality and achievement that communicate professional competence. The process of becoming certified engages a full circle of accountability to patients and families, along with professional colleagues. The American Nurses Credentialing Center (ANCC) offers 19 specialty certifications (ANCC, 2018).

What Is Accreditation?

The term *accreditation* is often confused with certification. Accreditation in higher education is a process by which a voluntary, nongovernmental agency or organization approves and grants status to institutions or programs (not individuals) that meet predetermined standards and criteria (US Department of Education, 2018). There are two types of accreditation in higher education and they are referred to as institutional or regional accreditation and programmatic or specialized accreditation. Institutional or regional accreditation refers to an entire university or college being accredited, indicating that all components of the institution contribute toward the institution or college's objectives and mission, whereas program or specialized accreditation refers to a specific discipline, department, or individual program of study within the university or college that is accredited (US Department of Education, 2018).

The ACEN, the CCNE, and the NLN CNEA are accrediting organizations that accredit nursing programs nationwide. Specifically, the ACEN accredits clinical doctorate/DNP specialist certificate, master's/post-master's certificate, baccalaureate, associate, diploma, and practical nursing programs (ACEN, 2018). The NLN CNEA accredits licensed practical nurse/licensed vocational nurse (LPN/LVN), diploma, associate, bachelor, master's, and clinical doctorate degree nursing programs (*NLN CNEA*, 2018), and the CCNE accredits baccalaureate and graduate programs, postgraduate APRN certificates, and nurse residency programs (CCNE, 2018).

Why should you be concerned about whether the nursing program you are attending, or thinking about attending, is accredited? Accreditation assures you, the student, and the public that the nursing program has achieved educational standards over and above the legal requirements of the state. It guarantees the student the opportunity to obtain a quality education. Accreditation is strictly a voluntary process.

Some graduate nursing programs require completion of an approved accredited undergraduate program as a prerequisite for admission to their master's or doctoral program. ACEN, CCNE, and the CNEA publish annually an official complete list of accredited programs.

NURSING EDUCATION: FUTURE TRENDS

Education is a lifelong process and an empowering force that enables an individual to achieve higher goals. Student access to educational opportunities is paramount to nursing education. A chapter on nursing education would not be complete without taking a look at the future.

The Changing Student Profile

Future nursing programs will need to be flexible to meet the learning needs of a changing student population. It has previously been stated that there is a growing population of nontraditional students—individuals who are making midlife career changes in part because of job displacement or job dissatisfaction. Minority individuals, foreign-educated students, and disadvantaged students are looking toward nursing education for career opportunities.

These changes mean that nurse educators will have to go further in addressing the needs of the adult learner. More programs will be needed that permit part-time study and allow students to work while attending school. One option may be for more night or weekend course and clinical offerings. There will continue to be a need for emphasis on remedial education such as developmental courses in math,

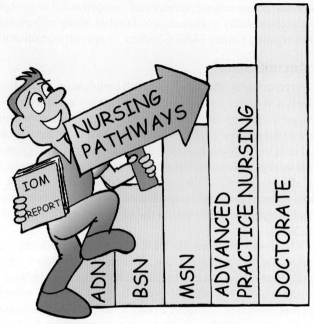

FIG. 7.3 The changing student profile.

English, and English as a second language. The diversity in the student population means increased diversity in the nursing workforce, which will contribute to quality health care for the nation's diverse population (Fig. 7.3).

Educational Mobility

Educational mobility will also need to be addressed further. A growing number of individuals in health care are seeking more education. The issue is not one of entry into practice but rather of how to best facilitate the return of these individuals to nursing school for educational advancement that fits their professional and personal needs. The growth of dual-enrollment nursing programs and web-based (online) courses may facilitate educational mobility.

A Shortage of Registered Nurses

According to the US Department of Health and Human Services, Health Resources and Services Administration (HRSA, 2017), there were approximately 2.8 million nurses employed in 2014, and it is projected that the number will increase to 3.9 million by 2030, which is a 39% increase nationally. Although these projections indicate that there will not be a nursing shortage nationwide, it is predicted that seven states will still be experiencing a nursing shortage. Even though these projections seem very positive, factors such as early retirement or increased demand may nullify any positive gains.

A Shortage of Qualified Nursing Faculty

Data on the nursing faculty shortage reported by the AACN in their *2015–2016 Salaries of Instructional and Administrative Nursing Faculty in Baccalaureate and Graduate Programs in Nursing* indicate that the "average ages of doctorally prepared faculty holding the ranks of professor, associate professor, and assistant professor were 62, 57, and 51 years, respectively" (AACN, 2017d, para 5).

There are fewer nurses entering the profession who are choosing a teaching role. Because of decreased numbers of new teachers, along with the number of current faculty retiring, the number of qualified faculty will continue to decline.

The ability to earn more in the clinical and private sector is also attracting potential nurse educators to leave academia. The American Association of Nurse Practitioners (AANP) gives the average salary of a nurse practitioner as $97,083 whereas the AACN reported that master's-prepared faculty had an annual income of $77,022 (AACN, 2017d, para 7). In addition, the shortage of nursing faculty was the primary reason that 64,067 qualified baccalaureate and graduate program applicants were not accepted into their respective nursing programs (AACN, 2017d, para 2).

Technology and Education

Educational learning will continue to change with advances in telecommunication and technology. Nurses and nurse educators will need education to implement these advances in the curriculum and in nursing practice. Cable television, the Internet, computer tablets, and smartphones have significantly extended the boundaries of the classroom; these technologies will facilitate the offering of courses to meet the lifestyle of the changing student population.

Changing Health Care Settings

There has been a major shift from inpatient to outpatient nursing services as health care and nursing focus on maintaining health rather than handling illness. However, with an increase in the age of the population, more inpatients have multiple chronic health problems. Society is now developing a variety of new health care settings. Are nurses educated for these new roles? What will the role of the advanced nurse practitioner be? Will there be enough nurses educationally prepared to meet these new challenges?

The Aging Population

There is a growing aging population. According to the Administration for Community Living (HHS ACL, 2018, p. 2), by 2040 there will be about 82.3 million older persons, over twice their number in 2000. The population age 65 and older has increased from 37.2 million in 2006 to 49.2 million in 2016 (a 33% increase) in just 10 years and is projected to more than double to 98 million by 2060. The older adult population represented 15.2% of the US population in 2016, but are expected to grow to 21.7% of the US population by 2040. The population age 85 and older is projected to double from 6.4 million in 2016 to 14.6 million in 2040 (a 129% increase!). Nursing educators need to address the provision of health care to the older adult population and continue to ensure its inclusion in nursing curriculum.

What great opportunities in nursing!

CONCLUSION

The future of nursing looks bright and exciting. With an increasingly diverse population, technological advances, changes in health care delivery, and increased demand for the RN services, nurses now have increased opportunities to chart their own destiny.

Nurses who have career plans and career goals will see the future trends in health care as a challenge and an opportunity for growth in roles such as case manager, independent consultant, nurse practitioner, nursing educator, nursing informatics specialist, policy maker, and entrepreneur. In contrast, nurses without career goals may find themselves displaced or obsolete. There has never been a more exciting time to be entering the profession of nursing than right now. Opportunities in nursing are wide open to those with the sensitivity and the creativity to embrace the future.

I challenge you to get out a piece of paper and put your educational goals down in writing. After you do this, set some deadlines for when you want to achieve these goals. Place this piece of paper in a prominent place where you will see it every day.

What's talked about is a dream,
What's envisioned is exciting,
What's planned becomes possible,
What's scheduled is real.

Anthony Robbins

RELEVANT WEBSITES AND ONLINE RESOURCES

Academic Progression in Nursing Program (APIN)
About APIN. http://www.academicprogression.org/about/

American Association of Nurse Practitioners
Planning your NP education. https://www.aanp.org/student-resources/planning-your-np-education

American Association of Colleges of Nursing
Your nursing career. http://www.aacn.nche.edu/students/your-nursing-career
List of schools that offer accelerated baccalaureate programs for non-nursing college graduates. http://www.aacn.nche.edu/leading-initiatives/research-data/BSNNCG.pdf
List of schools that offer entry-level or second-degree master's programs. http://www.aacn.nche.edu/leading-initiatives/research-data/GENMAS.pdf.

National Council of State Boards of Nursing
APRN Consensus Model: The Consensus Model for APRN regulation, licensure, accreditation, certification and education. https://www.ncsbn.org/aprn-consensus.htm

National League for Nursing
NLN overview. http://www.nln.org/about

Nursing's Centralized Application Service, Nursing CAS
Centralized application service for nursing programs. https://www.nursingcas.org/

BIBLIOGRAPHY

Accreditation Agencies Joint Statement on Academic Progression (2015). *Joint statement on national nursing education accreditation and academic progression.* Retrieved from http://www.academicprogression.org/resources/docs/Accreditation-Agencies-Joint-Statement-on-Academic-Progression.pdf.

Accreditation Commission for Education in Nursing (ACEN) (2018). *Nursing education accreditation.* Retrieved from http://www.acenursing.org/mission-purpose-goals/.

American Association of Colleges of Nursing (AACN) (2004). Position statement on the practice doctor in nursing. Retrieved from https://www.aacnnursing.org/News-Information/Position-Statements-White-Papers/Practice-Doctorate

American Association of Colleges of Nursing (AACN) (2013). *Competencies and curricular expectations for clinical nurse leader education and practice.* Retrieved from https://www.aacnnursing.org/Portals/42/AcademicNursing/CurriculumGuidelines/CNL-Competencies-October-2013.pdf.

American Association of Colleges of Nursing (AACN) (2017a). *Accelerated baccalaureate and master's degrees in nursing.* Retrieved from https://www.aacnnursing.org/Nursing-Education-Programs/Accelerated-Programs.

American Association of Colleges of Nursing (AACN) (2017b). *DNP fact sheet.* Retrieved from https://www.aacnnursing.org/News-Information/Fact-Sheets/DNP-Fact-Sheet.

American Association of Colleges of Nursing (AACN) (2017c). Fact sheet: Degree completion programs for registered nurses: RN to master's degree and RN to baccalaureate programs. Retrieved from https://www.aacnnursing.org/News-Information/Fact-Sheets/Degree-Completion-Programs.

American Association of Colleges of Nursing (AACN) (2017d). *Nursing faculty shortage.* Retrieved from https://www.aacnnursing.org/News-Information/Fact-Sheets/Nursing-Faculty-Shortage.

American Association of Nurse Anesthetists (AANA) (2016). *Certified Registered Nurse Anesthetists fact sheet.* Retrieved from https://www.aana.com/patients/certified-registered-nurse-anesthetists-fact-sheet.

American Association of Nurse Practitioners (AANP) (2018). *NP fact sheet.* Retrieved from https://www.aanp.org/all-about-nps/np-fact-sheet.

American College of Nurse-Midwives (ACNM) (2018). *Essential facts about midwives.* Retrieved from http://www.midwife.org/Essential-Facts-about-Midwives.

American Nurses Association (ANA) (1979). *The study of credentialing in nursing: A new approach.* Kansas City, MO: American Nurses Association.

American Nurses Credentialing Center (ANCC) (2018). Our certifications. Retrieved from https://www.nursingworld.org/our-certifications/.

Bureau of Labor Statistics (2017). *Occupational employment and wages: 29-1151 Nurse Anesthetists.* Retrieved from https://www.bls.gov/oes/current/oes291151.htm#nat.

Commission on Collegiate Nursing Education (CCNE) (2018). *About CCNE Accreditation.* Retrieved from https://www.aacnnursing.org/CCNE-Accreditation/About.

Commission on Nurse Certification (CNC) (2018). *CNL certification exam data.* Retrieved from https://www.aacnnursing.org/Portals/42/CNL/CNLStats.pdf.

Institute of Medicine (2010). *The future of nursing: Leading change, advancing health.* Retrieved from http://www.nationalacademies.org/hmd/Reports/2010/The-Future-of-Nursing-Leading-Change-Advancing-Health.aspx.

National Association of Clinical Nurse Specialists (NACNS) (2016). *Key findings from the 2016 Clinical Nurse Specialists census.* Retrieved from https://nacns.org/professional-resources/practice-and-cns-role/cns-census/.

National Council of State Boards of Nursing (NCSBN) (2010). *APRN Consensus Model FAQs.* Retrieved from https://www.ncsbn.org/APRN_Consensus_Model_FAQs_August_19_2010.pdf.

National League for Nursing. (NLN) (2016). *Percentage of students enrolled by type. Biennial survey of schools of nursing, Academic year*: (pp. 2015–2016). Retrieved from http://www.nln.org/docs/default-source/newsroom/nursing-education-statistics/percentage-of-students-enrolled-by-age-and-program-type-2016-(pdf).pdf?sfvrsn=0.

National League for Nursing (NLN) (2018). *Certification for nurse educators.* Retrieved from http://www.nln.org/professional-development-programs/Certification-for-Nurse-Educators.

National League for Nursing Commission for Nursing Education Accreditation (CNEA) (2018). Accreditation services. Retrieved from http://www.nln.org/accreditation-services/overview.

Schultz, M. J. (2016). Meeting current and future nursing needs through progression and innovation—the concurrent enrollment program at Maricopa Nursing. Unpublished manuscript.

Smiley, R. A., Lauer, P., Bienemy, C., Berg, J. G., Shireman, E., Reneau, K. A., & Alexander, M. (2018). The National Council of State Boards of Nursing (NCSBN) 2017 national nursing workforce survey [supplement]. *Journal of Nursing Regulation*, 9(3), 4–88.

Tri-Council for Nursing (2010). *Tri-Council for Nursing issues news consensus policy statement on the educational advancement of registered nurses.* Retrieved from https://www.aacnnursing.org/Portals/42/News/5-10-TricouncilEdStatement.pdf.

U.S. Department of Education (2018). Overview of accreditation in the United States. Retrieved from https://www2.ed.gov/admins/finaid/accred/accreditation.html#history

U.S. Department of Health and Human Services, Administration for Community Living (ACL) (2018). 2017 Profile of older Americans. Retrieved from https://acl.gov/sites/default/files/Aging%20and%20Disability%20in%20America/2017OlderAmericansProfile.pdf

U.S. Department of Health and Human Services, Health Resources and Services Administration (HRSA) (2017). *National Center for Health Workforce analysis. National and regional supply and demand projections of the nursing workforce* (pp. 2014–2030). Rockville: Maryland. Retrieved from *https://bhw.hrsa.gov/sites/default/files/bhw/nchwa/projections/NCHWA_HRSA_Nursing_Report.pdf.*

8

Nursing Theories

Ashley Zerwekh Garneau, PhD, RN

ⓔ http://evolve.elsevier.com/Zerwekh/nsgtoday/.

The only good is knowledge and the only evil is ignorance
Socrates (469–399 BC)

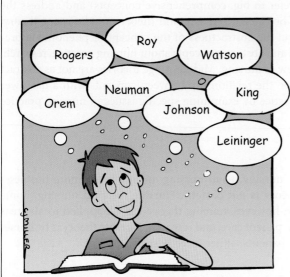

There are many nursing theories available to help guide my practice.

After completing this chapter, you should be able to:
- Identify the purposes of nursing theory.
- Distinguish between grand theory, middle-range theory, and practice theory.
- Describe the origins of nursing theory.
- Describe key concepts associated with nursing theory.
- Identify some of the more well-known and well-developed nursing theories.
- Discuss some of the main points of each of these theories.

Just mentioning the word theory, let alone nursing theory, can make many nurses' yawn reflexes start to work overtime. What is theory? Who are nursing theorists? What are the different nursing theories? Nursing theories are a way to organize and think about nursing, and the people who wrote theories are part of our nursing history. Theory provides an overall "theme" to what nurses do. In this chapter, the key words related to theory are defined, and the main elements of eight nursing theories are summarized. Buckle your seatbelts—we might be in for a bumpy ride. And no yawning!

NURSING THEORY

What Is Theory?

Quite simply, theories are words or phrases (concepts) joined together in sentences, with an overall theme, to explain, describe, or predict something. A more complex definition of a theory is "a set of interrelated concepts, definitions, and propositions that present a systematic way of viewing facts/events by specifying relations among the variables, with the purpose of explaining and predicting the fact event" (Kerlinger, cited in Hickman, 2003).

Theories help us understand and find meaning in our nursing experience and provide a foundation for direct questions whose answers offer insights into best practices and safe patient care. You might see theory referred to as a conceptual model or a conceptual framework in nursing textbooks and journals. Meleis offered a definition of nursing theory with the following: "an articulated and communicated conceptualization of invented or discovered reality in or pertaining to nursing for the purpose of describing, explaining, predicting or prescribing nursing care" (cited in Hickman, 2003, p. 16).

The bottom line is that words and phrases (concepts) are put together into sentences (propositions that show the relationships among the words/concepts), with an overall theme, to create theories. Theories also have some basic assumptions (jumping-off points; what is assumed to be true), such as the idea that nurses contribute to the patient's wellness and recovery from illness. Nursing theories also define four metaparadigms (metaparadigms refer to big, comprehensive concepts) and address the nursing process. Finally, nursing theories can be categorized as grand theory, middle-range theory, or practice theory. Each theory level is based on the abstractness of the concept or phenomena presented. For example, grand theories offer broad and abstract concepts about nursing practice, research, and education, which provide a more global view of nursing. Middle-range theories are not as abstract as grand theories; their focus is concentrated on the relationship between concepts with a narrower scope. Last, practice theories guide nursing practice by examining specific issues in nursing practice (Research for Best Practice Box 8.1).

What Nursing Theory Is Not

Nursing theory is *not* managed care, primary nursing, team nursing, or any other more business-related method of delivering care. Nursing theory is *not* obstetric nursing, surgical nursing, home health nursing, or any other nursing specialty; however, nursing theory can be applied to all areas of nursing, including administration, education, patient care, and research. Nursing theory is by nurses and for nurses, providing quality care to their patients, either directly or indirectly.

Why Theory?

Consider all that you do as a nurse. What you do is based on principles from many different professions, such as biology, sociology, medicine, ethics, business, theology, psychology, and philosophy. What is specifically based on nursing? Also, if nursing is a science (and it is), there must be some scientific basis for it. Furthermore, theory helps define nursing as a profession (Fig. 8.1).

Theory is a means to gather information, to identify ideas more clearly and specifically, to guide research, to show how ideas are connected to each other, to make sense of what we observe or experience, to predict what might happen, and to provide answers. A nurse is not a "junior physician," although for years nursing care has been based on the medical model. Because nursing is a

Practice Theory

Practice Issue

There are a limited number of studies reporting an examination of the use of a nursing theory to guide the care of school-age children with special health care needs in a school setting. Using Orem's Self-Care Deficit theory, Green (2012) discussed how school nurses can assist children with special health care needs in gaining independence with self-care and daily activities. Using Orem's Self-Care Deficit theory, researchers Wong, Wan, Choi, and Lam (2015) examined the relationship between basic conditioning factors (BCFs), self-care agency, and self-care behaviors in adolescent girls with dysmenorrhea. Findings from the study suggest that BCFs such as age, knowledge about medications used to treat menstrual pain (self-medication), and educational level of parents, along with self-care agency can influence an adolescent with dysmenorrhea to perform self-care measures associated with menstruation problems.

Implications for Nursing Practice

• Application of Orem's self-care deficit nursing theory can be used by school nurses to identify, plan, and implement nursing care measures that will assist children with special health care needs and their families in developing independence with self-care needs.

• School nurses can educate adolescent girls on common health-related issues such as menstruation, so that the adolescent is informed about self-care measures that can be used to alleviate associated symptoms of dysmenorrhea.

• In practice settings where vulnerable populations are present (such as school nursing), use of a nursing theory serves as an ideal theoretical framework for the nurse to identify self-care needs of the population and provide optimal nursing care with a goal of promoting self-care.

Considering This Information

Can you think of other vulnerable populations for which Orem's theory would be a theoretical framework to guide nursing practice?

References

Green, R. (2012). Application of the self-care deficit nursing theory to the care of children with special healthcare needs in the school setting. *Self-Care, Dependent-Care Nursing, 19*(1), 35–40.

Wong, C. L., Wan, Y., Choi, K. C., & Lam, L. (2015). Examining self-care behaviors and their associated factors among adolescent girls with dysmenorrhea: An application of Orem's self-care deficit nursing theory. *Journal of Nursing Scholarship, 47*(3), 219–227. https://doi.org/10.1111/jnu.12134.

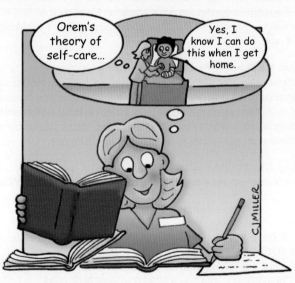

FIG. 8.1 Theory guides both research and nursing practice.

science (as well as an art) and a unique profession in its own right, nurses need nursing theory on which to base their principles of patient care (Critical Thinking Box 8.1; Research for Best Practice Box 8.2).

❓ CRITICAL THINKING BOX 8.1

What advantages and disadvantages do you see for using nursing theory in your nursing practice?

What Is the History of Nursing Theory?

In studying nursing theories and the people who created them, it is important to look at the background of the theorist and how life experiences, beliefs, and education influenced the resulting theory. What are the overall theme and main ideas of the theory, and how does the theorist define the four nursing metaparadigms (Box 8.1)?

🔍 RESEARCH FOR BEST PRACTICE BOX 8.2
Nursing Theory

Practice Issue

Although the focus of health care institutions in improving patient outcomes is based on evidenced-based practice, there is some beginning research that has investigated the use of a theoretical framework guided by nursing theory in examining patient perceptions in living and managing a medical condition.

Flanagan (2018) discusses that pain is a universal experience and persistent pain in older adults can be difficult to assess. Using Roy's adaptation model and the four adaptive modes (physiologic, self-concept, role function, and interdependence) can be useful as a model to assess factors that influence an older adult patient's experience and perception of pain.

Seah and Tham (2015) suggested that Roy's Adaptation Model could be used by nurses in managing patients with bulimia nervosa. The authors contended that Roy's Adaptation Model supports a multidisciplinary team approach in the context of providing patient care.

Implications for Nursing Practice

- Implementation of a nursing theory to examine patient and family experiences when faced with an illness or injury that may cause both physical and emotional life-altering changes can serve as a framework for nurses in guiding their practice.
- As part of the multidisciplinary health care team, nurses can assist patients and their families in adapting to the physiologic and psychosocial factors affected by a life-altering injury, chronic pain, and/or illness.
- Nursing theories can assist nurses in providing holistic nursing care.

Considering This Information

Do you feel it is important that a nursing theory guide your nursing actions? Which nursing theory fits your view of nursing practice?

References

Flanagan, N. M. (2018). Persistent pain in older adults: Roy's adaptation model. *Nursing Science Quarterly, 31*(1), 25–28. https://doi.org/10.1177/0894318417741095.

Seah, X. Y., & Tham, X. C. (2015). Management of bulimia nervosa: A case study with the Roy adaptation model. *Nursing Science Quarterly, 28*(2), 136–141. https://doi.org/10.1177/0894318415571599.

BOX 8.1   DEFINITION OF METAPARADIGMS

Person
Individuals, families, communities, and other groups who are participants in nursing and who receive nursing care.

Environment/Situation
The patient environment includes any setting and influencing factors that can alter the setting where the patient receives care. Factors influencing the environment include room temperature, family members' presence or lack of presence in the plan of care, work, and school.

Health
The patient's state of well-being. A patient's health is influenced by many physical and psychosocial factors.

Nursing
Nursing involves the use of the nursing process to assess, diagnose, plan, implement, and evaluate an individualized plan of care for providing patient care and education.

From Potter, P. A., Perry, A. G., Stockert, P., Hall, A., & Ostendorf, W. R. (2017). *Fundamentals of nursing* (9th ed., p. 42). St. Louis: Elsevier.

The four metaparadigms for nursing are nursing, person, health, and environment.

Florence Nightingale is considered to be the first nursing theorist. She saw nursing as "A profession, a trade, a necessary occupation, something to fill and employ all my faculties, I have always felt essential to me, I have always longed for; consciously or not. … The first thought I can remember, and the last was nursing work…" (Florence Nightingale as cited in Dunphy, 2015, p. 38). Now, you might not feel as dedicated as she, but Nightingale also stated, "Nursing is an art. … It is one of the Fine Arts; I had almost said, the finest of the Fine Arts" (Florence Nightingale, as cited in *Una and the Lion*, 1871, p. 6).

Nightingale had various influences, including her education (which was fairly comprehensive for a 19th-century English woman), her religion (Unitarianism), the history of the time (the Crimean War and invention of the telegraph), and her social status. The Unitarian belief involved salvation through health and wholeness, or our modern-day "holism." Nightingale believed that there was no conflict between science and spirituality. Science was necessary for the development of a mature concept of God (Dunphy, 2015). She also studied many other religions throughout her life, including Anglicanism, and considered starting a Protestant religious order of nuns.

Nightingale came from a very wealthy, prominent family and enjoyed traveling throughout Europe, one of the destinations being Kaiserwerth in Germany, where she observed and was moved by nuns caring for the ill. Nightingale felt a "calling" to care for others and began training with various groups, usually nuns who cared for the sick. When the Crimean War broke out, Nightingale was asked and volunteered to go to care for the wounded English soldiers. The Crimean War was the first war after the invention of the telegraph, so news of the war was more immediately circulated than had been previously experienced (Dunphy, 2015).

The overall theme of Nightingale's theory was that the environment influences the person. When she went to help soldiers during the Crimean War, her initial intent was to feed the soldiers healthy food, maintain cleanliness in the barrack hospital, and ensure proper sanitary and hygiene care (Dunphy, 2015) (Fig. 8.2). When soldier mortality rates fell, a legend was born!

Nightingale believed that nursing was separate from medicine and that nurses should be trained (although we prefer the word *educated*). She also believed that the environment was important to the health of the person and that the nurse should support the environment to assist the patient in healing (Dunphy, 2015).

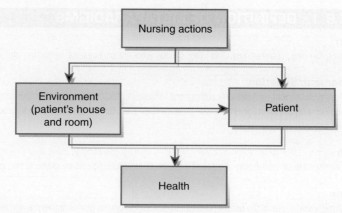

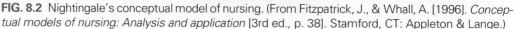

FIG. 8.2 Nightingale's conceptual model of nursing. (From Fitzpatrick, J., & Whall, A. [1996]. *Conceptual models of nursing: Analysis and application* [3rd ed., p. 38]. Stamford, CT: Appleton & Lange.)

To define the metaparadigms, Nightingale noted that the person is the center of the model and incorporated a holistic view of the person, someone with psychological, intellectual, and spiritual components. The nurse was a woman (because only women were nurses in Nightingale's day) who had charge of the health of a person, whether by providing wellness care, such as with a newborn, or by providing care to the sick. Health was the result of environmental, physical, and psychological factors, not just the absence of disease (Dunphy, 2015).

No other theories were identified or published until the 1950s when Peplau published her theory based on the interpersonal process. Other nurses were working on theories during that time and into the 1960s. In the 1970s, nursing was beginning to see itself as a scientific profession based on theoretical ideas. Nursing theory continues to influence health. For example, health care institutions seeking Magnet recognition are required to adopt a nursing theory or framework that guides nursing practice (Smith & Parker, 2015) (Table 8.1).

TABLE 8.1 NURSING THEORIES

YEAR	THEORIST	THEORY DESCRIPTION
1860	Florence Nightingale	Although her model did not have a specific name, the basic underpinnings revolve around how a person is influenced by the environment. Nursing was a "calling" to help the patient in a reparative process by directly working with the patient or indirectly by affecting the environment to facilitate health and recovery from illness.
1952	Hildegard Peplau	Interpersonal Relations Model—describes the four phases of the dynamic relationship between nurse and patient: orientation, identification, exploitation, and resolution.
1960	Faye Abdellah	Patient-Centered Approach—develops a list of 21 unique nursing problems related to human needs; promoted the use of a problem-solving approach to the practice rather than merely following physicians' orders. Responsible for changing the focus of nursing theory from a disease-centered to a patient-centered approach and moved nursing practice beyond the patient to include care of families and the elderly.
1961	Ida Jean Orlando	Theory of Deliberative Nursing Process—focuses on the interpersonal process between nurse and patient through a deliberative nursing process; most concerned with what was uniquely nursing.
1964	Lydia Hall	Core, Care, and Cure Model—model is depicted with three overlapping circles with the care circle representing the patient's body, the cure circle representing the disease that affects the patient's physical system, and the core circle representing the inner feelings and management of the person.

Continued

TABLE 8.1   NURSING THEORIES—cont'd

YEAR	THEORIST	THEORY DESCRIPTION
1966	Virginia Henderson	One of her main topics is the "unique functions of nurses." All of her materials provide a focus for patient care via 14 basic needs.
1966	Joyce Travelbee	Human-to-Human Relationship Model—believed that it was as important to sympathize as it was to empathize if the nurse and the patient were to develop a **human-to-human** relationship.
1969	Myra Estrin Levine	Conservation Model—focuses attention on the wholeness of the person, adaptation, and conservation, which is guided by four principles (conservation of energy, structure, personal integrity, and social integrity).
1970	Martha Rogers	Science of Unitary Human Beings—an abstract model addressing the complexity of the "unitary human being," which allows for the examination of phenomena (energy fields, paranormal) that other theories do not describe, as nurses promote synchronicity between human beings and their environment/universe.
1971	Dorothea Orem	Self-Care Nursing Theory—three interwoven theories of self-care, self-care deficit, and the nursing system help the nurse identify strategies to meet the patient's self-care needs.
1971	Imogene King	Theory of Goal Attainment—patient goals are met through the transaction between nurse and patient involving three systems (personal, interpersonal, and social).
1972	Betty Neuman	Neuman Systems Model—focuses on wellness and mitigating stress within three levels of prevention: primary, secondary, and tertiary.
1974	Sister Callista Roy	Roy's Adaptation Model—individual seeking equilibrium through the process of adaptation; identified six physiological needs (exercise and rest; nutrition; elimination; fluid and electrolytes; oxygenation and circulation; and regulation of temperature, senses, and endocrine system).
1976	Josephine Paterson and Loretta Zderad	Humanistic Nursing Theory—focuses on the nurse and the patient; dignity, interests, and values are of greatest importance; belief that there is more to nursing that is not explainable by scientific principles.
1978; 1991	Madeline Leininger	Theory of Culture Care Diversity and Universality—a grand theory that considers the impact of culture on the person's health and caring practices.
1979	Margaret Newman	Theory of Health as Expanding Consciousness—every person in every situation is ever-changing in a unidirectional, unpredictable, all-at-once pattern involving movement, time, space, and consciousness; emphasizes the importance of viewing patients in the context of their holistic patterns.
1979	Jean Watson	Theory of Human Caring—identifies 10 "carative" factors focusing on the interactions between the one who is caring and the one who is being cared for.
1980	Dorothy Johnson	Behavioral Systems Model—focuses on human behavior rather than the person's state of health; this theory helped clarify the differences between medicine and nursing.
1981	Rosemarie Rizzo Parse	Theory of Human Becoming—focuses on the human-health-universe; views nursing as a participation effort with the patient that focuses on health.
1983	Helen Erickson, Evelyn Tomlin, and Mary Ann Swain	Modeling and Role Modeling Theory—uses the understanding of the patient's world to plan interventions that meet the patient's perceived needs and that will help the patient achieve holistic health; focus is on the person receiving the care, not the nurse, not the care, and not the disease.
1984	Pat Benner	Professional-Advancement Model—applies the Dreyfus model of skill acquisition to nursing; area of concern is not how to do nursing but rather, "How do nurses learn to do nursing?"; identifies seven domains: practice-helping, teaching/coaching, diagnosing and monitoring, managing changes, administering and monitoring therapeutic interventions, monitoring quality care, and organizing to enact the work role.
1994	Karen Schumacher and Afaf Ibrahim Meleis	Transition Framework—formulated with the goal of integrating what is known about transition experiences across different types of transitions with nursing therapeutics for people in transition.
2001	Gladys L. Husted and James H. Husted	Symphonological Bioethical Theory—provides nurses and other health care professionals with a logical method of determining appropriate ethical actions.

Data from Fawcett, J. (2005). *Analysis and evaluation of contemporary nursing knowledge: Nursing models and theories.* Philadelphia: FA Davis; and Alligood, M. R. (2018). *Nursing theorists and their work* (9th ed.). St. Louis: Mosby.

Among the best-known and best-formulated theories or models are those by Dorothea Orem, Martha Rogers, Sister Callista Roy, Dorothy Johnson, Betty Neuman, Imogene King, Jean Watson, and Madeleine Leininger (see the *Definitions of the Metaparadigms* by these theorists in the *Evolve* website). Each theory has been around for more than 30 years, and each theorist has practiced nursing at the bedside, in the community, and in administration or education. At the end of this chapter are listed relevant websites and online resources related to each nursing theory and associated nursing theorist.

WHO ARE THE NURSING THEORISTS?

Selected Nursing Theorists
Dorothea Orem—Self-Care Nursing Theory
Orem's theory includes the overall theme of self-care. She sees the person as composed of physical, psychological, interpersonal, and social aspects. Nursing consists of actions that are designed to overcome or prevent self-care limitations (self-care deficits) or to provide care for someone who is unable to perform self-care. A nurse may need to do everything for the patient (wholly compensatory, such as for a patient who is under general anesthesia or a newborn), to do some things for the patient (partly compensatory, such as with a patient who is 2 days postop and may be able to do some things, but not everything, independently), or to educate the patient (supportive educative, such as with postpartum parents). Orem added that self-care requisites (food, water, air) are universal basic needs that individuals need to sustain life. Health, to Orem, is the internal and external conditions that permit self-care needs to be met (Hood, 2014). The environment is anything outside of, or external to, the person. Thus, in assessing a patient, a nurse using Orem's theory would ask, "What can the patient do for himself or herself? And what do I, as the nurse, need to do for the patient? What are the patient's self-care deficits (or things that he or she cannot do)? What nursing functions can be provided to the patient to assist in self-care and promote recovery?"

Orem's nursing process includes assessing the patient, deciding whether nursing care is needed, and, if so, determining which self-care deficits are present. Does the patient need wholly or partly compensatory or supportive-educative nursing care? The nurse needs to identify interventions and decide which interventions the patient can do (if any) and which interventions the nurse will do. The nurse describes which helping methods are used for the interventions (acting for or doing for another, guiding and directing, providing physical or psychological support, providing a therapeutic environment, or teaching) (Foster & Bennett, 2003). And all interventions fall under one of those five helping methods (Figs. 8.3 and 8.4).

Martha Rogers—Science of Unitary Human Beings
Martha Rogers was one of the most original thinkers of the nursing theorists. Her overall theme is that the person and the environment are one thing and cannot be separated. Rogers takes holism to a new level. The person, for Rogers, is an energy field that exhibits patterns (think of electrocardiogram [ECG] patterns, fetal heart rate patterns, biorhythms, auras). Health is an "index of field" (Rogers as cited in Hood, 2014, p. 141). Rogers, however, did not like to define the word *health* because she believed it was a value judgment (e.g., what your patient thinks is healthy about himself may not be what you think is healthy about the patient). The environment for Rogers was also an energy field that was interacting constantly with the energy field of the person (similar to what Nightingale thought). The role of nursing was to repattern the person and environment to achieve maximum health potential for the person. Although this may all sound a little far-fetched, many nurses, when first entering a patient's room in a hospital, will assess the patient and rearrange or clean up the room

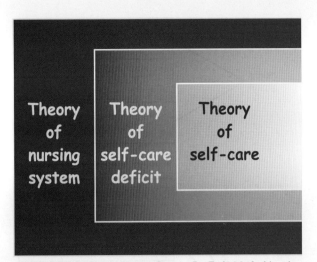

FIG. 8.3 Orem's self-care deficit model. (From Orem, D. E. [2001]. *Nursing concepts of practice* [6th ed., p. 141]. St. Louis: Mosby.)

to make things more convenient or therapeutic for caring for the patient. That is, the patient and environment are "repatterned" to achieve maximum health for the patient (Hood, 2014).

Rogers's theory is grounded in the science of physics and the ideas of matter and energy. Rogers was very interested in space travel and envisioned nurses as providing care for people on earth or in space. She felt that some pathologies were a result of our being earthbound (e.g., osteoporosis and arthritis) but that these diseases would not be an issue in outer space because of the changes in gravity. Rogers also believed in the value of nurses using creative therapies, such as touch, color, sound, motion, and humor. The use of complementary therapies (guided imagery, biofeedback, meditation, yoga, Reiki) fits very well with Rogers's ideas. The nursing care plan that Rogers developed, but was not sold on, included Pattern Manifestation Knowing-Assessment (our idea of *assessment*), Voluntary Mutual Patterning (whereby the nurse and patient pattern the environmental energy to promote health— or interventions), and Pattern Manifestation Knowing-Evaluation (our idea of *evaluation*) (Muth Quillen, 2003).

Rogers's theory, entitled "Principles of Homeodynamics," examines the wholeness of humans and their interactions with the environment. Under homeodynamics, three principles exist that further define the environmental conditions that humans experience, and they are resonancy, integrality, and helicy. Resonancy is the "continuous change from lower- to higher-frequency wave patterns in human/environmental fields" (from Rogers in *Nursing Science and the Space Age*, as cited in Alligood, 2014, p. 248).

Integrality looks at how human beings and the environment are continuously and simultaneously interacting. This interaction influences the changing life process that humans experience in their everyday activities. Helicy looks at the continuous and evolving pattern changes that exist between humans and their environment (Fig. 8.5).

Sister Callista Roy—Adaptation Model

Sister Callista Roy saw the person as a biopsychosocial being (yes, it does seem as if these theorists make up their own words) who is seeking equilibrium. Her overall theme was adaptation. The four

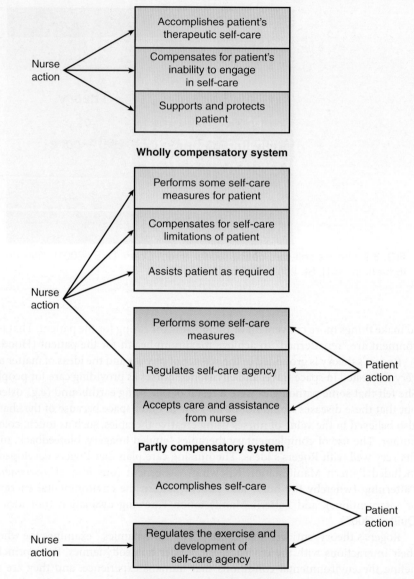

FIG. 8.4 Orem's basic nursing systems. (From Orem, D. E. [2001]. *Nursing concepts of practice* [6th ed., p. 351]. St. Louis: Mosby.)

adaptation modes represent the behavior responses exhibited by the individual and include "physiological-physical, self-concept–group identity, role function, and interdependence" (Tiedeman, as cited in Fitzpatrick & Whall, 2005, p. 152). As nurses, we are to assess how well the person is coping and adapting to stimuli. The stimuli could be any stressors that are making a person ill or causing the person to not adapt. The stimulus could be focal (the stimulus that is the greatest concern at the

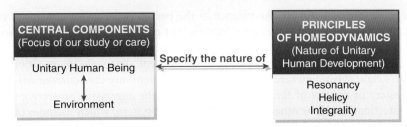

FIG. 8.5 Roger's science of unitary human beings. (From Fitzpatrick, J., & Whall, A. [1996]. *Conceptual models of nursing: Analysis and application* [3rd ed.]. Stamford, CT: Appleton & Lange.)

moment—e.g., labor pain), contextual (all other stimuli in the area that contribute to the effect of the focal stimulus, such as noise in the background), or residual (a stimulus that is unknown to the nurse but is bothering the patient—e.g., memories of past labors and births).

Health is defined as successful coping with stressors, and the environment is defined as the influences that affect the development of a person. Illness is unsuccessful coping. The nursing process is a problem-solving approach that encompasses steps to gather data, identify capacities and needs of the human adaptive system, select and implement approaches for nursing care, and evaluate the outcome of the care provided. In Roy's nursing process, she adds two assessment parts: (1) What is the stimulus? and (2) What is the person's response to the stimulus? The nurse's role is to influence stimuli to improve successful coping (Alligood, 2018) (Fig. 8.6).

Dorothy Johnson—Behavioral Systems Model

Dorothy Johnson was one of Roy's teachers at UCLA. Johnson's theme was balance; her theory is that the person is a behavior system and a biological system seeking balance (George, 1995). The environment is anything outside the person or behavior system. Health is balance or stability. The nurse's role

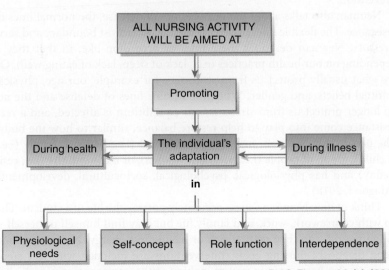

FIG. 8.6 Roy's adaptation model. (From Pearson, A., Vaughan, B., & Fitzgerald, M. [2005]. *Nursing models for practice* [3rd ed., p. 129]. Edinburgh: Butterworth & Heinemann.)

is to restore or maintain the balance in the person or behavior system. A visual example would be learning to use crutches after a leg fracture. The person needs to learn to balance (literally) on crutches but also needs to learn to "balance" the other aspects of his or her life that are affected by the broken leg.

Johnson views the nursing process as assessment, diagnosis, intervention, and evaluation. The person's eight subsystems are assessed. These subsystems are the achievement subsystem, which includes mastery or control of the self or environment; the aggressive/protective subsystem, which includes protecting oneself or others; the dependency subsystem, which includes obtaining attention or assistance from others; the eliminative subsystem, which includes not only physical elimination from the body but also being able to express one's feelings or ideas; the ingestive subsystem, which includes eating, as well as "taking in" other things such as pain medication or information; the affiliative subsystem, which includes relating to others or achieving intimacy; the sexual subsystem, which includes activities related to sexuality, such as procreating and sexual identity; and the restorative subsystem, which focuses on measures such as rest and relaxation to optimize mind and body restoration (Holaday, 2015) (Fig. 8.7).

> Consider how patients for whom you care would fall into each of these seven subsystems or which subsystems would most apply to the patients for whom you provide care.

Betty Neuman—Systems Model

Betty Neuman's conceptual model focuses on prevention, or prevention as intervention, as a response to stressors. Primary prevention is what a person does to prevent illness—for example, exercise, sleep 8 hours, eat a balanced diet. Secondary prevention is what is done when an illness strikes. For example, when a person with a myocardial infarction comes into the emergency department, what is done by the staff to prevent this person from dying or from having further heart damage? Tertiary prevention is what is done to rehabilitate a person after an illness or accident, such as cardiac rehabilitation or stroke rehabilitation. Tertiary prevention can move the person back to primary prevention again. The nurse's role is to help reduce the stressors through the three levels of prevention.

Neuman also talks about the flexible lines of defense, the normal lines of defense, and the lines of resistance. The flexible lines of defense are the outermost boundary and serve as the initial response to stressors. Neuman describes these lines as accordion-like, in that they can expand and contract depending on our health practices (e.g., lack of sleep, lack of eating well). Our normal lines of defense are what usually protect us from stressors—for example, our age, physical health, genetic makeup, spiritual beliefs, and gender. When the flexible lines of defense and the normal lines of defense can no longer protect us from stressors, our equilibrium is affected, and a reaction occurs. The lines of resistance come into play to help restore balance, similar to how the body's immune system works. The person, for Neuman, may be an individual (i.e., patient), family (i.e., parents of a chronically ill child), group of people (i.e., pregnant women), or a community (i.e., residents in an assisted-living facility) and has physiological, psychological, sociocultural, developmental, and spiritual variables (Alligood, 2018).

Think of how Neuman's ideas accurately portray the life of a student. The student struggles to keep up with coursework, work, and family life but may find himself or herself sleeping less, eating less or eating poorly, and then getting sick or having less energy. Neuman's nursing process has just three steps: diagnosis, nursing goals (interventions are included with this step), and nursing outcomes. Neuman also has a unique way of looking at the environment, which she identifies as the internal, the external, and the created environment. The created environment is developed by the patient

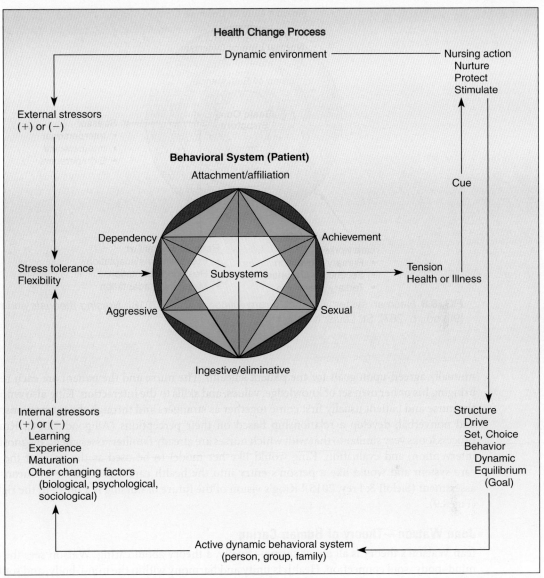

Health Change Process

Dynamic environment ———————— Nursing action
 Nurture
 Protect
 Stimulate

External stressors
(+) or (−)

Behavioral System (Patient)
Attachment/affiliation

Dependency   Achievement

Cue

Stress tolerance
Flexibility   Subsystems   Tension
 Health or Illness

Aggressive   Sexual

Ingestive/eliminative

Internal stressors
(+) or (−)
 Learning
 Experience
 Maturation
 Other changing factors
  (biological, psychological,
  sociological)

Structure
Drive
Set, Choice
Behavior
Dynamic
Equilibrium
(Goal)

Active dynamic behavioral system
(person, group, family)

FIG. 8.7 Johnson's behavioral systems model. (From Alligood, M. R. [2018]. *Nursing theorists and their work* [9th ed., p. 338]. St. Louis: Mosby.)

and serves as his or her protective device (Alligood, 2018). The created environment can be a healthy adaptation (e.g., someone relaxing through visualization), or it can be maladaptive (e.g., someone with a type of psychosis, such as schizophrenia) (Fig. 8.8).

Imogene King—Goal Attainment Model

The theme of Imogene King's theory is interaction and goal attainment. The person interacts with the environment, and health is a dynamic state of well-being. The nurse interacts with the patient to set

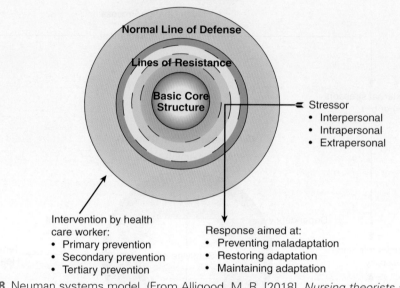

FIG. 8.8 Neuman systems model. (From Alligood, M. R. [2018]. *Nursing theorists and their work* [9th ed., p. 287]. St. Louis: Mosby.)

mutually agreed-upon goals for the patient's health. The nurse and the patient are each recognized as bringing his or her own set of knowledge, values, and skills to the interaction. King also emphasizes that the nurse and patient usually first come together as strangers and through the interactions, both verbal and nonverbal, develop a relationship based on their perceptions (Alligood, 2014). King's nursing process looks very similar to that with which nurses are already familiar: assessment, diagnosis, planning, intervention, and evaluation. King would like her model to be used as the basis of the U.S. health care system and would like a person's entry into the health care system to be by means of nursing assessment (Sieloff & Frey, 2015)! King's vision of the future of nursing is a move in the right direction (Fig. 8.9).

Jean Watson—Theory of Human Caring

Jean Watson's theory is all about caring—finally, a theory about caring. Watson sees the person as a mind–body–soul connection. Health is unity and harmony within the mind, body, and soul. The nurse comes in contact with the person during a "caring occasion" or "caring moment" and promotes restoration of a sense of inner harmony through Watson's 10 "carative" factors. To Watson, caring is a moral idea rather than an interpersonal technique (Alligood, 2014).

Here are Watson's 10 carative factors (with each one, see what nursing interventions you can identify):

1. The formation of a humanistic–altruistic system of values
2. The instillation of faith–hope
3. The cultivation of sensitivity to one's self and to others
4. The development of a helping–trust relationship
5. The promotion and acceptance of the expression of positive and negative feelings

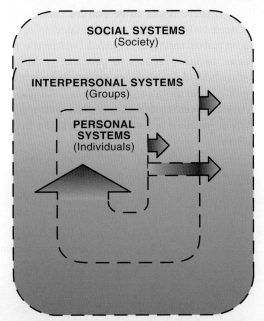

FIG. 8.9 King's goal attainment model for nursing. (From Pearson, A., Vaughan, B., & Fitzgerald, M. [2005]. *Nursing models for practice* [3th ed., p. 162]. Edinburgh: Butterworth & Heinemann.)

6. The systematic use of the scientific problem–solving methods for decision making
7. The promotion of interpersonal teaching–learning
8. The provision for a supportive, protective, and corrective mental, physical, sociocultural, and spiritual environment
9. Assistance with the gratification of human needs
10. The allowance for existential–phenomenological forces (Alligood, 2014)

Madeleine Leininger—Culture Care Theory

Madeleine Leininger's overall theme is culture. Leininger is the "Margaret Mead of the health field" and has traveled widely and studied many cultures. She sees the person as caring and capable of being concerned with the welfare of others. Nursing is a transcultural caring discipline and profession. Nurses need to be mindful of folk practices or generic health care practices. (Think of health care practices that were practiced when you were a child that would be considered folk or generic health care practices—e.g., Vicks VapoRub applied to your chest for a cold; depending on the illness, not drinking either hot or cold beverages; not sitting too close to the TV because it was "bad" for your eyes.) The nurse needs to be aware of and use culture care data that are influenced by religion, kinship, language, technology, economics, education (both formal and informal), cultural values and beliefs, and the physical (or ecological) environment. Leininger believes that there can be no curing without caring. Health is culturally defined (Alligood, 2014).

The health care professional needs to examine the prescribed health care requirements and decide if there can be culture care preservation or maintenance (where the relevant care values can be retained), or if there needs to be culture care accommodation or negotiation (where the cultural practices need to be adapted or negotiated to return the patient to health), or if culture care repatterning or restructuring is required (where the patient needs to change or significantly alter culturally based health practices to promote good health). Leininger's theory can be summarized in her Sunrise Model. Leininger replaced the word *model* with the term *enabler* "to clarify it as a visual guide for exploration of cultures" (Alligood, 2014b, p. 354). The upper half of the sunrise enabler (model) represents the various cultural factors that impact a person's views toward health. The lower half is for decision making between the health care professional and the person (Fig. 8.10).

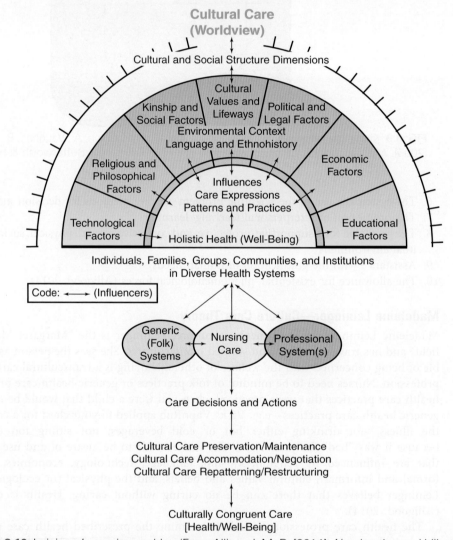

FIG. 8.10 Leininger's sunrise enabler. (From Alligood, M. R. [2014]. *Nursing theory: Utilization and application* [5th ed., p. 355]. St. Louis: Mosby.)

FUTURE OF NURSING THEORY

The future of nursing theory is at a turning point. We all understand that nursing theory, nursing research, and nursing practice form the foundation of nursing as a discipline. Many nursing programs and educators feel that it is not important to teach nursing theory and have dropped the content from the curriculum, so as a result, graduates from their programs do not see the importance of theory in practice. According to Karnick (2016), "As EBP increases in popularity, theory is not viewed as critical to nursing practice. In fact, theory is becoming passé in many baccalaureate programs and nonexistent in graduate education, especially the doctor of nursing practice programs (DNPs)" (p. 283).

With articles entitled, "Where have all the nursing theories gone?" (Parse, 2016); "Nursing theory: The neglected essential" (Karnick, 2013); and "Why teach nursing theory?" (Yancy, 2015), the literature speaks clearly to the concerns of the weakening of nursing theory in nursing curricula. Yancy (2015) states that as faculty move away from nursing models to guide curriculum development, "what constitutes nursing science will be lost and the unique contributions of nursing will be blurred" (p. 275). Dr. Calista Roy (2018), one of nursing's esteemed theorists, in a detailed personal narrative, discussed key issues in nursing theory development, challenges, and future directions. She notes that there is an imbalance among philosophical, conceptual/theoretical, and empirical inquiry in the nursing profession and proposes strategies for the profession to enhance nursing theory-based knowledge for practice by focusing on communication among various groups of stakeholders (American Academy of Nursing, Sigma Theta Tau, National League for Nursing, American Association of Colleges of Nursing, and so on) and creating a strategic plan across groups in a joint effort to resolve the crossroads dilemma. Will you be a part of the solution? Only time will tell.

CONCLUSION

In reviewing these nursing theories, you may find that some especially appeal to you and others do not. That is okay. What is important is to understand that nursing theories are a rich part of our nursing history and that they are a way to organize, deliver, evaluate, and ultimately improve the care we provide to the patient populations we serve (Critical Thinking Box 8.2).

> **? CRITICAL THINKING BOX 8.2**
>
> In reviewing the theories, which one would best fit in your clinical practice?
> Which theory most appeals to you and why?
> Which theory/theories would fit best with the following patient settings and why?
> * Perioperative patient
> * Obstetrical patient
> * Psychiatric patient
> * Nursing education
> * Managing a nursing unit
> * Community health
> * Organizing a computer-generated acuity form
> * Pediatric patients
> * Home health
> * Hospice care
> * Long-term care facility
> * Rehabilitative therapy

🔍 RESEARCH FOR BEST PRACTICE BOX 8.3

Future of Nursing Theory

Practice Issue

Given the changes facing health care in the 21st century, trends in nursing theory have been examined by Parse (2016) and Roy (2018), who both call for an examination of the importance of having nursing theory in nursing curriculum and practice.

Implications for Nursing Practice

- Based on their literature review, Im and Chang (2012) suggested that the profession of nursing continues to link nursing theory to research and practice and to expand use of nursing theory internationally and embrace international collaborative processes to gain awareness and understanding of international nursing perspectives. Im and Chang (2012) added that nursing theories remain in coexistence, so a multiple range of theories can be applied in various practice and academic settings.
- McCrae (2011) suggested that nursing theory in undergraduate curriculum is critical to advancing the practice of nursing.
- Karnick (2014) cautions that the discipline of nursing is on a slippery slope due to the increasing lack of nursing theory in nursing education.

Considering This Information

What are your thoughts about the inclusion of nursing theory in the curriculum? Was nursing theory content or a nursing theory course part of your nursing program curriculum?

References

Im, E. O., & Chang, S. J. (2012). Current trends in nursing theories. *Journal of Nursing Scholarship, 44*(2), 156–164. https://doi.org/10.1111/j.1547-5069.2012.01440.x.

Karnick, P. M. (2014). A case for nursing theory in practice. *Nursing Science Quarterly, 27*(2), 117. https://doi.org/10.1177/0894318414522711.

McCrae, N. (2011). Whither nursing models? The value of nursing theory in the context of evidence-based practice and multidisciplinary health care. *Journal of Advanced Nursing, 68*(1), 222–229. https://doi.org/10.1111/j.1365-2648.2011.05821.x.

Parse, R. R. (2016). Where have all the nursing theories gone? *Nursing Science Quarterly, 29*(2), 101–102. https://doi.org/10.1177/0894318416636392.

Roy, C. (2018). Key issues in nursing theory: Developments, challenges, and future directions. *Nursing Research, 67*(2), 81–92. https://doi.org/10.1097/NNR.0000000000000266.

Nursing theory has and hopefully will continue to guide nursing practice. Given the increasing complexity of the health care environment, nursing theory can contribute to the use of evidence-based nursing practice by linking theory with research and practice (Research for Best Practice Box 8.3).

🌐 RELEVANT WEBSITES AND ONLINE RESOURCES

Clayton State University
Nursing theory link page. http://www.clayton.edu/nursing/Nursing-Theory.

Current Nursing
Nursing theories. http://currentnursing.com/nursing_theory/.

Hahn School of Nursing and Health Science
Nursing theory and research. http://www.sandiego.edu/nursing/research/nursing-theory-research.php/.

Petiprin, A.
Nursing theory. http://www.nursing-theory.org/.

BIBLIOGRAPHY

Alligood, M. R. (2014). *Nursing theory: Utilization and application* (5th ed.). St. Louis: Mosby.

Alligood, M. R. (2018). *Nursing theorists and their work* (9th ed.). St. Louis: Mosby.

Dunphy, L. H. (2015). Florence Nightingale's legacy of caring and its application. In M. C. Smith & M. E. Parker (Eds.), *Nursing theories and nursing practice* (4th ed., pp. 37–54). Philadelphia: FA Davis.

Foster, P. C., & Bennett, A. M. (2003). Dorothy E. Orem. In University of Phoenix College of Health Sciences and Nursing (Ed.), *Theoretical foundations of nursing practice* (pp. 137–168). Boston: Pearson Custom Publishing.

George, J. B. (1995). *Nursing theories: The base for professional nursing practice* (4th ed.). Norwalk, CT: Appleton & Lange.

Hickman, J. S. (2003). An introduction to nursing theory. In University of Phoenix College of Health Sciences and Nursing (Ed.), *Theoretical foundations of nursing practice* (pp. 15–28). Boston: Pearson Custom Publishing.

Holaday, B. (2015). Dorothy Johnson's Behavioral system model and its application. In M. C. Smith & M. E. Parker (Eds.), *Nursing theories and nursing practice* (4th ed., pp. 89–104). Philadelphia: FA Davis.

Hood, L. J. (2014). *Leddy and Pepper's conceptual bases of professional nursing* (8th ed.). Philadelphia: Lippincott.

Karnick, P. M. (2013). Nursing theory: The neglected essential. *Nursing Science Quarterly*, *26*(2), 130–131. https://doi.org/10.1177/0894318413477210.

Karnick, P. M. (2014). A case for nursing theory in practice. *Nursing Science Quarterly*, *27*(2), 117. https://doi.org/10.1177/0894318414522711.

Karnick, P. M. (2016). Evidence-based practice and nursing theory. *Nursing Science Quarterly*, *29*(4), 283–284. https://doi.org/10.1177/0894318416661107.

Muth Quillen, S. (2003). Rogers' model: Science of unitary persons. In University of Phoenix College of Health Sciences and Nursing (Ed.), *Theoretical foundations of nursing practice* (pp. 309–323). Boston: Pearson Custom Publishing.

Nightingale, F. (1871). *Una and the lion.* Cambridge: Riverside Press.

Parse, R. R. (2016). Where have all the nursing theories gone? *Nursing Science Quarterly*, *29*(2), 101–102. https://doi.org/10.1177/0894318416636392.

Roy, C. (2018). Key issues in nursing theory: Developments, challenges, and future directions. *Nursing Research*, *67*(2), 81–92. https://doi.org/10.1097/NNR.0000000000000266.

Sieloff, C. L., & Frey, M. A. (2015). Imogene King's theory of goal attainment. In M. C. Smith & M. E. Parker (Eds.), *Nursing theories and nursing practice* (4th ed., pp. 133–151). Philadelphia: FA Davis.

Smith, M. C., & Parker, M. E. (2015). *Nursing theories and nursing practice* (4th ed.). Philadelphia: FA Davis.

Tiedeman, M. E. (2005). Roy's adaptation model. In J. J. Fitzpatrick & A. L. Whall (Eds.), *Conceptual models of nursing: Analysis and application* (pp. 146–176). Upper Saddle River, NJ: Prentice Hall.

Yancy, N. R. (2015). Why teach nursing theory? *Nursing Science Quarterly*, *28*(4), 274–278. https://doi.org/10.1177/0894318415599234.

9

Professional Image of Nursing

*Christa L. Steffens, EdD, MSN, RN**

ⓔ evolve.elsevier.com/Zerwekh/nsgtoday/.

Unless we are making progress in our nursing every year, every month, every week, take my word for it, we are going back.
Florence Nightingale

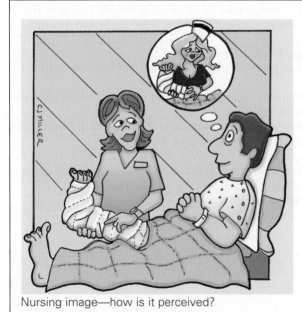

Nursing image—how is it perceived?

After completing this chapter, you should be able to:

- Discuss the effect of image on the public perception of nursing.
- Recognize the role of media in shaping the public perception of nursing.
- Describe different sociological models that characterize "professionalism."
- Apply Pavalko's characteristics as a framework to describe modern nursing practice.
- Identify the impact that nursing organizations have on professional practice.
- Describe the role of credentialing and certification in professional practice.

Nursing image—how is it perceived? What does it mean to be a professional nurse? How does the public view nursing? How does nursing define and view itself? What role does the public image of the nursing profession play in our current nursing climate? What do you do to further the image of a professional nurse?

*We would like to thank **Margi J. Schulta, PhD, RN, CNE, PLNC,** for her previous contributions to this chapter.

Historically, nurses have struggled to define the image of nursing and the professional role of the nurse. There are many different views and opinions, but nurses are definitely gaining ground when it comes to defining the profession of nursing. The annual Gallup survey for professions noted that for honesty and ethical standards, nursing has been rated at the top of the list for the past 16 years. In 2017, 82% of the American public rate the standards held by nurses as either high or very high; this rates the nursing profession 11 percentage points above any other profession (Brenan, 2017). The image of nursing is evolving and changing, with nursing being promoted and viewed as an intellectual, autonomous profession that demands a high level of commitment, focus, and a dedication to advancing education and scholarly activity.

Modern-day nursing has many dimensions, one of which includes the debate surrounding its identification as a profession. One ongoing challenge in nursing is to diligently foster and enhance the public image and the self-image of the nurse. In this chapter, the development of nursing into a profession is discussed, and the present and future dimensions of nursing's "image" are explored. The lasting impact of the 2010 Institute of Medicine report on *The Future of Nursing* and other significant position statements and reports on the profession will be discussed. Historical knowledge about our "rites of passage" provides an appreciation of the path nursing has taken as a profession and what the future of nursing may hold for the recent graduate in this complex and evolving health care world.

PROFESSIONAL IMAGE OF NURSING

What Do We Mean by the "Image" of Nursing?

Santa Filomena
Lo! in that hour of misery
A lady with a lamp I see
Pass through the glimmering gloom,
And flit from room to room.

Longfellow, 1857

Nursing has been identified as an "emerging profession" for at least 150 years. The historical context of nursing's image is often traced back to Florence Nightingale, the "founder of nursing." Florence Nightingale is recognized as a nurse, statistician, and writer who became known for her groundbreaking work during the Crimean War. Nurse Nightingale was also called the "Lady with the Lamp," as she was reported to have made rounds on her patients at night by the light of a lantern. International Nurse's Day is celebrated each year on her birthday, May 12, and the Nightingale Pledge is still recited by new nursing graduates around the world, often with the accompaniment of flickering candles in symbolic lamps. Even though much has been written about Florence Nightingale's many contributions, she is undeniably remembered as the pioneer of nursing education (Bostridge, 2008).

The professional image of nursing is dynamic and complex and has run the gamut from the virtuous Angels of Mercy of its professional origin all the way to sex symbols currently embodied as the Naughty Nurse. Over time, the image of nursing has made many other stops along a broad spectrum of stereotypes such as the doctor's handmaiden, the battle-axe, and mother figure among others (Darbyshire & Gordon, 2005; Gordon & Nelson, 2005; Kalisch, Begeny, & Neumann, 2007; Kalisch & Kalisch, 1983). However, of all the stereotypes nursing has struggled with, the Angel of Mercy seems to be the most pervasive. Afterall, who doesn't like to be thought of as an angel?

Gordon and Nelson (2005) explained the "virtue script" as an archaic frame of professional reference for nurses when all were associated with characteristics such as honesty, kindness, and virtue. Until the mid-19th century, respectable nurses existed only within the confines of the Church where fundamental modesty and a devotion to serving God placed them beyond reproach. The virtue script was born out of rejection of the notion that secular women caring for the sick were socially undesirable. Secular nursing pioneers, such as Nightingale, were often very virtuous and devout (Gordon & Nelson, 2005; Nelson, 2011). Such characteristics were congruous with those associated with nurses operating under a religious calling and served as a conduit to "transfer" an air of virtuosity to secular nurses. Thus, nursing became a suitable role for respectable women outside of the domestic domain.

While concepts of modesty and virtue served as a means to establish nursing as a socially acceptable occupation outside of the home, it also reinforced the socially inferior standing of women in existence prior to the late 20th century. Forced to downplay the knowledge and skill required to care for patients, nurses were expected to "say little and do much" (Gordon & Nelson, 2005; Nelson, 2011). While medicine and the scope of nursing practice have momentously advanced, the silent and humble nature of nursing has changed very little. The tendency to vacillate between a drive to solidify the professional and scientific standing of nursing yet desire to bask in the public admiration of a historically noble and selfless vocation makes portrayal of a consistent and accurate professional image difficult. Nurses must be willing to abandon the virtue script to continue to gain professional and scientific legitimacy within the current health care system.

The inherent silence among nurses has affected their professional visibility and may contribute to a lack of perceived value by society (Rezaei-Adaryani, Salsali, & Mohammadi, 2012). Despite a plethora of evidence connecting care of formally educated and technically skilled nurses with positive patient outcomes (Aiken et al., 2011), the profession continues to struggle against being marginalized. Gordon (2004) stated that "public communication is key to resolving the shortage of respect, recognition, and rewards" for the nursing profession (p. 278). Until nurses are willing to publicly challenge inaccurate portrayals within mass media, they will likely remain undervalued by society.

> I attribute my success to this—I never gave or took any excuse.
> *Florence Nightingale*

The image of professional nursing continues to evolve and is significantly affected by the media, women's issues and roles, and an ever-evolving high-technology health care environment.

Social media has been defined as "electronic tools that enhance communication, support collaboration, and enable users across the globe to generate and share content" (Thielst, 2013, p. 1). Social media has become a modality to rapidly disseminate information to the masses with the push of a button. The Pew Research Center reported that around 68% of American adults use a social media platform, which is an increase from 54% of the population noted in 2012 (Gramlich, 2018). Such statistics demonstrate how social media can be used to increase personal awareness of advances in health care, provide access to research and updates in evidence-based practices, or provide health information to a community (Ventola, 2014). In addition, one can create networks of professional contacts for reference and collaboration (Arrigoni, Alvaro, Vellone, & Vanzetta, 2016). Nursing education has also harnessed the power of social media. Some sources report as much as 53% of nursing schools are using social media tools to educate and recruit students (Peck, 2014). When used wisely, the positive effects of connecting patients and professionals from multiple disciplines seem infinite. However, if individuals are not mindful of the potential pitfalls of inappropriate use of social media, there can be serious professional repercussions.

As previously mentioned, social media has provided a way to rapidly communicate information to scores of people. When the contents of the communication are appropriate and propagate a professional image, it can be a major asset. However, when information that is inappropriate or unprofessional is made available to the public, long-standing personal and professional consequences may result. Social media sites like Facebook allow users to establish a social profile complete with photos, posts, and other personal information and permit other users to comment on the contents of the profile. The Pew Research Center found that approximately 53% of Facebook users did not understand how content on their news feed is influenced (Gramlich, 2018). The use of profanity, suggestive photos, or inflammatory comments pertaining to patients or an employer are regarded as extremely unprofessional and negatively affect one's personal image, and that of any associated personal or professional entities (Ventola, 2014). Any member of the nursing profession is a representative of the profession and should promote an appropriate image. If a nurse is unable to use discretion regarding the contents of a social media profile, the public is unlikely to believe him or her capable of demonstrating appropriate professional judgement (Peck, 2014). A recent Pew Research Center survey reported that even in the face of highly publicized data breeches, only 54% of Facebook users have adjusted their privacy settings in the past 12 months (Gramlich, 2018). To encourage development of a positive professional image, nurses must be vigilant about who is able to view their personal information and how they present themselves on social media. How nursing views itself in the evolution of the profession and how actively nurses are involved in the definition process will continue to determine the image and role of nursing in the future.

Recently, many have taken a more gender-neutral approach to recruiting and retaining men into nursing. The American Assembly of Men in Nursing (AAMN) has initiated the marketing campaign "Advancing Men in Nursing" with materials highlighting the camaraderie and opportunities available to men entering the profession. The professional, skilled, compassionate male image portrayed in posters and advertising is designed to break down the stereotypes typically associated with men in nursing (Stokowski, 2012). As more men enter the profession and there is a push to increase minorities in nursing, will the image of nursing change (Critical Thinking Box 9.1)?

? CRITICAL THINKING BOX 9.1

Think Quick!

Picture in your mind your image of a nurse—Did you just think of a female with tidy hair, a professional-looking uniform, serviceable white shoes, a stethoscope around her neck, a determined look in her eyes, an energetic walk, and a clipboard in hand? Or did you just envision a male nurse with many of those same attributes? The image of nursing is changing, and many media depictions now include men as nurses. There have always been men in nursing, but with the increasing respect for the profession, and the high touch, high technicality in the field of nursing, more men than ever are looking to become nurses. Indeed, many men who enter nursing are interested in fighting the same stereotypes that woman have battled through the years. The term "male nurse" is considered an unnecessary distinction, much like saying a "female physician"—the gender bias is simply not a critical element (Wilson, 2009). The first step in turning the tide of thought about gender in nursing is for members of the profession to alter their own perceptions.

Nurses should be thought of as autonomous and competent decision makers within their practice areas. Throughout the 1990s, a nationwide advertising campaign supported by the National Commission on Nursing Implementation Project produced radio and television ads that said, "If caring were enough, anyone could be a nurse." Nurses of America, an advocate organization sponsored by the National League for Nursing (NLN), implemented a very successful program directed toward improving the image of nursing as depicted on television, on radio, in print, and on lecture circuits. Consultants were contracted to work with executives, politicians, and celebrities to present nursing in a positive manner. This approach reinforced the image of the modern professional nurse as having critical thinking, evidence-based decision-making, and problem-solving skills.

At a nursing symposium in May 2012, it was noted that while the depiction of nurses in the media can affect how the public views nurses, it is truly up to each individual nurse to be proactive in presenting nursing as a respected profession (Muehlbauer, 2012). As noted by Groves (2007), accurate portrayals of nurses as professional members of the health care team are rare, but it takes time to change perceptions. The continued trend of building a positive, intelligent, competent, and professional image of nursing must continue. Nurses who are new to the profession need to be aware of the extraordinary challenges and opportunities that they will face. It is equally important for nurses to improve the self-image of the professional nurse. The behaviors and ethics displayed by nurses on a day-to-day basis can do much to elevate the present and shape the future image of nursing (Cohen & Bartholomew, 2008).

Nursing associations are working together to promote a positive image and to handle nursing shortage issues. Nurses for a Healthier Tomorrow, an alliance of 43 nursing and health care organizations, has launched a national media campaign that demonstrates, through print and broadcast media, the many opportunities for the career of nursing. One tangible example of this effort is the website www.nursesource.org. Sigma Theta Tau International, the international honor society for nursing, is the coordinator of Nurses for a Healthier Tomorrow. Review their website at www.nursingsociety.org. The American Nurses Association (ANA) published a flyer titled *Every Patient Deserves a Nurse*, along with other promotional materials for the lay public. The promotional message of these materials reinforces the positive image of nurses as patient advocates and critical resources both to patients and families, while also emphasizing the right of people to a safe health care environment.

In 2002, the Johnson & Johnson Company developed a nationwide campaign to support the nursing profession. This program, titled "The Campaign for Nursing's Future," was developed along with health care leaders and nursing organizations such as the National Student Nurse's Association (NSNA), the ANA, the American Organization for Nurse Executives (AONE), the NLN, and Sigma Theta Tau. The goal of this program is to increase the number of young adults entering nursing through raising the visibility of nurses of varied races, gender, and roles. The website for the campaign can be found at www.discovernursing.com. Since that time, nurses have made significant advances in promoting nursing to a more diverse population.

The negative images of nursing, those of the "naughty nurse" or the "Nurse Ratched" that are depicted in the media, are still prevalent, but these erroneous portrayals do offer professional nurses the opportunity to educate the public about what nurses truly do, or do not do. Nursing is not the only profession that struggles with a skewed media image. Some of these erroneous depictions may be related to the largely female population who seeks these professions; consider the sexual media images that are often illustrated by flight attendants, massage therapists, or secretaries. Other occupations that suffer from poor media portrayals include the "mad scientist" role (chemist or researcher), construction worker (often a sexual male image), or consider the negative images that both female and male lawyers are often faced with! Devaluation of the nursing profession by demeaning or comical images only extends the nursing shortage and further discourages talented people from entering the nursing profession. It is up to each individual to continue to display professional role modeling and provide public education on what nurses really do to empower the professional image of nursing (Cohen & Bartholomew, 2008).

> Do you feel most nurses portray a professional image? If so, what qualities do they possess to project this image? If not, what is lacking?

How can nurses change the image of nursing? How can the image of nursing become more congruent with the actual role the nurse plays in today's rapidly evolving health care environment? Nurses outnumber all other professions in health care. Mee (2006) suggests that nurses can promote the professional image of nursing by doing the following.

Patient Interactions

One by One. During the first 60 seconds that a patient sees the nurse, a lasting impression may be formed. Take a moment before meeting a new patient to portray confidence in your role and a respect for the patient from the beginning. Many health care institutions require nurses to wear nursing uniforms of a distinct color that separates them from nurse assistants and respiratory therapists.

Personal Interaction With the Public

Have a professional response ready in case someone asks about nursing. Present nursing's image positively, and relate what an important role nurses have in society as health care providers. Nursing advocacy starts with *you*! Every professional nurse has the responsibility to educate the public about what nurses do and the amount of education and dedication it takes to be a nurse. Believe in yourself, and project the image you want the public to see (Jacobs-Summers & Jacobs-Summers, 2011).

Public Speaking and Community Activities

Consider speaking at or visiting schools on Career Day. You don't have to be an expert at public speaking to discuss the role of the nurse with local community groups. A brief, interactive presentation at an elementary or high school can stimulate interest in nursing early—for both male and female students.

Participation in Political Activities

Increase the positive visibility of nurses through politics by becoming actively involved as a nurse lobbyist. Be aware of the current health care issues on the community, state, and national levels. Get to know the elected officials, and talk to them about the role of the nurse. This may be a valuable opportunity to present nursing in a very positive manner. Remember that most elected officials do not understand the role nurses play in health care (Mee, 2006).

The image of nursing continues to evolve as the many roles of nurses are portrayed through the media in the restructuring of health care environments and in a variety of settings, from emergency rooms to war zones. Studies continue to verify that competent nursing care affects mortality rates in critical care patients, and the future for many nursing jobs lies in the expanding role of nursing into emergency and disaster preparedness and integration of technology and informatics into practice settings (Health Resources and Services Administration [HRSA], 2010). The role and image of the nurse will continue to change as the many facets of health care delivery evolve during this century. The current nursing shortage will play a significant future part in the creation of the image and role of the nurse. How will nurses respond to these changes? How will you present yourself as a professional?

What Constitutes a Profession?

There are many ways to describe a "professional." What meaning does the word have for you as a graduate professional nurse? Controversy about the definition of the term *professional* as it relates to nursing is not a new issue. Strauss (1966), a noted sociologist, found the word *professional* used in reference to nursing in a magazine article published in 1892, titled "Nursing, a New Profession for Women." The nurses of the 20th and 21st centuries owe a great deal to Isabel Adams Hampton (later Isabel Hampton Robb) for her visionary focus in the late 1800s. She was an outstanding advocate for the professionalization of nursing. In the textbook *Nursing Ethics* (1900), she wrote:

> The trained nurse, then, is no longer to be regarded as a better trained, more useful, higher class servant, but as one who has knowledge and is worthy of respect, consideration, and due recompense.... She is also essentially an instructor; part of her duties have to do with the prevention of

disease and sickness, as well as the relief of suffering humanity.... These are some of the essentials in nursing by which it has become to be regarded as a profession, but there still remains much to be desired, much to work for, in order to add to its dignity and usefulness.

In Caplow's classic work from the early 1950s, *The Sociology of Work* (Caplow, 1954), several steps in the process of "becoming professional" were defined further, and the value of forming an association that defined a special membership was addressed. Caplow suggested that making a name change to clarify an area of work or practice would subsequently produce a new role. With the creation of this new role, the group would then establish a code of ethics and legal components for licensure to practice and educational control of the profession (Caplow, 1954). This process of becoming professional was taking place in nursing in 1897 with the establishment of the ANA. Other aspects of professionalization were also beginning to develop. For example, the *Code for Nurses* was suggested as early as 1926, although it was not written or published by the ANA until the early 1950s. Revisions were made in 1956, 1960, and 1976, with changes made in 1985 that included interpretative statements. In the summer of 2001 at the ANA convention, delegates again updated the code and changed the name to the *Code of Ethics for Nurses with Interpretive Statements*. The ANA deemed 2015 the Year of Ethics and issued an updated *Code of Ethics with Interpretive Statements* found at http://nursingworld.org/MainMenuCategories/EthicsStandards.

Almost 20 years after Caplow's work, Pavalko (1971) described eight dimensions of a profession. Pavalko's dimensions of a profession and their specific application to nursing are examined in more detail later in this chapter. Nursing continues to apply these dimensions to support nursing's move away from the occupational focus to a professional focus. Is nursing a profession or semi-profession?

By responding to the questions in Critical Thinking Box 9.2 (which presents Levenstein's model, a fourth model of professionalism), you will identify common themes in describing a profession. What are your thoughts about the nursing profession in light of these criteria?

❓ CRITICAL THINKING BOX 9.2

Levenstein's Characteristics of a Profession

What do you think about...
* The element of altruism
  How do you define caring in your clinical practice?
* Code of ethics
  Are you familiar with the ANA Code of Ethics?
* Collaboration with groups and individuals for the benefit of the patient
  What other groups do you work with in your clinical setting that affect the health needs of the patient and family?
* Colleagueship demonstrated by
  An organization for licensing
  * What is the role of the State Board of Nursing in your state?
  A group that helps ensure quality
  * Are you aware of the role of national nursing organizations that accredit nursing programs?
  * There are two national nursing organizations that accredit nursing programs; do you know what they are?
  Peer evaluations of practitioners
  * What is the role of job evaluations in terms of professional growth?
* Accountability for conduct and responsibility for practice decisions
  Who monitors professional conduct issues from a legal and ethical point of view?
  Does shared governance reflect more control of one's nursing practice?
* Strong research program
  Are you aware that a national center for nursing research is now operating in Washington, DC?

Others have written about professions and their development, but these sociological models present some logical characteristics for you to use to examine professionalism. According to Henshaw, a noted nursing leader and researcher, a profession includes "self-regulation and autonomy with ultimate loyalty and accountability to the professional group" (cited in Talotta, 1990). Nursing is a dynamic profession and continues to strive to enhance a professional image—which leads us to the next question.

Is Nursing a Profession?

Eunice Cole, a past president of the ANA, described nursing as a dynamic profession that has established a code of ethics and standards of practice, education, service, and research components. The standards for both the professional and practical dimensions of nursing are continually reviewed and updated. This next section examines the issues that challenge nursing as a profession by using Pavalko's eight dimensions to describe a profession.

1. A Profession Has Relevance to Social Values

Does nursing exist to serve self or others? Nursing historically had its roots in true altruism with lifelong service to others. As nurses, we focus not only on the treatment component of patient care as a part of our nursing practice but also on wellness and health promotion issues. The goal is to shift the focus of health care so that primary prevention becomes more valued. As this shift occurs, nurses will become increasingly important because of their ability to be teachers of health promotion activities and managers of wellness, which are activities that have an impact on social values.

2. A Profession Has a Training or Educational Period

According to Florence Nightingale, a nurse's education should involve not only a theory component but also a practice component. An educational process for any professional is critical because it transmits the knowledge base of the profession and, through research and other scholarly endeavors, advances the practice of the profession. The diversity of educational pathways for nurses has stimulated debate regarding the entry practice level for registered nurses. The Institute of Medicine report (2010), the OADN progression statement (2015), and the National League for Nursing (2011) all speak to the issue of advancing nursing education and entry into practice (see the end of this chapter for a list of relevant websites and online resources). Some questions surrounding the issues include the following:

- What changes will shape the future of associate degree nursing (ADN) programs?
- Will diploma or hospital-based nursing programs remain?
- How critical is it to complete a bachelor of science in nursing (BSN) program to handle the challenges of the health care environment, complex patient–family needs, and the expanding community-based settings for clinical work?
- Is a "ladder" approach or a concurrent enrollment program (CEP) to advanced education the best pathway for you?
- Will the practice doctorate in nursing (DNP) degree clarify or confuse advanced-practice roles in nursing?

These questions have been debated since the publication in 1965 of an ANA position paper that charged the profession with the goal of establishing nursing education at the baccalaureate level within 25 years. Almost 40 years have passed since then, and the issue continues to challenge the profession. The inability of nursing organizations and educational systems at all levels to come to agreement on this issue continues to affect the solidarity of the profession.

In the mid-1990s, some states (e.g., Maine and Idaho) engaged in debate about regulatory issues concerning the BSN as the entry credential. Beyond this generic-degree controversy are the issues associated with specialization: With the momentum from the AACN, the DNP has been established as the clinical practice degree for advanced practice. What should be the focus of the MSN degree or PhD degree? How will those degrees integrate into nursing education?

3. Elements of Self-Motivation Address the Way in Which the Profession Serves the Patient or Family and Larger Social System

In 1990, the Tri-Council of Nursing, along with the American Association of Colleges of Nursing, designed a "Nursing Agenda for Health Care Reform" to express collectively the views of nurses concerning health care. Endorsed by 39 major specialty nursing organizations, along with the ANA and the NLN, the Tri-Council emphasized a restructured health care system that would provide universal access to health care, direct health care expenditures toward primary care, and reduce costs.

Political activity is a way of translating social values into action. Nursing faces special challenges when, for example, nurses must go on strike for better pay and benefits or demonstrate a united front to gain federal funding rather than continuing a passive role in such issues. It is time for the nursing profession to define a new narrative that reflects how much the profession has changed, how critical nursing skills are to today's patient care, how the profession has stayed abreast of medical and technological innovation, and what nursing is going to look like in the future (Kaplan, 2000).

4. A Profession Has a Code of Ethics

Nursing, like other professions, has ethical dimensions. As noted earlier in the chapter, the nursing *Code of Ethics* published by the ANA dates to the 1950s. Key points of the code are provided in Box 9.1. The *Code of Ethics* is discussed in more detail in Chapter 19.

BOX 9.1   CODE OF ETHICS FOR NURSES

The ANA House of Delegates approved these nine provisions of the new Code of Ethics for Nurses at its June 30, 2001, meeting in Washington, DC. In July 2001 the Congress of Nursing Practice and Economics voted to accept the new language of the interpretive statements, resulting in a fully approved revised Code of Ethics for Nurses with Interpretive Statements, as follows:

1. The nurse, in all professional relationships, practices with compassion and respect for the inherent dignity, worth, and uniqueness of every individual, unrestricted by considerations of social or economic status, personal attributes, or the nature of health problems.
2. The nurse's primary commitment is to the patient, whether an individual, family, group, or community.
3. The nurse promotes, advocates for, and strives to protect the health, safety, and rights of the patient.
4. The nurse is responsible and accountable for individual nursing practice and determines the appropriate delegation of tasks consistent with the obligation to provide optimum patient care.
5. The nurse owes the same duties to self as to others, including the responsibility to preserve integrity and safety, to maintain competence, and to continue personal and professional growth.
6. The nurse participates in establishing, maintaining, and improving health care environments and conditions of employment conducive to the provision of quality health care and consistent with the values of the profession through individual and collective action.
7. The nurse participates in the advancement of the profession through contributions to practice, education, administration, and knowledge development.
8. The nurse collaborates with other health professionals and the public in promoting community, national, and international efforts to meet health needs.
9. The profession of nursing, as represented by associations and their members, is responsible for articulating nursing values, for maintaining the integrity of the profession and its practice, and for shaping social policy.

5. A Professional Has a Commitment to Lifelong Work

By this statement, Pavalko means that a professional sees his or her career as more than just a stepping stone to another area of work or as an intermittent job. Government data show that 83% of the nearly 2.9 million registered nurses work in health care (HRSA, 2010). Nursing constitutes the largest health care occupation, and more jobs are expected for registered nurses than for any other occupation. This faster-than-average growth is being driven by technological advances. Thus nursing as a career has great potential for financial rewards, involvement in a variety of professional endeavors, several different areas of practice, and a commitment to lifelong work.

6. Members Control Their Profession

Nurses are not entirely autonomous. Although nurses have the challenge to ensure that members of the profession honor the trust given them by the public, they also work under professional and legislative control. Among these controls are the 50 state boards of nursing, which regulate the scope of nursing practice within each state, and the professional practice standards that are supported both at local and national levels. In 1973, the ANA wrote the first *Standards of Nursing Practice* and since then has had a leadership role in the development of general and many specialty nursing practice standards. Moreover, specialty organizations maintain standards for certification.

Another publication by the ANA, *Nursing: Scope and Standards of Practice* (2015), discusses the use of nursing process and professional practice standards. The development of professional practice standards indicates to the larger social system that nursing can define and control its quality of practice. These national standards are incorporated into institutional standards to help guide nursing practice. Most recent publications by the ANA can be found on their website (www.nursingworld.org). The issue at hand, however, is that these professional practice standards authorize nurses to practice nursing. Nurses are expected to take responsibility for their own actions and not just follow orders without thinking critically.

Nurses practice in varied settings, and the advanced-practice nurse functions in a more autonomous professional role, such as the nurse-midwife, psychiatric clinical specialist, nurse practitioner, or certified nurse educator. In 1992, there were 100,000 advanced-practice nurses in the United States. Among practicing RNs, 55% achieved a baccalaureate or higher degree in nursing or a nursing-related field in 2010, compared with 27.5% in 1980 (HRSA, 2013). These changes represent the largest growing segment of specialty nursing practice. Advancing education and knowledge levels often allows for increased autonomy.

Most nurses in the United States work within a structured setting; three out of five jobs are in hospital, inpatient, or outpatient settings. Trends in those settings are slowly changing to give nurses a stronger voice. For example, nursing care delivery systems that have case management and shared governance reflect more progressive and autonomous environments (see Chapter 15). Nursing can control its scope of practice through professional organizations and published documents, along with an active voice in regulatory bodies, such as state boards of nursing.

7. A Profession Has a Theoretical Framework on Which Professional Practice Is Based

Nursing continues to be based in the sciences and humanities, but nursing theory is evolving. It was not until the 1950s that nursing theory was "born." In 1952, Dr. Hildegard Peplau published a nursing model that described the importance of the "therapeutic relationship" in health and wellness. Since then, other nursing theorists such as Martha Rogers, Sister Callista Roy, Dorothea Orem, and Betty Neuman have contributed to our evolving theory-based nursing science.

8. Members of a Profession Have a Common Identity and a Distinctive Subculture

The outward image of nursing has changed remarkably within the past 50 years. Nurses were once identified by how they looked rather than by what they did. The nursing cap and pin reflected the nurse's school and educational background. The modern-day trend emphasizes that it is not what is worn but what is done that reflects one's role in the nursing profession. The struggle to shift out of rigid dress codes was a major issue in the 1960s. Clothing and other symbols identify a subculture, and changes in that identification process occur slowly. What kind of image do you want to project as a professional nurse (Critical Thinking Box 9.3)?

? CRITICAL THINKING BOX 9.3

What Do You Think?

What Kind of Image Do You Want to Project as a "Professional"?
- Should nurses wear visible body jewelry, piercings, or have tattoos?
- Are the doctors on your unit called by their first or last names? How are *you* addressed in a professional setting?
- Are your credentials visible to indicate additional degrees or certifications? If not, why not? Is it the policy of the agency or facility where you work to display these?
- Are the nurses on your unit certified in their specialty areas? Is this recognized by your facility?
- What do your peers wear?
- Do you think scrubs look professional?
- Can a nurse wearing cartoon-character scrubs be taken seriously? Why? Why not?
- Should nurses leave the hospital in their scrubs and go run errands?
- What other professions are associated with a "uniform"?

Nursing colleagues reflect attitudes and values about the profession. Many schools of nursing have alumni associations, student nurse associations, and nursing honor societies or clubs on campus. These groups provide social interaction during the nursing education years and are great ways to network later in one's career. Belonging to a professional organization (such as the ANA) or a specialty organization helps professional nurses maintain certifications and network with peers, and it enhances collegiality and scholarship.

> "Nurses should choose optimism, making positive strides each day to celebrate who they are and the differences they make. Just a nurse—no, never."
> Melissa Fitzpatrick, 2001

When will the conflicts in educational preparation be resolved? How will we use further refinement and application of nursing theories in our clinical practice? What can nurses do to have more control of nursing practice regardless of the clinical setting? Will there be an increase in the percentage of people who are choosing nursing as a career? What are the forces that will help nursing "come together" and become not only a true profession but the largest and most powerful of all the health care professional groups? (Remember, there is always strength in numbers.)

NURSING ORGANIZATIONS

What Should I Know About Professional Organizations?

Nursing organizations have significant roles in empowering nurses in their emerging professionalism (Fig. 9.1). Yet many nurses do not belong to a national organization such as the ANA, or to their state

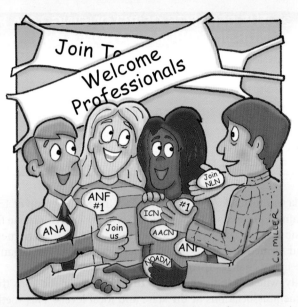

FIG. 9.1 There is a nursing organization to fit your needs.

affiliate organization, or even to specialty-focused groups such as the American Association of Critical-Care Nurses (AACN) or the National Black Nurses Association (NBNA). Of the 3.9 million registered nurses, membership in the constituent associations in ANA represents less than half of the nurses (ANCC, 2017; HRSA, 2010; NCSBN, 2018). During the past few years, researchers have examined the issue of belonging to a professional organization. Although there are no conclusive findings regarding why or how nurses choose nursing organizations, some have suggested that organizations representing nursing as a whole, such as the ANA and the NLN, do not meet the needs of the individual nurse practicing in today's changing health care environment.

Affiliation with a nursing organization to facilitate networking with colleagues is a valuable resource. As a recent graduate, you will need to examine your options for joining a professional group and then demonstrate your professional commitment by active participation. The question should be "Which ones should I join?" rather than "Should I join an organization?" (Box 9.2). In the next section, various organizations are reviewed, with historical notes to assist you in making the best choice as you begin your nursing career. A more complete directory of nursing organizations can be found on the *Evolve* website.

What Organizations Are Available to the Recent Graduate?

A few of these key professional organizations for individual and organizational membership are described in this section in alphabetical order. Many of these organizations publish a newsletter or professional journal, and most have websites. Individual memberships in your professional nursing organization and a specialty organization are great ways to maintain current knowledge about changes in your career field and create networking opportunities for both new graduate nurses and experienced nurses seeking to find a new position or to increase their knowledge (see Box 9.2).

American Nurses Association

The ANA is identified as the professional association for registered nurses. It was through the early efforts of Isabel Hampton Robb and others that the Nurses Associated Alumnae of the United States

BOX 9.2   THE BENEFITS OF BELONGING TO A PROFESSIONAL NURSING ORGANIZATION

- Representation and influence in the legislature
- Continuing education
- Develop leadership skills
- Participate in research
- Resources
- Personal benefits
- Networking
- Playing a part in reshaping the future of nursing

and Canada was formed. At the World's Fair in 1890, a group of 15 nursing leaders began discussions about forming a professional association. Six years later, alumnae from the training schools organized the professional association now known as the ANA. Canadian members split from the original group in 1911 and formed their own professional association. The organizational structure of the ANA has undergone many changes through the years.

Currently, when an individual joins the ANA, he or she joins the national organization along with the constituent associations at the state and local levels. This method geographically groups smaller clusters of members together according to their practice interests.

In 1974, the Employee Retirement Income Security Act (ERISA), an amendment to the Taft-Hartley Act, allowed professional nursing organizations to be considered labor unions. United American Nurses is the collective bargaining organization representing the ANA. After this significant event, some nursing administrators and managers withdrew their memberships from ANA because of the potential conflict of interest between professional affiliation and the workplace. However, this change generated the development of other major nursing organizations: the Center for the American Nurse (CAN) and the American Association of Nurse Executives (AONE).

The ANA has been at the forefront of policy issues and represents nursing in legislative activities. The cabinets and councils of the ANA have provided standards of practice for both the generalist and the specialist. The 1988 *Social Policy Statement* document defined nursing practice at both the generalist and specialist levels; this is echoed in the current 2010 *Social Policy Statement*. The certifying organization of the ANA is the American Nurses Credentialing Center (ANCC), which has certified more than 92,000 RNs in different practice areas at both the generalist and specialist levels, along with more than 125,000 advanced-practice nurses (ANCC, 2017). The ANCC, a subsidiary of the ANA since 1991, identifies its mission as improving nursing practice and promoting quality health care service through several types of credentialing programs. The ANCC has created a modular approach to certification that enables the nurse to be recognized for multiple areas of expertise, not simply for competency in a core clinical specialty. There are 12 specialty, 5 nurse practitioner certifications, 1 clinical nurse specialist certifications, and an interprofessional certification (ANCC, 2018). As a result of their "open door 2000" program, all qualified registered nurses, regardless of their educational preparation, can become certified as generalists in any of the following specialty areas: ambulatory care, informatics, gerontology, medical-surgical, pediatrics, pain management, professional development, nursing case management, and psychiatric-mental health nursing, to name a few (ANCC, 2018). Check out the available nursing specialty certifications at https://www.nursingworld.org/our-certifications/.

Have you considered attaining a specialty certification? If so, what certification would you like to obtain?

In addition to certifying individual nurses, the organization also accredits educational providers (i.e., organizations that issue continuing education credits for professional programs), recognizes excellence in magnet nursing services through the ANCC Magnet Recognition Program, and educates the public about credentialing and professional nursing. This organization is electronically linked on the home page of the ANA (www.nursingworld.org).

American Nurses Foundation and the American Academy of Nursing

Two other organizations associated with the ANA are the American Nurses Foundation, founded in 1955, and the American Academy of Nursing (AAN), founded in 1973. Briefly described, these organizations serve special purposes in support of research and recognition of nursing colleagues. The American Nurses Foundation was established as a tax-exempt corporation to receive money for nursing research. With the establishment of the National Nursing Research Institute, the focus has changed to one of support in the areas of policy making and research or educational activities. The AAN has a membership of more than 1500 nursing leaders and was established as an honorary association for nurses who have made significant contributions to the nursing profession. When a nurse is elected to the AAN, she or he is called a Fellow, and the credential following the nurse's name is FAAN. You may have had instructors who were faculty in the AAN, or you may be working with a nurse who is a FAAN. These nurses can provide valuable mentorship for the new graduate. The official publication of this organization is *Nursing Outlook*.

International Council of Nurses

The International Council of Nurses (ICN), established in 1899, is the international organization representing professional nurses. The focus of this nursing organization is on worldwide health care and nursing issues; it meets every 4 years and is headquartered in Geneva, Switzerland. The ICN has been involved in the development of ethical guidelines for the recruitment of nurses from low-income nations. Many European nations have adopted an ethical code and restrict their recruiting from 150 low-income nations (Anderson & Isaacs, 2007).

National League for Nursing

The NLN was established in 1952; however, the beginning of NLN can be traced back to the 1893 organization of the American Society of Superintendents of Training Schools for Nurses of the United States and Canada. Between the late 1800s and the early 1900s, seven nursing organizations formed and joined under the collective name and function of the NLN. One of the unique features of the NLN is that both individuals and agencies are members. The NLN adopted a strategic plan in 1995 to place community-based health care education and health care delivery at the center of its focus and activities (NLN, 1995). The NLN continues to foster improvement in nursing services and nursing education, and offers annual educational summits so that nursing faculty and leaders in all types of nursing education programs can come together. Non-nurses can also join the NLN, fulfilling its purpose of promoting the consumer's voice in some nursing policies. The NLN has a biennial convention and publishes *N&HC: Perspectives on Community* (called *Nursing and Health Care* before 1995), *NLN Update*, and numerous other publications that can be obtained by calling 800-669-1656 or by visiting their website at www.nln.org.

Before 1997, the NLN functioned as an accrediting body in all levels of nursing education. In 1997, the NLN created an independent organization called the National League for Nursing Accrediting Commission (NLNAC) to accredit educational and professional nursing programs. This organizational change was in response to new standards established by the US Department of Education (USDOE). This step was taken to separate accrediting activities from membership activities and to respond to the Higher Education Act Amendment of 1992. In 2013, NLNAC changed its name to the Accreditation Commission for Education in Nursing (ACEN) to maintain continued recognition by the USDOE as a Title IV Gatekeeper. This recognition by the USDOE ensures that nursing students enrolled in an accredited nursing education program continue to receive Federal Student Aid. Also during 2013, the National League for Nursing Commission for Nursing Education Accreditation (NLNCNEA) was established as another accreditation service of the NLN, which is **not** for Title IV purposes. Is your school an ACEN or CNEA-accredited institution? To find out, visit their websites at http://acenursing.org/ or http://www.nln.org/accreditation-services/.

National Student Nurses' Association

The NSNA is a fully independent organization with a membership of approximately 60,000 nursing students throughout the United States. NSNA mentors the professional development of future nurses and facilitates their entrance into the profession by providing educational resources, leadership opportunities, and career guidance.

The organization was formed in 1952. Becoming a member of the NSNA may be viewed as a way to begin the "professional" socialization process. There are local school chapters as well as state and national level memberships. Often, members of the NSNA serve on selected committees of the ANA and speak to the ANA House of Delegates regarding student-related issues. The quarterly journal, *Imprint*, is published by the NSNA. Visit their website at www.nsna.org.

Organization for Associate Degree Nursing

This group was organized in 1986 as an outgrowth of several state organizations. Texas was the first state to have a chapter, which was started in 1984. Membership in the Organization for Associate Degree Nursing (OADN) is open to AD nursing graduates, educators, and students. Individuals, states, agencies, and other organizations may also join. There are state and national chapters. The mission of this organization is to be the advocate for AD nursing education and practice while supporting advanced nursing education through academic progression. OADN strives to maintain eligibility for RN licensure for graduates of AD programs, to promote AD nursing programs in the community, to provide a forum for discussion of issues affecting AD nursing, to develop partnerships and increase communication with other health care professionals, to increase public understanding of the AD nurse, to participate at state and national levels in the formation of health care policies, and to facilitate legislative action supporting the activities of OADN. Visit their website at http://oadn.org/.

American Association of Colleges of Nursing

This organization is the national voice for university and 4-year college educational programs in nursing and has a membership of more than 500 colleges. The mission of the organization is to serve the public interest by assisting deans and directors in improving and advancing nursing education, research, and practice. This organization publishes a newsletter and a bimonthly nursing journal called the *Journal of Professional Nursing*. In the past few years, it has formed a subsidiary for credentialing purposes. That organization is the Commission on Collegiate Nursing Education (CCNE). This autonomous accreditation agency serves only baccalaureate and higher degree programs in the accreditation process. Additional information on either organization can be found at www.aacn.nche.edu.

American Board of Nursing Specialties

Significant growth in specialty practice in nursing has been evident since the late 1990s. Throughout the 1980s and 1990s, specialty organizations met annually as the National Federation of Specialty

Nursing Certifying Organization to discuss issues in certification and nursing practice. This organization dissolved, and many of the specialty organizations joined the American Board of Nursing Specialties (ABNS) in 1991. The ABNS was established to create uniformity in nursing certification; it now represents more than 25 specialty nursing organizations that promote specialty practice and address certification issues associated with specialty practice. The ABNS functions as a consumer advocate in promoting nursing certification.

As a recent graduate, are you interested in a particular specialty nursing practice area? How and when do you anticipate obtaining specialty certification? How will you include membership in a professional organization in your 5-year career-educational plan? Do you know the benefits of being a certified nurse? Do you work with nurses who are certified in their specialties?

American Assembly for Men in Nursing (Formerly Known as the National Male Nurses Association)

The purpose of AAMN is to recruit men into the profession of nursing, support men who are nurses in professional growth endeavors, and provide a framework for nurses to influence factors that affect men as nurses. At the time of this publication, the AAMN has chapters in 19 states (AAMN, 2018).

The American Red Cross

The American Red Cross is an international organization of approximately 190 Red Cross organizations around the world. Nurses of the American Red Cross pioneered public health nursing in the early 1900s. The American Red Cross is a voluntary agency that is supported by contributions and plays an important role in providing disaster relief and education in first aid and home health and in organizing volunteers to assist in hospitals and nursing homes. Nurse volunteers with the Red Cross play a significant role in assisting those who have been affected by natural disasters.

In summary, professional organizations play a significant role in enhancing the image of nursing. Their impact is seen in both educational and practice issues for generalist and specialist nurse roles. Organizations provide a voice for nursing in policy issues and serve to unite nurses as a group of professionals. Ultimately, it may be nursing organizations that will serve as the catalyst for change in the health care system, and their impact will be felt in the next century.

CONCLUSION

Throughout the past century, the image of nursing has undergone many changes. The portrayal of nurses in the media has impacted the public perception of both male and female professional nurses. How will nurses continue to refine, intensify, and manage the image of nursing for the future? Will the self-image of nursing change public perception? Nursing is defined as a profession. Participation in the political side of health care, active involvement in professional organizations, a dedication to furthering academic advancement through progression of all nurses, and a commitment to the improvement of nursing's self-image are all ways to meet the upcoming challenges both in the nursing profession and in this dynamic health care environment.

The questions will go on and on, and the answers will come from nurses in clinical practice, education, and research. These issues, which have a significant impact on nursing's professional image, must be resolved so nursing continues to move forward as a profession. As a recent graduate, you are the future of this exciting transition. The question to ask yourself is: What can I do to improve and maintain the image of nursing and the integrity of the profession? Change can and does begin with one person who is willing to step forward and make a difference. Is that you?

🌐 RELEVANT WEBSITES AND ONLINE RESOURCES

American Association of Colleges of Nursing
Joint statement on academic progression for nursing students and graduates. https://www.aacnnursing.org/News-Information/Position-Statements-White-Papers/Academic-Progression

Bureau of Labor Statistics. Occupational Outlook for Registered Nurses
http://www.bls.gov/ooh/healthcare/registered-nurses.htm#tab-1

Carnegie Foundation for the Advancement of Teaching
Book highlights from educating nurses: A call for radical transformation. http://archive.carnegiefoundation.org/elibrary/educating-nurses-highlights

Discover Nursing (Johnson & Johnson)
Information for nursing students and all nurses. https://www.discovernursing.com/

Institute of Medicine
The future of nursing: Leading change, advancing health. http://www.nationalacademies.org/hmd/Reports/2010/The-Future-of-Nursing-Leading-Change-Advancing-Health.aspx

BIBLIOGRAPHY

Aiken, L., Cimiotti, J., Sloane, D., Smith, H., Flynn, L., & Neff, D. (2011). The effects of nurse staffing and nurse education on patient deaths in hospitals with different nurse work environments. *Medical Care, 49*(12), 1047–1053. https://doi.org/10.1097/MLR.0b013e3182330b6e.

American Assembly for Men in Nursing (AAMN). (2018). *Advancing men in nursing.* Retrieved from http://www.aamn.org/.

American Nurses Association. (2015). *Code of ethics for nurses with interpretive statements.* Silver Spring, MD: ANA.

American Nurses Association. (2015). *Nursing: Scope and standards of practice* (3rd ed.). Silver Spring, MD: ANA.

American Nurses Association. (2010). *Social policy statement.* Kansas City, MO: ANA.

American Nurses Credentialing Center. (2018). *Our certifications.* Retrieved from https://www.nursingworld.org/our-certifications/.

American Nurses Credentialing Center. (2017). *2017 ANCC certification data.* Retrieved from https://www.nursingworld.org/~499e5e/globalassets/docs/ancc/2017-certification-data-for-website.pdf.

Anderson, B., & Isaacs, A. (2007). Simply not there: The impact of international migration of nurses and midwives—perspectives from Guyana. *Journal of Midwifery & Women's Health, 28*(6), 392–397. https://doi.org/10.1016/j.jmwh.2007.02.021.

Arrigoni, C., Alvaro, R., Vellone, E., & Vanzetta, M. (2016). Social media and nurse education: An integrative review of the literature. *Journal of Mass Communication & Journalism, 6*, 1. https://doi.org/10.4172/2165-7912.1000290.

Bostridge, M. (2008). *Florence Nightingale: The woman and her legend.* London: Viking Press.

Brenan, M. (2017). *Nurses keep healthy lead as most honest, ethical profession. GALLUP.* Retrieved from https://news.gallup.com/poll/224639/nurses-keep-healthy-lead-honest-ethical-profession.aspx.

Caplow, T. (1954). *The sociology of work.* Minneapolis: University of Minnesota Press.

Cohen, S., & Bartholomew, K. (2008). *Our image, our choice: Perspectives on shaping, empowering, and elevating the nursing profession.* Marblehead, MA: HCPro.

Darbyshire, P., & Gordon, S. (2005). Exploring popular images and representations of nurses and nursing. In J. Daly, S. Speedy, D. Jackson, V. Lambert, & C. Lambert (Eds.), *Professional nursing: Concepts, issues, and challenges* (pp. 69–92). New York: Springer Publishing.

Donelan, K., Buerhaus, P., Desroches, C., Dittus, R., & Dutwin, D. (2008). Public perceptions of nursing careers: The influence of the media and nursing shortages. *Nursing Economics, 26*(3), 143–150.

Gordon, S. (2004). Nurses and public communication: Protecting definitional claims. *Journal of Nursing Management, 12*, 273–278. https://doi.org/10.1111/j.1365-2834.2004.00486.x.

Gordon, S., & Nelson, S. (2005). An end to angels. *American Journal of Nursing, 105*(5), 62–69. https://doi.org/10.1097/00000446-200505000-00031.

Gramlich, J. (2018). *8 facts about Americans and Facebook. Pew Research Center.* Retrieved from http://www.pewresearch.org/fact-tank/2018/10/24/facts-about-americans-and-facebook/.

Groves, B. (2007). An image problem: From TV to silver screen. *The Record.* Retrieved from http://www.nursingadvocacy.org/news/2007/may/06_record.html.

Health Resources and Services Administration (HRSA). (2010). *HRSA study finds nursing workforce is growing and more diverse.* Washington, DC: HRSA. Retrieved from http://www.hrsa.gov/about/news/pressreleases/2010/100317_hrsa_study_100317_finds_nursing_workforce_is_growing_and_more_diverse.html.

Health Resources and Services Administration (HRSA). (2013). *The U.S. nursing workflow: Trends in supply and education.* Washington, DC: HRSA. Retrieved from https://bhw.hrsa.gov/sites/default/files/bhw/nchwa/projections/nursingworkforcetrendsoct2013.pdf.

Jacobs-Summers, H., & Jacobs-Summers, S. (2011). *The image of nursing: It's in your hands.* Retrieved from http://www.nursingtimes.net/nursing-practice/clinical-zones/educators/the-image-of-nursing-its-in-your-hands/5024815.article.

Kalisch, B. J., Begeny, S., & Neumann, S. (2007). The image of the nurse on the internet. *Nursing Outlook, 55*(4), 182–188.

Kalisch, B. J., & Kalisch, P. A. (1983). Anatomy of the image of the nurse: Dissonant and ideal models. *American Nurses Association Publications* (G-161), 3–23.

Kaplan, M. (2000). *Why isn't nursing more newsworthy? Medscape Nursing.* Retrieved from https://www.medscape.com/viewarticle/408390.

Mee, C. (2006). Painting a portrait: How you can shape nursing's image. *Imprint, 53*(5), 44–49.

Muehlbauer, P. (2012). How can we improve the way the media portrays the nursing profession? *ONS Connect,* (12), 21.

National Council of State Boards of Nursing (NCSBN). (2018). *Active RN licenses: A profile of nursing licensure in the U.S.* Retrieved from https://www.ncsbn.org/6161.htm.

National Organization for Associate Degree Nursing. (2012). *Joint statement on academic progression for nursing students and graduates.* Retrieved from https://www.oadn.org/leading-initiatives/apin-news/item/65-ana-joint-statement.

Nelson, S. (2011). The image of nurses—the historical origins of invisibility in nursing. *Texto & Contexto - Enfermagem, 20*(2), 223–224. https://doi.org/10.1590/S0104-07072011000200001.

Nursing-Informatics. (2003). *The in/visibility of nurses in cyberculture.* Retrieved from http://visiblenurse.com/visiblenurse1.html.

Pavalko, R. (1971). *Sociology of occupations and professions.* Itasca, IL: Peacock.

Peck, J. L. (2014). Social media in nursing education: Responsible integration for meaningful use. *Journal of Nursing Education, 19*, 1–6. https://doi.org/10.3928/01484834-20140219-03.

Peplau, H. (1952). *Interpersonal relationships in nursing.* New York: Putnam Press.

Rezaei-Adaryani, M., Salsali, M., & Mohammadi, E. (2012). Nursing image: An evolutionary concept analysis. *Contemporary Nurse, 43*(1), 81–89. https://doi.org/10.5172/conu.2012.2725.

Robb, I. H. (1900). *Nursing ethics: For hospital and private use.* Cleveland, OH: E. C. Koeckert.

Strauss, A. (1966). *The structure and ideology of American nursing: An interpretation in the nursing profession.* New York: Wiley.

Stokowski, L. A. (2012). Just call us nurses: Men in nursing. *Medscape Nurses.* Retrieved from http://www.medscape.com/viewarticle/768914_7.

Talotta, D. (1990). Role conceptions and professional role discrepancy among baccalaureate nursing students. *Image: Journal of Nursing Scholarship, 22*(2), 111–115. https://doi.org/10.1111/j.1547-5069.1990.tb00186.x.

Thielst, C. B. (2013). *Social media in health care: Connect, communicate, collaborate* (2nd ed.). Chicago: Health Administration Press.

U.S. Department of Health and Human Services, Health Resources and Services Administration, National Center for Health Workforce Analysis. (2014). *The future of the nursing workforce: National- and state-level projections, 2012–2025* (pp. 2012–2025). Rockville: MD: Author.

Ventola, C. L. (2014). Social media and health care professionals: Benefits, risks, and best practices. *Pharmacy and Therapeutics, (39)*7, 491-499, 520.

What's the big deal about naughty nurse images in the media? (2010). Retrieved from www.truthaboutnursing.org/faq/naughty_nurse.html.

Wilson, D. (2009). Meet the men who dare to care. Johns Hopkins Nursing, VII(2). Retrieved from http://web.jhu.edu/jhnmagazine/summer2009/features/men_in_nursing.html.

UNIT III

Nursing Management

10

Challenges of Nursing Management and Leadership

Peggy J. Black, MSN, RN, NE-BC*

ⓔhttp://evolve.elsevier.com/Zerwekh/nsgtoday/.

Leaders don't force people to follow—they invite them on a journey.
Charles S. Lauer

Outstanding leaders go out of their way to boost the self-esteem of their personnel.
If people believe in themselves, it's amazing what they can accomplish.
Sam Walton

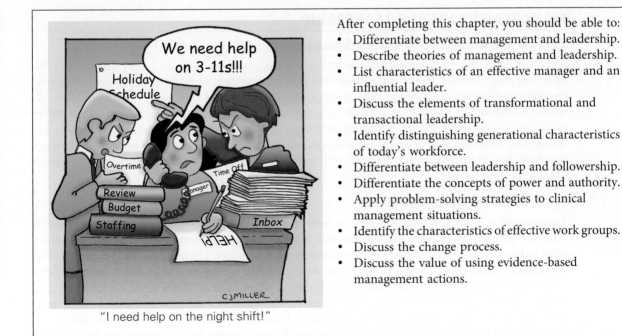

"I need help on the night shift!"

After completing this chapter, you should be able to:

- Differentiate between management and leadership.
- Describe theories of management and leadership.
- List characteristics of an effective manager and an influential leader.
- Discuss the elements of transformational and transactional leadership.
- Identify distinguishing generational characteristics of today's workforce.
- Differentiate between leadership and followership.
- Differentiate the concepts of power and authority.
- Apply problem-solving strategies to clinical management situations.
- Identify the characteristics of effective work groups.
- Discuss the change process.
- Discuss the value of using evidence-based management actions.

*We would like to acknowledge **Joann Wilcox, RN, MSN, LNC,** for her past contributions to the chapter.

As you move closer to meeting your goal of becoming a graduate nurse, give consideration to understanding the role of the nurse as a manager and as a leader. You might be thinking:

I do not want to be a manager; I am just a recent graduate!
OR
I want to take care of patients, not be a paper pusher!
OR
Am I ready to be followed by others?

Nursing, in any role, is a *people business. Management* is the process of effectively working with people. When you accept your first position as a recent graduate nurse, it is important to realize that you are becoming a part of a work group where members spend at least a third of their day interacting with each other. Therefore, registered nurses must be prepared to use varying levels of management skills, enhanced by interpersonal, followership, and leadership skills, to be effective in their role as a provider of patient care and as a member of the care team.

There are multiple levels of management that a registered nurse can practice. The specific level depends on the experience, competency, and defined role of the individual nurse. For example, as a recent graduate, you will have *primary management* responsibility for the patients for whom you will be providing care. This will include planning and coordinating the care with other nursing personnel, with health care staff, and with the patient and family members. Provision of this level of management is expected from all registered nurses who practice in the acute-care environment.

MANAGEMENT VERSUS LEADERSHIP

What Is the Difference Between Management and Leadership?

Although the terms *management* and *leadership* are frequently interchanged, they do not have the same meaning. A leader selects and assumes the role; a manager is assigned or appointed to the role. Leaders are effective at influencing others; managers, as providers of care, supervise a team of people who are working to help patients achieve their defined outcomes. Managers also have responsibility for organizational goals and the performance of organizational tasks such as budget preparation and scheduling. Although it is desirable for managers to be good leaders, there are leaders who are not managers and, more frequently, managers who are not leaders! So, let us discuss the actual differences in more detail.

The Functions of Management

Management is a problem-oriented process with similarities to the nursing process. Management is needed whenever two or more individuals work together toward a common goal. The manager coordinates the activities of the group to maintain balance and direction. There are generally four functions the manager performs: *planning* (what is to be done), *organizing* (how it is to be done), *directing* (who is to do it), and *controlling* (when and how it is done). All of these activities occur continuously and simultaneously, with the percentage of time spent on each activity varying with the level of the manager, the characteristics of the group being managed, and the nature of the problem and goal.

According to Norman (2018), planning is generally considered a basic management function and one on which managers should spend a significant part of their time. The foundation for all planning begins with the development of goals that reflect the mission and vision of the organization and defining strategies that will be implemented to meet and maintain that mission and vision. The next level of planning is used daily as a part of determining the requirements for accomplishing the work to be done and ensuring that what is needed is available. This planning must be congruent with the strategies for meeting the mission and vision of the organization. Along with this approach, a manager must also be able to plan for contingencies, which, if not addressed, will interfere with accomplishing what needs to be done. When managing a patient-care unit, which needs specific resources 24 hours a day, one can be certain that the unexpected will happen. Being prepared for the unexpected is a key function of a nurse manager.

Staff nurses practice the elements of planning as the plans of care for each patient are developed. For this process, the patient's current status and goals are assessed to determine what needs to occur during the time one is assigned to provide that care. The interventions needed are selected to advance the patient to the point of meeting his or her defined goals. This process of management of patient care uses the same planning skills as those used by someone who has the responsibility of managing staff.

Organizing occurs as the manager aligns the work to be done with the resources available to do that work (Norman, 2018). This requires knowledge of all parts of the work and a clear understanding of the competencies required of those who will be performing the assigned work. The manager must consider not only the licensing regulations but also the facility's policies when organizing the assignment of work. For example, licensing regulations may allow a licensed practical nurse to administer defined intravenous medications, but the facility policy may not allow that level of employee to perform that procedure. Another example would be that the licensing regulations for registered nurses do not specify that a newly licensed nurse cannot be assigned to work in a critical care unit. However, facility policy may state that registered nurses who wish to work in a critical care unit must have 1 year of other experience before being assigned to critical care service. Knowing this information prevents the manager from making decisions that may be unacceptable.

The next phase of management is providing direction or supervision. The manager retains accountability for ensuring the work is completed in a timely and competent manner. Additionally, staff members need to complete assigned work according to standards, policies, guidelines, and procedures with the understanding that the manager will provide sufficient observation and assessment of care being delivered to ensure that the care provided is safe and complete. When patient care falls below minimum standards, the manager has two actions to take. The first is to make certain the care and safety of the patient are addressed by ensuring the proper care is provided, and the second is to address the performance of the staff who did not provide the care as assigned. Managers need to be able to make decisions regarding the level of supervision needed by each staff member. Managers must also be able to motivate staff toward reaching their full competence to perform the assigned work with minimal observation and direction.

Staff nurses who are managing the care of patients need to have a clear understanding of the relevant policies, guidelines, and procedures related to the care provided and must be confident that they are competent to provide that care. The staff nurse must be cognizant of the expected outcomes of the care to be provided and how to determine if progress toward those outcomes is occurring. Actions to take when outcomes are not being met must be understood by the staff nurse who is managing the care.

Controlling is the last aspect of the planning function of the nurse manager. Most of the controls in health care facilities exist because health care is a highly regulated system, and much of what must be done is dictated by governments, insurers, evaluating agencies, health policy, and institutional policy. The effective manager needs to be cognizant of the regulations that affect his or her area of practice and must be able to clearly communicate the essence of these regulations to the staff. Staff members need to have a thorough understanding of regulations and the implications of noncompliance with these regulations. An example of external controls imposed because of regulations is the elimination of the use of certain dangerous abbreviations when a physician writes a medication order (see Chapter 11 for a list of abbreviations). This regulation is a part of The Joint Commission (TJC) Standards, as well as Standards from the Centers for Medicare & Medicaid Services (CMS). Although the initial focus of this regulation is on the physician, registered nurses may not implement an order that includes these eliminated abbreviations.

Control by the manager may also be demonstrated through data collected when reviewing quality of care to determine the level of compliance with standards and other quality monitors. These data give the manager the ability to validate observations, because these observations can represent the outcomes of care that has been provided. For instance, if the rate of hospital-acquired infections continues to be above the expected level, the manager has the information needed to implement and mandate interventions to reduce the number of infections.

> Florence Nightingale was an early nursing leader. What characteristics of a manager did she also demonstrate?

What Are the Characteristics and Theories of Management?

Active interest in management as a separate entity was first noted as part of the industrial revolution. The *traditional theory* developed at that time was based on the premise that there was a need to have the highest productivity level possible from each worker (Wertheim, n.d.). This theory is the basis for the hierarchy that has dominated much of management theory for almost two centuries. This type of management is also known as the bureaucratic theory of management, defined as "dividing organizations into hierarchies, establishing strong lines of authority and control." He [Weber, the author of this theory] stated that "bureaucracy is the basis for the systematic formation of any organization and is designed to ensure efficiency and economic effectiveness" (Mulder, 2017, p. 1). The manager who functions under the traditional theory follows rules closely and understands the concept of the division of labor and the chain-of-command structure. Historically, this kind of functioning was thought to be efficient and clear and was considered necessary to attain the most work from each employee. Throughout nursing history, this has been the theory on which the work of nurse managers was based. Since the mid-1990s, movement from this traditional theory has occurred, and more appropriate theories have been put into practice in multiple health care settings across the country.

Development of the *behavioral theory* of management (also called the *human-interaction* theory) followed the development of the traditional theory of management. This evolved as it became more evident that the humanistic side of management needed to be addressed (Hellriegel et al., 1999). Employees seeking recourse from some of the rules of hierarchy looked for assistance outside of their place of work, for instance, in the growing labor unions. Employers recognized the need to consider the human side of productivity to maintain a stable, satisfied workforce.

This was followed by the introduction of *systems theory*, which considers inputs, transformation of the material, outputs, and feedback (Hellriegel et al., 1999). Systems theory is implemented when consideration is given to the impact of decisions made by one manager on other managers or on parts of the system as a whole. This is important in health care, because it helped management move from making decisions in the traditional manner, in which departments functioned as though they were independent, to recognizing the interdependence of departments on each other. Recognizing that patients cannot be treated as though they are a number of separate and distinct parts has promoted the understanding and importance of systems theory. Behavioral theory, as it relates to management, considers the attitudes and needs of the employee, whereas systems theory examines the possible outcomes of all individuals affected by a decision.

The last theory of management to be considered is the *contingency theory*, which is also referred to as the *motivational theory* (Hellriegel et al., 1999). This theory focuses on the manager's ability to blend the elements of the earlier theories, use those elements to determine what motivates people to make choices, and thereby develop the most effective methods to complete the work that needs to be done. All of these theories are directed toward ensuring that employees are as productive and efficient as possible when working to meet the organizational goals or targets.

Consider how you might gain information about the management theory used in the facility in which you are seeking employment. What questions would you ask as a part of the interview process? Why is this important to you?

What Is Meant by Management Style?

You will experience a variety of management styles in your nursing practice. These styles follow a continuum from *autocratic* to *laissez-faire* (Fig. 10.1).

The *autocratic manager* uses an authoritarian approach to direct the activities of others. This individual makes most of the decisions alone without input from other staff members. Under this style of management, the emphasis is on the tasks to be done, with less focus on the individual staff members who perform the tasks. The autocratic manager may be most effective in crisis situations when structure and control are critical to success, such as during a cardiac arrest or code situation; however, this style of leadership is not effective for long-term use. In general, the autocratic manager will have a difficult time in motivating staff to become part of a satisfactory work environment, because there is minimal recognition of the contributions of staff to the work that needs to be done and minimal focus on the necessary relationships that make up the successful health care team. Many individuals,

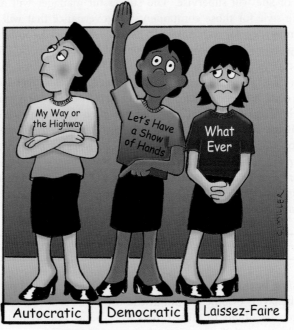

FIG. 10.1 Management styles.

particularly those from generations after the Baby Boomers, will not stay in a position in which autocracy is the major style of management.

On the other end of the continuum is the *laissez-faire manager*, who maintains a permissive climate with little direction or control exerted. This manager uses a hands-off approach and allows staff members to make and implement decisions independently and relinquishes most of his or her power and responsibility to them. Although this style of management may be effective in highly motivated groups, it may not be effective in a bureaucratic health care setting that requires many different individuals and groups to interact.

In the middle of the continuum is the *democratic manager*. This manager is people-oriented and emphasizes effective group functioning. The goals of the group are identified, and the manager is perceived as a group member who is also the group's organizer and keeps the group moving in the defined direction. The environment is open, and communication flows both ways. The democratic manager encourages participation in decision making; he or she recognizes, however, that there are situations in which such participation may not be appropriate, and the manager is willing to assume responsibility for a decision when necessary. The democratic style is a blend of autocracy and laissez-faire with assurances that the extreme ends of the continuum are rarely, if ever, necessary.

One example of a democratic manager following either the behavioral or contingency theory would be a manager who creates a Nurse Practice Committee on his or her unit. This committee would have some defined authority and responsibility to address specific items in the practice environment, such as schedules and practices on the unit. This type of committee supports the idea that staff and management are interdependent in governing the successful practice environment (McComiskey, 2017).

To be a successful manager working in a hierarchical organization, the nurse manager will need to adopt a democratic style of management, one that is flexible enough to adapt to the changing roles of nursing staff. The nurse manager should be willing and able to share power with the same people whom he or she will supervise. The successful manager will also need to acquire an element of laissez-faire style for those components of governance that will be under the auspices of the staff. It will be important for staff nurses to develop a balanced combination of autocracy and laissez-faire as they implement shared governance (stakeholder participation in decision making) that will include quality of care and peer review.

As is evident, the continuum of management styles ranges from what might be considered total control to complete freedom for subordinates. In choosing a management style, the manager must decide on levels of control and freedom and then determine which trade-offs are acceptable in each situation. Behaviors vary from telling others what to do to relinquishing to another group within the organization the authority for portions of the work to be done. As a new staff nurse, your initial involvement in management occurs when you manage the care of a group of patients. The next involvement may be as a part of the shared governance model that may be developing in your facility. As you gain experience and knowledge, it is important for you to develop an understanding of which style you should use, depending on what you hope to achieve.

> Look at managers on the units where you are assigned for clinical practice. How do they fit into these categories?

Leadership, in contrast, is a way of behaving; it is "a social process in which one individual influences the behavior of others without the use of threats or violence" (Ellis, 2016, p. 59) (Fig. 10.2). Leadership is the ability to cause others to respond, not because they have to but because they want to. Leadership is needed as much as management for effective group functioning, but each role has its place. The manager determines the agenda, sets time limits, and facilitates group functioning. The

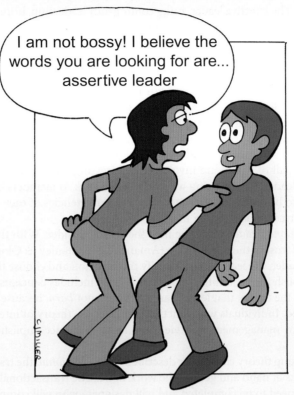

FIG. 10.2 Is this reflective of leadership?

leader "models change, establishes trust, sets the pace, creates the vision, [provides] focus, and builds commitment" (Manion, 1996, p. 148).

What Are the Characteristics and Theories of Leadership?

The many attempts to define what makes a good leader have resulted in a variety of studies and proposals. Researchers have tried to identify the characteristics or traits necessary to be a good leader. Several of these studies have defined the concept of a *born leader,* implying that the desired traits are inherited. This is often referred to as the "Great Man" theory, because it was first identified when leadership was generally thought to be a male quality, particularly as it related to military leadership (Amanchukwu, Stanley, & Ololube, 2015). With later research, it became clear that desired leadership traits could be learned through education and experience. It also became clear that the most effective leadership style for one situation was not necessarily the most effective for another and that the effectiveness of the leader is influenced by the situation itself. As leadership theories continue to develop, emphasis is more on what the leader does rather than on the traits the leader possesses.

Several other theories of leadership are worth discussing. The first is *contingency leadership,* which says that leadership should be flexible enough to address varying situations. Although this may sound complicated, it can be compared with your approach to patient care. As a nurse, you individualize a patient care plan based on the needs of the individual. Then the plan is implemented using available resources. The effective leader, using contingency leadership, brings the same flexible approach to each individual situation where leadership is required.

Situational leadership theory resulted from the study of the contingency theory. Under situational leadership theory, the leader attempts to function more closely in the situation being addressed. Blanchard and Hersey (1964) defined the situational leader as one who creates a positive atmosphere to maintain a good relationship with the team, has high expectations of the group, and maintains power but is flexible when necessary. A situational leader analyzes the needs of the current situation and then selects the most appropriate leadership style to address that particular situation. The selected style depends on the competencies of each employee who will be helping address the current situation. The authors state that a good situational leader may use different styles of leadership for different employees, all of whom are involved in addressing the same situation. This is not unlike what you, as a team leader, will be doing when assigning work to members of your work team. The assignments will need to be individualized based on the competencies of each member of the team to help ensure the patient-care goals can be met.

Interactional leadership is the next theory to consider. With this theory, the focus is on the development of trust in the relationship (Amanchukwu, Stanley, & Ololube, 2015). To be a successful interactional leader, the leader must identify the situation and choose the appropriate strategies and people to accomplish the goal. Interactional leadership includes concepts of behavioral theories, which begin to address the theory that leaders are *made* and not *born*, because the needed behaviors can be taught and learned. Individuals who function based on the theory of interactional leadership use democratic concepts of management and view the tasks to be accomplished from the standpoint of a team member.

Leadership theory can also be described as *transactional*; the transactional leader has a greater focus on the tasks at hand and getting the work done. The transactional leader will structure and clarify the tasks that need to be completed and will designate who will complete the tasks. Transactional leaders will discuss expectations and outcome with followers and will explain how the results are to be accomplished. Rewards will be given if the expectations and outcomes are achieved. The basis for the relationship between leader and follower is that punishment and reward motivate people. Transactional leaders seek equilibrium so the vision can be reached and intervene only when it appears that goals will not be attained (Asiri et al., 2016).

This leadership theory does not sound like one that many would be encouraged to embrace or follow, because the rewards are ultimately one-sided. However, the transactional approach to leadership still exists in most organizations, generally at the management level, because incentives are provided to gain a defined level of productivity. One may believe that this approach is closer to management than leadership, which may explain why it might not be effective at other levels in the organization. You can view a video about transactional versus transformational leadership here: https://youtube/ddt_IGMMOrI?t=75

Transformational leadership was introduced in the 1970s. This form of leadership occurs when the leader guides staff in knowing and understanding what their role is in the institution; the leader is willing to take risks, embraces change, and creates a positive work environment. The transformational leader is futuristic; has a strong, clear vision that has developed through listening, observing, and analyzing; and finally, truly buys into the vision to dramatically change the way things are currently done (Amanchukwu, Stanley, & Ololube, 2015).

As mentioned in an Institute of Medicine (IOM) report (2003b, 2004, and 2011), transformational leadership is the IOM's recommended leadership style, because this style focuses on change and how the leader adapts to change. A transformational leader does not view change as a barrier, but rather as an opportunity.

According to Sherman (2012), there are four key elements that characterize the transformational leadership style. The first element is idealized influence, meaning that the transformational leader is a "role model for outstanding practices which in turn inspires followers to practice at this same level." Inspirational motivation, the second element, is demonstrated by the leader being able to "communicate a vision" in a manner that others understand. Intellectual stimulation and individual consideration are the last two elements and address the fact that the leader values staff input and creativity while continuing to coach and mentor staff, recognizing there are both group and individual needs and issues to consider (Sherman, 2012, p. 64).

Characteristics of transformational leaders, according to Kouzes and Posner (2015), are that these leaders are courageous change agents who believe people will do what is right when provided direction, information, and support. They are also value-driven visionaries and lifelong learners; they lead by example and are individuals who can successfully handle the complexities of leadership. To accomplish their goals, they effectively change the traditional way of leading, which is often from the office, to leading from the place where the action is occurring.

Transformational leadership will be implemented when it is clear to the strong, visionary leader that current situation(s) cannot be "fixed" using the traditional methods that have worked in the past. In the early 1990s, Leland Kaiser, a renowned health care futurist, discussed transformational leadership, identifying the transformational leader as the primary architect of life in the 21st century. Many of the predictions made by Kaiser are now being recognized as part of transformational leadership. An example of this is what has occurred at Virginia Mason Medical Center, as the leadership of that organization took on the task of transforming health care at that facility (Kenney, 2011). The entire leadership team has worked together to ensure that this transformation occurred as envisioned.

If transactional leadership involves the use of leadership power over rewards and punishments, transformational leadership can be characterized as a process whereby the leader and followers work together in a way that changes or transforms the organization, the employees/followers, and the leader. It recognizes that real leadership involves transformation and learning on the part of the follower *and* leader. As such, it is more like a partnership, even though there are power imbalances involved.

Transactional leadership involves telling, commanding, or ordering (and using contingent rewards), whereas transformational leadership is based on inspiring, getting followers to buy in voluntarily, and creating a common vision. Transformational leadership is what most of us refer to when we talk about great leaders in our lives and in society.

The nurse shortage is a good example of a problem in which the solution will most likely be found by transformational leaders. It is evident that the old ways of fixing the nurse shortage have not been effective. Managers, lawmakers, and organizations have tried increasing wages, paying bonuses, recruiting foreign nurses, mandating staff-to-patient ratios, adding nurse-extenders, and implementing flexible shifts. None of these methods has had any long-lasting effects because they do not address the conflicts that have occurred as newer generations of nurses have reached the level where they want control of their practice as granted by education and licensure. A transformational leader understands the basis of these conflicts and develops a vision that will address the needs of the people involved in the conflict.

One might anticipate that the Chief Executive Officer and the Chief Nursing Officer of a hospital would both be transformational leaders. These leaders have a responsibility to see the bigger picture and to be able to describe that vision or picture to others. Porter-O'Grady (2003a) describes this type of leader as one who can "stand on the balcony" (p. 175). From this position, the leader can monitor the ebb and flow of the organization and determine in which direction the organization is moving. To be effective, the transformational leader must have a vision that can be put into words for others to understand. Check out the relevant websites and online resources at the end of the chapter for additional information on transformational leadership.

Although most leaders tend to lean toward one of the theories discussed here, fluctuations from one to another can occur, depending on the particular situation. In the health care setting, good leaders carefully balance job-centered and employee-centered behaviors and activities to meet both staff and patient needs effectively (Critical Thinking Box 10.1).

> ### ? CRITICAL THINKING BOX 10.1
>
> Consider your educational and clinical experiences. What leadership theories and styles have you observed? What management styles have you observed? Are there specific personality traits that enhance a person's performance in these two roles?

An effective leader works toward established goals and has a sense of purpose and direction. She or he must also be aware of how her or his behavior impacts the workplace. Emotions, moods, and patterns of behavior displayed by the leader will create a lasting impression on the behavior of the team involved. It is critical for the leader to be aware of this impact if she or he is going to be effective in managing and leading a team (Porter-O'Grady, 2003b). Rather than push staff members in many directions, the effective leader uses personal attributes to organize the activities and *pull* the staff in a common direction.

The most current theory addressing the changing environment in which we work is the *complexity theory* of leadership. The complexity theory addresses the "unpredictable, disorderly, nonlinear, and uncontrollable ways that living systems behave" (Burns, 2001, p. 474). This theory indicates that we need to look at systems, such as those in health care organizations, as patterns of relationships and the interactions that occur among those in the system.

Complexity theory is complex! However, the basis of the thinking can most easily be understood by comparing traditional ways of analyzing an organization to the ways in which this analysis would be accomplished using the complexity theory. The traditional method used to understand an organization is to "break a system into smaller bits and when we believe we understand the bits we put them all back together again and draw some conclusions about the whole" (IOM, 2011). Complexity theory examines the whole rather than the sum of its parts, because breaking a system apart removes all the impact of the human relationships that affect the whole.

Smyth (2015) asked, "Why do we struggle to achieve our goals in clinical outcomes, safety and financial performance in [health care facilities] when these facilities are chockfull of brilliant, well-intentioned people?" It is because those people bring factors such as varying levels of competence and performance and differing emotional states—all of which can have an unpredictable impact on the outcome. In general, most health care organizations work solely through hierarchies, which does not allow for the openness needed to achieve the best solutions to problems being addressed.

Following complexity theory, one understands that organizations are "organic, living systems" (Anderson et al., 2005) in which people act quickly and use knowledge sharing and patterns of relationships rather than the rules of a hierarchy. When leading according to the principles of complexity, change is understood as successful when accomplished by individuals as they adapt to variations in the environment and not as the linear managers dictate. "However, we are still mired in the hierarchical structures we have lived with for more than fifty years—going up and down the chain of command to make decisions …." (Smyth, 2015).

Although it was more than 35 years ago, Greenleaf (1977) developed the idea of a *servant leadership* model. This model focuses on others as its number-one priority—the need to serve others first. Service leaders are more focused on the concerns of others before themselves (Kouzes & Posner, 2015). This type of leadership promotes teamwork, collaboration, and total participation from the team. The defining qualities of a servant leader are the ability to listen and truly understand, the ability to be open-minded and nonjudgmental, and the ability to deal with ambiguity and complex issues. Other qualities include the ability to be a servant, help others, and teach before functioning as the leader.

As we complete the discussion on the theories and characteristics of leaders and managers, it becomes evident that there are more differences between these two groups than those briefly identified in the opening paragraph of this discussion. According to Walters (2016) the major differences are

- Leaders focus on effectiveness, and Managers focus on efficiency.
- Leaders ask what and why, and Managers ask how.
- Leaders deal with people and relationships, and Managers deal with systems, controls, and policies.
- Leaders initiate innovation, and Managers maintain the status quo.
- Leaders look to the horizon, and Managers look to the bottom line (pp. 1–2).

Management Requires "Followership"

Individuals can manage things, processes, and people. When thinking of nurse managers, it is generally assumed they are managing people who are managing the care of patients. When being managed, one is in the role of a follower—an essential role in the safe and effective delivery of patient care. The role of the follower is not always considered when discussing management functioning, but it is obvious that those who are expected to follow the direction of the manager are essential to the success of the manager.

Followership is "the ability to take direction well, to get in line behind a program, to be a part of a team and to deliver what is expected of you" (McCallum, 2013). There cannot be a truly effective leader without competent followers, because if the followers fail in the work they are doing, the manager will not be able to successfully complete the assigned work.

From the previous information, it appears there are significant differences between leadership and followership. Although this is true, the interconnections between these two functions make the differences almost irrelevant. "You can't have one without the other!" truly applies. They need each other to exist and to have a purpose. "You cannot be considered a leader if you have no one following you."

Although many believe that followers are subservient to leaders, leaders must be beholden to followers for both to be successful. Followers must have the ability to think critically and actively participate in the successful completion of the leadership directions/goals (Miller, 2007).

When assessing the success of a team or staff group, it is important to remember that, at times, individuals assume either leadership or followership roles or assume both leadership and followership roles during the completion of required tasks. A successful leader understands the role of followers and recognizes that followers should receive credit for the success of the team/group just as the leader receives this credit (Miller, 2007).

THE TWENTY-FIRST CENTURY: A DIFFERENT AGE FOR MANAGEMENT AND FOR LEADERSHIP

The face of leadership is changing, and this is very evident in nursing and health care. Changes in health care are altering some of the foundations of nursing practice. Shorter hospital stays and emerging therapeutics require less, but perhaps more intense, clinical time and challenge the need for certain nursing interventions that have become routine over time. Nurses are becoming increasingly frustrated with the reality that the nursing care they were taught to provide—and they feel they need to provide—is not possible given the decreased time spent with their patients (Porter-O'Grady, 2003c). This dissatisfaction may be compounded by the conflict between established nurses and upcoming generations of nurses. In general, younger generations of nurses have accepted the newer foundations of practice, whereas tenured staff often resist these changes. Thus, the task of learning how to bridge the gaps in a multi-generational staff must be added to the nurse manager's other responsibilities.

> "For the first time in history, five generations are working side by side, each with different leadership, communication and career development styles" (Moss, 2017, p. 1).

The generations that have retired or will soon retire in the nursing profession include those born during the 1920s, 1930s, and early 1940s, sometimes referred to as the Silent Generation or the Veteran Generation. This generation makes up less than 1% of the U.S. workforce and lead with a command-and-control style. The generations currently active in the nursing profession include the Baby Boomer Generation, born more or less between 1945 and 1960. This generation makes up about 27% of the workforce and are retiring daily. Generation X, born between 1960 and 1980, and the Millennial Generation (Generation Y), born between 1980 and 2000, make up between 35% and 37% of the workforce. Both of these generations like their independence and like direct communication with leader(s). The fifth generation in the workplace were born after 2000 and are referred to as Generation Z or Generation Now; however, this generation has the fewest individuals practicing in nursing. Some authors and social sources place Generation Z beginning as early as 1995 (Patel, 2007). Although they might not have completed nursing school, they could be in the health care field as nurse aides or technicians. This generation likes technology and best communicates via email and text messages (Moss, 2017).

The leadership of health care in the 21st century has been and will continue to be significantly affected by the diverse generations in today's workplace. These generational groups have major differences in communication styles, in what motivates them, in what turns them off, and in their workplace ideals (Clark, 2017). Great diversity also exists in the beliefs, attitudes, and life experiences of these various generations. Consequently, generational diversity has been recognized as one of the major factors precipitating conflict in the workplace. Box 10.1 lists the time frames of each generation and the percentage of each generation currently in the workforce.

> "Effective teamwork can be fostered in an environment that acknowledges the values, talents and work ethics of each generational cohort" (Clark, 2017, p. 386).

BOX 10.1   CHARACTERISTICS OF GENERATIONS

Silent or Veteran Generation: Born between 1925 and 1942—accounts for 1% of the current workforce
Baby Boomers: Born between 1943 and 1960—accounts for 27% of the current workforce
Generation X: Born between 1961 and 1979—accounts for 35% of the current workforce
Generation Y: Born between 1980 and 2000—accounts for 37% of the workforce
Generation Now/Gen Z: Born between 1995 and now—the newest group to the job market accounts for 1%–2% of the current workforce

From Moss, D. (2017). *5 generations + 7 values = endless opportunities*. Society for Human Resource Management. Retrieved from https://www.shrm.org/hr-today/news/hr-news/conference-today/pages/2017/5-generations-7-values-endless-opportunities.aspx.

The Silent or Veteran Generation

This oldest generation of nurses, which is also the group that is retiring or retired, was taught to rely on tried, true, and tested ways of doing things. Because of early experiences with economic hardship and living through the Great Depression of the 1920s and 1930s with their families, these nurses place high value on loyalty, discipline, teamwork, and respect for authority (Clark, 2017). Nurses from this generation have always worked within the hierarchy of management and diversity of leadership and are accustomed to the autocratic style of leaders and managers.

The Baby Boomers

The Baby Boomers make up the largest group of nurses working today, and fill the majority of nurse management positions today. Members of this group have a multitude of family responsibilities, frequently spanning three generations. In fact, this group is frequently referred to as the "sandwich generation," because these people are caught between caring for their children and caring for their own aging parents. Nurses in this group are very ambitious. They put in long hours and have a strong sense of idealism, both at home and at work. Baby Boomers value what others think, and it is important that their achievements are recognized. They have set and maintained a grueling pace between their family and employment responsibilities. This group has embraced technology as a method to increase productivity and to have more free time (Clark, 2017).

The individuals of the Baby Boomer generation are also most accustomed to working with autocratic leaders; they remain products of the hierarchical theory of leadership and management but are beginning to recognize and ask for some of the elements of the behavioral theory. They are also frequently challenged by nurses of younger generations, who see little value in hierarchical leadership in a system such as health care, which includes multiple groups and professions, some of whom have autonomy by licensure that is not recognized in a leadership hierarchy. By contrast, Baby Boomers are focused on building careers and are invested in organizational loyalty (Moss, 2017).

Generation X

Members of Generation X grew up in the information age; they are energetic and innovative. They are also hard workers, but unlike Baby Boomers, Gen X employees have little loyalty to, or confidence in, leaders and institutions. They value portability of their career and tend to change jobs frequently; they will stay in a position as long as it is good for them. This generation saw the downsizing of the 1990s, when organizational loyalty did not protect workers from loss of jobs or retirement. Thus, they tend to have little aspiration for retirement. The use of technology has initiated an expectation of instant response and satisfaction. Technology has shaped their learning style; they want immediate answers from a variety of sources (Clark, 2017). They want different employment standards, such as opportunities for self-building and responsibility for work outcomes. They want extensive learning and precepting, and they want their questions answered immediately.

Gen X nurses value their free time; therefore, flexible scheduling and benefits (daycare centers, liberal vacations, working from home) are important. They claim to be motivated by work that agrees with their values and demands (Clark, 2017). This group wants to work under motivational leadership with a democratic manager. If they do not find that kind of environment, they will have little reason to maintain employment in that institution.

Because most of the leaders and managers in health care are from the Baby Boomer generation, the conflict between these generations is certainly a significant contributor to the high turnover rate among younger nurses and the high rate of nurses finding employment outside of the hospital setting.

Generation Y

Members of Generation Y (also known as Generation Net, Nexters, or the Millennium Generation) were born between 1980 and 2000. This is the largest group, perhaps three times the size of Generation X; as such, this generation is having a formidable impact on the employment market. Those in their 20s and 30s are beginning to have an influence on how organizations are managed. This generation represents a large number of the children of the Baby Boomers. While the Baby Boomers were trying to master Windows and now the iPhone, these kids were playing with computers in kindergarten!

The impact of this generation is still being defined, but with the speed of generational changes, the impact of Generation Y may soon be integrated with the newest generation, currently labeled Generation Now. The Y Generation is smart and believes education is the key to success. For this group, diversity is a given, technology is as transparent as air, and social responsibility is a business imperative (Clark, 2017). Members of Gen Y are optimistic and interactive, yet they value individuality and uniqueness. They can multitask, think fast, and are extremely creative.

Managing this group will require a vastly different set of skills than exists in the market today. Generation Y nurses are not team players. They are in the driver's seat—they know that work is there for them if they want it. Focusing on understanding their capabilities, treating them as colleagues, and putting them in roles that push their limits will help managers recognize the potential of this group to become the highest-producing workforce in history (Clark, 2017). This is the most educated generation ever. Gen Y employees tend to change jobs frequently because they seek growth and expansion within the organization. If the opportunity to climb the corporate ladder is slow or nonexistent, they will move on to another job or organization (Clark, 2017). "They live in an era that offers instant gratification, instant information at the touch of a button. To [retain] a generation that sometimes has a short attention span, it's important to keep things constantly changing and evolving" (Fallon, 2016, p. 1). The hierarchy of health care leadership and management is generally not what they are seeking as a part of their employment because they will develop their own leadership position in whatever they are doing. How they function in the role of follower is still being determined, and the role of follower will likely be redefined by this fast-moving generation.

Generation Z or Generation Now

The newest generation is being called Generation Z or Generation Now. They have never lived without the Internet and other forms of rapid communication. This generation communicates through social media, such as Facebook, Twitter, Snapchat, and Instagram. LinkedIn is another avenue where young professionals connect and engage with like-minded people. "Social media is changing the way people communicate and is influencing their approaches to meeting their healthcare needs" (Flury, 2017, p. 272). This means they have never known a world without immediacy (Moss, 2017). The impact of this generation is already being felt in all aspects of our society and world. The way those in Gen Now/Gen Z think, act, find information, negotiate, and make decisions may make our present theories of leadership and management obsolete and just a part of our long history. Is this part of what Leland Kaiser envisioned when he talked about transformational leadership occurring when we were ready, or does Gen Now/Gen Z represent the emergence of a new leadership theory?

The challenge to nursing will be to develop a workplace, as well as a profession, that will be attractive to all these generations, particularly those who represent the mainstream of the workforce. Equally important is consideration by nurse leaders and managers of the unique differences that exist among the generations (Critical Thinking Box 10.2). According to Clark (2017), who has researched the different generations and the impact they have on health care organizations stated, "For healthcare organizations, these generational differences can enhance teamwork and improve patient care" (p. 394). Clark's research has validated the generational differences and the impact these differences are having on nursing. The key is to learn the art of compromise as these generations continue to learn to work together, and by understanding these generational differences, managers and leaders can "foster a work environment that embraces diversity and promotes productivity" (Clark, 2017, p. 394). Generation Z staff can show a new way to accomplish the work that is different from the task orientation of the older generations—both of which were, and are, appropriate for the system at the time. They perceive themselves to be leaders versus followers, which means management will need to do what can be done to "equalize" the perception of leaders and followers.

? CRITICAL THINKING BOX 10.2

What are the main issues, as stated by Clark (2017), of five generations in the workplace, and what are the implications?

Do employees understand customer needs?

Do employees understand how to interact with staff from the different generations?

How important is interaction among staff from different generations on patient satisfaction?

Do employees understand the workplace styles of different generations?

Example: A registered nurse from the Baby Boomer generation believes that when he/she gets a call to work on his/her day off, he/she should do this unless it is not possible from a family perspective. A registered nurse from Generation Y does not feel the same "level" of obligation to the workplace. The Baby Boomer "lives to work," whereas to Gen Y "works to live."

How does a leader address this difference to avoid an interstaff conflict?

How does the solution reflect staff understanding of patient satisfaction and outcomes, interaction with other staff members, and the differences among generations that are real and need to be respected and understood?

From Clark, K. R. (2017). Managing multiple generations in the workplace. *Radiologic Technology, 88*(4), 379–396. Retrieved from https://media.asrt.org/pdf/publications/RADT_Vol88_No4_Mammo.pdf#page=21.

Initially, there must be a focus on recruiting the younger generations into the health care fields, specifically into nursing. Emphasis must also be placed on retention of experienced nurses. These nurses are necessary to mentor the younger generations, and their experience is invaluable. Gurchiek (2016) works with young people and has outlined strategies for managing and motivating the younger generations (Boxes 10.2 and 10.3). Review these strategies—they are not new, nor are they exclusive to young employees. These strategies are applicable for every generation and every organization at any time (Critical Thinking Box 10.3).

? CRITICAL THINKING BOX 10.3

To what generation do you belong? How do your values regarding work and your personal characteristics fit that generation?

The changes in the way the younger generations relate to leadership and management may well be part of the reason more hospitals are becoming Magnet certified. Magnet is a comprehensive program relating to many aspects of nursing and nursing practice, but the basis for most of the success of the program is the acceptance of a change in the way practice is governed and controlled. Magnet facilities demonstrate a true implementation of shared governance in which the nursing staff has control of the clinical practice of nursing and practice aspects of the work environment (HCPro, 2016).

Up to this point, leadership has been considered primarily as a part of management. In 2004, and then expounding on the role in 2007, the American Association of Colleges of Nursing (AACN) created a group to develop a position of clinical nurse leader (CNL). As defined by the AACN (2018), the CNL is a master's degree–prepared registered nurse who focuses on:

- Care coordination
- Outcomes management

BOX 10.2   MOTIVATIONAL STRATEGIES FOR GENERATIONS X AND Y

1. Let them know that what they do matters.
   - When was the last time a letter from a patient who was very pleased with the care on a unit was shared with the staff? When was the last time management sat down with all of the unit personnel to tell them they are doing a good job? When was the last time the Chief Executive Office complimented the staff on a job well done?
2. Tell them the truth.
   - When did the managers on a unit acknowledge to the staff exactly what was going on? For example, the surgery schedule is going to be heavy this next week, there are going to have a lot of new admissions, and a lot of patients who will be going home. Acknowledge that the work level is going to increase, and ask whether any of the staff have suggestions for improving the coordination and workload assignments.
3. Explain why you are asking them to do it.
   - When a difficult time is anticipated, explain to the staff what is happening and why. Maybe a particular area of the hospital is overloaded and additional staff are being pulled from their regular units to help. These patients must be accommodated and cared for—this is why the hospital is there, and maintaining patient census is what pays the bills.
4. Learn their language.
   - When was the last time the unit manager, head nurse, or other manager actually sat down with the staff (all levels) to find out who they are and what they like to do? What are their priorities? Their family situations? What do they do on their days off?
5. Look for rewarding opportunities.
   - When did a staff member handle a particularly difficult patient situation very well with acknowledgment at that time given to the staff member? Give positive feedback when opportunities arise. Do not wait for a performance evaluation to do so.
6. Praise them in front of their peers and other staff.
   - Acknowledge a job well done at a staff meeting or in the presence of people who are important to that person.
7. Make the workplace fun.
   - Making the hospital work environment fun can sometimes be a little difficult, but there are opportunities for humor if we just look for them. Patients share a lot of humor with the staff. Is the staff encouraged to share that humor with the rest of the unit personnel? When something funny happens to staff, are they encouraged to laugh and share with others?
8. Model behavior.
   - Does the behavior of the unit manager or head nurse model the behavior the manager is expecting others to exhibit? What about confidentiality? Is it expected of the personnel? Does the manager practice it as well?
9. Give them the tools to do the job.
   - What about effective communication skills or, perhaps, good customer service skills? The health care industry is in the business of providing a service for the customer—the patient. Training is offered for the technical skills—new equipment, procedures, policies—but what about training for the skills necessary to handle people? How about skills to deal effectively with the angry patient, the difficult doctor, the outraged family (Clark, 2017)?

These strategies are from Gurchiek, K. (2016). *What motivates your workers? It depends on their generation*, Society for Human Resource Management. Retrieved from https://www.shrm.org/resourcesandtools/hr-topics/behavioral-competencies/global-and-cultural-effectiveness/pages/what-motivates-your-workers-it-depends-on-their-generation.aspx.

BOX 10.3   MOTIVATIONAL STRATEGIES FOR GENERATION Z OR GENERATION NOW

In addition to Box 10.2, consider these strategies specific to Generation Z:
1. Look at where they are going for information.
   - They are always on the lookout for something new. It is the job of the leader or manager to stay current to keep up with them.
2. Make your message relevant.
   - They know when they are being "talked to." They consider their time precious, and they want you to use their time wisely.

- Transitions of care
- Interprofessional communication and team leadership
- Risk assessment
- Implementation of best practices based on evidence
- Quality improvement (para 1).

The rationale for this position is that with the changing health care needs of this society, the CNL is critical to successfully addressing the many significant clinical issues facing the system during a time when resources are becoming limited. Having a highly prepared individual in the clinical setting is meant to positively impact the current patient safety issues by identifying and managing risk while meeting standards of quality clinical care.

As stated by Tornabeni and Miller (2008), "Improved patient care requires more nurses, better educated nurses and revised systems and environments for delivering patient care" (pp. 608–609). Many factors support this need; it is known that with shorter lengths of stay and increasing complexity of care and treatment, stability in the delivery of nursing care is essential for reaching the defined outcomes of that care. Stability in nursing care delivery must also be accomplished so that use of available resources is maximized, while patient handoffs and risks are minimized as these outcomes are reached.

This role is a combination of a bedside nurse, case manager, clinical educator, and team leader. The introduction of the CNL role also addresses a long-standing complaint about acute-care nursing practice. Within the clinical setting, the two major opportunities for advancement were to assume a management position or become a clinical educator. Both essentially remove individuals from the bedside, which is the heart of our practice. With this new clinical role, nurses who wish to advance to a different role while providing direct patient care now have the opportunity to do so.

To understand the success of the CNL role, consider this example: Performance measures were identified for the staff of a surgical unit as a part of a quality review program. These performance measures involved antibiotic use and venous thromboembolism prophylaxis. To effectively transform the nurses' thought processes and gain buy-in to this performance improvement, the need for a cultural change was identified. A CNL was made available to assist the staff in understanding the need for this change and the benefits that would come about after this change was implemented. The CNL is a transformational leader who uses more than one style of leadership to motivate his or her employees to perform at a level of excellence (AACN, 2018).

POWER AND AUTHORITY IN NURSING MANAGEMENT

Do You Know the Difference Between Power and Authority?

Having power means that one can effect change and influence others to meet identified goals. Having authority relates to a specific position and the responsibility associated with that position. The individual with authority has the right to act in situations for which she or he is held responsible within the institutional hierarchy. This is a role most often assumed as a part of management.

Power and responsibility always go hand in hand!

What Are the Different Types of Power?

There are many different types of power, so let us discuss those that are most common. *Legitimate power* is power that is connected to a position of authority. The individual has power as a result of the position. The head nurse has legitimate power and authority as a result of the position held.

Reward power is closely linked with legitimate power in that it comes about because the individual has the power to provide or withhold rewards. If supervisors have the power to authorize salary increases or scheduling changes, then they have reward power.

Coercive power is power that is derived from a fear of consequences. It is easy to see how parents would have coercive power over children based on the threat of punishment. This type of power can also be used with staff members when, for example, there is the threat of receiving unfavorable assignments. However, when considering the characteristics of the upcoming generations, this sort of power may not be effective with them.

Expert power is based on specialized knowledge, skills, or abilities that are recognized and respected by others. The individual is perceived as an expert in an area and has power in that area because of this expertise. For instance, the enterostomal therapist has expertise in the care of individuals who have had ostomies. Therefore, staff nurses seek out the therapist as a resource and use the expert's knowledge to guide the care of these patients. The CNL is another example of a nurse-expert who acts as a resource for others.

Referent power is power that a person has because others closely identify with that person's personal characteristics; they are liked and admired by others. Individuals who have knowledge that is needed by others to function effectively in their roles possess *information power*. This type of power is perhaps the most abused! An individual may, for example, withhold information from subordinates to maintain control. The leader who gives directions without providing needed information on the rationale or constraints is abusing information power.

Leadership power is the "capacity to create order from conflict, contradictions, and chaos" (Sullivan & Decker, 2012). This is possible when the staff or people involved in the conflicts trust a leader who can influence people to respond because they want to respond!

Leaders and managers need to understand the concept of power and how it can be used and abused in working with others. Nurses, on the whole, need to identify ways to increase their power within the health team. Graduate nurses need to be aware of and willing to implement methods and resources to increase their personal power. As they gain experience in the staff nurse role, they can develop expert power by increasing competency in their roles and clinical skills.

> If you really want to see the best use of power, see a nurse who is actually providing the care that a patient needs and how many times he or she has to manage the system, massage the system, and find ways through the system just to get good care for patients. That's power.
>
> **Beverly Malone, PhD, RN, FAAN**

Refining interpersonal skills that enhance the ability to work with others can expand many types of power, such as information, referent, and leadership power. These skills include clearly and completely communicating information that people need to know while gaining support for work to be done through delegating or by encouraging staff to step forward to do what's necessary to accomplish the stated goals. Demonstrating a willingness to give and receive feedback while providing positive communication is also important when working to develop and enhance power in working with others.

It is also important to recognize what detracts from power. Impressing others as disorganized, either in personal appearance or in work habits, engaging in petty criticism or gossip, and being unable to say *no* without qualification are some of the behaviors that can detract from power.

Today there is much discussion in nursing about the importance of power and the concept of *empowerment*. To *empower* nurses is to provide them with greater influence and decision-making opportunities in their roles. The realization of greater power in the profession depends on the willingness of administrators to allocate this power and of nurses to accept it, along with the accompanying responsibility.

There are some people in the health care system who believe that nurses are powerless—among these people are many nurses. Part of this perception of powerlessness is related to the fact that minimal time is spent learning leadership skills and more than 50% of nurses are not educated at the baccalaureate level where most of the leadership skills are discussed and practiced.

It is essential that nurses, who spend more time than others at a patient's bedside, feel confident in identifying "activities that can improve patient care or help the unit run more smoothly" (Garner, 2011). The growth in the number of Magnet hospitals is making a significant difference and decreasing the number of nurses who are hesitant to let their power show!

The basis for practice in Magnet-credentialed facilities is the empowerment of staff to make decisions that directly affect the practice of registered nurses who are providing direct care. This is accomplished through the development of a culture that supports the decentralization of management, power, and authority anywhere that registered nurses are providing care. A clearly delineated structure for making appropriate decisions and clearly communicating them must be in place and accessible to all registered nurses in the organization. The responsibility for monitoring compliance and outcomes is also shared by the registered nurse staff rather than leaving this important function solely to management.

MANAGEMENT PROBLEM SOLVING

How Are Problem-Solving Strategies Used in Management?

Management is a *problem-oriented process*. The effective manager analyzes problems and makes decisions throughout all the planning, organizing, directing, and controlling functions of management. Problem solving can be readily compared with the nursing process (Table 10.1). This is because the nursing process is based on the scientific method of problem solving. The two are essentially the same, as can be seen by comparing the steps of one with the other.

As with the nursing process, problem solving does not always flow in an orderly manner from one step to the next. Throughout the process, feedback is sought, which may indicate a need to alter the plan to reach the desired objective. The most critical step in either process is identifying the problem (identified as the *nursing diagnosis* in the nursing process). Frequently, the originally identified *problem* may be too broad or unclear. Only the symptoms of the problem may be seen initially, or there may be several overlapping problems. If an approach is used to relieve only the symptoms, the problem will still exist. The good manager will guide the process of identifying the problem by asking questions such as "What is happening?" "What is being done about it?" "Who is doing what?" and "Why?" It is important to differentiate among facts and opinions and to attempt to break down the information to its simplest terms. Think of it as being a detective looking for every clue!

TABLE 10.1 NURSING PROCESS VERSUS PROBLEM SOLVING	
NURSING PROCESS	**PROBLEM SOLVING**
Assessment	Data gathering
Analysis/nursing diagnosis	Definition of the problem
Development of plan	Identification of alternative solutions
Implementation of plan	Implementation of plan
Evaluation/assessment	Evaluation of solution

After the problem is clearly identified, the group should *brainstorm* all possible solutions. Often the first few alternatives are not the best or most practical. Identifying a number of viable alternatives usually provides more flexibility and creativity. All possible solutions must fall within existing constraints, such as staff abilities, available resources, and institutional policies. The more complex the problem, the more judgment is required. In some cases, the problem may extend beyond the manager's scope of responsibility and authority; therefore, it may be necessary to seek outside help.

After identifying all the alternatives, each must be evaluated based on the changes that would be required in existing policies, procedures, staffing, and so forth, and the effect these changes would have. Ask "What would happen if …" questions to clarify the short- and long-term implications of each alternative. Keep in mind that the perfect solution is not possible in most situations.

Problem solving represents a choice made among possible alternatives that are thought to be the best solutions for a particular situation. At its best, problem solving should involve ample discussion of the possible solutions by those who are affected by the situation and who possess the knowledge and power to support the possible solution. After an alternative is selected, it should be implemented unless new data or perspectives warrant a change. Feedback should be sought continuously to provide ongoing evaluation of the effectiveness of the solution. Remember that simply choosing the best alternative does not automatically ensure its acceptance by those who work with it!

Evidence-Based Management Protocols and Interventions

Just as nurses are expected to practice using evidence-based protocols and interventions for clinical decision making, managers are expected to use management practices that are based on demonstrated outcomes. This may be difficult to accomplish, because management practices are often deeply embedded in the culture of an organization. Making a change to practices that are known to work from practices that may have worked in the past may be viewed as a challenge to the core philosophy of that organization.

> *If a manager is guided by the best logic and evidence and if they relentlessly seek new knowledge and insight, from both inside and outside their organizations, to keep updating their assumptions, knowledge and skills, they can be more effective.*
>
> **Pfeffer & Sutton, 2006**

To accomplish this, the manager needs to develop a commitment to searching for, and using, processes and solutions that are factually based, so the decisions that are made lead to the intended outcomes (Pfeffer & Sutton, 2006). It is believed that there is much peer-reviewed information regarding managing organizations that is not used because of the desire to do things as they have always been done—knowing that they do work some of the time.

The example provided in an article in the *University of California Riverside Human Resources Workplace Health and Wellness* relates to the use of stand-up meetings versus the traditional sit-down meetings. Evidence indicates that during stand-up meetings it took 33% less time to make decisions (Bowles & Chobdee, 2018). Using this model could save an organization many hours a year that could be put to another productive use or could be eliminated from the payroll. However, very few organizations use this model for meetings, even in the face of the clear evidence regarding the impact it would have on the organization.

Appropriate hand washing between patient encounters is a problem that has affected health care since the 1850s. The solution sounds simple—wash your hands between patient encounters—but history demonstrates that having leaders/managers who require this solution has not been effective. Random surveys of staff in health care facilities demonstrate that rates of hand washing average "about 38.7%" (World Health Organization [WHO] in Armellino et al., 2012).

A study conducted in 2009 to 2010 by Armellino et al. used "remote video auditing with and without feedback" to determine the rate of hand hygiene among the staff in an intensive care unit (2012, p. 1). The prefeedback period demonstrated a hand hygiene rate of less than10%. The visualization of performance with feedback resulted in a hand hygiene rate of 81.6%. The evidence from this study demonstrates that staff are more compliant when they know they are being observed and when they receive feedback regarding these observations.

Although this study pertained to hand hygiene, the elements of observation and feedback can be assumed to increase compliance with other aspects of practice that require minimal variation in the practice. Secondarily, one can take this evidence a bit further and correlate the infection rate in this intensive care unit during the period in which the 81.6% hand hygiene compliance occurred. Consider what changes in patient status and hospital costs would be noted if an 81.6% hand washing compliance resulted in a major reduction in hospital-acquired infections.

One would expect health care providers to have the routine down pat *and* to set the highest standard for compliance. Unfortunately, that's not the case. Experts estimate that health practitioners comply with recommended hand hygiene procedures less than 50% of the time—contributing to some dire consequences. Nearly two million hospitalized patients in the United States develop infections each year, and the most common transmitters of health care-associated pathogens are the contaminated hands of health care workers. Eighty thousand patients die from these infections each year (Goldmann, 2018, para 2).

A study conducted by Garcell, Arias, Miranda, Jimenez, and Serrano (2017) used direct observation for hand hygiene compliance, because it is the standard practice recommended by the WHO to monitor compliance. They used nurses who were specifically trained in what measures to observe and record. The observations were conducted on seven units. The findings indicated that the greatest areas of compliance were among health care providers who came in contact with blood or body fluids (80%) and after patient contact (85%). The lowest area of compliance was washing hands before patient contact (34%). Handwashing compliance before the observations ranged from 58.6% to 70%, and due to the observations, compliance ranged from 85.1% to 91.6%.

Although this study pertained to hand hygiene, the elements of observation and feedback can be assumed to increase compliance with other aspects of practice that require minimal variation.

What other aspects of practice can you think of that can be measured using direct observation? Using regular feedback?

Nurses who are prepared to practice using evidence-based clinical information may find that using these same skills and approaches to management is the norm. This will require a collaborative working relationship with the tenured management staff, who may see this result in a shift of power to the staff who do use evidence-based management practices as a regular part of decision making.

Frequently, implementing the solution to a problem causes several other problems to arise. This can be avoided if the selected solutions are evidence based and if they are tested before implementation to identify any areas that may be negatively affected by the new solution. This testing should be a formal process that follows the steps of a failure modes and effects analysis, which is meant to identify and address risk points that may not have been evident when the solution was selected. Many of you will be given the opportunity to work with others to complete an analysis of new procedures, for example, before that new procedure is fully implemented. If problems arise after the analysis, testing, and implementation, the new problems should not be allowed to impede the implementation process. Instead, pause and consider each problem individually, solve it, and then return to the plan that was tested. The old adage "If at first you don't succeed, try, try again" is most appropriate when applying the problem-solving process, but using evidence-based solutions should keep repeat trials to a minimum. Remain positive, confident, and flexible! Let us apply the process to an actual problem.

John is the head nurse on a busy medical-surgical unit with 32 patients. Staff members have complained to him that too much time is being spent during the morning change-of-shift report. After asking questions and seeking additional information, John determines that a clearer definition of the problem is that the night charge nurse does not give a clear, concise report. Researching the peer-reviewed literature for solutions that address end-of-shift communication and involving the night charge nurse in the problem-solving process help define the problem. Is it because the nurse does not have adequate knowledge of how to give a change-of-shift report? Or is it a flaw in the report system that does not allow for adequate communication to occur?

Can you see how, after the problem has been clarified, it becomes more amenable to an acceptable, and perhaps even easy, solution?

How Are Problem Solving and Decision Making Related?

By definition, problem solving and decision making are almost the same process, with one very notable difference. Decision making requires the definition of a clear objective to guide the process. A comparison of the steps of each illustrates this difference (Table 10.2). Although both problem solving and decision making are usually initiated in the presence of a problem, the objective in decision making may not be to solve the problem but only to deal with its results. It is also important to distinguish between a good decision and a good outcome. A *good outcome* is the objective that is desired, and a *good decision* is one made systematically to reach this objective. A good decision may or may not result in a good outcome. Although it is desirable to have both good decisions and good outcomes, the good decision maker is willing to act, even at the risk of a negative outcome.

Susan is the evening charge nurse on a medical unit that has a total of 24 patients. One of the patients is terminally ill and seems to be having a particularly difficult evening. The patient requires basic comfort measures but little complex care. Susan has a choice of assigning the patient to another registered nurse or delegating care to a nursing assistant. If she assigns the registered nurse, the workload for the other staff will be heavier, and she herself will be assigned to the terminally ill patient, to provide the care that cannot be delegated to the nursing assistant. Susan decides to assign the registered nurse because this patient requires the emotional and physical support best provided by a registered nurse. During the shift, the registered nurse spends time sitting with the patient. Close to the end of the shift, the patient dies. Was this a good decision with a bad outcome or a good decision with a good outcome?

Decision making is values based, whereas problem solving is traditionally a more scientific process. Efforts to acquire evidence-based information as one is identifying alternative solutions to problems

TABLE 10.2 PROBLEM SOLVING VERSUS DECISION MAKING

PROBLEM SOLVING	DECISION MAKING
Define problem	Set objective
Identify alternative solutions	Identify and evaluate alternative decisions
Select solution and implement	Make decision and implement
Evaluate outcome	Evaluate outcome

move the decision-making process into the scientific arena. Nurses will continue to make decisions based on personal values, life experiences, perceptions of the situation, knowledge of risks associated with possible decisions, and their individual ways of thinking, but these factors will be influenced by the availability of information and solutions that have been scientifically tested. Because of these variables, two individuals given the same information and using the same decision-making process may arrive at different decisions, but the probability of different decisions should be lower after evidence-based information is available.

In today's ever-changing health care environment, it is important for nurses and nurse managers to be effective in both problem solving and decision making. The good manager will evaluate the problem-solving or decision-making process based on criteria that provide a view of the big picture. These criteria include the likely effects on the objective to be met, on the policies and resources of the organization, on the individuals involved, and on the product or service delivered.

The quality of patient care depends on the ability of the nurse to effectively combine problem solving with decision making. To do so, nurses must be attuned to their individual value systems and understand the effect of these systems on thinking and perceiving. The values associated with a particular situation will limit the alternatives generated and the final decision. For this reason, the fact that nurses typically work in groups is beneficial to the decision-making process. Although the process is the same, groups generally offer the benefits of a broader knowledge base for defining objectives and more creativity in identifying alternatives. It is important for nurses to understand the roles of individuals within the group and the dynamics involved in working in groups to take full advantage of the group process. Chapter 11 focuses on communication, group process, and working with teams.

What Effect Does the Leader Have on the Group?

The leader's philosophy, personality, self-concept, and interpersonal skills all influence the functioning of the group. A leader is most effective if members are respected as individuals who have unique contributions to make to the group process. Can you remember our earlier discussion of the characteristics of a good leader? The ability to influence and motivate others is particularly important in the group process.

Whenever the combination of people in a group is altered, the dynamics are changed. If the group is in the working phase, it will revert to the initiating phase when a new person or persons are added and will remain there until they have been assimilated into the group and a new dynamic has been formulated. The most effective groups are those that have had consistent membership and are highly developed. These groups demonstrate friendly and trusting relationships; the ability to work toward goals of varying difficulty; flexible, stable, and reliable participation of members; and productivity with high-quality output. Leadership within these groups is democratic, and the members feel positive about their participation and the outcomes of the group process. Now let us apply these principles to a real situation!

When you graduate and accept a nursing position, you will become a new nurse in the work group, causing it to regress to the initiating phase. This is your opportunity to demonstrate to the members of the group that you are worthy of being included in the group. If this is your first nursing position, you will also demonstrate to the group that you are worthy of entering the nursing profession. During this time, you may experience feelings of loneliness, isolation, and distance that accompany the initiating phase. However, your feelings of pride, excitement, eagerness, and accomplishment should quickly eradicate those feelings of distance, because there is much to gain and much to offer when entering a new group with common goals.

Put your energy into forming supportive professional relationships, including the social aspects of these relationships. Seek and use feedback and ask for help in areas that are not as familiar to you, such as priority setting. As you contribute your individual talents to the group, you will move from being a dependent new person to full group membership. It is important that you do not underestimate the length of time that may be needed to accomplish this task! Group processes proceed very slowly in some cases, and it may be 6 months or more before you are accepted as a full member of the work group. Do not be discouraged! Instead, use this opportunity to gain information regarding what you can offer to the next new member of the group and what you can do to make transitioning from school to practice a positive experience.

Management skills come with experience in nursing, so do not be too hard on yourself during the transition phase. Identify experienced staff nurses who are effective at managing the care of their assigned patients and identify nurse managers who have the skills you would like to incorporate into your management style. Look at the positive side of working with staff nurses and various nursing managers as a means to assist you in the development of your personal management style. Develop the ability to think like a manager as you perform your assignments—always look at the big picture.

THE CHALLENGE OF CHANGE

How many times have you heard staff nurses complain about how powerless they feel about the lack of control they have over their work environment? They say they are frustrated with the amount and quality of patient care they are able to deliver and that staffing patterns are placing undue stress on them. Some will talk about leaving the acute-care environment to try some other aspect of nursing (perhaps home health) as a less stressful option. Why do they run from a situation, rather than thinking about how they can act to change it? Do they feel powerless to do so? Is it easier to withdraw and escape?

One thing we all know is that change is inevitable, particularly in today's health care delivery system. Economic factors have taken center stage, and cutbacks in all aspects of health care services are occurring. Additionally, the Patient Protection and Affordable Health Care Act of 2010 has brought changes to many aspects of health care. A major aspect of this act is that health insurance companies cannot set lifetime and yearly limits on what they spend for your medical coverage (HealthCare.gov, 2019). Consider the kinds of changes that this situation can create on an almost immediate basis. Are you prepared to accept the challenges ahead while continuing to provide quality care as a part of your professional obligation? Change can be like a truck with no driver at the wheel: It moves slowly and steadily toward you (see Fig. 10.3). You have three options: you can move out of the situation and perhaps miss some opportunities; you can just stand there and withdraw, doing what you are told just to avoid conflict; or you can start to run with it, jump on, and try to steer it in a positive direction.

So, how do you begin to direct the change that is on the horizon? The first thing to know about the change process is that it, too, has similarities to problem solving and the nursing process. Let us lay them out and compare the two processes (Table 10.3).

Does the information in Table 10.3 look familiar? Maybe it is not that hard to take control and be a change agent! The first thing you need to know about the change process is that resisting change is a natural response for most people. All of us are most comfortable in our state of equilibrium, where we feel in control of what we are doing. To handle change effectively, it is important to understand that every change involves adaptation. It requires a period of transition in which the change can be understood, evaluated in light of its impact on the individual, and, one hopes, eventually embraced.

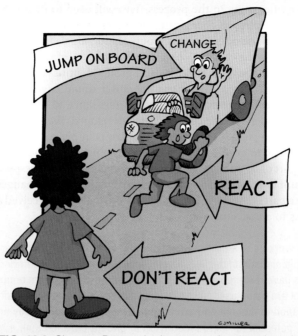

FIG. 10.3 Change: React, don't react, or jump on board.

TABLE 10.3 NURSING PROCESS VERSUS CHANGE PROCESS

NURSING PROCESS	CHANGE PROCESS
Assessment	Recognition that a change is needed; collect data
Identification of possible nursing diagnoses	Identification of problem to be solved
Selection of nursing diagnosis	Selection of one of possible alternatives
Development of plan	Implementation of plan
Implementation of plan	Implementation of plan
Evaluation	Evaluation of effects of change
Reassessment	Stabilization of change in place

There are various reasons for people's resistance to change and understanding them will help you to implement the change process more effectively. Here is a list of the most common factors that cause resistance to change:

- A perceived threat to self in how the change will affect the individual personally
- A lack of understanding regarding the nature of the change
- A limited ability to cope emotionally with change
- A disagreement about the potential benefits of the change
- A fear of the impact of the change on self-confidence and self-esteem

Kurt Lewin (1947) sought to incorporate these concepts in his Change Theory. He identified three phases in an effective change process: *unfreezing*, *moving*, and *refreezing*. In the *unfreezing phase*, all of the factors that may cause resistance to change are considered. Others who may be affected by the change are sought out to determine if they recognize that a change is needed and to determine their interest in participating in the process. You will need to determine whether the environment of the institution is receptive to change and then convince others to work with you.

The *moving phase* occurs after a group of individuals has been recruited to take on responsibilities for implementing the change. The group begins to sort out what must be done and the sequence of actions that would be most effective. The group identifies individuals who have the *power* to assist in making the plan succeed. *(What types of power would be most effective?)* The group also attempts to identify strategies to overcome the natural resistance to change—and how to achieve a cooperative approach to implement the change. Once developed, the plan is then put into place.

The *refreezing phase* occurs when the plan is in place and everyone involved knows what is happening and what to expect. Publicizing the ongoing assessment of the pros and cons of the plan is an important part of its ultimate success. Be certain someone is responsible for continuing to work on the plan so that it does not lose momentum. Finally, make the changes stick—or *refreeze*. This will make the change a part of everyday life, and it will no longer be perceived as something new. Now let us apply this process to a real situation!

Taneeka is working in a medical-surgical unit at a 200-bed acute-care hospital. She constantly hears her peers complaining about the lack of adequate nursing staff, and during the previous 3 months, two full-time staff nurses have resigned. To cover the unit, part-time staff from temporary agencies and from the hospital staffing pool are being used to supplement the remaining regular staff. Because these staff members have little orientation to the unit and are frequently assigned where they are needed the most, the continuity of care and a potential for increased errors in patient care became a major concern.

Rather than continuing to complain about the situation or considering leaving, Taneeka decided to act and try to steer the change truck. She approached a few of the nurses and initiated a discussion about the changes in staffing and how scheduling had become a nightmare for the charge nurse. She enlisted the support of several members of the staff to begin problem solving possible solutions. They agreed that increased staffing was probably not a possible immediate solution and agreed to work within the constraints that they had.

Several of the pool nurses were receptive to requesting that their assignment be limited to this one unit, and they agreed to schedule their hours to complement each other. This, in essence, would add a shared full-time position, at no additional cost, and would also provide consistency of patient care. When the proposal was presented to administrators, they agreed to support the idea based on its economic and patient-centered benefits.

Who Initiates Change and Why?

Another aspect to consider when evaluating change is to determine who wants the change and why. Is it the system? Is it management? Is it you, the nurse? Or is it the patient? There should be a specific rationale for change, and the identified change should be carefully planned, implemented, and evaluated to ensure the outcome is as anticipated. By identifying who is initiating the change and the reason for the change, the implementation plan can be better defined and understood, particularly regarding how implementation will affect the staff or the system.

The Change Truck—how will you respond?

React—move out of the way. Let the truck (change) pass you by. However, opportunities may be missed.

Do not act—just stand there and let the truck run over you. It will leave you behind and, more than likely, in worse shape than when you started.

Act—start running when you see it coming. Pace the truck until you can decide when to jump on and steer it in the direction you want to move.

System

The most common reason for change is that what you did before is no longer effective. For example, the electronic medical record is largely replacing the handwritten medical record system, because the old system does not allow integration of the information in the record. The handwritten record generates volumes of paper and is not adequate to keep pace with the number of patients and the need to access key information quickly from various individuals both inside and outside of the traditional hospital (home health nurse or hospice nurse at the patient's home).

Management

Change frequently occurs when new regulations are developed by agencies that license or approve the facility. This provides a new perspective regarding how the system currently operates and what part of the system needs to be changed to comply with the new regulation. A significant change in almost all areas of the hospital occurred with the implementation of the Health Insurance Portability and Accountability Act of 1996 (HIPAA) regulations. Employees at all levels needed to know the answers to these questions: "How will the implementation of HIPAA change my job? Do I know how to respond to a request for information?" (Critical Thinking Box 10.4).

? CRITICAL THINKING BOX 10.4

What changes have you made in your life?

How long did one situation last before it changed again?

You have just learned to deal successfully with the changes associated with being a student. Now you are facing the challenge of change again as you prepare for your role as a practicing registered nurse.

Patient

When customers are not satisfied, something within the system needs to change. What are the specific patient problems, and how can they be resolved? The fact that medical errors continue to occur at a high rate is of concern to patients or to people who may become patients. This has been publicized in the mainstream media for several years with minimal evidence that errors have been reduced. A continued high rate of medical errors makes the public want change and expect the system, management, and staff to create the solutions to this problem. Does change at this level require the use of transformational leadership and evidence-based decisions?

Yourself

Sometimes we impose change on ourselves. We may or may not like it, but we see a need for some aspect of change to occur (Table 10.4). Who has ever enjoyed being transferred to a different unit if the one we are working on is slated to close? Stop to consider how you are going to implement the change. How will your work environment be affected? If change involves other employees, include them as a part of that change. Gain the power that comes from working as a team.

Only when you feel threatened by a change will you go through the steps (i.e., resistance, uncertainty, assimilation, transference, integration) to conquer it (Wilson, 1996) (Fig. 10.4). All change will elicit some type of resistance. It is up to you to increase the impetus for change while decreasing resistance. The decision to be involved with change will help steer you in a direction that will be most beneficial.

TABLE 10.4 EMOTIONAL PHASES OF THE CHANGE PROCESS

EMOTIONAL PHASE	CHARACTERISTICS	INTERVENTIONS
Anxiety	The employee is not sure what will happen next and not sure what change will look like.	Explain how changes will affect the status quo.
Happiness	The employee feels good about the chance to get rid of things that don't work.	Listen to the employee about what they thought didn't work; correlate how the change will be better.
Threat	The employee is not sure how the change will affect her/him.	Explain how changes will affect them.
Fear	The employee is fearful of how the change will force him/her into a new way of thinking and doing things.	Validate fear and explain how the change will be a better solution.
Anger	The employee blames others for forcing the change and demonstrates envy, resentment.	Be assertive and assist with problem solving. Encourage the employee to determine the source of his or her anger.
Guilt	The employee is angry at her- or himself for not coping well.	Listen to the employee; validate feelings as normal, and identify some coping strategies with them.
Despair	The employee feels confused and apathetic; no energy left; nothing seems to work; sorrow, self-pity, and feelings of emptiness.	Encourage quiet time for reflection as inner search for identity and meaning occurs.
Hostility	The employee shows aggression toward him- or herself, others, and the change; diffused energy; feelings of powerlessness and insecurity and a sense of disorientation.	Encourage quiet time for reflection as inner search for identity and meaning occurs.
Acceptance	The employee becomes emotionally detached from the situation; begins to make sense of the change; some renewal of energy and willingness to take on new roles or assignments resulting from change.	Allow the employee to move at their own pace. Explain again the importance and the effects of the change.
Moving forward	The employee exerts control and is ready to make the change happen; positive attitude; willingly expends energy to explore new events that are occurring; reunification of emotions and cognition.	Assume a directive management style; assign tasks; provide direction.
Other emotions may include:		
Denial	The employee denies the reality that change will occur; experiences negative changes in physical health and emotional and cognitive behavior.	Actively listen, be empathetic, and use reflective communication.
Disillusionment	The employee decides the change isn't for her/him and leaves.	Offer stress-management programs or allow the employee to move on.

Adapted from Hills, R. (2016). The 12 emotional stages of change. Retrieved from https://peopledevelopmentmagazine.com/2016/10/06/12-emotional-states-change/.

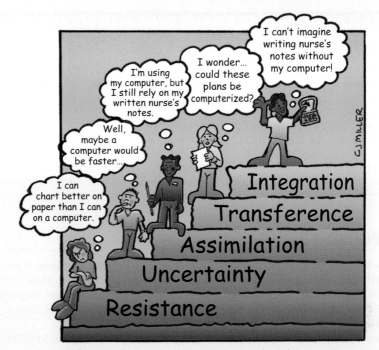

FIG. 10.4 Five steps toward conquering change.

CONCLUSION

As a new graduate, you will be facing many transitions, including the transition from a "newbie" providing direct care for assigned patients, to managing the care for a group of patients, to a team leader role where you are managing the care of a group of patients through a team of staff members. You may also be appointed to a formal management position or may assume the role of an informal, but powerful, leader. All of these phases or roles require the characteristics of a leader who can influence others, including patients, to respond because they want to respond.

Think about the characteristics of your generation—will these influence your management style as you consider how you will positively engage with all the members of your staff? How will you contribute to resolving some of the differences in the nursing environment? Will you research the literature to find those actions that have proven effective, or will you do what has always been done? Understanding management and leadership along with your generational characteristics will facilitate the development of a leadership and management style that is a reflection of you. Improving your ability to reach out to those outside the organization through communication and the literature will provide you with the tools to build effective nursing management practices while leading a successful team.

⊕ RELEVANT WEBSITES AND ONLINE RESOURCES

7 Great Leadership Traits
https://www.youtube.com/watch?v=2IEp4TVpxgA

Institute for Healthcare Improvement (IHI Open School)
L101: Introduction to health care leadership. http://www.ihi.org/education/ihiopenschool/Pages/default.aspx

Leadership Styles: Which Type of Leader Are You?
https://youtube/ddt_IGMMOrl?t=75

Sherman, R. O.
Becoming a transformational nurse leader. http://www.emergingrnleader.com/transformational-nurse-leader/

BIBLIOGRAPHY

Amanchukwu, R. N., Stanley, G. J., & Ololube, N. P. (2015). Management: A review of leadership theories, principles and styles and their relevance to educational management. *Management, 5*(1), 6–14. https://doi.org/10.5923/j.mm.20150501.02. Retrieved from https://www.researchgate.net/publication/283081945_A_Review_of_Leadership_Theories_Principles_and_Styles_and_Their_Relevance_to_Educational_Management.

American Association of Colleges of Nursing. (2018). Clinical nurse leader (CNL). Retrieved from https://www.aacnnursing.org/CNL.

Anderson, R. A., Crabtree, B. F., Steele, D. J., & McDaniel, R. R. (2005). Case study research: The view from complexity science. *Qualitative Health Research, 15*(5), 669–685.

Armellino, D., Hussain, E., Schilling, M., Senicola, W., Eichorn, A., & Dlugacz, Y. (2012). Using high-technology to enforce low-technology safety measures: The use of third-party remote video auditing and real-time feedback in healthcare. *Clinical Infectious Diseases Advance, 54*(1), 1–7. https://doi.org/10.1093/cid/cir773. Retrieved from http://www.ncbi.nlm.nih.gov/pubmed/22109950.

Asiri, S. A., Rohrer, W. W., Al-Sumrimi, K., Da'ar, O. O., & Ahmed, A. (2016). The association of leadership styles and empowerment with nurses' organizational commitment in an acute health care setting: A cross-sectional study. *BMC nursing, 15*(38). https://doi.org/10.1186/s12912-016-0161-7.

Blanchard, K., & Hersey, P. (1964). *Management of organizational behavior: Leading human resource.* New York: Morrow.

Bowles, L., & Chobdee, J. (2018). Standing meeting guidelines. *UC Riverside Human Resources Workplace Health & Wellness.* Retrieved from https://wellness.ucr.edu/Standing_Meeting_Guidelines.pdf.

Burns, J. (2001). Complexity science and leadership in healthcare. *Journal of Nursing Administration, 31*(1), 474–482.

Clark, K. R. (2017). Managing multiple generations in the workplace. *Radiologic Technology, 88*(4), 379–396.

Cordeniz, J. (2002). Recruitment, retention, and management of generation X: A focus on nursing professional. *Journal of Healthcare Management, 47*(4), 237–249.

Ellis, P. (2016). Leadership skills: The ethically active manager. *Wounds UK, 12*(1), 58–60.

Flury, C. (2017). Social media as a leadership tool for nurse executives. *Nursing Economics, 35*(5), 272–275. Retrieved from https://www.nursingeconomics.net/necfiles/2017/SO17/272.pdf.

Fallon, N. (2016, November 14). The modern millennial: Management tips for employers. *Business News Daily.* Retrieved from https://www.businessnewsdaily.com/9565-managing-modern-millennials.html.

Garner, C. (2011). Powerlessness is bad practice: Any nurse can be a facilitator of change. *American Sentinel University: The Sentinel Watch.* Retrieved from http://www.americansentinel.edu/blog/2011/04/11/facilitating-change-white-paper/.

Garcell, H. G., Arias, A. V., Miranda, F. R., Jimenez, R. R., & Alfonso Serrano, R. N. (2017). Direct observation of hand hygiene can show differences in staff compliance: Do we need to evaluate the accuracy for patient safety? *Qatar Medical Journal*, 1. https://doi.org/10.5339/qmj.2017.1. (2). Retrieved from https://www.ncbi.nlm.nih .gov/pmc/articles/PMC5514426/.

Goldmann, D. (2018). The sound of two hands washing: Improving hand hygiene. *Institute for Healthcare Improvement*. Retrieved from http://www.ihi.org/resources/Pages/ImprovementStories/ SoundofTwoHandsWashing.aspx.

Gurchiek, K. (2016). What motivates your workers? It depends on their generation. *Society For Human Resource Management*. Retrieved from https://www.shrm.org/resourcesandtools/hr-topics/behavioral-competencies/ global-and-cultural-effectiveness/pages/what-motivates-your-workers-it-depends-on-their-generation.aspx.

HCPro. (2016). Shared governance nursing training program. Retrieved from http://www.hcpro.com/NRS-328056-868/Shared-Governance-Nursing-Training-Program.html.

HealthCare.gov. (2019). Ending lifetime & yearly limits. Retrieved from https://www.healthcare.gov/health-care-law-protections/lifetime-and-yearly-limits/.

Hellriegel, D., Jackson, S., & Slocum, J. (1999). *Management* (8th ed.). Reading, MA: Addison-Wesley.

Institute of Medicine. (2011). *Keeping patients safe: Transforming the work environment of nurses*. Washington, DC: National Academies Press.

Kenney, C. (2011). *Transforming health care*. New York: Taylor & Francis Group.

Kouzes, J. M., & Posner, B. Z. (2015). Leading figures: Developing your leadership style with Kouzes and Posner leadership framework. Retrieved from http://leadingfigures.com/resources/DevelopingYourLeadershipStyle WithKouzesAndPosner.pdf.

Kovner, C. T., Brewer, C. S., Fatehi, F., & Jun, J. (2014). What does nurse turnover rate mean and what is the rate? *Policy, Politics, and Nursing Practice*, *15*(3-4), 64–71. https://doi.org/10.1177/1527154414547953.

Lewin, K. (1947). Group decisions and social change. In Newcomb, T. M. , & Hartley, E. L. (Eds.), *Readings in social psychology*. New York: Henry Holt.

Manion, J. (1996). *Team-based health care organizations*. Gaithersburg, MD: Aspen Publishers.

McCallum, J. (2013). Followership—the other side of leadership. *Ivey Business Journal*. Retrieved from http:// iveybusinessjournal.com/publication/followership-the-other-side-of-leadership/.

McComiskey, F. (2017). The fundamental managerial challenges in the role of a contemporary district nurse: A discussion. *British Journal of Community Nursing*, *22*(10), 489–494. https://doi.org/10.12968/ bjcn.2017.22.10.489.

Miller, M. (2007). Transformational leadership and mutuality. *Transformation*, *24*(3/4), 180–192.

Moss, D. (2017). 5 generations + 7 values = endless opportunities. Society for Human Resource Management. Retrieved from https://www.shrm.org/hr-today/news/hr-news/conference-today/pages/2017/5-generations-7-values-endless-opportunities.aspx.

Mulder, P. (2017). Bureaucratic theory by Max Weber. Retrieved from https://www.toolshero.com/management/ bureaucratic-theory-weber/.

Norman, L. (2018). What are the four basic functions that make up the management process? Retrieved from: https://smallbusiness.chron.com/four-basic-functions-make-up-management-process-23852.html.

Patel, D. (2017). 8 ways Generation Z will differ from Millennials in the workplace. Retrieved from https://www .forbes.com/sites/deeppatel/2017/09/21/8-ways-generation-z-will-differ-from-millennials-in-the-workplace/ #343f331b76e5.

Pfeffer, J., & Sutton, R. (Jan. 1, 2006). Evidence-based management. *Harvard Business Review*. http:// www.connectthedotsconsulting.com/documents/Confidence%20in%20Decision%20Making,%20esp% 20Women/HBR%20on%20Making%20Smart%20Decisions/Evidence-Based%20Mgmt-HBR% 20Jan2013.pdf.

Porter-O'Grady, T. (2003). A different age for leadership. Part 1: New context, new content. *Journal of Nursing Administration*, *33*(2), 105–110.

Porter-O'Grady, T. (2003). A different age for leadership. Part 2: New rules, new roles. *Journal of Nursing Administration*, *33*(3), 173–178.

Porter O'Grady, T. (2003). Researching shared governance: A futility of focus. *Journal of Nursing Administration*, *33*(4), 251–252.

Sherman, R. O. (2012). What followers need from their leaders. *American Nurse Today*, *7*(9), 62–64.

Smyth, R. (2015). Applying complexity theory to healthcare delivery is not complicated. *Forbes/Pharma & Healthcare*. Retrieved from http://www.forbes.com/sites/roysmythe/2015/01/08/applying-aspects-of-complexity-theory-to-health-care-delivery-its-not-complicated/.

Stanley, J., Gannon, J., Gabuat, J. et al. (2008). The clinical nurse leader: A catalyst for improving quality and patient safety. *Journal of Nursing Management*, *16*(5), 614–622. https://doi.org/10.1111/j.1365-2834.2008.00899.x.

Stetler, C. B., Ritchie, J. A., Rycroft-Malone, J., & Charns, M. P. (2014). Leadership for evidence-based practice: Strategic and functional behaviors for institutionalizing EBP. *Worldviews on Evidence-Based Nursing*, *11*(4), 219–226. https://doi.org/10.1111/wvn.12044.

Sullivan, E., & Decker, P. (2012). *Effective leadership and management in nursing* (8th ed.). Prentice-Hall.

Tonges, M., Baloga-Altieri, B., & Atzori, M. (2004). Amplifying nursing's voice through a staff-management partnership. *Journal of Nursing Administration*, *34*(3), 134–139.

Tornabeni, J., & Miller, J. (2008). The power of partnership to shape the future of nursing: The evolution of the clinical nurse leader. *Journal of Nursing Management*, *16*(5), 608–613. https://doi.org/10.1111/j.1365-2834.2008.00902.x.

Walters, N. (2016). 17 of the biggest differences between managers and leaders. *Business Insider*. Retrieved from https://www.businessinsider.com/biggest-differences-between-managers-and-leaders-2016-3.

Wertheim, E. G. (n.d.). Historical background of organizational behavior. *College of Business Administration, Northeastern University*. Retrieved from https://www.scribd.com/doc/6926402/Historical-Background-of-Organizational-Behavior.

Wilson, P. (1996). Empowerment: Community economic development from the inside out. *Urban Studies*, *33*(4-5), 617–630.

Building Nursing Management Skills

Jessica Maack Rangel, MS, RN, ASPPS

http://evolve.elsevier.com/Zerwekh/nsgtoday/.

Example is not the main thing in influencing others; it is the only thing.
Albert Schweitzer

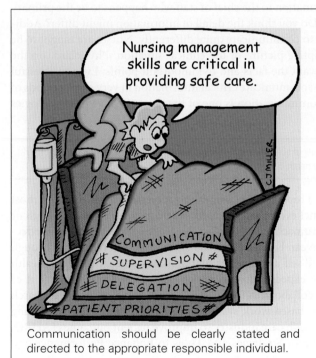

Communication should be clearly stated and directed to the appropriate responsible individual.

After completing this chapter, you should be able to:
- Analyze effective communication as it relates to eliminating harm.
- Analyze Team STEPPS 2.0 Tools as an evidence-based teamwork system to optimize patient outcomes.
- Assess current methods of safe communication, including transcription of prescriber's orders.
- Use a standardized hand-off communication tool (SBAR or I-SBAR-R) for exchanging patient information.
- Discuss strategies to manage and prioritize your time in the clinical setting.
- Identify criteria for supervising and delegating care provided by others.

The entry-level nurse is expected to demonstrate competence as a manager of patient care and the inter-professional team caring for the patient. The process of building nursing management skills encompasses effective communication, management of prioritization in the clinical setting, and management of other members of the interprofessional health care team to maintain patient safety and eliminate preventable harm. The topics in this chapter will be helpful in your development of management skills that keep patients safe while you are a student as well as during your transition period as a new graduate.

COMMUNICATION AND PATIENT SAFETY

We have all learned different ways of communicating. Our tone, inflections, and decibel level are all learned. Roles with perceived authority differences have a significant impact on how we communicate, if we communicate, and how much information we communicate. This is called an authority gradient—that is, the balance of decision-making power or the steepness of command hierarchy in a given situation (AHRQ, 2018b). *Silence Kills* is an older research study, which found that health care workers had seen colleagues cutting corners, making mistakes, and demonstrating incompetence; however, fewer than one in ten discussed their concerns with those coworkers (Vital Smarts, 2005). The new graduate nurse might feel even more reluctant to speak up to an expert nurse if she or he saw a potential mistake. Consider where perceived authority gradients exist between physician and nurse, supervisor and direct report, expert and novice. How and to what degree information is shared will vary. This is why team building and simulation are so important: to break down perceived barriers to communicate effectively. Consider how you might share information regarding a patient's condition with a colleague with whom you have worked and whom you trusted; then consider how you might communicate this same information to the chief of staff who happens to be the primary physician on the case and who is in a hurry. Do you think the detail of information might differ? Additionally, nurses and physicians are educated to communicate quite differently. Nurses are taught to be broad in their narrative. They give a descriptive picture of the clinical situation. Physicians, on the other hand, learn to be very concise—they want the facts and the important points. Even in stressful situations, nurses must find effective ways to communicate critical information in very short periods of time to keep their patients safe. I-SBAR-R communication is one of the most effective methodologies for the transfer of succinct information.

> Communication failures are the root cause for the majority of sentinel events (an unexpected occurrence that reaches the patient and results in severe temporary or permanent harm or death (Schumacker, 2015).

A 2015 study by The Joint Commission (TJC) reported that communication failure was the third most frequent root cause of sentinel events. Sentinel events are unexpected occurrences involving death or serious physical or psychological injury (Schumacher, 2015). The integration of teamwork and effective communication into day-to-day practice can help to eliminate errors that lead to harm. Through exercises in teamwork, cultural sensitivity, and self-awareness/situational awareness techniques, health care providers learn skill sets that promote expeditious and appropriate care. The Department of Defense (DoD) Patient Safety Program in collaboration with the Agency for Healthcare Research and Quality (AHRQ) developed an evidence-based work system in 2007 that focused on improving communication and teamwork skills in the health care industry to improve patient outcomes (AHRQ, 2017). The result was Team STEPPS 2.0—Team **S**trategies and **T**ools to **E**nhance **P**erformance and **P**atient **S**afety (Box 11.1).

Communication challenges in practice were identified early by TJC as well as other accrediting bodies. The National Patient Safety Goals were developed for implementation beginning in 2003 and are updated yearly with the expectation of full implementation and compliance as a condition of accreditation. Failures in communication involved *incomplete* communication among caregivers. TJC issued a National Patient Safety Goal: *Improve staff communication*. Specifically, "Get important test results

---

BOX 11.1   TEAM STEPPS

Team STEPPS 2.0 provides higher-quality safer patient care by:
- Producing highly effective medical teams that optimize the use of information, people, and resources to achieve the best clinical outcomes for patients.
- Increasing team awareness and clarifying team roles and responsibilities.
- Resolving conflicts and improving information sharing.
- Eliminating barriers to quality and safety.

---

to the right staff person on time" (TJC, 2019). It is now an expectation that health care settings have embedded a standardized approach for handing off communication, including passing information regarding orders and test results to keep patients safe.

How Can I Improve My Verbal Communication for Patient Safety?

Let us focus on a couple of communication techniques that can improve the accuracy of the care we provide. First, TJC notes that there is a big difference between verbal orders and telephone orders. Orders received verbally (with the health care provider present) should never be accepted except in an emergency or during a procedure where the health care provider is in a sterile procedural environment and read-back verification techniques are utilized to assure accuracy. There is too much opportunity for transmitting and transcribing the order incorrectly. Telephone orders are acceptable because the health care provider is simply not present to input the orders unless he or she has access to the electronic health record (EHR), where computerized prescriber order entry (CPOE) is available expeditiously. To make this even safer, practice a "read back." In other words, handwrite or input into the EHR the order or test results given to you and read it back to the verify accuracy of the orders and confirm that they were understood correctly. Many medication errors have been directly attributed to the failure to communicate information *at the point of transition*. Specifically, any hand-off of communication is a point of vulnerability, whether it is a telephone communication, a communication of a critical test result, or a transition in the level-of-care report. All have been shown to be critical points in the patient's care. Points of transition in communication encompass all disciplines. Distractions and interruptions play a large role in medication errors and other health care errors.

Consider how often we miscommunicate outside of health care with each other and think of the implications for the clinical setting. You are asked to stop by the store and pick up bread, eggs, and milk, but you forgot to pick up the milk because you relied on your memory. There are lots of factors that may have led you to forget the third item. You had other things on your mind; you were tired from your shift; or you were interrupted by a phone call. Such variables that can interfere with our performance and accurate communication are called "human factors," and they often influence the communication transition between different parties. These are the very same factors that can and do affect your ability to recall information you just received and act on it appropriately.

How much more effective would it have been had you actually *written down* what you were asked to bring home and then *read that list back* to the person who gave it to you? Fatigued, distracted, worried, or sleepy—had you repeated the written list back to the other person, chances are the milk would have made it home too! This is precisely how to manage the verbal and telephone transmission of information from caregiver to caregiver (Box 11.2).

CHAPTER 11 Build

BOX 11.2   SAFETY STEPS FOR VERBAL AND PHONE ORDERS
Step 1: Order is communicated verbally.
Step 2: Order is documented verbatim.
Step 3: Documented order is read directly back to the person who gave it for confirmation that it is accurate and understood correctly.

It's that simple! This process minimizes errors of omission and commission and eliminates the need to rely on memory to recall an order accurately. Your patients' lives depend on it!

How Can I Improve My Written Communication for Patient Safety?

The next communication concern is how we write and document in the EHR to communicate essential information. Legibility and clarity are nonnegotiable essentials. Remember, the written or typed word is another point of transmission that has proved to be a root cause of many catastrophic errors. How often has a medication ordered at 5.0 mg been mistaken for 50 mg because the decimal point was too light to be noticed? Consider instead .5 mcg being mistaken for 5 mcg. The resultant overdose could have devastating consequences. When numbers are being documented, the trailing "0" *must be eliminated* to avoid the confusion between 5.0 mg and 50 mg. Likewise, the insertion of the "0" before the decimal is crucial to differentiate 0.5 mcg from 5 mcg. In 2003, TJC released a Sentinel Event Alert that is still being addressed today regarding these very documentation issues, which have led to grave miscommunications. This TJC alert includes strategies to eliminate harm.

Additionally, the Institute for Safe Medication Practices (ISMP) has a detailed list of abbreviations, symbols, and dose designations that have frequently been misinterpreted, leading to harmful medication errors (ISMP, 2019). Check the ISMP's List of Error-Prone Abbreviations, Symbols, and Dose Designations at the ISMP's website (https://www.ismp.org/recommendations/error-prone-abbreviations-list). Although the EHR has helped to mitigate many of these issues, the risk is ever present.

Furthermore, many written abbreviations used to designate dosage frequency must be eliminated. Abbreviations such as qd for "daily" have become targets for clarification because they can easily be misunderstood (qd has been mistaken for qid, meaning "four times a day"). Plain language in documentation and patient materials has helped to eliminate these errors. Many facilities have disallowed the use of these "unsafe" or "unapproved" abbreviations because of their potential for causing errors that can lead to harm for a patient.

Organizations within the health care delivery system will have their own abbreviations, acronyms, and symbols that should not be used. These abbreviations and symbols may be in addition to the recommendations from TJC and other accrediting bodies. It is imperative to become familiar with the approved abbreviations, symbols, and acronyms that can be used. TJC has mandated that these dangerous abbreviations be eliminated from any documentation, printed or written, when patient-care issues are being communicated (Critical Thinking Box 11.1, Table 11.1).

? CRITICAL THINKING BOX 11.1

What happens when an unsafe abbreviation is found in a patient order?
- Step 1: Notify the prescriber of the order containing the unsafe abbreviation.
- Step 2: Ask for a clarifying order to clear any misinterpretation of the order.
- Step 3: Document the clarification.

TABLE 11.1 THE JOINT COMMISSION OFFICIAL "DO NOT USE" LIST OF ABBREVIATIONS[a]

DO NOT USE	POTENTIAL PROBLEM	USE INSTEAD
U, u (unit)	Mistaken for "0" (zero), the number "4" (four) or "cc"	Write "unit"
IU (International Unit)	Mistaken for IV (intravenous) or the number 10 (ten)	Write "International Unit"
Q.D., QD, q.d., qd (daily)	Mistaken for each other	Write "daily"
Q.O.D., QOD, q.o.d., qod (every other day)	Period after the Q mistaken for "I" and the "O" mistaken for "I"	Write "every other day"
Trailing zero (X.0 mg)[b]	Decimal point is missed	Write X mg
Lack of leading zero (.X mg)		Write 0.X mg
MS	Can mean morphine sulfate or magnesium sulfate	Write "morphine sulfate"
MSO_4 and $MgSO_4$	Confused for one another	Write "magnesium sulfate"

[a]Applies to all orders and all medication-related documentation that is handwritten (including free-text computer entry) or on preprinted forms.
[b]**Exception:** A "trailing zero" may be used only where required to demonstrate the level of precision of the value being reported, such as for laboratory results, imaging studies that report size of lesions, or catheter/tube sizes. It may not be used in medication orders or other medication-related documentation.
From The Joint Commission. (2016, 2004). Official "Do Not Use" List. Retrieved from https://www.jointcommission.org/topics/patient_safety.aspx

Once again, it's that simple! However, one more word of caution must be added for written communication when a nurse is dealing with patients. Cultural variants of the written word must be acknowledged and minimized. Consider a prescription for a primarily Spanish-speaking patient that reads, "Take once daily for 5 days." The word *once* in Spanish means eleven! Interpretive services must be accessed if the language spoken and written is not the patient's primary language. Consider that most pharmacies will even print the medication directions in the patient's primary language if requested. Direct and succinct written and verbal communication in a language that is clearly understood by the patient is essential to appropriate and safe care. Remember that just because the patient can speak English does not mean that the patient can *read* English or any language at all. It's important to use a Team STEPPS 2.0 strategy "check back." A check back is a closed-loop communication strategy used to verify and validate information exchanged (AHRQ, 2018a). Simply put, ask the patient to repeat back to you what he or she understood—for example, discharge instructions, how to take a medication, how to do a dressing change, and so forth. The Centers for Medicare & Medicaid Services (CMS) requires organizations to provide language services for all patients who need them (Critical Thinking Box 11.2).

❓ CRITICAL THINKING BOX 11.2

Role-play with a partner the transcription of verbal prescriber orders and the reading back of those orders for clarity and accuracy. Can you identify any potential miscommunications?

Health care literacy has become a focal point across the nation. This is the degree to which individuals have the capacity to understand their health care information. It is staggering how many patients simply do not understand their health care instructions, consents, or medication administration directions. The National Library of Medicine (2012) has reported that the reading abilities of adults are typically three to four grade levels behind the last year of school completed. A high-school graduate typically has a seventh- or eighth-grade reading level. Therefore it is essential for the health care provider to ask patients to repeat back what they understand about their condition, medications, education, and discharge instructions (a check back). As a health care professional, you now speak a language that is unfamiliar to those outside of health care. Consider that you and the patient's physician may refer to the patient's high blood pressure condition as hypertension. Does the patient realize that hypertension and high blood pressure are the same things, or does he or she think that hypertension is a "hyper" condition in which the person cannot sit still? You might be surprised when you hear what the patient understands about his or her own condition!

Transcribing Written Orders

In the process of providing safe patient care, it is essential that prescriber orders be communicated clearly and correctly to the health care team. The prescriber order must clearly indicate what is to be done, when it should be done, and how often it should be done. All orders must include the patient's identifying information and the current date and time. Table 11.2 provides a summary of the various types of orders. The process for transcribing orders may involve other health team members, such as the unit secretary, but it is the nurse's responsibility to verify that the orders are input correctly regardless of how the order was transcribed. This involves making sure that the order has been clearly understood and documented accurately. If any component of the order is not clear, the prescriber should be contacted for clarification (Box 11.3).

The CPOE is an electronic means for entering a prescriber order. This system has the benefit of reducing errors by minimizing the ambiguity of handwritten orders as well as intercepting errors when they most commonly occur—at the time the order is written. The system also has the added benefit of allowing a new order to be entered from multiple locations. This, in turn, decreases the need for telephone orders, as the person writing the order can use any computer terminal within the system to do so (and sometimes smartphone technology is utilized to facilitate remote order entry). The CPOE system is integrated with other patient information, including laboratory information, diagnostic results, and medication records. Even with all the advantages of the EHR, in the event the systems shut down, best practices related to the transcription of orders, accuracy of orders, and legibility of orders cannot be forgotten. Keep in mind that not all health care settings have CPOE available.

TABLE 11.2 **TYPES OF WRITTEN ORDERS**

TYPE	DESCRIPTION
One-time-only order	An order for a medication or procedure to be carried out only one time.
PRN order	An order to be carried out when the patient needs it, not on a scheduled basis. For example, a PRN pain medication order.
Standing order	A health care provider's routine set of orders for a specific procedure or condition. For example, a surgeon may have standing preoperative and/or postoperative orders for an abdominal surgery patient.
STAT order	An order that is to be implemented immediately. Usually, it is a one-time order. The term is derived from the Latin word *statim*, which means "immediately."

BOX 11.3 **STEPS IN TRANSCRIBING ORDERS**

1. Read all of the order(s).
2. Determine whether all request forms (laboratory, medication, diagnostic test) and/or contacts have been initiated.
3. Review notes for order entries.
4. Follow institutional policy for rechecking orders and signing off.

COMMUNICATING WHEN IT IS CRITICAL—WHAT DO YOU NEED TO DO?

Critical Patient Tests

Communication of critical test results is yet another vulnerable time when errors can occur. Critical test results warrant expeditious communication to the responsible licensed caregiver without delay. This includes not only critical laboratory values but also other diagnostic test results specifically defined by the institution. The primary goal is to transmit the critical information to the person who can most quickly stabilize the patient. Documentation of how this was accomplished is essential to promoting and providing validation that the critical test result was communicated and, if needed, acted on.

On occasion nurses are notified of a critical test result without passing that communication along to the health care provider who has the scope and authority to act on the result. Assumptions are sometimes made that the health care provider is aware of the test result or that notifying the nurse is enough. The health care provider in this case is the individual who is able to act on the result of the test. The nurse is NOT that person. The prescriber who ordered the test IS.

> "When in doubt, call it out" to the health care provider and document the results of that conversation when you are clarifying ambiguous orders.

Managing critical information regarding a patient's test result is all about getting the information to the right person. What should be done if you cannot reach the prescriber who ordered a test with critical results? As a nurse, you may find it necessary to initiate the chain-of-command or chain-of-resolution procedure or policy. Most institutions have a process that identifies a step-by-step method of whom to contact in case the health care provider cannot be reached. The nurse continues to care for the patient, documenting the care that has been provided and all attempts that were made to contact the health care provider. Finally, the nurse is responsible for determining that resolution has occurred and for documenting the resolution in the medical record. It is vital that you become aware of the chain-of-command or chain-of-resolution policy at your place of employment and understand situations that warrant its initiation. Merely documenting in the patient's chart that you tried to notify the health care provider does not take responsibility for the patient's current health status away from you. You are the advocate for the patient and are responsible to assure communication has taken place.

Critical Hand-Off Communication

It is the standard of care as well as accrediting bodies' expectations that health care facilities must implement a standardized approach to communications. The implementation of a hand-off communication tool helps to reinforce to clinicians that they have a responsibility to provide succinct, accurate information and safe, high-quality care throughout the patient's period of hospitalization through to a safe discharge, thus making the patient's hospital journey a safe one.

One of the communication modalities that is often employed in the health care setting is called "I-SBAR-R Communication," mentioned earlier. Originally this tool was called SBAR, and now it has been updated to I-SBAR-R to reinforce the importance of patient safety goal 2 (read-back communication) and patient identification. Integrating I-SBAR-R techniques into your communication with other team members will organize your discussion and promote patient safety (Grbach, 2008).

Scenario: Mrs. Smith is an 84-year-old patient who was admitted with a diagnosis of uncontrolled diabetes. It's 2:00 a.m. and the nurse notices that the patient is in respiratory distress. She assesses Mrs. Smith and calls the health care provider:

"Dr. Brown, I'm Nancy Jones, RN **(I)**, and I've been caring for Mrs. Jane Smith, an 84-year-old female in room 302 who was admitted tonight and is experiencing increased shortness of breath and is very anxious. **(S)**

"She's never had an episode like this before. She has no history of respiratory distress, asthma, or COPD. She was sitting up in bed and had a sudden onset of shortness of breath. She does have a history of thrombophlebitis. **(B)**

"She is breathing 42 breaths a minute. Her pulse oximeter is showing an oxygen saturation of 86% on room air. She has bilateral breath sounds with some expiratory wheezes in all lobes. Her skin is pale, cool, and clammy. She is oriented but very anxious. She is afebrile, pulse of 120, and blood pressure of 92/60. Her glucose is 130. She is sitting up in bed; compression stockings are in place. **(A)**

"I've called a rapid response team. Would you like me to obtain arterial blood gases or administer some oxygen? Could you come in and see her?" **(R)**

Dr. Brown says, "Thanks for the update on Mrs. Smith's condition. Please initiate oxygen at two liters per nasal cannula. Let's order arterial blood gases. I'll be in within the next hour to see her but call me with any changes or concerns." **(R)**

"I will place the order for arterial blood gases to be drawn and administer oxygen at two liters per nasal cannula and will call you back with any changes or concerns." **(R)**

Imagine how differently this conversation could have gone had the nurse not had an organized manner to communicate this urgent situation, especially in the middle of the night when the health care provider may have been asleep!

I-SBAR-R provides a common and predictable structure and can be used in virtually any clinical setting. Use of I-SBAR-R also refines critical thinking skills; *before* communication is delivered, the person initiating the communication makes an assessment of the patient and provides a recommendation for ongoing care. I-SBAR-R is a communication strategy that helps to organize critical information and focus on it (Box 11.4). Additionally, the use of a standardized communication and reporting method may help alleviate the anxiety that students and new graduate nurses experience during hand-off communication (Kostiuk, 2015). A recent initiative from TJC encourages the use of the acronym SHARE to promote effective hand-off communication (Box 11.5).

Shift Change—So Much to Say ... So Little Time

Any time there is an exchange of information, there is a possibility for miscommunication either by omission (forgetting to share something important) or by simply focusing on the things that are not as essential as others (the patient's nephew who is coming to visit versus the pending critical test result).

BOX 11.4 SITUATION-BACKGROUND-ASSESSMENT-RECOMMENDATION (I-SBAR-R) TOOL

I = Identification: Identify yourself and your patient (two identifiers are used).
S = Situation: What is happening at the present time?
B = Background: What are the circumstances leading up to this situation?
A = Assessment: What do I think the problem is?
R = Recommendation: What should we do to correct the problem?
R = Read-Back or Response: Receiver acknowledges information given: What is his or her response?

From Grbach, W. (2008) *Reformulating SBAR to "I SBAR R," QSEN.* Retrieved from http://qsen.org/reformulating-sbar to i sbar r/.

BOX 11.5   HAND-OFF COMMUNICATION

Benefits of the Hand-off Communications Targeted Solutions Tool

- Facilitates the examination of the current hand-off communication process.
- Provides a measurement system that produces data that support the need for improving the current hand-off communication processes.
- Identifies areas of focus, such as the specific information needed for the transition that is being measured.
- Provides customizable forms for data collection.
- Provides guidelines to determine the most appropriate hand-off communication processes.

The Joint Commission Hand-off Communication Acronym: SHARE

To improve effective patient hand offs, The Joint Commission recommends following the "SHARE" acronym, which stands for:

- **S**tandardize critical content:
  - Provide details of patient's history and status when speaking with receiver
  - Identify and stress key information and critical elements about patient when talking with the receiver
  - Synthesize patient information from disparate sources prior to passing it on to the receiver
  - Develop and use key phrases to help standardized communications
- **H**ardwire within your system:
  - Develop and use standardized forms and tools and methods, e.g., checklists, SBAR tool
  - Establish a workspace or setting that is conducive for sharing information about a patient, e.g., zone of silence
  - Have patient present during hand-off discussion between sender and receiver
  - State expectations about how to conduct a successful hand-off
  - Focus on the system, not just the people
  - Identify new and existing technologies to assist in making the hand-off successful and complete, e.g., electronic medical records, PDAs
  - Ensure access to electronic medical record is available to all staff caring for patient
  - Integrate process into electronic medical record application
  - Provide post-acute staff with access to hospital information systems (if part of the same health care system)
  - Examine the work flow of health care workers to ensure a successful hand-off
- **A**llow opportunity to ask questions:
  - Use critical thinking skills when discussing a patient's case
  - Share and receive information—as an interdisciplinary team—about the patient at the same time, e.g., "pit crew"
  - Expect to receive all key information and critical elements about the patient from the sender
  - Collect sender's contact information in the event there are follow-up questions
  - Scrutinize and question the data
- **R**einforce quality and measurement:
  - Demonstrate leadership's commitment to implement successful hand-offs
  - Utilize a sound measurement system to determine the real score in real time
  - Hold staff managing patient's care responsible
  - Monitor compliance of standardized form, tools, and methods for hand-off between sender and receiver
  - Measure the specific, high-impact causes of a poor hand-off and target solutions to those causes
  - Use data as the basis for a systematic approach for improvement
- **E**ducate and coach:
  - Teach staff on what constitutes a successful hand-off
  - Standardize training on how-to conduct a hand-off
  - Engage staff—real time performance feedback; just-in-time training
  - Make successful hand-offs an organizational

From The Joint Commission. (2010). *Joint Commission Center for Transforming Healthcare tackles miscommunication among caregivers*. Retrieved from http://www.centerfortransforminghealthcare.org/assets/4/6/CTH_Hand-off_commun_set_final_2010.pdf; and The Joint Commission. (2012). *Center for Transforming Healthcare released a new hand-off communications Targeted Solutions Tool* (TST). Retrieved from http://www.centerfortransforminghealthcare.org/center_transforming_healthcare_tst_hoc/

How can the nurse possibly begin to decide what is important to discuss in the short amount of time provided for the change-of-shift report? With a standardized method to hand off or communicate the care of the patient to another clinician, a miscommunication of information is less likely. This means for the nurse that any time a report is transferred from one person to another (even a colleague who covers another for a break), the adopted method for communicating information must be followed.

Some of the most critical elements in a change-of-shift report using the patient's medical record include

- Two patient identifiers (typically name and date of birth)
- Current medical diagnoses
- Health care provider or providers on the case
- Pertinent medical/social history
- Current physical condition (review of systems)
- Resuscitation status (no resuscitation, full resuscitation)
- Nutritional status (nutritional intake, nothing by mouth [NPO], supplements)
- Pending or critical issues and tests

When appropriate, a bedside report that involves the patient and his or her significant family members, as consented and appropriate, has demonstrated greater satisfaction and improved outcomes for the patient because the patient is an active member of her or his own health care team: patient-centered care! This provides the opportunity for the patient and family to greet the oncoming caregiver and for both caregivers to assess the patient together, especially where there may be skin integrity issues or wounds involved. When I-SBAR-R guidelines are consistently used, the shift report and patient transfer are organized, thorough, and also concise. Furthermore, important information is not forgotten, and the transition of care is then more complete and safer for everyone involved.

How Can I Deal With All the Interruptions?

Interruptions are among the major threats to effective time management and patient safety. Studies have found that interprofessional health care team members are distracted and interrupted as frequently as once every 2 minutes. It was concluded that *each* interruption resulted in a 12.7% increased risk of a medication error (Beyea, 2014). Not only is time taken away from goal-directed activities, but clearly interruptions create patient safety hazards! Of course, some interruptions are inevitable, but they are manageable. Begin by recognizing when *you* are permitting interruptions. Do you start one task and then begin another rather than concentrating on completing the first? Do you respond to added distractions (e.g., television, ringing telephones, and chatty colleagues) at times when task completion is required? When possible in nonemergency situations, use your time-management strategies and communication skills to remain focused on the task at hand. Colleagues and visitors will accept that you may need to get back to them when you have finished what you are doing. Write down when and where you can reach them and then follow through.

Responding to interruptions can also mean that you are doing your job caring for your patient's needs. For example, when you are interrupted to answer a patient's call light or answer a physician's telephone call, you are caring for your patient. These activities are part of your nursing responsibilities. They may not be of an urgent nature and can be delayed a short time, or they may be urgent and necessitate an immediate response; either way, you will have to handle them eventually. Rather than feeling that you have been interrupted, remind yourself that what you are doing is accomplishing part of your job. There are many aspects of your job that you cannot control, but you can always choose how to respond.

Evidence has demonstrated that medication administration and shift report are critical times to minimize interruptions. To signify the need not to interrupt the caregiver engaging in these critical tasks, facilities are employing various strategies to alert others that the nurse is involved in a critical task. Many clinical settings have created a "no-interruption zone" around medication administration/dispensing areas and educate visitors on honoring this time for the sake of patient safety. Others have tried having the staff wear brightly colored vests while giving report or medicating patients until the task is complete. In this way everyone, from the physician to the families, is aware that the caregiver is engaged in a critical task that requires his or her full attention (Pape & Richards, 2010). However, there are exceptions to when interrupting the nurse or health care provider is necessary regardless of the task in which the individual is engaged. The following emergency situations (which include but are not limited to a deteriorating patient, initiating a rapid response, a patient or family expressing a critical need) are just a few examples of when encountering an interruption is warranted.

Working with your team and creating a list of those tasks that are best served by minimal interruptions can facilitate effective teamwork. Prioritizing what is most important will keep you and your colleagues on task.

Everyone needs some totally uninterrupted time to relax, refocus, and reenergize. During clinical experience or while you are at work or at home, spend a few minutes in a quiet place by yourself (e.g., the nurses' lounge, the chapel, an empty patient room, a bedroom at home) to evaluate what is happening or what should happen next. Practice mindfulness.

What Skills Do I Need to Use the Telephone Effectively?

Many nurses spend time on the telephone talking with physicians, patients, their families, and other health care personnel. Here are some tips for making telephone communication productive. It is honoring of others' time and priorities to ask the person you are calling if this is a convenient time to talk based on the urgency. If you anticipate that your conversation will involve complex information, make notes ahead of time so that you can keep your conversation as focused and brief as possible. Try organizing your conversation in the I-SBAR-R communication format. After discussing detailed, critical information on the telephone, it is wise to follow up with a documented communication to the other person. This helps clarify and confirm the information discussed. If your telephone conversation requires a follow-up action, you must document that.

It is difficult to focus on a telephone conversation if you are doing something else at the same time. Your communication will be more effective if you do one thing at a time. (Case in point: How often do you pass people on the road who are driving recklessly only to find that they are talking on a cellular telephone or texting?) Recent graduates often experience a challenge when they are communicating with other health care professionals, especially on the telephone. Box 11.6 highlights some helpful tips.

BOX 11.6 TIPS FOR COMMUNICATING WITH HEALTH CARE PROVIDERS ON THE TELEPHONE

1. Use the I-SBAR-R technique.
2. Say who you are right away.
3. State your business briefly but completely.
4. Ask for specific orders when appropriate.
5. If you want the health care provider to assess the patient, say so.
6. If the health care provider is coming, ask when to expect him or her.
7. If you get cut off, call back.
8. Document all attempts to reach a health care provider. If you cannot reach a health care provider or get what you need, notify your chain of command or chain of resolution.

MANAGING TIME IN THE CLINICAL SETTING

One of the main sources of job dissatisfaction reported by nurses is too little time to provide their hands-on care. This "limited time" to provide patient care has been exacerbated by changing nurse-to-patient ratios, the increase in numbers of patients, and the higher acuity of these patients. In response to this issue, nurses must develop competent skills in time management and priority setting. Nurses can use several techniques to maximize the time spent in providing patient care. It is important to determine which patients require the most time. Then ask yourself whether they require time that can be delegated to someone else or whether they need the time because they are the most unstable and ill patients. It is essential to communicate any concerns regarding unsafe patient assignments through the chain of command or chain of resolution so that care can be safely managed and patients receive the care they need (Critical Thinking Box 11.3, Fig. 11.1).

> **? CRITICAL THINKING BOX 11.3**
>
> Develop a flow sheet to organize your time and patient care for your clinical schedule. Obtain an assignment for an RN on one of the units to which you are assigned for clinical. Can you prioritize and delegate this RN's assignment appropriately?

> Request consistent patient assignments whenever possible. This allows you to develop relationships with your patients and their families and promotes time management because you become familiar with the special needs of these patients.

Get Organized Before the Change-of-Shift Report

Develop your own work organization sheet or use one provided by the agency to document information you will need to begin coordinating care for a group of patients. Modify this form as you discover

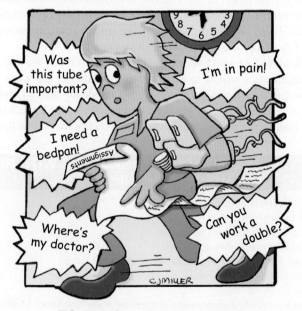

FIG. 11.1 Can you work overtime?

Name: *Susan*

Time	Activities	Room 416	Room 417	Room 418
7–8	✓ MAR Shift report ✓ vitals	✓ Bld sugar 7:30 insulin	I.V. @ 125/hr. turn ✓ pulses	7:45 pre-op NPO ✓ consent form
8–9	assessments meal trays	meds x3-9 up for meals	meds x2-9 If leg dsg. assist c̄ meal	To OR
9–10		shower chg bed ✓ pain meds	complete bath ✓ pulses turn	
10–11	Chart			Chg bed
11–12	meal trays lunch	up for meals ✓ Bld sugar insulin?	turn ✓ pulses assist c̄ meal	
12–13	Chart assessment	meds x2-12	IVPB-12	Return fm OR? N.G. suction I.V.
13–14		diabetic teaching	turn ✓ pulses If. leg dressing change	
14–15	I & O's IV's report info			

FIG. 11.2 Work organization sheet.

areas that require improvement. Avoid distractions as you receive a report and begin to fill out your time management (or work organization) form. Get the information needed to plan the care for your patients and begin to organize your shift activities (Fig. 11.2).

Prioritize Your Care

Setting priorities has become difficult in light of the dichotomy between the expected outcomes of efficiency, safety, and satisfaction against the perceived limitations of resources, including time. Priority setting is not only based on patient needs but also is influenced by the needs of the organization and the accountability of the nurse. Priorities are established and reprioritized throughout the day according to patients' assessed needs and unscheduled interruptions, both minor and emergent. Plan your day around the patient you perceive to be the sickest. This is the patient who is at the greatest risk for harm if you do not address his or her needs first.

> Prioritize patients by using the ABCDE (airway, breathing, circulation, disability, exposure) system or Maslow's hierarchy of needs. Of highest priority are the patients with problems or potential problems related to the airway. Next are those having difficulty with breathing and then those with circulation problems. When you are using Maslow's hierarchy of needs to assist with prioritization, you must meet physiological needs first: that is, resolve any difficulty with oxygenation first. Be flexible and reprioritize as emergencies occur.

Prioritize your patients after you receive report and immediately proceed to the patient you have placed highest on your priority list. Remember that your prioritization may change as you complete your initial assessments. Additional modifications will be made according to the location of patients' rooms to avoid wasted time and movement. When you first enter a patient's room, introduce yourself, perform hand hygiene measures, and complete a quick environmental assessment. Think about any supplies you will need when you return to the room. Complete the focused assessment, validate the safety of your patient, and proceed to your next patient. After you have completed your initial rounds, reassess your initial prioritization, modify according to your assessments, and plan your day. Utilize your peers and other interprofessional members of your health care team as needed to provide safe care. This includes all team members helping each other to provide optimal care. The Team STEPPS 2.0 tactic of cross-monitoring is an error-reduction strategy that involves:

- Monitoring actions of other team members
- Providing a safety net within the team
- Ensuring that mistakes or oversights are caught quickly and easily
- Watching each other's back

For example, a characteristic assignment for the day could be
- A patient who is 1 day postoperative and wants something for pain
- A geriatric patient with dysphagia who is vomiting
- A patient with diabetes who is angry about the care given by the last shift
- A geriatric patient whose bed is wet because of urine incontinence

Which of these patients needs your immediate attention and which tasks could be expeditiously completed by delegating? Most likely the one who is vomiting needs the nurse's attention first because this patient is at increased risk for aspiration. Next is probably the patient who is in pain. You could possibly delegate the bath and bed change of the geriatric patient who has soiled the bed with urine. Ask the charge nurse to visit with the angry patients. Assisting your colleagues in their assignments if yours are completed is another mutual support technique in Team STEPPS 2.0 called task assistance, also known as "no one sits until we all sit."

Identify the busiest times on the unit; do not schedule a dressing change when medications are due to be given. If you have dressing changes for several patients, start with the cleanest and progress to the more contaminated wounds (Critical Thinking Box 11.4).

? CRITICAL THINKING BOX 11.4

How do the efficient nurses on your clinical unit prioritize their time and their patients' needs?

Watch those nurses who always seem to get everything done and done well and who still enjoy nursing. Ask them about their secrets of time management and try out some of their tips.

Organize Your Work by Patient

By organizing your work by patient, you maximize the number of tasks that can be accomplished with each visit to the patient. The nurse thinks strategically: "How can I multitask or accomplish several objectives in one visit to the patient?" By using this technique, the nurse can combine assessment, the administration of medications, and teaching during one patient visit (see Fig. 11.2).

Another way to organize and coordinate the needs of the patient is by implementing hourly rounds. This is where the caregivers (both nursing and ancillary help) can alternate visiting patients every hour to verify that patients' needs are met proactively. This is often referred to as meeting the "three Ps":

THREE Ps OF NURSING ROUNDS

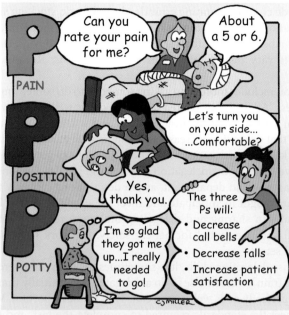

FIG. 11.3 "Three Ps" of hourly rounds.

pain, position, and potty. Is the patient in pain? Does the patient need assistance in changing position? Does the patient need assistance in toileting? When this strategy is implemented, patients use call bells less, have fewer falls, and express greater satisfaction. It also helps the nurse to prioritize tasks with minimal interruptions (Fig. 11.3).

MANAGING OTHERS

Communicating and getting along with other health care team members can be challenging at times. Most people are easygoing, straightforward, and supportive. They add to your energy and ability to function effectively and contribute to team goal attainment. However, if you experience a phone call or visit from someone who just wants to talk when you are busy, you may need techniques to set a boundary. Tell that person, "Now is not a good time. Could we discuss this later?" or even "I've got a commitment. Could we postpone this conversation until tomorrow?" Some individuals set up barriers to organizational accomplishment through negative thinking, chronic lateness, poor crisis management, dependency, aggression, and similar unproductive behaviors. These barriers may have to be communicated to the chain of command or chain of resolution to mitigate any impact on patient care. On occasion, exhibitions of such behavior in relation to a crisis may occur. However, when people use these behaviors as their everyday modus operandi (method of operating), they interfere with the attainment of individual and organizational goals. Even in the best of human relationships, conflict and emotions are inevitable. To protect your time and achieve your goals, it may be necessary to work with your leadership and health care team members to stay focused. Learning to say no and using assertive communication can help as well. It is essential to set clear boundaries while demonstrating respect for both yourself and the other person.

What About Delegating and Time Management?

You may have seen nurses performing nonnursing activities during your clinical experience; these would include cleaning, running errands, clerical work, stocking supplies, and other tasks. The appropriate delegation of nonnursing tasks can give the nurse more time for patient care. Even some patient care tasks can be delegated after verifying the training and competence of unlicensed personnel. These requirements vary in different states and institutions. Review Chapter 14 for more specifics on delegation.

Delegation includes more than asking someone to do something. The American Nurses Association (ANA) states, "All decisions related to delegation, as well as assignment, are based on the fundamental principles of protection of the health, safety and welfare of the public" (ANA, 2012). This definition emphasizes that delegation increases the responsibility and accountability of the registered nurse (RN). Be sure you know the delegation rules and regulations of your state's nursing practice act. Additionally, you will have to know the delegation policies and job descriptions of nursing team members in your employing agency and department, as job descriptions can vary from one department to another.

Nurses are taught to anticipate and meet the needs of others. Because of this, nurses tend to have great difficulty in sharing and delegating the many responsibilities given to them. Delegation is a learned skill and is essential for patient safety, for work to be successful, and to help others grow in their skill sets.

To increase delegation skills, it is sometimes necessary to overcome the myth of perfection. When you teach or train someone else to do a delegated task, initially that person may not be able to perform the activity perfectly or as well as you can. That is not important. What is important is that the person is able to meet the standards required to complete the task and to delegate appropriately to others. With experience, most people will improve in their skills (and may even surpass you). Simulation and team-building practice can help with this. You are not only helping them grow but are freeing up your time to tend to more complex tasks (Critical Thinking Box 11.5).

❓ CRITICAL THINKING BOX 11.5

On your clinical unit, how many levels of personnel provide patient care? How is the nursing care of patients delegated?

Determine which patients are the most stable and whose positive progress can be anticipated. The stable patients with predictable progress should be the first whose care is delegated. The care of unstable, unpredictable patients should only be delegated to an RN. An RN should also be assigned to any patient who is undergoing a procedure or treatment that may cause him or her to become unstable.

When you are working with unlicensed assistive personnel (UAP), you can delegate to them such activities as have specific, unchanging guidelines. For example, feeding, dressing, bathing, obtaining equipment for the nursing staff, picking up meal trays, refilling water containers, straightening up cluttered rooms—all of these activities should have guidelines according to institutional policies, should fit within the job description, and should be followed by the UAP. To the extent possible, involving the UAP in bedside reports is optimal.

Patient teaching and discharge planning are also the responsibility of the RN. RNs are responsible for determining the patient's learning needs and establishing a teaching plan. It is also the RN's responsibility to coordinate and implement the discharge planning. The RN should request input from all interprofessional health care team members who have assisted in providing care for the patient or who have been otherwise involved (e.g., dietary management, physical therapy) in the patient's care. After the RN has implemented the teaching plan, it is important that the other RNs, licensed practical nurses, vocational nurses, and UAP be aware of what the patient has been taught so that they can follow up and report any pertinent observations to the RN (Critical Thinking Box 11.6). Thorough discharge planning that is understood by the patient and family can prevent unnecessary readmissions and harm to the patient.

> **? CRITICAL THINKING BOX 11.6**
>
> Determine how and to whom patient care is delegated on your current clinical unit. What guidelines are implemented? Is it within the nursing scope of practice?

Nursing care makes a difference in patient outcomes. This care is more than performing tasks. It incorporates assessment, care planning, and the initiation of interventions, interprofessional collaboration, and outcome evaluations. It includes patient and family teaching, therapeutic communication, counseling, discharge planning, and teaching. To maximize the impact that nursing care can have on patient outcomes, nurses must develop and integrate multiple strategies to promote effective time management.

Supervising and Evaluating the Care Provided by Others

To meet the demanding and complex needs of the public for safe and good-quality patient care, it is imperative that the use of all nursing resources be maximized. The licensed practical nurse and other unlicensed personnel can function as extensions to the RN as providers of care if definitive supervision and evaluative guidelines are established. State boards of nursing are responsible for articulating those guidelines.

> Unlicensed personnel: An individual not licensed as a health care provider; a nursing student providing care that is not a part of his or her nursing program.

Supervision entails providing direction, evaluation, and follow-up by the RN for nursing tasks that have been delegated to unlicensed personnel. The following criteria apply to the RN who functions in a supervisory capacity:

- Provide directions with clear expectations of how the task is to be performed.
- Verify that the task is being performed according to standards of practice.
- Monitor the task being performed; intervene if necessary.
- Evaluate the status of the patient.
- Evaluate the performance of the task.
- Provide feedback as necessary.
- Reassess the plan of care and modify it as needed.

These criteria apply to RNs who delegate nursing care for patients with acute conditions or those patients who are in an acute-care environment. The continued growing need for unlicensed personnel, as well as the role of the practical nurse in providing care, will require the RN to serve in the supervisor and evaluator roles and to be accountable and responsible for those assigned nursing tasks.

It is never easy to provide constructive feedback regarding a deficiency or an area needing improvement; however, sandwiching the constructive feedback between layers of recognition and positive reinforcement makes the communication more palatable and effective. Keep in mind that when you are providing constructive feedback, you are simply providing your evaluation of an individual's performance, not his or her character. Here's an example of how a supervisor effectively used the "sandwich" method for providing constructive feedback.

Carrie is a new graduate who has completed the first 6 weeks of employment. She is consistently tardy and delays shift reports. When Carrie arrived in the supervisor's office for her evaluation, the supervisor was very nice in her approach to talking with her. The supervisor reviewed with Carrie the progress she has made in orienting to the unit and managing the care of a group of patients. Carrie was pleased with the recognition of her progress. Next, the supervisor addressed Carrie's tardiness on the unit and how it had affected the shift report. Carrie acknowledged this as a problem and discussed the situation, making some suggestions to alleviate the problem. The supervisor was supportive of Carrie's suggestions and her initiative to examine the tardiness issue.

When you are providing constructive feedback, you should:
- Actively listen to the individual's perception of the situation
- Focus on the facts
- Provide an opportunity for the individual to self-reflect
- Support the individual

When you are providing constructive feedback, you should not:
- Argue with the individual's perception of the event
- Reprimand, scold, or belittle the individual
- Offer unsolicited personal advice (e.g., "This is what I think you should do…")
- Coerce or make intimidating statements to demonstrate your authority

CONCLUSION

Building nursing management skills that promote patient safety is a new task for the graduate nurse. The implementation of self-management and the management of others' skills in the clinical setting is challenging. By using effective communication, time management, prioritization in the clinical setting, and managing other members of the health care team, the new graduate can begin to grow professionally and personally. See the additional relevant websites and online resources listed here for developing your management skills further.

After your clinical schedule has been organized, you will become a more effective nurse and will begin to have the time to provide safe nursing care, which leads to positive patient outcomes.

⊕ RELEVANT WEBSITES AND ONLINE RESOURCES

American Nurses Association
Developing delegation skills. Retrieved from http://nursingworld.org/MainMenuCategories/ANAMarketplace/ANAPeriodicals/
 OJIN/TableofContents/Vol152010/No2May2010/Delegation-Skills.html.

The Joint Commission
Sentinel event policy and RCA2. Retrieved from https://www.jointcommission.org/sentinel_event.aspx.

BIBLIOGRAPHY

Agency for Healthcare Research and Quality (AHRQ). (2018a). *TeamSTEPPS™. 2.0 Curriculum.* Retrieved from https://www.ahrq.gov/teamstepps/instructor/index.html.
Agency for Healthcare Research and Quality (AHRQ). (2018b). *Patient safety network glossary 2018.* Retrieved from http.psnet.ahrq.gov/glossary.

Agency for Healthcare Research and Quality (AHRQ). (2017). *About TeamSTEPPS.* Retrieved from https://www .ahrq.gov/teamstepps/about-teamstepps/index.html.

American Nurses Association. (2012). *ANA's Principles of Delegation by Registered Nurses (RN) to Unlicensed Assistive Personnel (UAP).* Retrieved from https://www.nursingworld.org/~4af4f2/globalassets/docs/ana/ ethics/principlesofdelegation.pdf.

Grbach, W. (2008). *Reformulating SBAR to "I-SBAR-R."* Retrieved from http://qsen.org/reformulating-sbar-to-i-sbar-r/.

Institute for Healthcare Improvement (IHI). (2018). *Medication reconciliation to prevent adverse drug events.* Retrieved from http://www.ihi.org/Topics/ADEsMedicationReconciliation/Pages/default.aspx.

Institute for Safe Medication Practices (ISMP). (2019). *Recommendations: List of error-prone abbreviations.* Retrieved from https://www.ismp.org/recommendations/error-prone-abbreviations-list.

Beyea, S. (2014). *Interruptions and distractions in health care: Improved safety with mindfulness.* Retrieved from https://psnet.ahrq.gov/perspectives/perspective/152/Interruptions-and-Distractions-in-Health-Care-Improved-Safety-With-Mindfulness?q=Interruptions+and+Distractions+in+Health+Care+Improved +Safety+with+Mindfulness.

Kostiuk, S. (2015). Can learning the ISBARR framework help to address nursing students' perceived anxiety and confidence levels associated with handover reports? *Journal of Nursing Education, 54*(10), 583–587. https://doi .org/10.3928/01484834-20150916-07.

National Library of Medicine. (2012). *Health literacy.* Retrieved from https://nnlm.gov/initiatives/topics/health-literacy.

Pape, T., & Richards, B. (2010). Stop "knowledge creep." *Nursing Management, 41*(2), 8–11. https://doi.org/ 10.1097/01.NUMA.0000368559.85028.e3.

Schumacher, P. (2015, April 29). Patient safety: Sentinel event statistics released for 2014. *Joint Commission Online.* Retrieved from https://www.jointcommission.org/assets/1/23/jconline_April_29_15.pdf.

The Joint Commission (TJC). (2019). *National patient safety goals.* Retrieved from https://www.jointcommission .org/assets/1/6/2019_HAP_NPSGs_final2.pdf.

The Joint Commission (TJC). (2018a). *Handoff communications.* Retrieved from https://www .centerfortransforminghealthcare.org/news/press/handoff.aspx.

The Joint Commission (TJC). (2018b). *Facts about the do not use abbreviation list.* Retrieved from https://www .jointcommission.org/about_us/patient_safety_fact_sheets.aspx.

The Joint Commission (TJC). (2016). *Sentinel event statistics data—event type by year (1995 - Q2- 2016): Most commonly reviewed sentinel event types.* Retrieved from https://www.jointcommission.org/assets/1/18/Event_ type_2Q_2016.pdf.

The Joint Commission. (2015). *Sentinel event data root causes by event type 2004-Q2 2015.* Retrieved from http:// www.jointcommission.org/assets/1/18/Rootcauseeventtype.pdf.

The Joint Commission (TJC). (2014). *Advancing effective communication, cultural competence, and patient and family-centered care: A roadmap for hospitals.* Retrieved from https://www.jointcommission.org/roadmap_ for_hospitals/.

VitalSmarts. (2005). *Silence kills: The seven crucial conversations for healthcare.* Retrieved from https://www .vitalsmarts.com/resource/silence-kills/.

Westbrook, J. I., Woods, A., Rob, M. I., Dunsmuir, W. T., & Day, R. O. (2010). Association of interruptions with an increased risk and severity of medication administration errors. *Archives of Internal Medicine, 170*(8), 683–690. https://doi.org/10.1001/archinternmed.2010.65.

12

Effective Communication, Team Building, and Interprofessional Practice

JoAnn Zerwekh, EdD, RN
and Ashley Zerwekh Garneau, PhD, RN

ⓔ http://evolve.elsevier.com/Zerwekh/nsgtoday/.

To effectively communicate, we must realize that we are all different in the way we perceive the world and use this understanding as a guide to our communication with others.
Anthony Robbins

High-functioning teams require collaboration between physicians, nurses, pharmacists, social workers, clinical psychologists, case managers, medical assistants, and clinical administrators.
Department of Veterans Affairs, 2010, p. 2

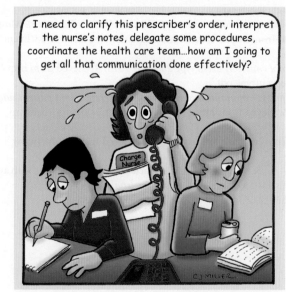

Communication should be clearly stated and directed to the appropriate, responsible individual.

After completing this chapter, you should be able to:
- Describe the basic components of communication.
- Identify effective ways of communicating with the health care team
- Describe an assertive communication style
- Apply effective communication skills in various nursing activities
- Identify different types of groups and explain group process
- Discuss team building, group problem solving, and interprofessional practice
- Analyze components of interprofessional practice

Communication is like breathing—we do it all the time, and the better we do it, the better we feel. At times communication can be so subtle that others are not able to understand the communicator. Communication between people in everyday life is an exercise in subtleties and interpretations. The more personal the information, the more indirect and obscure the message becomes. In nursing, indirect communications and obscure terminology can make the difference between life and death. When you say, "I want to be clear when I communicate with others," it is no different from washing windows. The clearer the window, the better we see. Communicating with the health care team and teaching patients what they need to know is part of the foundation of nursing care (Critical Thinking Box 12.1).

? CRITICAL THINKING BOX 12.1
Try This …

1. In how many different ways can you communicate this sentence to change its meaning or tone? "I do not care how you've done that procedure before; do it my way now."
2. The instructor says to you, "Come to my office at 2:00 p.m. There's something I want to talk to you about." What are some possible interpretations of this message?
3. A patient's spouse says to you, "I do not need your help when we go home." How many possible explanations can you come up with regarding the meaning of the communication?
4. During hand-off report, the nurse says to you, "I bet your shift today will be a memorable one—your newly admitted patient is quite the character." How might this message be interpreted?

COMMUNICATION IN THE WORKPLACE

Sharing information with the health care team can require a variety of approaches. This communication on a daily basis may involve delegation of a nursing procedure to nursing personnel, clarification of a prescriber's orders, reevaluation of a patient-care assignment of another health care team member, or coordination of various hospital departments (e.g., radiology, dietary, pharmacy, surgery, laboratory) to provide nursing care. Create role-playing situations with your peers by taking turns acting in the supervisor and subordinate roles (Critical Thinking Box 12.2).

? CRITICAL THINKING BOX 12.2
Try This …

Role-play these situations with your classmates. Try taking turns acting in the supervisory and subordinate roles.
1. The charge nurse has asked the team leader and the nurse caring for Mr. Smith to provide an update on his progress and anticipated discharge date.
2. You are the team leader giving bedside reports to two nursing assistants and one LPN who will be working on your team today.
3. You are caring for a patient who has been newly diagnosed with type 2 diabetes. You discuss the patient's care and discharge plan with the dietitian, social worker, and patient's wife.
4. You are a nursing supervisor on a telemetry unity. On a couple occasions you have noticed a staff nurse's unpleasant body odor but have not said anything to the nurse hoping that the body odor issue was an isolated event. During rounds today, a patient informed you that the nurse's body odor was making her feel nauseated and she would like to be assigned another nurse. You inform the nurse of the body odor concern.

How Can I Communicate Effectively With My Supervisor?

Upward communication with supervisors takes on a formal nature. It is important to learn and use the appropriate channels of communication. For example, you may share information with your designated team leader on the unit. The team leader shares information with the nursing supervisor or nurse manager, who shares information with the assistant vice president of nursing, who shares information with the vice president of nursing, and so on. From this example, you can see the communication approach taken with the appropriate chain of command.

Do you remember the game you played as a child in which someone whispers a secret to the next person, and each person repeats the secret down the line until the last person speaks the secret aloud? The secret may have started out as "Jenny was out picking berries today so she can bake a pie." By the end of the line, it may have become "Jenny is so allergic to cherries that she breaks out into hives." The point is that messages can become very distorted when they travel through the chain of command in the upward flow of communication. Hosley and Molle (2006) say that when communicating with your supervisor, it is important to present your concerns or needs clearly, explain how the issue makes you feel, explain how the issue has affected you, and suggest a solution to the issue that benefits both your needs and the needs of the larger unit. It is also important to listen objectively to the response of the supervisor, because there may be good reasons for granting or not granting the request.

Hosley and Molle (2006) offer the following tips for talking to your supervisor:
1. Keep your supervisor informed of potential or upcoming issues/problems.
2. If a problem is developing, make an appointment to talk it over (especially if you think the meeting will be longer than 15 minutes). Scheduling an appointment demonstrates courtesy in terms of the supervisor's time and minimizes interruptions during the meeting.
3. Be organized. Have specific information available, especially written documentation of facts. Focus on resolving the problems, not just the problems. List on a piece of paper what items/issues you would like to discuss so as to keep you focused during the meeting.
4. State the facts. Avoid blaming others, exaggerating, and using overly dramatic expressions. Keep the conversation focused on your needs.
5. Use "I" statements, and explain what you think in a professional manner.
6. Do not share the details of your conversation with others who do not have a stake in the issue.

How Can I Communicate Effectively With Other Nursing Personnel?

When you speak with other professional nurses and health care team members, you communicate using a lateral, or horizontal, flow of information (Merlino, 2017). This type of communication is best achieved in a work climate that promotes a sense of trust and respect among colleagues. Ideally, professional nurses should view themselves as equals in their interactions with members of other health care disciplines, and their approach to communication should be a lateral one. The basis of this communication is the ability of the nurse to see himself or herself as competent and worthy of being an equal to physicians, social workers, dietitians, and others. Gaining this self-confidence is a major goal of every recent graduate. Using effective communication practices, as described in this chapter, and communication reporting tools (see Chapter 11 for information on hand-off communication) will help you to achieve that goal.

Even a recent graduate will soon be providing direction to licensed nursing personnel and unlicensed assistive nursing personnel (see Chapter 14 for further information on delegation). It is important to remember that these people also have needs for satisfaction and self-esteem. Directions do not have to be given in the form of authoritative commands unless an emergency calls for immediate action in a prescribed way. Marquis and Huston (2014) suggest that when you provide direction, you must think through exactly what you want done, by whom, and when. You must get the full attention of the other person so that you will know that he or she hears you accurately. You should provide clear, simple instructions in step-by-step order, using a supportive tone of voice. Before the other person goes to do the task, ask for feedback to verify that he or she has accurately heard your instructions. Follow-up is necessary to make sure that your directions were followed and to find out what happened in case something more must be done. Involving personnel who are at other levels of nursing care in the planning and evaluation of patient care will increase those associates' sense of responsibility for the outcomes and will help you to seem less authoritarian. Refer to the checklist in Critical Thinking Box 12.3 to identify areas needed for growth.

? CRITICAL THINKING BOX 12.3

Facilitation Skills Checklist

Directions: Periodically during the clinical experience, use this checklist to identify areas needed for growth and progress made. Think of your clinical patient experiences. Indicate the extent of your agreement with each of the following statements by marking the scale: **SA, strongly agree; A, agree; NS, not sure; D, disagree; SD, strongly disagree.**

	SA	A	NS	D	SD
1. I maintain good eye contact.	SA	A	NS	D	SD
2. Most of my verbal comments follow the lead of the other person.	SA	A	NS	D	SD
3. I encourage others to talk about feelings.	SA	A	NS	D	SD
4. I am able to ask open-ended questions.	SA	A	NS	D	SD
5. I can restate and clarify a person's ideas.	SA	A	NS	D	SD
6. I can summarize in a few words the basic ideas of a long statement made by a person.	SA	A	NS	D	SD
7. I can make statements that reflect the person's feelings.	SA	A	NS	D	SD
8. I can share my feelings relevant to the discussion when it is appropriate to do so.	SA	A	NS	D	SD
9. I am able to give feedback.	SA	A	NS	D	SD
10. At least 75% or more of my responses help to enhance and facilitate communication.	SA	A	NS	D	SD
11. I can help a person to list some possible alternatives.	SA	A	NS	D	SD
12. I can help a person to identify some goals that are specific and observable.	SA	A	NS	D	SD
13. I can help a person to specify at least one next step that might be taken toward the goal.	SA	A	NS	D	SD

Adapted from Myrick, D., & Erney, T. (2000). *Caring and sharing* (2nd ed.). Minneapolis: Educational Media Corporation (p. 168).

WHAT DOES MY IMAGE COMMUNICATE TO OTHERS?

Remember the old saying "Do not judge a book by its cover."

Unfortunately we know that most people do not follow that suggestion. People develop impressions about us from the way we look, sound, talk, and act. Often we are less careful about the messages we send with our appearance and behavior than we are when we choose our words. But our image may speak louder than our words. Think about it. Would you feel comfortable accepting nutritional advice from a nurse who was morbidly obese? How would you like it if your instructor criticized your professionalism while wearing dirty shoes, a wrinkled uniform, bright red nail polish, and four earrings in each earlobe? What would you think about a physician whose progress notes contained many misspelled words and poor grammar?

Your credibility is enhanced by good communication. Your image will help you communicate your professional credibility. Maintaining personal hygiene and grooming is essential. Your appearance at work should conform to the norms for professionals in your work setting; save your individuality for your personal time away from work.

Another aspect of your image is your depth and breadth of knowledge of your particular area in nursing. However, you must also be familiar with a wide variety of subjects so that you can have conversations with people beyond nursing. When people find that they have interests in common with you, they become more willing to communicate.

Flexibility is necessary for effective communication with different kinds of people. This means that you are willing and able to adapt your behavior to relate more comfortably or effectively with others. Flexibility is part of a positive image and says to people that you are willing to accept responsibility for changing your behavior to meet the professional needs or requirements of others. Take an inventory of your appearance, knowledge, and attitude. If you are not sure what kind of image you are communicating, ask several trusted friends.

How Do Gender Differences Influence Communication Styles?

Men and women view their work environments from different perspectives (Mindell, 2001; Vengel, 2010). Men often see the world from a logical, sequential, focused perspective. Women often tend to see the big picture and to seek solutions based on what makes people feel comfortable. Subtle communication differences can create barriers to open, healthy communication between men and women in the workplace. Within the workplace, the dominant communication style is direct, confident, and assertive. This style may be more familiar to men, because they are often raised hearing more aggressive, direct language from their parents, whereas many women may be more used to a soft, supportive tone of voice and choice of words. Cultural values learned in childhood also play a role in the communication style a person chooses. This style may have to be modified to make interactions more successful. A woman who is communicating with a man may have to be more direct and assertive than usual, whereas a man may have to learn to be less aggressive in many situations.

To summarize, men and women have innately different communication styles, often developed from their childhood experiences and environment. To be successful in the workplace, we all have to learn as much as we can about communication differences, identify our own styles, and have the flexibility to use other communication techniques as situations warrant.

What Should I Know About the "Grapevine"?

> The grapevine is like the tabloid newspapers. Would you bet your job on the accuracy of a rumor? So when in doubt, check the facts out!

In addition to formal messages, communication can be informal. This type of communication flows upward, downward, and horizontally and is known as the *grapevine*. Whereas some people think of this kind of communication as gossip, others say it is the way things really get done. No matter how we describe the grapevine, we know that it flourishes in all settings. People enjoy the satisfaction of the social interaction and recognition associated with the grapevine. It also provides information to employees that may not be easily obtained in any other way. It may be the quickest way to find out what the supervisor really values or what new job openings are available (Marquis & Huston, 2014) (Fig. 12.1).

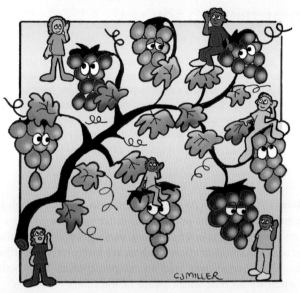

FIG. 12.1 What should you know about the grapevine?

Mindell (2001) provides the following tips for controlling the grapevine:

1. Provide factual information to answer questions before they are asked. Few employees get all the information they feel they need.
2. Communicate face to face whenever possible. Do not trust the accuracy of messages conveyed through a third party.
3. Whenever rumors are running through the grapevine, hold a meeting to provide information and answer questions.
4. Do not spread rumors. Make sure you have all the facts from their source.
5. Enlist the support of respected leaders to spread the truth.
6. Address significant issues as soon as possible with your manager so that negative feelings can be defused.
7. Make sure that what is put in writing is clear and accurately understood.

How Can I Handle Cultural Diversity at Work?

Giger (2013) tells us that culture is a pattern of values and beliefs reflected in the behaviors we demonstrate. Whenever a group of people spend an extended period of time together, that group develops a culture. Each of us comes from a cultural background, and we have beliefs, values, and behaviors that result from that background. In our workplaces, we will encounter many different types of people coming from diverse cultural backgrounds. To communicate effectively, we must understand our own culture as well as the other person's culture. In addition, we must acknowledge and adhere to the cultural norms or rules that have developed in our workplace.

We must be aware of stereotypes that may interfere with our ability to see people as individuals. If we view people according to stereotypes, we might limit the way in which we perceive their communication. Even positive stereotypes involve assumptions about people that may be inaccurate and thus may limit the nurse's ability to use all of his or her work skills effectively (Critical Thinking Box 12.4).

? CRITICAL THINKING BOX 12.4
Try This ...

As you go about your work, take note of the various people you interact with and your reactions to them. Write these observations down so that you can reflect on them later. What kinds of thoughts come to mind when you see a female executive, an older woman, or a handsome man dressed in a suit? What kinds of thoughts come to mind when you see people of ethnic origins that differ from your own? How do your initial impressions affect the way you communicate with each of these people?

Now picture yourself in the homes of five of your patients. Choose people from different cultural backgrounds. How are their homes different? In what ways do their homes reflect their culture? How does the family communicate in the home? What do you need to know about each culture so that you can provide culturally congruent care effectively while avoiding any stereotyped beliefs?

According to Arredondo (2000), communication goes through many filters when a person interacts with someone whom he or she perceives as different. Some of those filters are related to culture, gender, education level, age, and experience. When messages go through these filters, the messages may change because the actual communication symbols are interpreted according to a person's own cultural values and beliefs. This change may lead to misperceptions and misinterpretations. Communication is improved when we become more aware of the filters we use.

Within the work culture, people often communicate using jargon, inside jokes, or slang unique to the work setting. Acronyms are an example of jargon that health care workers understand but patients may not. It may seem to patients and their families that we are speaking in a code or foreign language. To interact effectively, we must speak clearly, avoid jargon or slang, and keep our communications short and to the point. Long explanations with lengthy terminology can be confusing to people who are not familiar with the health care culture.

Differences in the cultural backgrounds of workers can be a real asset. Sometimes we may have to provide care to patients who speak languages other than English, and we may have to enlist the skills of a medical interpreter to translate or interpret, especially when cultural values influence the interpretation of the patient's behavior. We must understand and respect cultural differences in patients. We can learn how to do this by interviewing the patient in a culturally competent manner (see Chapter 21 for more information on conducting a cultural assessment). Respect and empathy enhance communication with people from other cultures, whether those people are patients or coworkers (Giger, 2013).

COMPONENTS OF EFFECTIVE COMMUNICATION

How Can I Communicate Effectively in Writing?

Communication takes place not only when words are spoken but also when they are written and then read by someone else. A big part of a nurse's overall effectiveness depends on the ability to write effectively. This includes written treatment plans, progress notes, job descriptions, consultation requests, referrals, and memos. Some of you may even write articles for nursing journals or chapters for textbooks!

Mindell (2001) provides some guidelines for writing. First, determine whether you have to write in a formal way. Most upward communication must be formal, which means that you should use proper titles, format, grammar, spelling, and punctuation. Never allow something you have written to be sent without careful proofreading. Nothing creates a negative impression faster than sloppy work, misspelled words, or poor grammar. If you must, ask someone else to do this proofreading and make sure that it is done well. Take the time to make necessary revisions before sending your written work to others.

Also decide what your purpose is before you write (Marquis & Huston, 2014). This will help you to organize your thoughts so that everything you write helps to meet your purpose. Learn to write exactly what you mean. Choose words that are clear and specific. Often this means simple, small words. Be careful to use technical words only when you are sure you are choosing the correct words and that your reader will understand you. Keep your sentences short and simple, with only one idea in each sentence.

> Try using the KISS principle: Keep It Short and Simple.

When you learn to be clear and concise, you will write the essential information without many lengthy phrases. Your readers will be very grateful if they can follow your thoughts easily. Make sure the first sentence in each paragraph identifies the key point for that paragraph. The reader should not have to guess what you are trying to say. Use a format that guides the reader. This means that main points on each page are easy to locate visually and concepts are identified by headings or titles. Remember, how well you write strongly influences how you are evaluated. What you put down on paper makes a lasting impression, and people will make judgments about your credibility and professionalism for a long time after you have actually written the words.

How Can I Learn to Speak Effectively?

From giving a change-of-shift report to another nurse, to explaining your plans for a new protocol on the unit, to the organization's administration, you will have many opportunities speaking to individuals or an entire audience! Even now as a student, you may have the opportunity to make a presentation to your peers.

> The first step in making effective presentations is to develop a positive attitude. *Accentuate the positive!*

Many of us let our anxiety intimidate us when it comes to public speaking. However, public speaking can be a great chance to show off your skills, your ability to be creative, and your willingness to be a star entertainer. Think of your presentation as a wonderful opportunity to have the attention of others on just you, even if only for a few minutes (Arredondo, 2000).

> The second guiding principle in making good presentations and speaking in front of an audience is practice. *Practice makes perfect!*

A well-planned rehearsal gives you a chance to see how long it will take to say what you want, and it will help you feel more comfortable saying the words easily. Here are some tips on presentation preparation from Kushner (2004) and Peoples (1992).

Analyze Your Audience

What do they already know, and what do they need to know? Have a few objectives for what you want your audience to receive from your presentation.

Do Your Homework

Know enough about your subject to make your talk clear and believable. Make sure you can answer at least a few questions.

Plan the Presentation

This includes making an outline of the content and the teaching strategies you might use. Visual aids or activities may be used to involve the audience in active participation. Visual aids should keep the presentation focused and organized. They should help you hold your audience's attention. **(Plus, you are more likely to persuade with visual cues.)**

Add Spice to the Presentation

The more active your audience's participation, the longer they will pay attention. Choose at least one presentation strategy that involves them, such as question/answer, role-playing, or small-group discussion. Highlight visually on slides or using other types of media the key points you want your audience to remember. Pecha Kucha is an innovative format for developing presentations. A Pecha Kucha is essentially a slide-show presentation where you show 20 slides, each for 20 seconds (Pecha Kucha, 2019). Check out the following video from University of North Dakota for details on developing a Pecha Kucha (https://www.youtube.com/watch?v=32WEzM3LFhw) (Fig. 12.2). **Use an attention grabber at the beginning** to make sure your audience is listening. This may be a friendly greeting, a stimulating question, a startling statistic, a relevant story, or a quote by an expert. Then, in brief and concise words, tell your audience the purpose of the presentation and what it will cover.

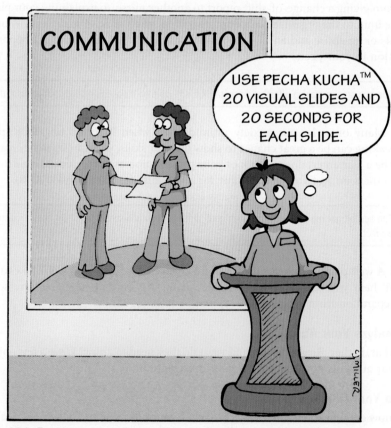

FIG. 12.2 Engage your audience. (From https://www.pechakucha.org/contact.)

Create Cheat Sheets

Cheat sheets are your clues—jot down the first couple of words around a topic to help you remember what to say or what questions to ask, or include small pictures or drawings to jog your memory during the presentation in case you stumble and fumble with your thoughts and words. If the speech or presentation is an important one and is fairly formal, you may want to prepare a script. This means that you write out exactly what you will say and have it typed double-spaced, with a wide margin on the left side. Here you can write notes to yourself about when to use your visual aids or when to pass out materials for the audience. Even if you choose to write a script, **be sure to memorize the first 2 minutes of what you are going to say!**

The Closing

In your closing, review what you have said, summarize the benefits or implications of what you have said, and reiterate any action you want taken. **(Design your closing *first*, because it is the most important part of the formal presentation. It may sound crazy to work backward, but the closing is what the audience will hear last and remember. Write it out and memorize it!)**

Final Details

Be familiar with the room and equipment you will use prior to the presentation. Determine that everything you need is there before you begin. Make sure that the spelling on your visual aids and handouts is correct. Speak with confidence and enthusiasm while making as much eye contact as you can. Walk around the room and use your hands and arms to make dramatic gestures. They add energy and interest. Most important—relax and have some fun. If you make a mistake, learn to laugh at yourself and move on. Your audience will forgive you. They may not be any more comfortable with public speaking than you are and will generally reach out and be supportive of you.

What Listening Skills Do I Need to Develop?

Listening effectively is one of the most powerful communication tools you can have. It is more than just hearing the words of others. Listening involves concentrating all your energy on understanding and interpreting the message with the meaning the sender intended. Of the four verbal means of communication—writing, reading, speaking, and listening—listening requires most of our communication time, yet we often pay the least attention to our listening skills (Mindell, 2001). It has been estimated that people actually remember only one-third of the messages they have heard, although they spend 70% of their time listening (Marquis & Huston, 2014).

> Did you know? People speak at 100 to 175 words per minute, but they can listen intelligently at 600 to 800 words per minute (Poskey, 2013).

There are reasons why people are not good listeners (Arredondo, 2000). We simply do not pay enough attention; we hear what we want to hear and filter out the rest. Listening requires concentration, and that means doing nothing else at the same time. Some people think of listening as a passive behavior; they want to be in control by talking more. We think a lot faster than people speak, so we often think way ahead, think about other things, or daydream. Maybe too many distractions are interfering with listening, such as background noises (text messages and other alert sounds made by mobile devices) or movements.

One of the most problematic reasons for ineffective listening is that people allow their emotions to dictate what they hear or do not hear. If the message is making demands on us to do more, change what we do, or do better, we may stop listening and start dealing with our own feelings of anger, guilt, or anxiety. We may start planning our own defensive response while the other person is still talking.

Think about situations where you've had difficulty listening, understanding, or remembering what was said. Consider these examples:

■ A psychiatric patient who has recently been admitted displays acutely psychotic thought processes by talking rapidly in pressured speech, using words and phrases so loosely connected that the whole conversation is disorganized and incomprehensible.

■ A charge nurse spends 5 minutes screaming at her team leader, criticizing everything she has done that day, and then asks the team leader to carry out a very specific and detailed change in the prescriber's orders for a patient.

■ Another nurse asks you to hang an intravenous solution for the patient in Room 1253 while you are writing a progress note in a patient's chart. When you finish, you cannot remember the room number where you agreed to hang the intravenous solution.

It becomes essential to develop effective listening skills (Arredondo, 2000). Here are some tips.

Make Sure You Can Hear What Is Being Said

Move closer, eliminate distracting noises, and most important of all, do not talk. You cannot hear someone else when you are talking.

Focus Your Attention on What Is Being Said

Actively concentrate by analyzing the key points as they are being made. Take notes. Do not do anything else while you are listening except to concentrate on hearing and understanding what is being said.

Recognize and Control Your Emotional Response to What Is Being Said

Focus on hearing and seeing accurately what is being communicated. You will have time to ask questions and explore your feelings after the other person finishes. As Vertino (2014) pointed out, if you feel threatened during communication with others, step back and take a few minutes to calm down before responding.

Make the Decision to Listen and Accept the Other Person's Needs and Feelings, Whatever They Are

Improved understanding of the other person is gained through listening, and this understanding will help you to be more effective in solving problems and eliminating negative feelings.

Pay Attention to Nonverbal Communication as You Listen to the Words

Much of a message's meaning is communicated through the sender's tone of voice, facial expressions, and body movements. You must listen with your eyes and your ears.

Fight Off Distractions

Do not let the speaker's style of communicating, his or her mannerisms, or other interruptions such as telephone calls or another person vying for your attention break your concentration.

Take Notes

If a lot of factual, important information is being shared, take notes—but just jot down key words or numbers or the note-taking itself will become a distraction. You may also ask the speaker to put in writing what he or she has said.

Let the Speaker Tell the Whole Story

Make it a point not to interrupt. Don't assume you know what is going to be said. Don't formulate criticisms as you listen.

React to the Message, Not the Person

Ask yourself, "Are my feelings or biases interfering with my listening?" Seek clarification of your understanding by verifying what you have heard.

Respond Positively to the Feelings Being Communicated

Empathy and acceptance will make it easier for the communication to continue. Maintain a positive attitude about listening. Recognize that listening is necessary for success. Allow yourself to hear all sides of an issue.

Identify the characteristics of your listening skills in Critical Thinking Box 12.5.

? CRITICAL THINKING BOX 12.5

Try This …

Develop a listening action plan.
1. I listen most effectively when …
2. I have difficulty listening when …
3. My best listening skills are …
4. To improve my listening skills, I will …

How Can I Use Nonverbal Communication Effectively?

Nonverbal communication uses movements, gestures, body position, facial expressions, and voice tone to transmit messages (Varcarolis, 2017). To convey confidence and leadership ability, it is necessary to learn to use certain nonverbal signals effectively. Here are some tips.

Make Eye Contact With the Person With Whom You Are Talking

This helps the person interpret your message more favorably and says that you are giving your full attention to the conversation.

Stand Up Straight, With Shoulders Back

You may want to lean slightly forward toward the other individual to convey your interest. Stand with your toes pointed slightly outward and slightly apart and approximately 18 in to 4 ft from the person you are talking to so that you do not invade his or her personal space. Avoid personal remarks unless you know the person well and it is a casual conversation.

To Suggest Confidence, Use an Assertive Voice Without Pauses

Avoid a whining, nagging, or complaining tone. You may have to listen to your recorded voice to gain some insight into how you sound to others.

Watch for Distracting Behaviors

Avoid negative behaviors that detract from your verbal messages—nodding constantly, yawning, playing with your hair, checking messages on your phone, looking away from the other person, or constantly shifting your weight from one foot to the other. When you use your hands in gestures, keep your forearms up and the palms of your hands open. Avoid making a fist or shaking a pointing finger at the other person.

How Can I Communicate Effectively by Using Technology?

Many of us use technology as a modality for making communication easier. Although cell phones, e-mail, text messaging, tablets, and other mobile devices may be conveniences, they must be used thoughtfully to make a positive contribution to your overall image as an effective communicator. Believe it or not, there is an actual term for communicating properly online—*netiquette*. Deep and Sussman (1995) give the following netiquette tips.

Do Not Misuse or Overuse E-mail and Text Messaging

Review the tips for the effective use of e-mail and text messaging. If you need to send a long document or detailed message, use e-mail.

Learn to Use Computer Software

Using technology can make not only your work but also your communication easier and more effective. Integrated computer systems on hospital units, electronic health record systems, passive infrared tracking of patients and nurse locations along with enhanced nurse-call systems, wireless in-house telephone systems, and web-based electronic grease boards to track patients throughout their days of scheduled surgeries, diagnostic tests, and so forth can be viewed on computer monitors in patients' rooms or from large display monitors strategically located throughout a department (Bahlman & Johnson, 2005).

When You Send E-mail Messages

If you are sending messages by e-mail, be sure to perform a grammar and spell check, and read your words carefully before sending them. Because you are sending words without the benefit of clarifying nonverbal communication, the likelihood of being misinterpreted is greater. Make sure your messages are as clear as they can be. Include your name and the subject in the e-mail note.

Do Not Send an Emotional Outburst in an E-mail

These messages can seem more hostile than you intended, and you can alienate or anger many people. If you would not say these words in person, then do not send them by e-mail (Box 12.1).

When You Leave a Voice Mail Message for Someone, Speak Slowly and Distinctly

This is especially important when you are leaving your telephone number so that the other person can return your call. It is frustrating to receive a message but not be able to understand the name or have to replay the message to get all of the digits in the phone number. Make your voice mail message brief but complete, saying when you called, what you want the other person to do, and when you can be reached.

If You Are Using Call Waiting, Do Not Leave Callers on Hold

Explain to the first caller that you must briefly answer another call, then take the number of the second caller, with the assurance that you will call back as soon as you finish your first call. This interruption should last no longer than 10 seconds. Be sure to write down the telephone number of the second caller so that you do not forget it by the time you finish the first call.

BOX 12.1 TIPS FOR USING E-MAIL EFFECTIVELY

1. Stop, think about what you want to say, *then write.*
   - Be sure to determine whether an e-mail is the appropriate communication medium. E-mail is meant for quick, simple communication. Ask yourself whether a phone conversation or face-to-face meeting would be more appropriate.
2. Include a descriptive subject line.
   - In the subject line of the e-mail note, place a description of what the e-mail is about. Be specific—for example, Quarterly QA Report or Case Study Assignment—Informatics.
3. Make your e-mail note easy to read.
   - Use short paragraphs, usually no more than two or three paragraphs at most—get to the point, quickly. Consider that most people have a limited attention span with e-mail, especially if they are receiving a lot of messages.
   - Have ample white space on the page. Usually five to seven lines of text are best for a paragraph.
   - Use bullets or numbers to guide the reader.
   - Carefully choose your font size, type, and color. Using a bright color (such as purple) may not convey as professional a tone as a standard black or navy font would. Very large fonts (14-point or more) might make your message seem "loud" and accusatory. A sans serif font, such as Arial or Tahoma 10–12 point, is easier to read on the computer screen than a serif font such as Times Roman.
4. Be precise, concise, and clear.
   - Use a conversational writing style.
   - If responding to multiple questions embedded in a large e-mail, copy the questions into your e-mail and write your answers next to them using a different font color.
   - When replying to a message, include enough of the original e-mail note to provide context to your response.
   - If in doubt, spell it out—limit your use of jargon or abbreviations.
   - Always spell check and proof your e-mail before you send it.
5. Demonstrate netiquette—be professional and maintain appropriate online tone.
   - Do not type in all CAPS! Capitals can be used for emphasis, but all caps looks like you're yelling at the person. If you emphasize everything, then nothing ends up seeming more important than the rest.
   - Do not type in all lowercase—this violates the rules of English grammar and usage. Keep in mind that you are not texting a friend.
   - If a communication is upsetting to you, keep calm and collected. Your emotional state can slip into an e-mail without notice, in the form of curt sentences, skipped pleasantries, and blunt comments.
   - Remember, unlike telephone and personal conversations that fade from the memory with time, impulsive e-mail responses have "staying power"—meaning the e-mail is readily available in e-mail boxes, can be printed out, distributed to others, and attain a level of importance that was never intended.
   - A word about flaming (which is the expression of extreme emotion or opinion in an e-mail message, often derogatory); be polite and pleasant, and consider whether you want to respond to a flaming e-mail.
6. Be careful with attachments.
   - Open attachments only if you trust the source, because attachments can contain executable files that can spread viruses and slow down processing.
   - Consider the size of the attachments—large files (greater than 1000 KB or 1 MB) can clog up networks and rapidly fill your Inbox. Many servers prohibit the sending and receiving of large e-mail file attachments.
   - Use spam filters and delete chain e-mails or other scams—do not open the document or have the viewing pane open, because this can perpetuate the spam.
7. Watch humor.
   - Find different ways to express emotion, body language, and intonation, when warranted. Use smileys, also called emoticons, to convey feelings in your message; however, be careful not to overuse them.
   - As in any setting, humor can be misconstrued, so be extra careful and exercise good taste and discretion before transmitting any humor.
8. Include a signature.
   - Include a signature with your e-mail, usually no more than four to six lines of text. Remember, this part of your message is the last thing the receiver will read.
   - Include your name, title, contact information, and e-mail address or URL. Many e-mail programs can be set up to attach automatically a default signature or signature file to the end of all your outgoing messages (including replies).

Continued

BOX 12.1   TIPS FOR USING E-MAIL EFFECTIVELY—CONT'D

9. Review your message before sending.
   - Remember, e-mail is not confidential; do not send personal or sensitive e-mail, because there is no "secure" e-mail system.
   - Review and proof your message before clicking "Send."
   - Read your message aloud; you are more likely to catch typos and grammatical errors when you are "hearing" them.
10. Respond to e-mail.
   - Make an effort to respond to e-mail within 24 hours. Otherwise, use the auto-reply function to inform the person when you will respond.
11. Text messaging.
   - Keep in mind that most agencies do not want you texting during your clinical work. Check with faculty about using your smart phone in the clinical area.

When You Call Someone, Ask if He or She Has Time to Talk, and Offer to Call Back at a More Convenient Time if Necessary

People appreciate this courtesy and will be more likely to have a positive conversation with you if it is conveniently timed and is respectful of their busy schedules.

If You Are Conducting a Conversation or a Meeting With a Speaker Phone or by Means of a Teleconference, Make Sure That Each Party to the Call Is Introduced to the Others

Do not use the speaker phone unless you are including a group in the conversation. Even with a conference call, there should be some structure to the discussion, including an agenda or a specified purpose and time for the call. Learn how to "mute" a conversation, especially when there is considerable background noise.

When You Must Send a Personal Message, Especially a Reminder or a Thank-You Note, the Most Powerful Way Is to Send a Handwritten Note

This conveys the importance you connect with the message and continues the interpersonal aspect of the communication. If you must communicate something that you expect will have a significant emotional impact, do it face to face. This communication style also gives you an opportunity to read the other person's nonverbal communication and offers a chance to negotiate a comfortable understanding once your message has been received.

GROUP COMMUNICATION

What Is Group Process?

When we discuss the dynamics and communication patterns of groups, it is important to note that personality conflicts may develop during the different cyclical phases of the group. In **forming** the group, think back to orientation day for nursing school. You sit surrounded by some people you have never seen before and some you have known from your prenursing classes. A common bond is that you are all there for well-defined reasons, including finding out who is in your clinical group and who the instructors will be. Of course, the orientation is mandatory. You sit in the auditorium or classroom talking, listening, and watching those around you, playing your part in a form of controlled pandemonium. The pandemonium can actually be considered the storming phase. In the **storming** phase, you begin to act out the roles you normally portray in the presence of your peers as you discuss your fears, fantasies, and hopes for the successful completion of your nursing program (Tuckman & Jensen, 1977).

Next, you are divided into clinical groups. You now begin to reevaluate the personality composition of the new groups. As you begin to react to your new relationships, you start to exhibit personality traits to establish the role you would like to be identified with in the group setting. Unfortunately your unconscious defense mechanisms surface in the form of competitive conflict or one-upmanship within the group, and your hope is that your response will secure the role you would like to have within the group. It is at this time that **norming** begins to develop among members of the group, with the help of the instructors. Norming occurs during the development of mutual goals and guidelines that help to redefine people's behavioral roles in the group. This can lead to agreement and activities that will help to establish a purposeful clinical experience involving interdependence and flexibility.

During the **performing** phase, everyone knows one another; all are able to work together and to trust one another. The group works together and makes changes in a seamless way because there is a high degree of comfort among the group members that funnels all of the energy of the group toward the task at hand—getting through nursing school. Later Tuckman and Jensen (1977) added the final stage, **adjourning,** which has been called *deforming* and *mourning* by others. This phase is about completion and disengagement, both from the tasks and from the group members. You may have experienced or will experience the adjourning phase as you move from one clinical group to another or during the transition from student to graduate, as you are nearing completion of your nursing program.

Groups can be multipurpose and multidynamic, as are the basic role choices of each participant in a group. When people are working within a group, the real fun and excitement start when group members begin responding to and dealing with the unconscious and semiconscious defense mechanisms of the individuals who are using these mechanisms in the roles they play in the group. The responses of the defensive individual tend to be unproductive, time-consuming, and inappropriate to the harmony and overall function of a group effort. In my years of nursing and group participation, the following tend to be my favorite dysfunctional group personalities.

The **self-servers,** who feel that the rules of the group do not apply to them. They show up late. They are usually unprepared to work. At times they will walk in and out of the group for superficial reasons while appearing preoccupied with unrelated work or issues from outside of the group. When they do participate, their contributions are of little consequence. If they refuse to be functional members of the group, they may have to be asked to leave the group.

The first response of a **critical conservative** to a creative suggestion can be, "No, it won't work," or "But it's always been done this way," or "How can you people succeed if you've never done this before?" They seem to have a criticism for any suggestion other than their own. If it is not done their way, it just is not right. They are obsessively negative and fearful of changes. It is important to recognize the lessons of experiences and outcomes, but it is equally important to find new approaches to old problems.

The **motor mouths** talk just to hear themselves talk. They interrupt at any given moment to make statements or deliver a verbose response, possibly because they feel they have been quiet for too long. Even when another person is talking, motor mouths will talk over the speaker's words just to be the center of attention. These people may begin to make a statement, only to ramble in and out of the group's issue, and end up talking about unrelated issues that are usually about themselves. I suggest redirecting their conversation to focusing on the issue and periodically asking them for a short critical assessment of the issues in question.

The **mouse** is the silent observer who is fearful of voicing an opinion. Usually the mouse sits transfixed, watching other individuals take risks and responsibility for their input to the group. The mouse nods his or her head at appropriate times and answers questions in one or two words. The mouse may be a real addition to the group, especially if others in the group are able to find ways to engage and encourage the mouse to voice opinions and feelings about the group issues. It is important to remember that these people may be some of the best observers and listeners; ask them for their input. You may find them to be valuable assets to your team. Regardless of where you choose to work or the type of care delivery system you are in, these group members are always there!

How Can You Improve Communications in Group Meetings?

Nurses participate in many meetings, from patient-care conferences to more formal committee meetings. Communication within a group of people can be an opportunity to influence the quality of care provided to patients. When you participate as a member of a group, the following are positive behaviors that will help you to communicate effectively and will also help the group to accomplish its tasks more efficiently:

1. If you are the meeting organizer, provide an agenda to the group a few days prior to the meeting, so that each member has an opportunity to review the meeting agenda items and come prepared to participate in the meeting (Riley, 2017).
2. Come prepared. Bring all the "stuff" you need.
3. Ensure that a group member will serve as the recorder and write up the meeting minutes to be disseminated to the group. Riley (2017) suggests that this role be rotated among group members.
4. Listen. Be open to other viewpoints.
5. Keep on track. Do not visit or chit-chat or bring other work to do.
6. Present your ideas or opinions. Ask other members for theirs.
7. State disagreements in a professional manner. Be able to back them up.
8. Clarify as needed. Do not assume.

All of us have been to and participated in meetings that were disorganized, confusing, and a waste of time. Critical Thinking Box 12.6 will help you to identify some unpleasant group meeting experiences and give you the opportunity to change future meetings.

？ CRITICAL THINKING BOX 12.6

Try This …

Think of particularly unpleasant experiences you have had at meetings. You might think about meetings involving your clinical group or study group. Develop a list of ideas about what was wrong with those meetings.

The key to effective meetings is the planning and organization that occur before the meeting is actually held. An effective technique using de Bono's (1999) Six Thinking Hats can spur a group meeting to better productivity and problem solving (Box 12.2). Planning should allow the facilitator to think through what the meeting is for, who should attend, and how it should run. There should be a clear purpose for every meeting and every item on the agenda. Every item should require some action by the group with clear expectations as to what is to be completed before the next meeting (Riley, 2017). If making a telephone call or sending a memo could achieve the purpose in another way, then a face-to-face meeting may not be necessary.

If you are making a formal presentation, some audiovisual equipment will be necessary, and chairs will have to be arranged so that everyone can see the presenter and the audiovisuals. If the meeting is for discussion and decision making, a table at which everyone can sit face to face will be more effective, and someone will have to take meeting minutes. Look at Fig. 12.3. This type of note taking clarifies who is responsible for what activities. At the conclusion of the meeting, summarize the decisions and identify the plan of action. At the end of the meeting, the time for the next meeting should be established. All members should receive a copy of the meeting minutes.

BOX 12.2   EDWARD DE BONO'S SIX THINKING HATS: LOOKING AT A DECISION AND WORKING THROUGH A PROBLEM CONSIDERING SIX POINTS OF VIEW

Six Thinking Hats is an important and powerful technique created by Edward de Bono that can be used as an effective group process tool in meetings that get bogged down with diverse views and adamant positions. It offers a strategy to "think outside the box" by challenging the group to think or see all sides of an issue. Each "Thinking Hat" represents a perspective or way of thinking. During a meeting, a "different color hat" can be put on or taken off to indicate the type of thinking the person is using. By putting on a different hat in a particular sequence, problem solving is encouraged.

White Hat: Neutral, Objective, Concerned With Facts and Figures—The Fact Hat
Used to think about facts, figures, and other objective information (think of a scientist's white lab coat).
- What facts and data are available?
- What facts would help me further in making a decision?
- How can I get those facts?

Red Hat: The Emotional View—The Emotional Hat
Used to elicit the feelings, emotions, and other nonrational but potentially valuable senses, such as hunches and intuition (think of a red heart). Encourages people to express their feelings without the need for apology, explanation, or attempt to justify them.
- How do I really feel?
- What is my gut feeling about this problem?

Black Hat: Careful, Cautious—The "Devil's Advocate" Hat
Used to discover why some ideas will not work, this hat inspires logical negative arguments (think of a devil's advocate or a judge robed in black). Helps you to see problems in advance (spot flaws in thinking), prepare for potential difficulties, and prepare contingency plans to counter the issues.

- What are the possible downside risks and problems?
- What is the worst-case scenario?
- What are the weak points of the plan? It allows you to eliminate them, alter them, or prepare contingency plans to counter them.

Yellow Hat: Sunny and Positive—The Optimistic Hat
Used to obtain a positive, optimistic outlook, this hat sees opportunities, possibilities, and benefits of a decision (think of the warming sun). Keeps you going when the going gets tough.
- What are the advantages?
- What would be the best possible outcome?

Green Hat: Associated With Fertile Growth, Creativity, and New Ideas—The Creative Hat
Used to find creative new ideas (think of new shoots sprouting from seeds).
- What completely new, fresh, innovative approaches can I generate?
- What creative ideas can I dream up to help me see the problem in a new way?
- Are there any additional alternatives or can this be done in a different way?
- Could there be another explanation?

Blue Hat: Cool, the Color of Sky—The Organizing Hat
Used as a master hat to control the thinking process (think of the overarching sky, or a "cool" character who's in control).
- Review my thoughts—it suggests the next step for thinking.
- Sum up what I have learned and think about what the next logical step is—asks for summaries, conclusions, and decisions.

From deBono, E. (1999). *Six thinking hats*. MICA Management Resources. Retrieved from http://www.debonogroup.com/six_thinking_hats.php. Reprinted with permission of the McQuaig Group. Copyright© 1985. All rights reserved. No photocopying or reproduction of this material without consent.

TEAM BUILDING AND INTERPROFESSIONAL PRACTICE

What Is Team Building?

Team building is "the process of influencing a group of diverse individuals, each with their own goals, needs, and perspectives, to work together effectively for the good of the project such that their team will accomplish more than the sum of their individual efforts could otherwise achieve" (Wideman, 2017). Another definition of a team is "a small number of people with complementary skills who are committed to a common purpose in performance of common goals, for which they hold themselves

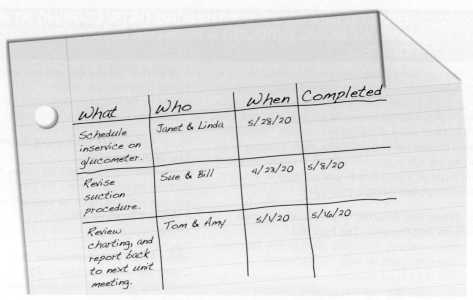

FIG. 12.3 Action time line for meetings.

mutually accountable" (Katzenbach & Smith, 2003, p. 45). Katzenbach and Smith state that the right mix of attributes is needed in three categories that help ensure a highly complementary and functional team. The three categories described are interpersonal skills, problem-solving and decision-making skills, and technical or functional expertise (Critical Thinking Box 12.7).

❓ CRITICAL THINKING BOX 12.7

Think About …

Try to assess and come to your own conclusion regarding the following hypothetical problem by picturing the *who, what,* and *why* before you read what the experts in the field would say.

You will be responsible for the care of your critically ill parent during his or her stay in the hospital during the next 2 months. Assemble a team of your nursing peers to deliver care to your parent. The care will be based on the highest level of difficulty because of the serious nature of the diagnosis.

- What nurses would you choose to help you?
- Why would you choose those specific nurses?
- What qualities would you want them to have when they are caring for your family member?
- What skill level would you want them to possess to carry out the overall treatment plan?
- If some of them lacked the skill levels to meet the treatment plan criteria, what would be an appropriate approach to this inadequacy?

Teams are a formal way to actualize collaboration. Collaboration is at the heart of successful decision making. Collaboration among team members leverages skills, time, and resources for the benefit of the team and that of the organization. If you examine the word *collaboration*, you will see that "co-labor" is the core of the word—meaning "working together toward some meaningful end."

There are many health care professionals who play an integral role in providing quality patient care. Think about what health care professionals you would be collaborating with in the following patient scenario.

You are providing care to a patient with a diagnosis of chronic bronchitis and heart failure. The patient requires nebulizer treatments and has orders for continuous positive airway pressure (CPAP). Arterial blood gases have been ordered, and the lab has just called you to confirm that the patient is in the room. A physical therapy (PT) evaluation and a low-sodium cardiac diet have been ordered by the cardiologist. The patient's spouse is concerned that she will be unable to provide care for her husband after discharge, as she works full time and they have no family nearby to care for him during the day while she is at work.

Well, how many health care professionals did you come up with?

It is a fact that as a nurse you will be part of the health care team. This will require you and other health care professionals to collaborate, communicate, and coordinate delivering safe and effective patient care. Not only will you need to have an understanding of nursing practice, but you must have a foundational understanding of the responsibilities and roles of other health care professions because they will be part of the health care team that you are working with.

What Is Interprofessional Practice?

As its name implies, interprofessional practice involves health care professionals across disciplines working together in providing patient care. The World Health Organization (WHO) offers the following definition of interprofessional practice—that it exists "When multiple health workers from different professional backgrounds work together with patients, families, caregivers, and communities to deliver the highest quality of care across settings" (WHO, 2010, p. 13). Regardless of what type of health care setting you work in as a professional nurse, you will be working with others, including patients and their families as well as the community at large. As you know by now, collaborating and communicating with others is a skill, and it takes time and deliberate practice to develop.

During your clinical rotation, have you communicated with other nonnursing health care professionals (respiratory therapist, registered dietitian, physical therapist, social worker, radiologist technician, phlebotomist, etc.) involved in your patient's care? If you answered "no" to this question, you are not alone. Nevertheless, it is not too early to begin honing your interprofessional practice skills. In fact, you can begin right now while you are still in your nursing program by engaging in learning experiences and activities with students from other health care disciplines on your campus (Research for Best Practice Box 12.1).

When Nurses Work Together as an Interprofessional Team, Everyone Involved Benefits!

In health care, the imperative is on the quality of care and interprofessional teams, as reported by the Institute of Medicine (2003) and other leaders in health care education (Interprofessional Education Collaborative Expert Panel [IPEC], 2011). It is also clear that interprofessional teamwork is essential in care delivery outcomes and cost control (Fig. 12.4).

One of the most important ingredients in the team approach to delivering patient-centered care is a positive psychological and emotional bond among members of the team; it helps to develop more cohesiveness among the individuals of the team. Without a positive cohesive bond, there can and will be limits to the overall quality and function of the team. You as nurses are the unknown intervening variables that either make or break the quality of the team-nursing concept. You and your colleagues, as an interprofessional team, have the skills necessary to handle the multitudes of problems associated with care delivery. You may want to ask yourselves:

RESEARCH FOR BEST PRACTICE BOX 12.1

Interprofessional Collaborative Practice Using Human Patient Simulation

Practice Issue

The current health care climate requires health care professionals to work together as an interprofessional team. Health professions students from various disciplines (nursing, respiratory care, dentistry, medicine, physical therapy, etc.) have limited opportunities in the clinical practice setting for engaging in team-based experiences to further their knowledge and understanding of interprofessional practice. Considering this, health education programs are exploring various learning opportunities for students across health care arenas to work together as a routine part of their education. As the IPEC has pointed out, "The goal was, and remains, to help prepare future health professionals for enhanced team-based care of patients and improved population health outcomes" (IPEC, 2016, p. 1). Although didactic and laboratory instruction is essential to foundational concepts and skills in each respective health education program, interprofessional education is difficult to employ in these learning environments. However, the use of human patient simulation offers health professions students an opportunity to collaborate and communicate with each other during a simulated clinical patient scenario.

Rossler and Kimble (2016) conducted a study examining readiness for interprofessional learning and collaboration among prelicensure nursing, respiratory therapy, health administration, and physical therapy students. The authors' findings suggested that all students gained an appreciation and understanding of their role in working on a team as well as the responsibilities of each team member outside of their discipline. Student participants also reported that the simulation experience gave them an opportunity to practice interprofessional communication. Lee and colleagues (2018) conducted a systematic review of the use of simulation in interprofessional education among health care disciplines. The authors noted that when more than two health care professions were represented in an interprofessional simulation, students participating in the interprofessional simulation reported a greater sense of collaboration and understanding of how interprofessional collaboration is essential to providing patient care.

Implications for Nursing Education and Practice

- Nursing and allied health programs can introduce students to interprofessional practice concepts through human patient simulation.
- Rotating team roles among students will assist students in acquiring knowledge of the various responsibilities of each team member's role.
- The implementation of interprofessional practice activities can improve communication and collaboration among health care professionals.

Considering This Information

Can you identify additional activities or educational opportunities for promoting interprofessional practice?
  What potential challenges do you feel may surface when you are working with other health professions students?
  How can you overcome these challenges?

References

Interprofessional Education Collaborative (IPEC). (2016). *Core competencies for interprofessional collaborative practice: 2016 update.* Washington, DC: Interprofessional Education Collaborative.

Lee, C. A., Pais, K., Kelling, S., & Anderson, O. S. (2018). A scoping review to understand simulation used in interprofessional education. *Journal of Interprofessional Education & Practice, 13*, 15–23. https://doi.org/10.1016/j.xjep.2018.08.003.

Rossler, K. L., & Kimble, L. P. (2016). Capturing readiness to learn and collaboration as explored with an interprofessional simulation scenario: A mixed-method research study. *Nurse Education Today, 36*, 348–353.

- Are you as an individual mentally and emotionally prepared for providing team-based care?
- Can you reflect and make changes on your individual performance as well as the overall team's performance in care delivery?
- Is your attitude about yourself and your peers conducive to support interprofessional teamwork?
- Are you willing to make difficult decisions in directing team care delivery and be accountable?

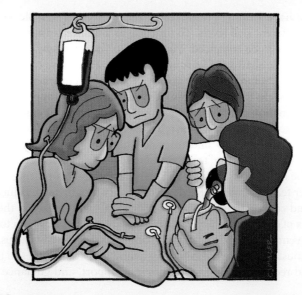

FIG. 12.4 When nurses work as a team, everyone benefits.

- Are you willing to relinquish control of those under your direction when necessary?
- Are you adaptable to changing your role on a team and in different health care settings?

Nurses read and do research to help formulate problem solving and innovative approaches in the establishment of functional care-delivery models. What is frequently left out of the equation is the extent of the role that management is willing to play in helping to ensure the success of the new ideas. Is management willing to share control and leadership to help ensure a successful outcome in nurse-managed teams? I have been witness to the creation of nursing leadership roles—some consisting of team nursing care delivery, decentralization of authority, and shared governance—only to have them fail because of limitations and perceived liabilities placed on the nursing staff by management. At other times, failures were caused by the last-minute intervention of management, usurping the managerial authority of the nursing teams. Some other factors responsible for group or team failure are:

- Nursing staff being unprepared or lacking the interpersonal communication skills needed to work with other staff members in a unified team setting.
- Nurses unwilling to move in and out of leadership roles to ensure the unity of the group and best possible outcomes.
- Management being pressured by upper management for faster adaptation to cost-cutting policies, which usually causes communication between management and nursing to consist of veiled threats, innuendoes, mixed messages, and other subtle negative forms that affect the morale of the nursing staff.
- Nursing supervisors and administrative staff who appear to support shared governance but are unwilling to relinquish actual control of the nursing staff.

Actions always speak louder than words. Work toward transparent communication with administrators. Try to meet them halfway and find out what they are willing to do to support your teams or groups. How much interest do they have in the actual quality of health care delivery? Are they interested in learning the dynamics of your role as a nurse or the role of the interprofessional team? Let them know what type of support you need from them. Explain to them the importance of mutual respect and support in the overall quality of nursing care.

When you are forming a team, realize that perfection is an illusion created in the mind of a critic. All of us have different skill levels. To function as a unified team, you will have to work with peers whose skills may have to be enhanced. You can help your peers by working side by side with them to build confidence while sharing in learning situations. Find ways to make the learning situations enjoyable, show a sense of humor, and give positive reinforcement whenever possible. Fear and guilt undermine confidence and destroy the cohesiveness of a team or group.

In the formation of any team or group, the mental and emotional stability of the individuals who make up the team or group will be reflected in the quality of their work under stress and their ability to focus during care delivery and to establish a working rapport with the other team members. It is important for the stronger team members or group members to provide support and guidance as needed. The attitude of the stronger members of the team can go a long way in building confidence in the other team members. The level of quality for any team is increased substantially by the level of comfort and camaraderie among the individuals who make up the team.

The mix of complementary skills and experience can also help to give strength to the overall group. Taking inventory of technical and communication skills helps identify where weaknesses and strengths must be considered before assigning individual duties to the team members. All team members should receive learning opportunities, support, and guidance to strengthen the cohesiveness of the team.

Realizing the importance of collaborative practice in health care, leaders from dentistry, nursing, medicine, osteopathic medicine, pharmacy, and public health united to develop the Interprofessional Education Collaborative (IPEC) to advance interprofessional education and practice (IPEC, 2011). In 2011, the IPEC board developed core competencies for interprofessional collaborative practice to foster curriculum development across health professions disciplines. The 2011 report identified four competency domains and related subcompetencies for improving interprofessional collaboration and practice; these include values/ethics for interprofessional practice, roles/responsibilities, interprofessional communication, and teams/teamwork (IPEC, 2011). In 2016, the IPEC Board updated the original report to include the four competencies within a singular domain of interprofessional collaboration. The IPEC 2016 update also addresses health system changes that have taken place since the release of the original report, specifically focusing on its triple aim (improving the experience of care, improving the health of populations, and reducing the per capita cost of health care) and the implementation of the Patient Protection and Affordable Care Act in 2010 (IPEC, 2016, pp. 1–2). Their report continues to note that high-functioning interprofessional teams in health care must exhibit features of good team function in all four key competencies.

Working on a team will require you to have an understanding of your own role as well as other health care professionals who are part of your team. Recognizing each team member's role is vital to ensuring that the health care needs of the patient are being met. It will be important for the team members to effectively communicate with one another to make sure that high-quality patient-centered care and continuity of care are delivered (Box 12.3 and Fig. 12.5).

ASSERTIVE STYLES OF COMMUNICATION

All of us have a style or way of communicating with others that is often based on our own personality and self-concept. In other words, the kind of people we are and the way in which we see ourselves influence the process of communication. This style can be divided into three common types: passive or avoidant, aggressive, and assertive (Marquis & Huston, 2014). The following are some characteristics of each style:

BOX 12.3 BASIC ROLES OF GROUP MEMBERS

The following are some roles that individuals adopt when participating in a group. Each member may adopt more than one role.

- Encourager—To be a positive influence on the group
- Harmonizer—To make/keep peace
- Compromiser—To minimize conflict by seeking options
- Gatekeeper—To determine the level of group acceptance of individual members
- Follower—To serve as an interested audience
- Rule maker—To set standards for group behaviors
- Problem solver—To solve problems to allow the group to continue its work
- Leader—To set direction
- Questioner—To clarify issues and information
- Facilitator—To keep the group focused
- Summarizer—To state the current position of the group
- Evaluator—To assess the performance of the group
- Initiator—To begin group discussion

From Riley, J. B. (2017). *Communication in nursing* (8th ed.). St. Louis: Elsevier (p. 248).

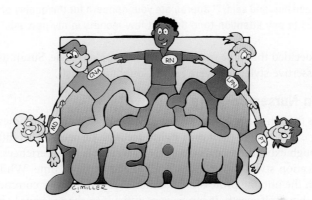

FIG. 12.5 We work as an interprofessional team!

People who tend toward **passive** or **avoidant behavior** let others push them around. These people do not stand up for themselves, do what they are told regardless of how they feel about it, are not able to share their feelings or needs with others, and have difficulty asking for help. They tend to feel hurt, anxious, or angry at others for seeming to take advantage of them.

Aggressive behavior means that a person puts his or her own needs, rights, and feelings first and communicates that in an angry, dominating way; attempts to humiliate or "put down" other people; conveys a righteous, superior attitude; works at controlling or manipulating others; is seen by others as punishing, threatening, demanding, or hostile; and shows no concern for anyone else's feelings.

Assertive behavior means that a person stands up for himself or herself in a way that does not violate the basic rights of another person; expresses true feelings in an honest, direct manner; does not let others take advantage of him or her; shows respect for other's rights, needs, and feelings; sets goals and acts on those goals in a clear and consistent manner and takes responsibility for the consequences of those actions; is able to accept compliments and criticism; and acts in a way that enhances self-respect.

See if you can match the person with his or her style after you have read the descriptions.

■ *Jane*

Jane is a very shy, quiet senior nursing student who can't think straight when her instructor asks her questions in the clinical area. She wishes she could be more like her classmates, who seem to find it easy to talk about their experiences during clinical conference. During her evaluation, her instructor says she doesn't know enough theory and can't handle the pressures of the clinical unit. Jane says nothing and signs her evaluation. When she gets back to her room alone, she cries uncontrollably.

■ *Susan*

Susan is a senior nursing student who is highly verbal with her classmates. She is known to be opinionated, and in every conference with her clinical group she finds a chance to criticize someone. She blames the nursing staff on the clinical unit for making her look bad by giving her too much work to do and not enough time or help. When her instructor tells her she has not integrated sufficient theory in her written assignments, she says, "It's not my fault; you should have told me sooner."

■ *Mark*

Mark is a senior nursing student who is described by his clinical group as goal-oriented and confident. He wrote learning objectives for himself at the beginning of the last clinical experience and brought them with him, along with a self-evaluation for his final evaluation conference. He listened to his instructor's suggestions, thanked her, and said, "I appreciate your concern for the quality of my nursing skills. I'm aware now of what I need to pay attention to in the first few months in my new job."

If you decided that Jane used a passive or avoidant style, Susan used an aggressive style, and Mark used an assertive style, you were right. Congratulations!

How Can Nurses Be More Assertive?

It seems as though many nurses do not consistently act or communicate in an assertive way. Some have a hard time believing in their own rights, feelings, or needs. This difficulty may have started in childhood through exposure to many negative statements or experiences. It is important to recognize that communication style is learned and reinforced through time. While you are in nursing school and working in the nursing profession, additional experiences or comments may reinforce those negative messages about self-worth. It can be very difficult to change your behavior, especially when it involves taking risks. The first step is to recognize what the barriers are. What is it that prevents you from being more assertive? Is it previously learned behavior, or are you afraid of the repercussions of assertive communication? Check the list in Box 12.4. If this list includes statements you feel are true, then you have identified some roadblocks to your ability to develop more assertive communication.

Look over this list of barriers to assertive communication and think about yourself. Do any of these explain your feelings? The development of assertiveness takes self-awareness and practice. It will help

---

BOX 12.4   **BARRIERS TO ASSERTIVENESS**

Barriers to practicing assertiveness include the following misconceptions:

- Using an assertive communication style may threaten others.
- If you don't have anything nice to say, don't say anything.
- If you feel uncomfortable when presenting your position or stating your feelings, you are nonassertive.
- Assertiveness should come easily and spontaneously.
- Health care facilities do not promote or support assertive behavior.
- You cannot be assertive and consider another person's feelings and behavior at the same time.
- Assertive behavior is just another way of complaining.
- If I am assertive, I will lose my job.
- There is no difference between assertiveness and aggressiveness.

you if you identify and accept your position right now with regard to assertiveness so that you can make a plan to develop this skill.

What Are the Benefits of Assertiveness?

Assertive communication is the most effective way to let other people know what you feel, what you need, and what you are thinking. It helps you to feel good about yourself and allows you to treat others with respect. Being assertive helps you to avoid feeling guilty, angry, resentful, confused, or lonely. You have a greater chance to get your rights acknowledged and your needs met, which leads to a more satisfying life.

What Are My Basic Rights as a Person and as a Nurse?

As an adult human being, you have some legitimate rights. You may have to do some work to allow yourself to believe in your rights. You may have learned other values that make it difficult to accept the validity of these rights. But belief in your own value as a separate individual and confidence in the positive concepts associated with assertiveness as a communication style will help you to believe in your rights.

Consider the rights and responsibilities of the nurse. The issue of rights can become one-sided. When nurses consider rights, responsibilities must also be included. These rights are yours as a registered nurse; acquiring them and holding them are your responsibility (Chenevert, 1997).

How Can I Begin to Practice Assertive Communication?

There are a variety of ways to learn to be more assertive in your communication style, but they all involve self-awareness and practice. It may not feel totally comfortable at first, but as you work at it, assertive communication will come more naturally.

> Changing one's behavior requires a conscious decision.

At first, it is helpful to practice being assertive by yourself. Rehearse what you might say by talking to yourself while looking in a mirror. After you feel more comfortable, ask a friend to help you practice. The two of you can role-play some assertive conversations. You may even want to video or audio record your practice so you can get an idea of how you look and how you sound. If sharing your feelings with your instructor or charge nurse makes you extremely uncomfortable, set the situation aside. You can work on it after you are more confident. You should practice being assertive in a situation in which there is minimal risk to you, so you can experience success. Share your feelings and practice being assertive with someone with whom you are comfortable. Personal risk should be at a minimum. When you are ready, try out your new assertive communication skills in a mildly uncomfortable situation you would like to change. Pay attention to how you feel. Ask for feedback from the other person. You will then be able to evaluate your progress and decide what other information you may need in order to continue your practice.

What Are the Components of Assertive Communication?

Assertive communication is a technique used to get one's needs met without purposely hurting others. It incorporates the principles of therapeutic communication, active listening, and a willingness to compromise. When you use these skills, you will be able to express yourself more effectively during challenging situations and handle confrontation in a professional manner. When you are confronted by a situation that provokes anger, take a deep breath, pull yourself away, get your emotions under control, and then approach the individual privately in a nonthreatening manner. The following are some hints for using assertive communication:

- Use "I" statements: "I am really upset about …."
- Describe the behavior that has upset you and focus on the present: "You have been texting and talking on your personal cell phone on the unit several times in the past 2 days."
- Discuss the consequences of the behavior: "This behavior is contrary to the agency policy and could result in …."
- State how the behavior needs to be modified and the time frame for this change: "You must immediately stop this interruption to your work and only use your cell phone off the unit while on your breaks."

The following strategy is a way to think about expressing your feelings and needs that will assist you to communicate assertively: **I feel … about … because …**

Let us look at an example:

- I feel tired and cranky, because I'm not paying enough attention to my family's needs.
- I feel hurt and angry about Dr. Jones yelling at me in front of others because I need to feel competent and respected at work.

These statements are most successful when you maintain direct eye contact, stand up straight, and speak in a clear, audible, firm tone of voice. After expressing your own feelings and needs, it is helpful to seek clarification of the other person's feelings or needs. This can be done with the following questions: "How do you feel about that?"

"What were you thinking and feeling at that time?"

"How would that affect you?"

With skillful listening and clear communication, the problem can be defined without placing blame or putting down the other person. Notice the use of "I" messages—that indicates willingness to accept responsibility for the process of defining the problem and negotiating a workable solution. To find a compromise, you have to be willing to meet the other person halfway. You may agree to try it your way one time and the other person's the next. Or you may both agree to change or give up something. You may do something for him or her if he or she does something else for you. Remember that in the work setting you cannot always have things exactly as you want them. You must be willing to change and compromise (Riley, 2017).

When to Use Assertive Communication

Here are some examples of situations in which assertive communication would be helpful.

■ *Communicating Expectations*

Supervisor: "You're being pulled to the orthopedic unit today because they're short-staffed."

Nurse: "I expect to be oriented into the unit and the equipment before I give nursing care because I haven't worked on that unit in more than a year."

■ *Saying No*

Physician: "Come with me right now. I need some help doing a procedure on Mr. Smith."

Nurse: "I can't come with you right now. Let me have the nursing assistant get Mrs. Anderson back to bed, and I'll help you then."

■ *Accepting Criticism*

Head nurse: "It seems to me that you are having difficulty updating your nursing care plans and getting the changes on the electronic medical record before the end of the shift."

Nurse: "I have been falling behind on updating my care plans in the electronic medical record. I need to work on better time management. Do you think you could help me with that?"

■ *Accepting Compliments*

Home care patient's spouse: "My wife feels very comfortable when you are here taking care of her. It's obvious you know what you're doing."

Nurse: "Thank you. Your feedback is important to me."

■ *Giving Criticism*

Nurse: "I want to talk with you about your care of Mrs. Samuelson. I found her sitting in a wheelchair alone in the hallway. It is your responsibility to make sure that she is not left alone, so that nothing happens to her."

Aide: "I do not think that's my job."

Nurse: "We talked about your responsibilities of caring for Mrs. Samuelson this morning when you received your assignment. If you have difficulty in carrying out this assignment, I expect you to ask for help."

■ *Accepting Feedback*

Head nurse: "I wanted to tell you that I have noticed an improvement in your communication with Dr. Turner. He has not complained about his patient's care for 2 weeks, and yesterday he told me that he had a positive discussion with you about home health care options for Mrs. Atkins."

Nurse: "Thank you. I have been working very hard at not responding angrily to his sarcastic comments and criticisms."

■ *Asking for Help*

Nurse: "I am having a hard time with Mr. Jones. He seems to have a way of pushing my buttons, so I get angry. It is hard for me to ask for help because I expect myself to care for all patients without difficulty."

Community health nurse supervisor: "Mr. Jones can be a difficult patient. Can I help you?"

Nurse: "Yes. I need help in understanding why I get so angry at him, and I want to know how to handle him in a more positive way."

Remember that you must evaluate how your assertive communication feels to you and seek feedback from others about how you are being interpreted. You need to know whether people perceive you as aggressive rather than assertive. It may mean modifying your communication to make sure you are standing up for yourself without violating the rights of others.

It should also be noted that some situations will not be resolved just because you communicated assertively. Finding a workable solution is a process involving other people who must take responsibility for their own feelings and needs. When others are unable to acknowledge their feelings, to listen, or to negotiate a compromise, your assertive communication may make you feel better about yourself, but it may not produce an immediate solution. But keep trying. Persistence pays off.

Remember, too, that there are some situations in which you must simply follow orders (i.e., carrying out a prescriber's orders and following a facility's policies and procedures). Sometimes you must put aside your own needs to meet the needs of the patients for whom you are caring. However, your judgment will improve as you gain experience, and you will recognize ways to communicate your needs and feelings with the goal of improving the processes and procedures used in your work setting.

CONCLUSION

Interpersonal skills, effective communication, group process, team building, and interprofessional practice are important for the nurse because they form the foundation for creating an effective working environment and delivering high-quality care. Well-planned, well-executed, and well-validated communication, along with a caring and positive attitude, will foster motivation, success, and satisfaction for the nurse in both the student role and as a new graduate.

Now that you have learned more about communicating effectively, try doing the student exercise in Critical Thinking Box 12.8, and review the relevant websites and online resources that follow. Happy communicating!

CRITICAL THINKING BOX 12.8
Communication Exercise

Directions: Use the following situations to reflect on key points covered in this chapter. Think of a way to communicate effectively in each situation. You may want to consider your own individual solutions and then role-play or discuss your ideas with a group of your classmates.

1. Develop a list of 10 patients who are hospitalized on your unit. For each patient, provide some personal information, a diagnosis, and some data about his or her progress during the previous 24 hours. Use the information you have listed to give a change-of-shift report to the four staff members who will be caring for these patients during the next 8 hours.

2. You have asked to speak to Dr. Sanders about your concerns in caring for one of her patients who has required much physical care since she was discharged from the hospital. Dr. Sanders has a reputation for being cold, aloof, and sarcastic. You have never spoken directly to her alone before.

3. You are a member of the home health care agency's procedures committee. After attending the last meeting, you have been given the responsibility for drafting a revision to the procedure used when controlled substances are being administered. You know that you need more information before you can begin your work. Send a memo to at least three different members of the agency staff identifying what information you would like them to provide. Make a follow-up phone call to make sure that they received the memo.

⊕ RELEVANT WEBSITES AND ONLINE RESOURCES

American Academy of Communication in Health Care
https://www.achonline.org/

American Association of Colleges of Nursing
Interprofessional education. https://www.aacnnursing.org/Interprofessional-Education.

Interprofessional Education Collaborative (IPEC)
What is Interprofessional Education (IPE)? https://www.ipecollaborative.org/about-ipec.html

Interprofessional Professionalism Collaborative
http://www.interprofessionalprofessionalism.org/

BIBLIOGRAPHY

Arredondo, L. (2000). *Communicating effectively.* New York: McGraw-Hill.

Bahlman, D. T., & Johnson, F. C. (2005). Using technology to improve and support communication and workflow processes. *Association of Perioperative Registered Nurses Journal, 82*(1), 65–73.

Chenevert, M. (1997). *Pro-nurse handbook* (3rd ed.). St. Louis: Mosby.

Deep, S., & Sussman, L. (1995). *Smart moves for people in charge.* Reading, MA: Addison-Wesley.

Giger, J. N. (2013). *Transcultural nursing* (6th ed.). St. Louis: Elsevier/Mosby.

Hosley, J., & Molle, E. (2006). *A practical guide to therapeutic communication for health professionals.* St. Louis: Elsevier/Saunders.

Institute of Medicine. (2003). *Health professions education: A bridge to quality.* Washington, DC: The National Academies Press.

Interprofessional Education Collaborative (IPEC). (2016). *Core competencies for interprofessional collaborative practice: 2016 update.* Washington, DC: Interprofessional Education Collaborative.

Interprofessional Education Collaborative Expert Panel (IPEC). (2011). *Core competencies for interprofessional collaborative practice: Report of an expert panel.* Washington, DC: Interprofessional Education Collaborative.

Katzenbach, J. R., & Smith, D. K. (2003). *Wisdom of teams.* New York: Harper Business.

Kushner, M. (2004). *Presentations for dummies.* New Jersey: Wiley Publishing.

Marquis, B., & Huston, C. (2014). *Leadership roles and management functions in nursing: Theory and application* (8th ed.). Philadelphia: JB Lippincott.

Merlino, J. (2017). *Communication: A critical healthcare competency.* Retrieved from https://www.psqh.com/analysis/communication-critical-healthcare-competency/.

Mindell, P. (2001). *How to say it for women: Communicating with confidence and power using the language of success.* Paramus, NJ: Prentice Hall.

Peoples, D. A. (1992). *Presentations plus.* New York: John Wiley & Sons.

Pecha, Kucha. (2019). *Pecha Kucha 20 × 20.* Retrieved from https://www.pechakucha.org/.

Poskey, M. (2013). *Effective communication: Easier said than understood.* Retrieved from https://www.irmi.com/articles/expert-commentary/effective-communication.

Riley, J. B. (2017). *Communication in nursing* (8th ed.). St. Louis, MO: Elsevier.

Tuckman, B., & Jensen, M. (1977). Stage of small group development revisited. *Group and Organization Studies, 2,* 419–427.

Varcarolis, E. M. (2017). *Essentials of psychiatric mental health nursing* (3rd ed.). St. Louis: Elsevier.

Vengel, A. (2010). *The influence edge: How to persuade others to help you achieve your goals.* San Francisco: Berrett-Koehler Communications.

Vertino, K. (September 30, 2014). Effective interpersonal communication: A practical guide to improve your life. *OJIN: The Online Journal of Issues in Nursing. 19*(3). https://doi.org/10.3912/OJIN.Vol19No03Man01 manuscript 1.

Wideman, M. (2017). *Wideman comparative glossary of project management terms v5.5. (Source PMK87).* Retrieved from http://www.maxwideman.com/pmglossary/PMG_T00.htm.

World Health Organization (WHO). (2010). *Framework for action on interprofessional education & collaborative practice.* Retrieved from http://apps.who.int/iris/bitstream/10665/70185/1/WHO_HRH_HPN_10.3_eng.pdf?ua=1.

13

Conflict Management

JoAnn Zerwekh, EdD, RN

(e)http://evolve.elsevier.com/Zerwekh/nsgtoday/.

Everything that irritates us about others can lead us to an understanding of ourselves.
Carl Jung

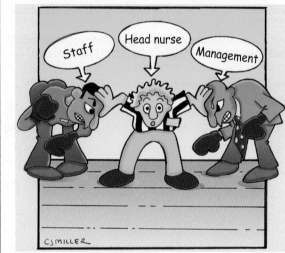

There is a better approach to conflict resolution than fighting it out.

After completing this chapter, you should be able to:
- Identify common factors that lead to conflict
- Discuss five methods to resolve conflict
- Discuss techniques to use in handling difficult people
- Discuss solutions and alternatives in dealing with anger
- Identify situations of sexual harassment in the workplace and discuss possible solutions

Can you imagine a world without conflict? Why, it would be a world without change! Conflict is inevitable wherever there are people with differing backgrounds, needs, values, and priorities.

A stereotypical perspective of conflict related to nursing is that "nice" nurses avoid conflict. According to Beauregard et al. (2003), although caricatured images of the nurse may encompass the "old" battle-ax, the control freak, the naughty nurse, or the doctor's handmaiden, the primary perception of the nurse by the public is one of the caring angel who is gentle and kind. Conflict within the nursing profession has traditionally generated negative feelings, to the extent that many nurses use avoidance as a coping mechanism because of their feeling that the "public's stereotypical image of them demanded that they be 'nice,' self-sacrificing, and submissive nurses and that if they engaged in conflict they would be branded emotional or unfeminine women" (Kelly, 2006, p. 27).

The presence of conflict in a situation is not necessarily negative but may, in fact, have some positive results. As a process, conflict is neutral. Following are some possible outcomes of conflict:

- Disturbing issues are brought out into the open, which may avert a more serious conflict.
- Group cohesiveness may increase as individuals resolve issues.
- New leadership may develop as a consequence of resolution.
- The results of conflict can be constructive, occurring when productive outcomes are achieved, or destructive, leading to poor communication and creating dissatisfaction.

CONFLICT

What Causes Conflict?

Let us look at some common factors of conflict as they relate to nursing.

Role Conflict

When two people have the same or related responsibilities with ambiguous boundaries, the potential for conflict exists. For example, a nurse on the shift from 11 p.m. to 7 a.m. may be uncertain whether he or the nurse on the shift from 7 a.m. to 3 p.m. is responsible for weighing a patient.

Communication Conflict

Failing to discuss differences with one another can lead to problems with communication. Communication is a two-way process; when one person is unclear in a communication, the process falls apart. A recent graduate may find that with a busy schedule, numerous patient demands, and a shortage of time, it is easy to forget to notify a patient's family of a change in visiting hours—a great annoyance to the family members who arrive only to find that they cannot visit.

Goal Conflict

We all have unique goals and objectives for what we hope to achieve in our places of employment. When one nurse places his or her personal achievement and advancement above everyone else's, conflict can occur. An example of this can be seen in the new graduate nurse who pursues an advanced nursing degree immediately following graduation; the experienced nurse in the unit may feel that the new graduate nurse requires a minimum length of time at the bedside before advancing his or her education.

Personality Conflict

Wouldn't it be great if we got along with everyone? Of course, we all know that there are just some people with whom we have a difficult time. The situation is all too familiar, and many times we may find ourselves with such thoughts as "I'll try to overlook her negative, lousy behavior; after all, she doesn't have much of a family life." Trying to change another person's personality is like guaranteeing an unhappy ending to a story.

Ethical or Values Conflict

During a cardiac arrest, a graduate nurse has a conflict with the physician's order of "no code" on a young adolescent patient. She has difficulty taking care of the adolescent, because he reminds her of her younger brother, who died tragically in an automobile accident.

Conflicts in nursing may fit into one or more of the aforementioned categories. Consider some common areas of conflict among nursing staff, including scheduling days off, determining vacation leave, assigning committees, patient care assignments, and performance appraisals, to name just a few.

What Are Common Areas of Conflict Between Nurses and Patients—and Between Nurses and Patients' Families?

Guttenberg (1983) identifies five common areas of conflict among nurses and their patients and families.

1. **Quality of care.** This is by far the most common area of conflict and the easiest to remedy. Families are typically concerned with how well their loved one is being cared for, how friendly the nurses are, how well the hospital or home health services are provided and coordinated, and how flexible the hospital is with visiting hours and meeting patients' special needs.

2. **Treatment decisions.** This area of conflict often arises between the family of an older adult and the nurse. A physician may order a treatment with which the family does not agree. In this situation it is very important that the nurse not defend the physician's orders or attempt to persuade or convince the family that the physician or nurse knows what's best for the patient. In these situations, the issue is rarely the treatment itself but rather the family's wish to decide what is right for the loved one. Be sure to clarify the orders and explain to the family that you are supposed to carry them out unless the family negotiates directly with the physician to change them. Conflict may also exist between the nurse and physician regarding the care of older adults. For example, a physician may decline to perform a medical procedure on an older patient owing to his or her advanced age or preexisting comorbidities.

3. **Family involvement.** For example, when a young adult is diagnosed with cancer, numerous issues may arise concerning the presence of family members during procedures and the extent of their involvement in the overall care. Such issues are based on the family's real need to feel significant and adequate in meeting the young adult's needs.

4. **Quality of parental care.** This can become an issue when nurses are unhappy with how parents are participating in their child's care. It is helpful to offer parenting classes that can encourage parents to meet other parents and can model positive parenting techniques. Fear of being a bad parent by not responding to every cry an infant makes is a good example of an area where the nurse can educate the parents on responding to their infant's physical and emotional needs.

5. **Staff inconsistency.** This is another issue that is easily prevented. Make sure that staff members on each shift are consistent in enforcing hospital policies and that they notify other shifts of any attempts at manipulation by family members or patients.

According to Cochran and Elder (2015), poor management of conflict has been shown to impact patient safety negatively.

CONFLICT RESOLUTION

What Are Ways to Resolve Conflict?

Unresolved conflicts waste time and energy and reduce productivity and cooperation among the people with whom you work. In contrast, when conflicts are resolved, they strengthen relationships and improve the performance of everyone involved (Kim, Nicotera, & McNulty, 2015). The key to managing conflict successfully is tailoring your response to fit each conflict situation instead of relying on one particular technique. Each technique represents a different way to achieve the outcome you want and to help the other person achieve at least part of the outcome that he or she wants. How do you know which technique to use? That depends on the following questions:

- How much power do you have in this situation compared with the other person?
- How much do you value your relationship with the person with whom you are in conflict?
- How much time is available to resolve the conflict?

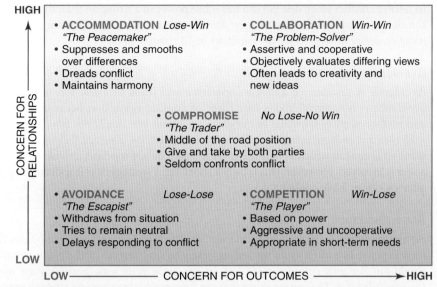

FIG. 13.1 Model for conflict resolution. (Modified from Douglas, E., & Bushardt, W. [1988]. Interpersonal conflict: Strategies and guidelines for resolution. *Journal of American Medical Record Association, 56*[2], 18–22; Sullivan, E., & Decker, P. [1988]. *Effective management in nursing.* Menlo Park, CA: Addison-Wesley.)

An example of a model for conflict resolution can be found in Fig. 13.1. This model incorporates several views of conflict resolution. Filley (1975) described three basic strategies for handling conflict according to outcome: win-win, lose-lose, and win-lose. Various others have identified the following five responses to resolve conflict: competition, accommodation, avoidance, compromise, and cooperation. In a study, the prevalent style for conflict resolution used by nursing students was compromise, followed by avoidance (Hamilton, 2008). As noted in this research study, compromise attempts to meet the needs of individuals on both sides of a conflict, whereas collaboration, which may take more time, offers the best avenue or approach to settling the conflict—an approach that will satisfy both participants (win-win solution). A research study by Iglesias and Vallejo (2012) examined predominant conflict-resolution styles used by a sample of Spanish nurses in two work settings, academic and clinical, in order to determine differences between these environments. The findings indicate that conflict management styles varied according to work setting, with nurses in an academic environment most frequently using the compromising style and nurses in the clinical environment most frequently using the accommodating style.

Let us look at an example and apply the model.

Suppose that the charge nurse on your unit had posted the vacation schedule for the month of December. You, as a recent graduate, have asked to be off during the week of Christmas. You notice on the schedule that none of the recent graduates has received the Christmas holidays off. You feel that this is unfair because you will not have an opportunity to be with your family during the Christmas holidays. How can you resolve this conflict?

Competition

This is an example of the *win-lose* situation. In this situation, force—or the use of power—occurs. It sets up a type of competition between you and your charge nurse. Typically competition is used to resolve conflict when one person has more power in a situation than the other. *In the given situation, the charge nurse refuses your request for Christmas vacation, explaining that the staff members with more seniority have priority for vacation at Christmas time.*

Avoidance

Avoidance is unassertive and uncooperative and leads to a *lose-lose* situation. In some situations, avoidance is not considered a true form of conflict resolution because the conflict is not resolved and neither party is satisfied. *In the given situation, you would not have approached the charge nurse with the Christmas schedule issue.* Usually, both persons involved feel frustrated and angry. There are some situations in which avoiding the issue might be appropriate, as when tempers are flaring or much anger is involved. However, this is only a short-term strategy; it is important to get back to the problem after emotions have cooled.

Accommodation

Accommodation is the *lose-win* situation, in which one person accommodates the other at his or her own expense but often ends up feeling resentful and angry. *In the given situation, the charge nurse would put her own concern aside and let you have your way, possibly even working for you during the scheduled slot. The charge nurse loses and the graduate nurse wins, which may set up conflict among staff and other recent graduates.* When is accommodation the best response? Is it when conflict would create serious disruption, such as arguing, or when the person with whom you are in conflict has the power to resolve the conflict unilaterally? In this response to conflict, differences are suppressed or played down while agreement is emphasized.

Compromise

Compromise or bargaining is the strategy that recognizes the importance of both the resolution of the problem and the relationship between the two people. Compromise is a moderately assertive and cooperative step in the right direction, in which one creates a *modified win-lose* outcome. *In the given situation, the charge nurse compromises with you by allowing you to have Christmas Eve off with your family but not the entire week.* The problem lies in the reduced staffing that will occur for a short period. The compromise may not be totally satisfactory for either party, but it may be offered as a temporary solution until more options become available.

Collaboration

Collaboration is the strategy that involves a high level of concern for the problem, the outcome, and the relationship. It deals with confrontation and problem solving. The needs, feelings, and desires of both parties are taken into consideration and re-examined while searching for proper ways to agree on goals. Collaboration is a *win-win* solution with a commitment to resolve the issues at the base of the conflict. It is fully assertive and cooperative. *In the given situation, you and the charge nurse discuss the week of Christmas and the staffing needs and agree that you will work the first half of that week and the charge nurse will work the second half of that week. You also agree to be there the first part of the week to complete the audit on the charts from the previous week for the charge nurse. In this situation both people are satisfied and there is no compromise regarding what is most important to each. That is, the charge nurse gets her audit completed and the recent graduate is able to spend half of Christmas week with her family.* What is your particular style for resolving conflict? (Critical Thinking Box 13.1.)

❓ CRITICAL THINKING BOX 13.1

Conflict Questionnaire

Directions: Consider situations in which you find that your wishes differ from those of another person. For each of the following statements, think how likely you are to respond to each situation in the manner described. Check the rating that best corresponds to your response.

	VERY UNLIKELY	UNLIKELY	VERY LIKELY	LIKELY
1. I am usually firm in pursuing my goals.				
2. I try to win my position.				
3. I give up some points in exchange for others.				
4. I feel that differences are not always worth worrying about.				
5. I try to find a position that is between others' and mine.				
6. In approaching a negotiation, I try to consider the other person's wishes.				
7. I try to show the logic and benefits of my position.				
8. I always lean toward a direct discussion of the problem.				
9. I try to find a fair combination of gains and losses for both of us.				
10. I attempt to work through our differences immediately.				
11. I try to avoid creating unpleasantness for myself.				
12. I might try to soothe others' feelings and preserve our relationship.				
13. I attempt to get all concerns and issues out immediately.				
14. I sometimes avoid taking positions that create controversy.				
15. I try not to hurt the other's feelings.				

SCORING: Very unlikely = 1; Unlikely = 2; Likely = 3; Very likely = 4.

	ITEM:	ITEM:	ITEM:	
COMPETING	1 _____	2 _____	7 _____	TOTAL _____
COLLABORATING	8 _____	10 _____	13 _____	TOTAL _____
COMPROMISING	3 _____	5 _____	9 _____	TOTAL _____
AVOIDING	4 _____	11 _____	14 _____	TOTAL _____
ACCOMMODATING	6 _____	12 _____	15 _____	TOTAL _____

(From Thomas, K. W. [1977]. Toward multidimensional values in teaching: The example of conflict behaviors, *Academy of Management Review, 2*, 487.)

What Are Some Basic Guidelines for Choosing the Technique to Use?

In some situations, certain techniques and responses work best. You may have to use accommodation or avoidance when you lack the power to change the situation. When you have conflict in a relationship that you value, it might be more helpful to use accommodation, compromise, or collaboration.

When there is no immediate, pressing sense of urgency to solve an issue, any of the five techniques can be used. However, when you are facing an emergency situation or a rapidly approaching deadline, your best bet is to use competition or accommodation. Just remember the following key behaviors in managing conflict:

1. Deal with issues, not personalities.
2. Take responsibility for yourself and your participation.
3. Communicate openly.
4. Avoid placing blame.
5. Listen actively.
6. Sort out the issues.
7. Identify key themes in the discussion.
8. Stay focused in the present; don't dwell on the past.
9. Weigh the consequences.
10. Identify resolution options.
11. Develop an outcome and obtain consensus.

Suppose that you follow all of these suggestions and you still are confronted with that difficult situation or that difficult person. Read on.

DEALING WITH DIFFICULT PEOPLE

What Are Some Techniques for Handling Difficult People?

Now that we have discussed conflict-management techniques, we are ready to look at techniques for handling difficult people. How do you deal with an abusive physician or supervisor? How do you react when someone constantly complains and gripes about something? How do you handle the know-it-all who will not even listen to your thoughts about an issue? (See Research for Best Practice Box 13.1 for suggestions on managing difficult employees.)

I am sure that you, if you have not already, will in the near future run into a "Sherman tank" (Fig. 13.2). According to Bramson (1981), Sherman tanks are the *attackers*. They come out charging and are often abusive, abrupt, and intimidating. But more important, they tend to be downright overwhelming.

Remember Dr. Smith, who flew into a tirade because you forgot to have a suture removal set at his patient's bedside at 8 a.m. sharp? Remember how you felt? "My heart was beating so loud I could hear it, and I was sure everyone else around could hear it too. I was so furious at him for the comments he made."

In understanding Sherman tanks, it is important to realize that they have a strong need to prove to themselves and others that their views are right. They have a very strong sense of what others ought to do but often lack the caring and the trust that would be helpful in getting things done. They usually achieve what they want, but at the cost a lot of disagreements, lost friendships, and uncomfortable relationships with their coworkers. Sherman tanks are often very confident and tend to devalue those who they feel are not confident. Unfortunately they demean others in a way that makes them look very self-important and superior. How do you cope with a Sherman tank? The most important thing is to keep your fear and anger under control and to avoid an outright confrontation about who is right and who is wrong. The following are some specific things you should do:

■ Do not allow yourself to be run over; step aside.
   ■ Stand up for yourself. Defend yourself, but without fighting. Seek support when warranted.

Managing Difficult Employees

Practice Issue

Nurse managers are often faced with a difficult employee. The difficult employee's negative conflict behavior affects team performance effectiveness, job satisfaction, and turnover intention. According to Pareto's 80/20 rule, 20% of employees/workers will cause 80% of the problems, which means that a small number of issues are responsible for a large percentage of the effect.

In an environment of team collegiality, there is less negative conflict; increased commitment to the organization; and greater satisfaction, autonomy, and control over practice. In professional practice environments, nurses experience constructive conflict approaches and effectiveness is enhanced in the workplace.

It is part of the nurse manager role to create an environment that facilitates professional practice. This type of environment requires that employees are socialized to their nursing role. In these professional practice environments, the unique preferences, perspectives, opinions, concerns, and choices of the individuals are recognized and valued. During nursing school, professional role socialization ("think like a nurse") is initiated and later solidified during the early years of practice, when the new graduate incorporates knowledge, skills, attitude, and affective behavior associated with carrying out the expectations of the nursing role.

Additionally, nurse managers may encounter conflict among employees in which the nurse manager must serve as a mediator among the employees involved in an argument or disagreement. The role of a mediator is to help disputants in coming to a resolution or agreement. The mediator helps the parties involved by "defining problems, enumerating priorities, exploring alternatives, and facilitating resultant negotiations" (Cheng, 2015, p. 311).

Implications for Nursing Practice

Effective role socialization occurs when the nurse engages in actions that benefit other nurses and/or patients and families by helping, supporting, and encouraging mutual goal accomplishment and/or well-being.

- There must be positive interdependence among the nursing staff.
- Nurses must understand and use constructive conflict-management skills.
- Mediation techniques should be employed when disputes arise between employees and/or patients and their families.
- There must be a high level of trust among the nursing staff.
- Prosocial behavior should be noted among staff, with the feeling of "sink or swim together" versus "you sink and I swim."
- Do not procrastinate in dealing with difficult employees, patients, or their families.
- A high basic self-esteem is noted among nursing staff in an empowering, healthy workplace environment.
- The conflict negotiation strategy used may be collaboration (win-win) or mediation.

Considering this Information

How might you use some of the strategies listed in this chapter to handle a difficult employee? What types of activities are you involved in as a student that promote a positive professional practice environment? What essential skills would be important for a nurse to possess to serve as a mediator?

References

Arnold, E., Pulich, M., & Wang, H. (2008). Managing immature, irresponsible, or irritating employees. *Health Care Manager, 27*(4), 350–356.

Cheng, F. K. (2015). Mediation skills for conflict resolution in nursing education. *Nurse Education in Practice, 15*(4), 310–313. https://doi.org/10.1013./j.nepr.20115.02.005.

Cornett, P. A., & O'Rourke, M. (2009). Building organizational capacity for a healthy work environment through role based professional practice. *Critical Care Nursing Quarterly, 32*(3), 208–220.

Cornett, P. A. (2009). Managing the difficult employee: A reframed perspective. *Critical Care Nursing Quarterly, 32*(4), 314.

Hader, R. (2008). Workplace violence survey 2008: Unsettling findings. *Nursing Management, 39*(7), 13–19 326.

Middaugh, D. J. (2015). Managing the 80/20 rule. *Medsurg Nursing, 24*(2), 127–129.

Rondeau, A. (2007). *57% of managers time is spent dealing with difficult staff.* Retrieved from http://www.selfgrowth.com/articles/57_of_Managers_Time_is_Spent_Dealing_With_Difficult_Staff.html.

Siu, H., Laschinger, H. K. S., & Finegan, J. (2008). Nursing professional practice environments: Setting the stage for constructive conflict resolution and work effectiveness. *Journal of Nursing Administration, 38*(5), 250–257.

U.S. Equal Employment Opportunity Commission. (2009). *Fact sheet: Sexual Harassment.* Retrieved https://www.eeoc.gov/eeoc/publications/upload/fs-sex.pdf.

U.S. Equal Employment Opportunity Commission. (2016). *Select Task Force on the Study of Harassment in the Workplace: Executive Summary.* Retrieved https://www.eeoc.gov/eeoc/task_force/harassment/report.cfm#_Toc453686298.

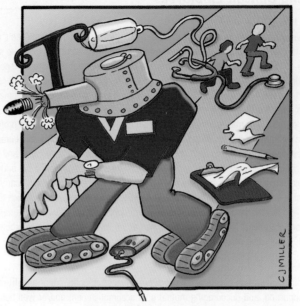

FIG. 13.2 Sherman tank.

- Give such a person a little time to run down and express what they might be ranting about.
- Sometimes it is necessary to be rude; get in your word in any way you can.
- If possible, try to get the person to sit down. Be sure to maintain eye contact with him or her while you state your opinions and perceptions forcefully and assertively.
- Do not argue or try to cut the person down.
- When he or she finally hears you, be ready to be friendly.

Next to the Sherman tanks are the *snipers* (Fig. 13.3). They are the pot-shot artists—not as openly aggressive as the Sherman tanks. Their weapons are their innuendoes, their digs, and their nonplayful teasing, which is definitely aimed to hurt you. Snipers tend to choose a hidden rather than a frontal attack. They prefer to undercut you and make you look ridiculous. So, when you are dealing with snipers, remember to expose the attack—that is, "smoke them out." Ask very calmly questions like these:

"That sounded like a put-down. Did you really mean it that way?" Or you might say, "Do I understand that you don't like what I'm saying? It sounds as if you are making fun of me. Are you?"

When a sniper is giving you criticism, be sure to obtain group confirmation or denial. Ask questions or make statements such as, "Does anyone else see the issue this way?" "It seems as though we have a difference of opinion," or "Exactly what is the issue here? What is it that you don't like about what occurred?" One way to prevent sniping is by setting up regular problem-solving meetings with that person.

Also difficult to cope with are the *constant complainers*. These people often feel that they are powerless, so they draw attention—but seldom action—to their problem. A complainer points out real problems but does it from a very unconstructive stance. Coping with a complainer can be a challenge. First, it is important to listen to the complaints, acknowledge them, and make sure you understand what the person said by paraphrasing it or checking out your perception of how the person feels. Do not necessarily agree with the person, with a complainer, it is important to move into a

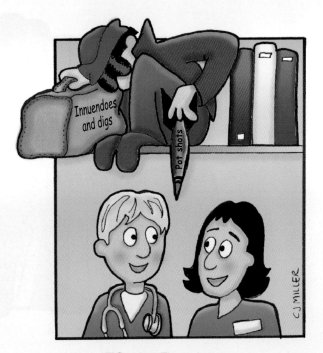

FIG. 13.3 The sniper.

problem-solving mode by asking very specific, informative questions and encouraging him or her to submit complaints in writing. For example, try communicating with the constant complainer in the following manner:

"Did I understand you to say that you are having difficulty with your patient assignment?"
"Would it be helpful if I went to the pharmacy for you, so that you could complete your chart on your pre-operative patient?"

Next are the maddening ones: the *clams* (Fig. 13.4). The clams have an entirely different tactic from the previous three. They just refuse to respond when you need an answer or want to have a discussion. It might be helpful to try to read a clam's nonverbal communication. Watch for wrinkled brows, a frown, or a sigh. How to deal with clams? Try to get them to open up by using open-ended questions and waiting very quietly for a response. Do not fill in their silence with your own conversation. Give yourself enough time to wait with composure. Sometimes a little "clamming" of your own might be helpful, as by using the "friendly, silent stare," or FSS. The way to set up the FSS is to have a very inquisitive, expectant expression on your face with raised eyebrows, wide eyes, and maybe a slight smile—all nonverbal cues to the clam that you are waiting for a response. When clams finally open up, be very attentive. Watch your own impulses—do not bubble over with happiness just because he or she has finally given you two moments of attention. Avoid the polite ending; in other words, get up and say, for example:

"This was important to me. I'm not going to let this issue drop. I'll be back to talk to you tomorrow at 2 o'clock." Do not be the nice guy and say, "Thanks for coming in. Have a nice weekend. I'll see you tomorrow."

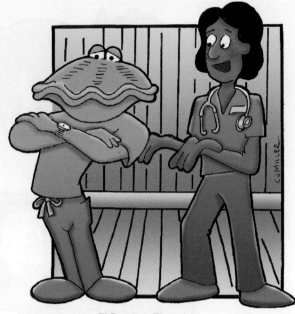

FIG. 13.4 The clam.

Be very direct and tell the clam what you are going to do, especially if the desired discussion did not occur.

What Is Anger?

Anger is something we feel. When we become angry, we usually assume that it's because we are upset about what someone has done or said. Often we want to pay that person back or take out our anger on them. When anger arises, it is often difficult to see beyond the moment, because the target of anger is usually consumed with thoughts of revenge for the wrongdoing that has occurred. Weiss and Cain (1991) state that, "Anger is often a cover-up emotion … that disguises what is really going on inside you." But anger is a signal, and according to Lerner (1997), it is "one worth listening to" (p. 1). She goes on to say that

> Our anger may be a message that we are being hurt, that our rights are being violated, that our needs or wants are not being adequately met, or simply that something is not right. Our anger may tell us that we are not addressing an important emotional issue in our lives, or that too much of ourselves—our beliefs, values, desires, or ambitions—are being compromised in a relationship. Our anger may be a signal that we are doing more and giving more than we can comfortably do or give. Or our anger may warn us that others are doing too much for us, at the expense of our own competence and growth. Just as physical pain tells us to take our hand off the hot stove, the pain of our anger preserves the very integrity of our self. Our anger can motivate us to say "no" to the ways in which we are defined by others and "yes" to the dictates of our inner self. (p. 1)

No matter what, when feelings of frustration, disappointment, or powerlessness take over, there is no doubt that anger is in the making. Anger seems to begin in situations fraught with threats and anxiety.

Anger has two faces. One is *guilt,* which is anger aimed inward at what we did or did not do, and the other is *resentment,* which is anger directed toward others at what they did or did not do.

> The following is true about both guilt and resentment: They both accumulate over time and lead to a cycle of negative energy that poisons our relationships and stifles our personal growth.

There is another side of the coin, however. If feelings of anger signify a problem, then venting anger does not necessarily solve it. Actually, if change and successful resolution do not occur, venting anger may serve to maintain it. Tavris (1984) suggests that we learn two things about handling anger: first, how to think about anger, and second, how to reduce the tension. More about this later in the chapter.

Box 13.1 shows a summary of different anger styles. Just think about anger from a cardiovascular point of view. Most authorities consider anger to be among the most damaging and dangerous emotions because your pulse and blood pressure become elevated, sometimes to dangerous heights.

What Is the Solution for Handling Anger?

> Change the image of it!

Stop

Appraise the situation. Don't do a thing. You are at a pivotal point. You have two ways to go: one is to become angry and the other is to reevaluate the situation. Try to look at a way to reinterpret the annoying comment. Consider the following example:

"Who does that charge nurse think she is to treat me like I'm a dummy!" or "How could someone be so thoughtless as to not remember my birthday!" You can reinterpret these and say to yourself, "Maybe if she weren't so unhappy, she wouldn't have considered doing such a thing" or "Maybe that person is having a rough day." The important thing here is to empathize with the person and try to find justifications for the behavior that was so annoying to you.

Look

When concept of yourself or another is about to be or has been attacked—what *shoulds or musts* have been violated? In other words, what has just occurred that has led you to feel angry with yourself or with another?

After receiving the end-of-shift report and making patient rounds, a recent graduate goes into a patient's room to take vital signs. Within moments the patient has a cardiac arrest. Two hours later, while completing her charting, the recent graduate states guiltily, "I should have taken those vital signs earlier. It just must be the first thing I do when I get on the unit. I should have been on top of this. I must do better." Notice the self-criticism in the recent graduate's comments. Guilt, like resentment, can be a habit. It demonstrates—too clearly—how we respond to a situation in a negative manner. To help you get in touch with these feelings, try eliminating the words "must" and "should" from your vocabulary for just an hour. It is surprising to find out how frequently we use these terms.

Change

How do you change the image? One of the ways is to use humor. Humor makes the anger (guilt and resentment) tolerable. Remember that it is difficult to laugh and frown at the same time. (It takes only 15 facial muscles to laugh but twice that many to frown.) If reappraising the situation and using humor both fail as ways to manage your anger, some suggest venting the anger—for example, by getting mad, yelling, shouting, telling someone off, or breaking things. Although this might make us feel better momentarily, in the long run such outbursts make us feel worse.

BOX 13.1 ANGER CHARACTERISTICS AND TRIGGERS

What Is Your Anger Style?

Passive Characteristics
- Avoidance—no eye contact or avoiding communicating with others; "silent treatment or cold shoulder"
- Withdrawing emotionally
- Becoming ill or anxious
- Sitting on the fence and not making a decision
- Talking about frustrations but showing no feelings
- Doing little or nothing or putting things off to thwart others' plans
- Not feeling anger when something is wrong

Aggressive Characteristics
- Acting out or lashing out at another person; out-of-control behavior
- Bullying
- Incivility—offensive, intimidating, or hostile action
- Explosive sudden outburst and release of feelings
- Taking anger out on someone or something else (i.e., kicking the dog, breaking things)
- Violence—getting physical or hurting people
- Bringing up old grievances

Passive-Aggressive Characteristics
- Resenting and blaming others; opposition to the demands of others
- Hidden action to get back at someone; conscious revenge
- Procrastination and intentional mistakes in response to others' demands; intentional inefficiency; "forgetting" to do things and using forgetfulness as an excuse
- Cynical, sullen, or hostile attitude
- Frequent complaints about feeling underappreciated or cheated; being self-deprecating

What Are Red Flags and Long-Standing Issues That Trigger Anger?
- Experiencing feelings of insecurity, being discounted and/or threatened, humiliated, rejected
- Having to wait a long time for a person or an appointment
- Getting caught in traffic congestion or crowded buses, airplanes, or other similar frustrating situations
- Joking comments made about sensitive topics
- Friends borrowing items and not returning them or returning them in disrepair
- Friends borrowing money and not paying you back
- Being wrongly accused of some action or comment
- Having to clean up after someone who does not keep things as tidy as you expect
- Having a neighbor who plays loud music or is engaged in other behavior that is inconsiderate
- Being placed on hold for long periods of time while on the telephone
- Having your computer crash and losing valuable data
- Being given wrong directions when asking for assistance
- Having money or property stolen
- Being taken for granted by family and friends

(Valentine, P. E. [2001]. A gender perspective on conflict management strategies of nurses. *Journal of Nursing Scholarship, 33*[1], 69–74. Vivar, C. [2006]. Putting conflict management into practice: A nursing case study. *Journal of Nursing Management, 14,* 201–206. doi: https://doi.org/10.1111/j.1365-2934.2006.00554.x.)

Why does this method of venting anger, that is, letting it all hang out, make us feel worse? First, think of all the physiological changes that are occurring in your body: blood pressure, pulse, and respirations increase; the muscles contract; and adrenalin is released. Sound familiar? It is the "fight or flight" adrenal response. Can it be healthy to maintain a constant state of stress and readiness to respond? Another disadvantage of an uninhibited outburst of anger is that it may lead the other person to retaliate.

It might be important to recognize the difference between venting and acknowledging our anger. A typical expression of anger might be something such as the following:

"Hey, you turkey, what do you think you're doing? Don't you know how to put that catheter in? Are you stupid or something? Either you figure it out or you get out of here. You hear me?"

This approach is insulting, demeaning, and accusatory. It is also likely to lead to some type of provocative response. In contrast, when we acknowledge our feelings, we make statements such as *"I feel angry about …"* or *"I feel hurt about …"* or *"I feel guilty about …"* The use of "I" statements is our first step toward taking responsibility for ourselves by owning up to our own feelings instead of blaming others.

Venting anger simply does not work unless you want to intimidate those around you, coerce them into submission with a hot temper, or, even worse, look childish while ranting, raving, and beating the floor or each other with foam bats. So what does work? *Face it, embrace it, and erase it!*

First, acknowledge the anger *(face it)*: Ask, "What am I feeling? Anger? Guilt? Rage? Resentment?"

Second, identify the provoking or triggering situation *(embrace it)*: Ask, "What caused this feeling? Whose problem is it?"

Third, determine what changes must occur *(erase it)*: Ask, "What can I change? Can I accept what I cannot change?" Then take action and let go of the rest. Other ways to handle anger and remove yourself from the vicious cycle of guilt and resentment are in the following sections.

> Move.

Get Active

Try exercise or anything involving physical activity, such as walking, aerobics, and running. Clean the garage or a kitchen drawer. If you are sitting, get up. If you are in bed, move your arms around. Just get active and do something!

> Focus.

Refocus on Something Positive

Think of your cup as half full, not half empty. Look at the problematic situation: "My charge nurse won't give me Christmas off. However, I am not scheduled to work either Christmas Eve or New Year's Eve. So by working Christmas Day, I'm assured of the other days off."

> Breathe.

Pay Attention to Your Breathing

Slow it down. Take deep, slow breaths, feeling the air move through your nose and down into your lungs. Check out your body for areas of tenseness. Often anger can be felt as tightness in the chest and abdomen.

Conflict is an inevitable part of our day-to-day experience. How we negotiate and handle conflict and anger may not always be easy. You might be thinking right now, "This looks good on paper, but in real life, it's not that easy to put into practice." If you're feeling this way, take a risk and try changing your approach and viewpoint.

> The important thing is learning about yourself.

How do you cope with conflict? How do you handle difficult people? How do you respond when angry?

SEXUAL HARASSMENT IN THE WORKPLACE

In today's world, sexual harassment as a source of conflict has been taken seriously, as evidenced by the widespread visibility and increased recognition of the issue. The US Equal Employment Opportunity Commission (EEOC) reported that between the years 1995 to 2016, at least 3085 employees in medical and surgical hospitals filed claims of sexual harassment, as reported by *BuzzFeed News* using EEOC data (Vo, 2017). The following lists the number of claims filed in selected areas of the health care industry as stated by Rege (2017), using the same dataset:

- Other miscellaneous ambulatory health care services—1911
- Nursing care facilities—1530
- Medical laboratories—436
- Physicians' offices (excluding mental health specialists)—382
- Home health care services—314
- Direct health and medical insurance carriers—254
- Offices of other miscellaneous health care practitioners—140
- Specialty hospitals—81
- Psychiatric and substance abuse hospitals—73
- Ambulance services—51
- Other outpatient care centers—5

The restaurant industry is the only industry surpassing all others in claims (10,057 of them) (Rege, 2017). Having examined more than 170,000 claims, Vo (2017) notes that overall, women filed 83%, men filed 15%, and the remaining 2% didn't specify a gender. Some studies show that more than 80% of individuals who experience harassment never file a formal complaint at their places of work. Nearly three out of four individuals who experience harassment (sexual or otherwise) never even raise the issue internally, as documented in the US EEOC Task Force's executive summary (2016). They postulate that the reasons for failing to report the harassing behavior or to file a complaint is that the victims fear that they won't be believed, there will not be any action on their claim, or that social or professional retaliation will occur.

Harassment in the workplace will not stop on its own; it is on all of us to be part of the fight to stop workplace harassment. According to the EEOC (2016), we cannot be complacent bystanders and expect our workplace cultures to change by themselves. For this reason they suggest exploring the launch of an *It's on Us* campaign for the workplace.

The potential impact of harassment on nursing students both in the classroom and in the practice area is significant. According to Dowell (1992), nursing administrators and educators must be proactive in writing and implementing policies regarding sexual harassment. Valente and Bullough (2004) concur that employers should outline consequences and infractions of sexual harassment in their policies as well as provide ongoing education about what constitutes sexual harassment and enforce a "no tolerance" policy.

The issue of sexual harassment came to the forefront during the 1991 confirmation hearings of Supreme Court Justice Clarence Thomas (Allen, 1992). A once-secretive problem is now openly discussed in newspapers and by the media. As awareness about sexual harassment increased, we all realized how little we knew about it and what we could do about it. The majority of cases involve women who report being harassed by men, but the reverse has also occurred. In nursing, the stereotypical situation of sexual harassment involves a nurse (i.e., a woman) and a doctor (i.e., a man) because of the large number of nurses who are women. However, with the increase in the number of men entering the nursing profession, there is the potential for men to experience sexual harassment in the workplace. Roth and Coleman (2008) agree that actual and perceived barriers exist that prevent men from entering the nursing profession. In an effort to remove existing barriers and attract more men, the authors recommend that the image of men in nursing and the media's depiction of male nurses should be showcased as positive, and that increasing staff diversity by recruiting men within the nursing workforce should be embraced by both the public and by nursing itself (Fig. 13.5).

What Is Sexual Harassment?

The US Supreme Court recognized claims for sexual harassment as a form of discrimination based on sex under Title VII of the Civil Rights Act of 1964. According to Friedman (1992), "sexual harassment refers to conduct, typically experienced as offensive in nature, in which unwanted sexual advances are made in the context of a relationship of unequal power or authority" (p. 9). He goes on to explain that victims of sexual harassment are subjected to sexually oriented verbal comments, unwanted touching, and requests for sexual favors. The typical problem, known as *quid pro quo harassment*, arises when unwelcome sexual advances have been made and an employee is required to submit to those demands as a condition either of employment or of promotion. "Hostile work environment" has been used as a legal claim to show that "the atmosphere in the work (or other) environment is so uncomfortable or offensive by virtue of sexual advances, sexual requests, or sexual innuendoes that it amounts to a hostile environment" (Friedman, 1992, p. 16). Hershcovis and Barling (2010) succinctly state, "Sexual

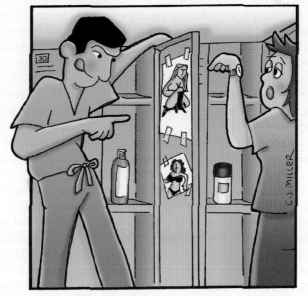

FIG. 13.5 Sexual harassment.

harassment has been described in terms of its three subcomponents: gender harassment, unwanted sexual attention, and quid pro quo" (p. 875). Let us look at hypothetical examples of how sexual harassment can affect nursing.

Samantha, a recent graduate, was receiving continued requests from a male patient to provide him with a complete bed bath. However, when a male nurse was assigned to this patient the following day, the patient reported to the male nurse that he was capable of bathing himself and proceeded to take a shower.

Lisa, the evening charge nurse, was quite excited that Tom, a recent graduate, was going to work on her unit. Lisa pursued Tom by repeatedly asking him for assistance with patient care. And when she called him into her office, she would touch him inappropriately.

According to the US EEOC, sexual harassment can occur in a variety of circumstances, including but not limited to the following:

- The victim as well as the harasser may be a woman or a man. The victim does not have to be of the opposite sex.
- The harasser can be the victim's supervisor, an agent of the employer, a supervisor in another area, a coworker, or a nonemployee.
- The victim does not have to be the person harassed but could be anyone affected by the offensive conduct.
- Unlawful sexual harassment may occur without economic injury to or discharge of the victim.
- The harasser's conduct must be unwelcome (EEOC, 2009).

What Can I Do About It?

There are two ways to handle this type of workplace conflict: informally and formally through a grievance procedure. Start with the most direct measure. Ask the person to STOP! Tell the harasser in clear terms that the behavior makes you uncomfortable and that you want it to stop immediately. Also, you might want to put your statement in writing to the person, keeping a copy for yourself. Tell other people, such as family, friends, personal physician, or minister, what is happening and how you are dealing with it. Friedman (1992) suggests keeping a written journal of harassing events, including all attempts to try to stop the harassment. The need to exercise power and control, rather than sexual desire, is frequently the motive of the sexual harasser (perpetrator). If sexual harassment is occurring as a result of miscommunication and misinterpretation of actions and is primarily driven by sex, not power, then telling the perpetrator to stop will often clear up any misconceptions. However, if the perpetrator is power-driven, the harassment will continue as long as he or she views the victim as passive, powerless, and frightened. What may be most difficult for the recent graduate is facing the fear that surrounds threats of job insecurity or public embarrassment (Friedman, 1992).

If a direct request to the perpetrator to stop does not work, then an informal complaint may be effective, especially if both parties realize a problem exists and want it to be solved. The goal of the informal method is to stop the harassment but not to punish the perpetrator. This method helps the person filing the complaint to maintain a harmonious relationship with the perpetrator. According to Friedman (1992), "a formal grievance usually requires filing a written complaint with an official group such as a hearing" (p. 65). This is a legal procedure that is guided and regulated by federal and state laws specific to this type of grievance. Before a 1991 amendment to the Civil Rights Act (Title VII), the means of correcting this bad situation—making it right or compensating the victim for difficulty encountered—were quite restricted. What has occurred as a result of this act is that victims of intentional discrimination may now seek compensatory and punitive damages. Each state has an EEOC, which has as its specific charge the enforcement of Title VII.

Unfortunately you may be faced with sexual harassment and conflict in the workplace. It is important to learn to deal with your feelings and to be aware of actions to take in case this happens to you. When this type of situation is resolved in a constructive, positive manner, it will enable you to feel better about your ability to manage conflict.

Prevention of sexual harassment is an important strategy that must be addressed in the workplace and in schools and universities. Dowling (2018) identifies four strategies that are applicable across many settings:

1. Build and sustain a culture of leadership and accountability.
2. Develop and maintain antiharassment policies and procedures.
3. Implement compliance training.
4. Establish workplace civility training and bystander intervention training.

According to the EEOC, harassment in the workplace will not stop on its own—it's on all of us to be part of the fight to stop workplace harassment. We cannot be complacent bystanders and expect our workplace cultures to change themselves. For this reason, we suggest exploring the launch of an *It's on Us* campaign for the workplace (EEOC, 2016).

CONCLUSION

Most of us have experienced conflict. Building effective conflict-management skills is key to working with patients, staff, and physicians. Various models exist to provide a framework for effective conflict resolution; the "win-win" model of *collaboration* is the strategy that aims for the highest level of resolution and is fully assertive and cooperative in approach. It requires creative nursing management and understanding to recognize and acknowledge that conflict will exist whenever human relationships are involved. This must be tempered with open, accurate communication and active listening by maintaining an objective—not emotional—stance as conflict resolution strategies are implemented. Review the Relevant Websites and Online Resources.

🌐 RELEVANT WEBSITES AND ONLINE RESOURCES

Community Tool Box
Section 6. Training for Conflict Resolution. http://ctb.ku.edu/en/table-of-contents/implement/provide-information-enhance-skills/conflict-resolution/main.

Conflict Resolution Network
http://www.crnhq.org/.

How to Deal With Difficult People
https://managementhelp.org/interpersonal/difficult-people.htm

MindTools
Conflict resolution. Resolving conflict rationally and effectively. http://www.mindtools.com/pages/article/newLDR_81.htm.

Program of Negotiation (Harvard Law School)
Series of articles on conflict resolution. http://www.pon.harvard.edu/?p=34983/?mqsc=E3519589

Segal, J., & Smith, M
Conflict resolution skills. http://www.helpguide.org/articles/relationships/conflict-resolution-skills.htm.

Webne-Behrman, H
8 steps for conflict resolution. https://www.ohrd.wisc.edu/home/HideATab/FullyPreparedtoManage/ConflictResolution/tabid/297/Default.aspx.

BIBLIOGRAPHY

Allen, A. (1992). Equal opportunity in the workplace. *Journal of Postanesthesia Nursing, 7*(2), 132–134.

Beauregard, M., et al. (2003). Improving our image a nurse at a time. *Journal of Nursing Administration, 10,* 510–511.

Blancett, S. S., & Sullivan, P. A. (1993). Ethics survey results. *Journal of Nursing Administration, 23*(3), 9–13.

Bramson, R. (1981). *Coping with difficult people.* New York: National Press Publications.

Cochran, A., & Elder, W. B. (2015). Effects of disruptive surgeon behavior in the operating room. *American Journal Surgery, 209,* 65–70.

Dowell, M. (1992). Sexual harassment in academia: Legal and administrative challenges. *Journal of Nursing Education, 31*(1), 5–9.

Dowling, R. A. (2018). Four strategies to prevent sexual harassment in your practice. *Urology Times, 2,* 20–22. Retrieved from http://www.urologytimes.com/business-urology/four-strategies-prevent-sexual-harassment-your-practice.

Filley, A. C. (1975). *Interpersonal conflict resolution.* Glenview, IL: Scott Foresman.

Friedman, J. (1992). *Sexual harassment: What it is, what it isn't, what it does to you, and what you can do about it.* Deerfield Beach, FL: Health Communications.

Guttenberg, R. M. (1983). How to stay cool in a conflict and turn it into cooperation. *Nurse Life, 3*(3), 25–29.

Hamilton, P. (2008). Conflict management styles in the health professions. *Southern Online Journal of Nursing Research, 8*(2), 2.

Hershcovis, M. S., & Barling, J. (2010). Comparing victim attributions and outcomes for workplace aggression and sexual harassment. *Journal of Applied Psychology, 95*(5), 874–888. https://doi.org/10.1037/a0020070.

Iglesias, M., & Vallejo, R. (2012). Conflict resolution styles in the nursing profession. *Contemporary Nurse, 43*(1), 73–80. https://doi.org/10.5172/conu.2012.43.1.73.

Kelly, J. (2006). An overview of conflict. *Dimensions of Critical Care Nursing, 25*(1), 22–28.

Kim, W., Nicotera, A., & McNulty, J. (2015). Nurse's perceptions of conflict as constructive or destructive. *Journal of Advanced Nursing, 71*(9), 2073–2083. https://doi.org/10.1111/jan.12672.

Lerner, H. (1997). *The dance of anger: A woman's guide to changing the patterns of intimate relationships.* New York: Harper & Row.

Libbus, M. K., & Bowman, K. G. (1994). Sexual harassment of female registered nurses in hospitals. *Journal of Nursing Administration, 24*(6), 26–31.

Roth, J., & Coleman, C. (2008). Perceived and real barriers for men entering nursing: Implications for gender diversity. *Journal of Cultural Diversity, 15*(3), 148–152.

Tavris, C. (1984). Feeling angry? Letting off steam may not help. *Nurse Life, 4*(5), 59–61.

Valente, S. M., & Bullough, V. (2004). Sexual harassment of nurses in the workplace. *Journal of Nursing Care Quality, 19*(3), 234–241.

Vo, L. T. (2017). We got government data on 20 years of workplace sexual harassment claims. *BuzzFeed News.* https://www.buzzfeednews.com/article/lamvo/eeoc-sexual-harassment-data#.reAEQ4VD1.

Weiss, L., & Cain, L. (1991). *Power lines: What to say in problem situations.* Dallas: Taylor.

14

Delegation in the Clinical Setting

*Ruth I. Hansten, MBA, PhD, RN, FACHE*_R

Let whoever is in charge keep this simple question in her head (not how can I always do the right thing myself but) how can I provide for this right thing always to be done?

Florence Nightingale

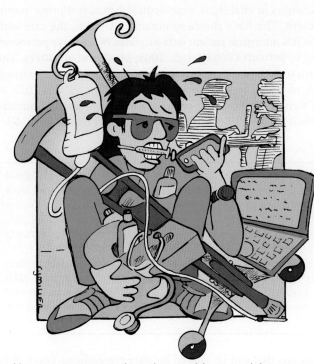

Nurses must recognize when and how to delegate and assign care tasks.

After completing this chapter, you should be able to:

- Define the terms *delegation, assignment, supervision,* and *accountability.*
- Apply the five rights of delegation in nursing practice.
- Delegate tasks successfully based on individualized patient-centered outcomes.
- Apply the "four Cs" of initial direction for a clear understanding of your expectations.
- Provide reciprocal feedback for effective evaluation of the delegate's performance.

Expert teamwork can make (or break) patient-care results and our own job satisfaction. As you review the multitude of team members you work with, how do you determine the best use of the resources they have to offer? What is your role as the registered nurse (RN) on the team in terms of making these decisions? Your ability to effectively delegate and assign the tasks that must be done—based on desired patient outcomes—will go a long way toward determining the success of your efforts. As nursing leads the way to better health care across the care continuum, RNs will supervise additional innovative roles of team members as they strive to provide leadership, working to provide cost-effective, high-quality care for everyone in a digital and robotic era (NCSBN, 2016a).

WHAT DOES DELEGATION MEAN?

State boards of nursing and professional associations, such as the American Nurses Association (ANA) and the National Council of State Boards of Nursing (NCSBN), have clarified definitions of the terms related to clinical leadership. Clinical delegation has been with us since the dawn of nursing, but team-work has taken on new meaning as many types of assistive personnel have been added to our care delivery models (Kalisch & Schoville, 2012; NCSBN, 2016a). Current evidence points to the conclusion that inappropriate care assignments, delegation, and supervision may be leading to missed care and untoward clinical outcomes (Bittner & Gravlin, 2009; Bittner et al., 2011; Gravlin & Bittner, 2010; Hansten, 2014a, 2014b; Kalisch, 2015; Kalisch et al., 2009, 2011; Scruth & Pugh, 2018). Researchers reviewing the failure to rescue (FTR), a situation in which a patient is deteriorating but the symptoms are not noted before death, indicate that changes in vital signs, neurological status, and urine output may occur up to 3 days before the final event. The RN's choice of nursing assistants, the care with which they are supervised, and how well the RN interprets patient data provided by assistive personnel may be either life-threatening or lifesaving to patients (Bobay et al., 2008; Mushta et al., 2017). The practice gaps and key causes that bring harm to patients, constituting clear evidence of lack of nursing knowledge and competence, include "lack of professional responsibility" in 73% and also "lack of intervention" in 47% of the 2016 NCSBN's analysis of nursing errors reported by boards of nursing (Zhong, 2016). The crucial clinical supervisory role of nurses impels us to perfect our skills in dele-gation, supervision, and accountability.

> **Delegation:** is "… the process for a nurse to direct another person to perform nursing tasks and activities." The National Council of State Boards of Nursing (NCSBN) describes this as the nurse transferring authority, whereas the ANA calls this a transfer of responsibility. Both mean that a registered nurse (RN) can direct another individual to do something that that person would not normally be allowed to do. Both papers stress that the nurse retains accountability for the delegation" (NCSBN, 2005, p. 1). The National Council of State Boards of Nursing's Model Nurse Practice Act (2012) simplified the definition of delegation to "transferring to a competent individual the authority to perform a selected nursing task in a selected situation."
>
> **Assignments:** "… the routine care, activities, and procedures that are within the authorized scope of practice of the RN or Licensed Practical Nurse/Vocational Nurse (LPN/VN) or part of the routine functions of the unlicensed assistive personnel (UAP) …included in the course work taught in the … basic education program" (NCSBN, 2016a, pp. 6–7). The nurse who assigns must maintain the responsibility to be sure that the work is done correctly and completely and retains accountability for the overall nursing care of that patient (NCSBN, 2016a, p. 7).

As you can see, these are generic definitions that can be altered by state regulations. You will be selecting the task and the situation in which to delegate or assign work. You will make a decision to delegate based on your assessment of the desired patient outcome and the competency of the indi-vidual to whom you are assigning a task. These real-time decisions in a constantly changing clinical landscape require complex critical thinking skills. In the pages ahead, we discuss steps that use the "five rights" to assist you in this practice, making it easier for you safely maximize your team's efforts.

> **Supervision:** The "provision of guidance or oversight by a qualified nurse for the accomplishment of a nursing task or activity with initial direction of the task or activity and periodic inspection of the actual act of accomplishing the task or activity" (NCSBN, 2012, p. 1).

Nurses are often confused regarding supervision. This responsibility does not belong to only the one with the title of *manager* or *house supervisor*; rather, the expectation by law is that any time you delegate or assign a clinical task to someone else, you will be held accountable for the initial direction you give and the timely follow-up (periodic inspection) to evaluate the performance of the task. This clinical care supervision should not be confused as the hiring or progressive discipline of employees that your manager or department director would perform.

The Delegation Process

In order to determine when and how an RN should delegate, the ANA, the NCSBN, and your own state's nursing practice acts offer decision-making support. See Fig. 14.1 for a decision tree guiding the delegation by RNs to UAP (ANA, 2012). Some state boards and professional associations offer similar decision trees for your assistance.

After it is determined that the RN is able to delegate through **assessment and planning**, the RN must **communicate**. Initial direction and ongoing discussion must be a two-way process involving the nurse who assesses the nursing assistive personnel's understanding of the delegated task and the nursing assistive person who asks questions regarding the delegation and seeks clarification of expectations.

Surveillance and supervision are ongoing through the episode of care. The purpose of surveillance and monitoring is related to the nurse's responsibility for patient care within the context of a patient population. The nurse supervises the delegation by monitoring the performance of the task or function and assures compliance with standards of practice, policies, and procedures. Frequency, level, and nature of monitoring vary with the needs of the patient and the competence of the team member.

Evaluation and feedback can be the forgotten steps in delegation and should include a determination of whether the delegation was successful, how the assignment was completed, and the patient results, to determine the effectiveness of the delegation (NCSBN, 2016a, p. 8; NCSBN & ANA, 2005, pp. 7–9).

> Delegation, assignment, and supervision are integrated processes: After you delegate or assign, you must supervise. You remain accountable for the total nursing care of your patients.

WHO IS ACCOUNTABLE HERE?

One of the biggest questions concerning teamwork and delegation is the issue of personal accountability. The definition of delegation already notes that the nurse is accountable for the total nursing care of the individuals. What does this really mean?

> **Accountability:** "Being answerable for what one has done and standing behind that decision and/or action" (Hansten & Jackson, 2009, p. 79).
> **Accountability:** "to be answerable to oneself and others for one's own choices, decisions, and actions as measured against a standard…" (ANA, 2015, p. 41).

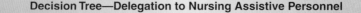

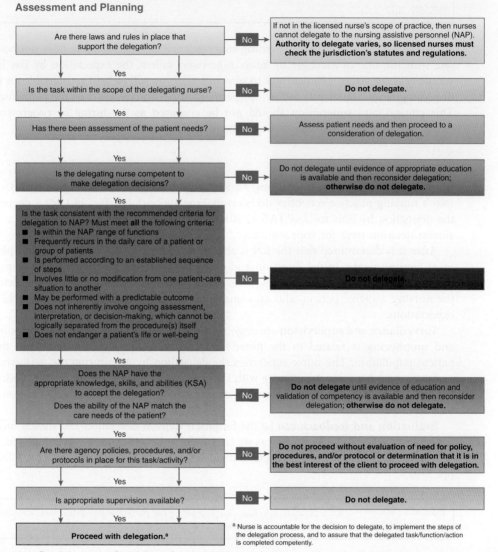

FIG. 14.1 Decision tree for delegation by registered nurses. (American Nurses Association. [2012]. ANA's Principles for Delegation by Registered Nurses to unlicensed assistive personnel (UAP). http://www.nursingworld.org/MainMenuCategories/ThePracticeofProfessionalNursing/NursingStandards/ANAPrinciples/PrinciplesofDelegation.pdf, p. 12.)

Some nurses equate accountability with "I am the one to blame." No wonder some nurses are afraid to delegate if someone else might make a mistake and they are going to take the blame! Let's not forget that accountability also means taking the credit for the positive results we achieve through the actions and decisions we make, as well as our freedom to act because of our licensure. Our individual choice to take action (personal accountability) is based on our professional knowledge and judgment, unleashing the art and science of nursing as applied to real-time individual patient and family situations using the gifts and skills of team members each day (Samuel, 2006). An important reminder about accountability before you take the weight of the world on your shoulders is the following statement:

> The delegate is accountable to "accept activities based on their own competency level, maintain competence for delegated responsibility, [and] maintain accountability for delegated activity" (NCSBN, 2016a, p. 6).

It is important to focus on what you are accountable for in this process and to let the delegate also assume his or her own level of accountability. It's also true that the delegate's level of education or experience may mean "they don't know what they don't know," so you must use your comprehensive understanding of the patient and his condition to guide you to ask the right questions to instruct the delegate and keep patients safe. The RN is accountable for the following:

- Assessing the patient's needs
- Assessing when to delegate/assign activities
- Planning the desired outcome
- Assessing the competency of the delegate
- Giving clear directions and obtaining acceptance from the delegate
- Following up on the completion of the task
- Providing feedback to the delegate

What if the delegate makes a mistake in completing the task? For what are you accountable? Let us consider the following example:

> It is 8.00 a.m. on your busy medical-surgical unit. You did not include your assigned nursing assistant in the shift report at the bedside with the off-going night shift, planning to offer your team member a quick verbal report and written assignment later. As you begin to administer a pain medication, you hear a shout and the sounds of someone hitting the floor. The patient in question was a two-person assist and your nursing assistant had attempted patient toileting alone. The whiteboard in the room and the electronic medical record (EMR) had not been updated during report to reflect "two-person assist for ambulation."
> - What are you accountable for?
> - Did you delegate correctly?
> - What do you do now?

Based on a review of the previous guidelines, we can say that you did not delegate or assign appropriately. Your communication, although planned, was delayed and incomplete, placing both your nursing assistant and your patient in unwarranted peril. Your system of communication on your unit also lacked verbal and written immediate instruction for all nursing assistants, including updating the patient whiteboards and/or EMR during bedside shift report. You are accountable for correcting the clinical effects and system origins of this error: immediate patient assistance, discussing the error with your supervisor, documenting the fall, talking with your nursing assistant about how you could best improve the timeliness and accuracy of your delegation and assignment, following up with your unit council or quality leaders to review the gaps in unit communication and change-of-shift processes that provided the opportunity for delayed communication. After caring for your patient in the middle of what could be a life-threatening event, your nursing assistant may need some reassurance and support as together you determine how you could better offer enough detailed information so that she could safely begin shift activities.

For more on the *how-to*s, read on as we discuss the Five Rights of Delegation.

The Five Rights of Delegation

1. The right task
2. Under the right circumstances
3. To the right person
4. With the right directions and communication
5. Under the right supervision and evaluation (NCSBN, 2005, p. 2; updated and affirmed NCSBN, 2016a, p. 8)

THE RIGHT TASK

The first part of any decision regarding delegation is the determination of what needs to be done and then the assessment of whether this is a task that can be delegated to someone else. However, personal barriers in the nurse can prevent letting go of tasks. Some suffer from "supernurse syndrome" and believe that no task should be delegated because no one can do it better, faster, or easier than the nurse can (Fig. 14.2). Others labor under the idea that never delegating tasks or gathering data will somehow ensure patient safety; they believe that their martyrdom (and overtime) is respected by their peers. Others fear offering direction and feedback and want assistive personnel to "just do their jobs" without any input from the RN; they do not fully understand the RN's and team members' accountability for the tasks being performed. These issues, along with role confusion, may lead to the omission of care

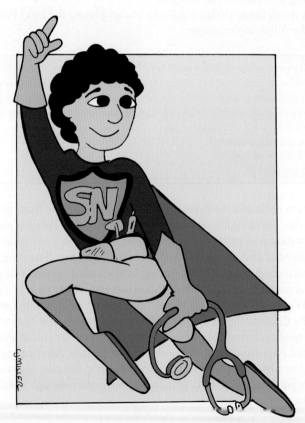

FIG. 14.2 Many nurses suffer from "supernurse syndrome."

(Hansten, 2014a, pp. 70–72; Scruth & Pugh, 2018, pp. 172–174). In its alarming report, *To Err Is Human*, the Institute of Medicine (IOM) provided statistical data on the frequency of medical errors and sentinel events occurring within the health care system, reporting between 44,000 and 98,000 sentinel events as preventable adverse events (IOM, 2000). The Agency for Healthcare Research and Quality (AHRQ) report (2018) shows that the untiring efforts of nurses and other health care quality professionals saved about 8000 lives between 2014 and 2016 as well as $2.9 billion in costs; however, there has been an increase in pressure ulcers and catheter-associated urinary tract infections. Patient hydration, positioning, hygiene, and nutrition tasks can be carried out by assistive personnel under the licensed nurse's supervision; but when improper delegation or follow-up occurs, care omissions can create an environment for the development of pressure ulcers and other patient safety issues (Hansten, 2014a; Kalisch, 2015). If the nurse cannot humanly "do it all," then care tasks can be missed, resulting in patient harm (Laws & Hughes, 2018, pp. 4–5).

In comparison, other nurses may be all too eager to delegate the least desirable tasks to someone else. A word of caution is necessary here: if we focus only on making task lists for others to do, we eliminate the very core of our purpose. Remember, your role as the RN on the team involves the coordination and planning of care, with your primary focus on identifying, with the patient and the physician, the desired outcomes for your patients. Once determined, interventions will be readily apparent, and decisions regarding possible delegation of these tasks must be made.

Reflection: Do I personally tend toward being a "supernurse" or "supermartyr," wanting to do everything myself, because I won't let go of nursing tasks? Or do I tend to be a "dumper" who would rather let the assistive personnel do all messy or difficult tasks? Or do I tend to be afraid to give direction and correct others for fear of not being "liked"? What kind of feedback could I ask for that would help me to monitor my tendencies and improve my leadership?

WHAT CAN I DELEGATE OR ASSIGN?

Fortunately there are several reference sources to help you in making this determination. The first thing we recommend looking at is the nurse practice act for your state. Each state board of nursing has a nurse practice act that guides nursing decisions about what to delegate to nursing assistive personnel. Be sure you become familiar with your state's nursing practice statute, regulations, rules, policies, care standards, and advisory opinions.

> Considering this, a professional registered nurse (RN) *can delegate* or *assign*
> - Discrete tasks or data retrieval based on patient condition and planned outcome
> - Tasks that the delegate is competent to do and is allowed to do according to your state regulations and organizational job descriptions and skills checklists
> - Tasks that the competent delegate has also agreed to do and understands preferred outcome, parameters, and how and when to report to the delegating RN

Your state board of nursing or nursing quality assurance commission has likely addressed the issue of delegation or assignment and developed rules, advisory opinions and/or standards of practice that may offer information regarding who can do what. The scope of practice for each care-provider level usually includes a description of the processes that may be performed at that level. In an attempt to clarify the role of the LPN/LVN, the NCSBN constructed the Practical Nurse Scope of Practice White Paper (NCSBN, 2005) asking nursing education programs, regulatory agencies, and practice settings to educate nursing professionals about the differences in LPN and RN roles and to articulate clearly the LPN and RN scope of practice regulations.

However, variation continues among state nurse practice acts, administrative codes, and practices along portions of the care continuum from ambulatory care to long-term care for both LPN/VN roles and various health care assistant roles, such as certified medication aides (NCSBN, 2016b, pp. 7–8; NCSBN, 2017a, p. S13).

Traditionally, their clinical experience has given students opportunities to observe how RNs communicate and delegate tasks to LPNs. However, clinical site availability in settings where LPNs are employed has dramatically decreased, preventing students from observing the delegation of tasks by the RN to the LPN (Garneau, 2012). Therefore decreased clinical site experience coupled with unfamiliarity regarding the scope of practice regulations for the LPN also contributes to ineffective delegation (Mole & McLafferty, 2004; NCSBN, 2006; Nhongo, 2018).

> If you work with licensed practical nurses (LPNs) or licensed vocational nurses (LVNs), consult your specific state's rules and regulations along with your organization's job descriptions. LPN practice varies from state to state.

The NCSBN Model Rules (2017a) states that the LPN/VN practices "under the supervision of an RN, advanced practice registered nurse (ARNP), licensed physician or other authorized healthcare provider" (pp. 1, 3.1.2); he or she participates and collaborates in nursing care. This role is not one that allows independent practice and is designed for amplifying nursing care for stable, predictable conditions at both the site and with the patient. A key distinction between RNs and LPNs is related to the first step of the nursing process: assessment. The LPN collects data during the health history and physical examination, whereas the RN conducts a comprehensive physical assessment and develops a plan of care for the patient based on assessment findings. Moreover, the RN initiates and provides patient teaching and discharge planning and also evaluates the patient's response to the plan of care and his or her understanding of the information provided (NCSBN, 2019a). The LPN contributes to the development and/or updates the plan of care and reinforces patient teaching and discharge instructions (NCSBN, 2016b). In the midst of health care payment reform and attempts to connect all parts of the care continuum for the provision of better health care for entire populations, state practice rules for care providers may be changing quickly. For example, more states have recently promulgated rules related to certified medication aides in long-term care or community settings. These aides are certified nursing assistants (CNAs) who may, with additional training and certification, administer some routine medications, functioning under the supervision of an RN (or possibly LPN, depending on the state). In addition, community health care lay assistants are often deployed out of medical homes (ambulatory care clinics) or public health departments. These workers, following procedural rules, may function as case finders or perform such tasks as checking vital signs or making home checks in the community. An RN or a physician supervises these community health aides. Medical assistants (MAs) in ambulatory clinics not always specifically addressed by state practice regulations and have functioned under the direct supervision of physicians in their offices, but currently their roles are regulated in some states. Creative roles will emerge in the future as states and municipalities attempt to find better, more cost-effective ways to deliver care. RNs should remain tuned in to their state's health division's regulatory changes as new roles and responsibilities emerge. *Whatever roles may be designed to assist them, RNs remain accountable for the nursing care of their patients, even though those whom they supervise may be the individuals completing the tasks.* One of the causes of disciplinary action that is listed in many nurse practice codes under "professional misconduct" is "delegating to an unlicensed person activities that can only be performed by licensed professionals" or "failure to adequately supervise or monitor those to whom care has been delegated" (Brous, 2012, p. 55; NCSBN, 2017a, p. 17).

The next place to look is in your organization, obtaining a copy of the job description, nursing responsibilities, and the skills checklist for each care provider. This will give you a very specific list of tasks from which to work; but remember, there are other considerations. Even if the skills checklist includes ambulation of patients, it is up to you to determine whether this individual patient's condition and the specifics of this assistant's competency match. It may not be advisable to delegate the first ambulation of a postoperative total hip replacement patient to the new patient care assistant (PCA) (Critical Thinking Box 14.1).

? CRITICAL THINKING BOX 14.1

In Your Organization, Could You Delegate the Following Tasks?

	YES	NO
Bladder retention catheter insertion	☐	☐
Taking vital signs	☐	☐
Feeding a patient	☐	☐
Hygienic care	☐	☐
Medication administration	☐	☐
Discontinuing an intravenous line	☐	☐
Teaching insulin administration	☐	☐

If you have questions and need clarification for your state, go online to your board of nursing to consult statutes, rules, regulations, and advisory opinions or call your nursing regulatory body for assistance. (See www.ncsbn.org for links to your state's nursing regulatory commission of board of nursing.) Be aware that your state may have introduced or passed a bill that may affect your practice in relation to residents of neighboring states. In early 2018, a total of 29 states had passed legislation approving enhanced interstate compact licensure regulation legislation designed to allow nurses to practice across state lines because of e-consultation, telenursing, or other technology that would broadcast nursing practice across state borders (NCSBN, 2019b).

Beyond the law, your employer will have job descriptions and skills checklists that may clearly define the role of the caregiver. If you have not seen these documents, be sure to review them soon. This is the baseline for determining "who does what" and selecting the right task to delegate. Because many organizations develop creative assistant roles to leverage the professional judgment of RN personnel, the scope of practice of each role will be defined first by law. If the organization extends the role of a patient care technician to include preoperative teaching, you want to be aware that this is clearly an RN function and by statue, standards, or state administrative code is not allowed to be delegated to the technician.

> A job description or policy should never supersede the state legal limits of the scope of practice.

Is There Anything I Cannot Delegate?

Again, your first resource is the law. Many states are very specific in their descriptions of what duty cannot be delegated and belongs only to the RN's scope of practice. The NCSBN reminds us that:

"Nursing is a knowledge-based process discipline and cannot be reduced solely to a list of tasks. The licensed nurse's specialized education, professional judgment, and discretion are essential for quality nursing care.... While nursing tasks may be delegated, the licensed nurse's generalist knowledge of client care indicates that the practice-pervasive functions of assessment, evaluation, and nursing judgment must not be delegated" (NCSBN, 1995, p. 2). The NCSBN reiterated in their 2016 National Guidelines for Delegation that "the practice pervasive functions of clinical reasoning, nursing judgment, or critical decision-making cannot be delegated" (NCSBN, 2016a, p. 6).

According to nurse-attorney Joanne P. Sheehan, nurses cannot delegate the following:

- In-depth assessments that identify needs and problems and diagnose human responses
- Any aspect of planning, including the development of comprehensive approaches to the total care plan (This does not preclude other team members from collaborating and offering information.)
- Any provision of health counseling, teaching, or referrals to other health care providers (*Author's note: in some states standardized or preapproved patient education materials can be offered by LPN/LVNs.*)
- Therapeutic nursing techniques and comprehensive care planning (Sheehan, 2001, p. 22) (Critical Thinking Box 14.2).

💡 CRITICAL THINKING BOX 14.2

Where to Look to Determine the Right Task

- State nurse practice act, rules, policies, advisory opinions
- Employee job description
- Skills checklist
- Demonstrated competency

With the right task selected according to state scope of practice, the policies in your agency, and your assessment of the situation, there is still work to be done.

Do Not Delegate
- Professional nursing judgment, clinical reasoning, and critical decision-making.
- The registered nurse (RN) nursing process: Data gathering and some tasks or interventions can be delegated (see Right Task) but the comprehensive assessment, nursing diagnosis, care planning, evaluation, and care coordination may not be delegated.
- With patient education, there is some variance by state regulation, but patient education planning and comprehensive patient education are generally reserved for RNs.

THE RIGHT CIRCUMSTANCES

Next, "Right Circumstances—appropriate patient setting, available resources, and consideration of other relevant factors" (NCSBN, 1995, p. 2) suggests that the staffing mix, community needs, teaching obligations, and the type of patient receiving care should also be considered. The clinical condition of the patient must be assessed and must be stable (NCSBN, 2017b, p. 8). Different rules for delegation may apply regarding what and how an RN must delegate in-home care, long-term care, or care in community settings for the developmentally disabled or group boarding homes for assisted living (Hansten et al., 1999; Hansten & Jackson, 2009).

Emergency departments may have different rules for delegation to UAPs with additional emergency training. Other settings—such as correctional facilities, ambulatory care clinics, or assistive living long-term care—may have state rules related to medication aides (MAs), or other technicians (Research for Best Practice Box 14.1).

RESEARCH FOR BEST PRACTICE BOX 14.1

Delegation and Supervision

Practice Issue

Changes in health care reimbursement and care delivery reforms would indicate that nurses are fantasizing if they believe they will be able to practice effectively without proficient delegation skills. Nurses will have to exhibit expert leadership at the point of care so as to use our nation's human and material resources cost-effectively to improve the health of our communities. Compounding the fractures that can occur in teamwork when multiple individuals must communicate in a complex situation, early discharges, advances in technology, increased registered nurse (RN) autonomy, better-informed consumers, and expanded legal definitions of liability all increase the need to use the best delegation and supervision techniques (Croke, 2003; Laws & Hughes, 2018).

A study geared to understand the critical thinking processes of nurses in delegation showed that nurses often expect assistive personnel to have a higher degree of knowledge and skill than they possess or were licensed to perform, such as the nursing process, prioritizing, and assessment (Bittner & Gravlin, 2009; Hansten, 2014a). Nurses report difficulty with delegating because of the structure of care delivery, with multiple assistive personnel reporting to multiple RNs, and challenges in how to communicate what needs to be done as well as how to follow up without offending coworkers (Standing & Anthony, 2008). However, difficulties with delegating appropriately mean that there is missed care, leaving hospitalized patients in jeopardy because of the consequences of omissions—such as hospital-acquired pressure ulcers, infections, and errors as well as FTR deteriorating patients (Kalisch, 2015; Kalisch et al., 2009; Scruth & Pugh, 2018). Many insurers will not reimburse these hospital-acquired conditions and errors, and they cost the patient/family and health care organizations billions per year nationally (Virkstis et al., 2009).

Review of care issues involving cases in which the five rights of delegation and supervision were not followed showed that problems were related to the RN's failure to provide the right direction or communication (13.9%) or supervision (12.4%). A total of 60.6% of deficiencies were related to the UAP not following through with a task that was delegated or not following unit/department procedures (Standing et al., 2001).

To help nurses learn how to work effectively within teams at their work sites, organizations have provided in-depth education in applying the principles of delegation at work, and they have combined that training with a consistent care delivery structure. At the end of 16 weeks of instructor-guided self-study, professional practice skills have improved up to 37% and the use of supervision checkpoints by RNs with team members has doubled in frequency (Hansten, 2008a, 2009, 2014a,b).

Implications for Nursing Practice

- There is a need for ongoing education for nurses regarding team leadership skills and unit practices that create care delivery models supporting nurses in delegating and supervising effectively in highly complex work (Hansten, 2005, 2009, 2014a, 2014b; Nhongo et al., 2018; Standing & Anthony, 2008).
- Each health care team must create a care delivery model that includes a clear plan for the day, proper times for initial direction and ongoing supervision, and updating of clinical and performance information (Hansten, 2008a, 2008b).
- Communication lapses have been a frequently reported root cause of sentinel events from 2013 to 2015 (2015a). The Joint Commission's (TJC) National Patient Safety Goals have included a need to develop a standardized approach to hand-off communication. Although many hospitals have interpreted the term *hand off* to consist of the information shared between shifts and at patient transfer, the need for accurate, ongoing updating of patient data *during* a team's shift or episode of care would also apply. Ongoing root cause analysis of sentinel events shows that the communication lapses continue to be problematic unless the organization has trained the employees in face-to-face standardized critical content in all communications with other team members throughout the care continuum (TJC, 2019).
- Missed care resulting from poor-quality delegation and supervision skills and unclear assignments can result in health care–acquired conditions that will no longer be paid for by insurers. These conditions cost the patients and their families more than dollars, such as untoward pain and suffering. The reimbursement losses and costs from poor quality can provide the motivation to sink scarce funds into the development of delegation and teamwork skills (Bittner et al., 2011; Hansten, 2014b; Kalisch, 2015).

Continued

Q RESEARCH FOR BEST PRACTICE BOX 14.1—cont'd

Considering This Information

What education and orientation processes are in place in your organization to promote effective delegation and supervision? If these processes are not present now, how can you be involved in their development? What unit processes could be created that would help teams collaborate throughout the shift?

References

Alfaro-LeFevre, R. (2019). *Critical thinking, clinical reasoning, and clinical judgment* (7th ed.). Philadelphia, PA: Elsevier.

Bittner, N., & Gravlin, G. (2009). Critical thinking, delegation, and missed care in nursing practice. *Journal of Nursing Administration, 39*(3), 142–146.

Bittner, N., Gravlin, G., Hansten, R., & Kalisch, B. (2011). Unraveling care omissions. *Journal of Nursing Administration, 41*(12), 510–512.

Croke, E. (2003). Nurses, negligence, and malpractice. *American Journal of Nursing, 103*(9), 9.

Hansten, R. (2005). Relationship and results oriented healthcare: Evaluate the basics. *Journal of Nursing Administration, 35*(12), 522–525.

Hansten, R. (2008a). *Relationship & results oriented healthcare planning & implementation manual.* Port Ludlow, WA: Hansten Healthcare PLLC.

Hansten, R. (2008b). Why nurses still must learn to delegate. *Nursing Leadership, 10,* 19–25.

Hansten, R. (2009). A bundle of best bedside practices. *Health Care Management, 28*(2), 111–116.

Hansten, R. (2014a). Coach as chief correlator of tasks to results through delegation skill and teamwork development. *Nurse Leader, 12*(4), 69–73.

Hansten, R. (2014b). *The master coach manual for the relationship & results oriented healthcare program.* Port Ludlow, WA: Hansten Healthcare PLLC.

Kalisch, B. (2006). Missed nursing care. *Journal of Nursing Care Quality, 21*(4), 306–313.

Kalisch, B. (2015). *Errors of omission: How missed nursing care imperils patients.* Silver Spring, MD: American Nurses Association.

Kalisch, B., & Begeny, S. (2005). Improving nursing unit teamwork. *Journal of Nursing Administration, 35*(12), 550–556.

Kalisch, B., Landstrom, G., & Williams, R. (2009). Missed care: Errors of omission. *Nursing Outlook, 57,* 3–9.

Laws, L., & Hughes, C. (2018). Errors of omission in nursing care and its impact on patient care. *Texas Board of Nursing Bulletin, 49*(2), 4–5.

Nhongo, D., Hendricks, J., Bradshaw, J., & Bail, K. (2018). Leadership and registered nurses (RNs) working after-hours in residential aged care facilities (RACFs): A structured online literature review. *Journal of Clinical Nursing.* https://doi.org/10.1111/jocn.14565.

Scruth, E., & Pugh, D. (2018). Omission of nursing care: An international perspective. *Clinical Nurse Specialist, 32*(4), 172–174. https://doi.org/10.1097/NUR.0000000000000380.

Standing, T., & Anthony, M. (2008). Delegation: What it means to acute care nurses. *Applied Nursing Research, 21,* 8–14.

Standing, T., Anthony, M., & Hertz, J. (2001). Nurses' narratives of outcomes after delegation to unlicensed assistive personnel. *Outcomes Management for Nursing Practice, 5*(1), 18–23.

The Joint Commission. (2015a). *Sentinel Event Data Summary,* 2015. Retrieved from http://www.jointcommission.org/sentinel_event.aspx.

The Joint Commission. (2015b). *Hand-off Communications Targeted Solutions.* Retrieved from http://www.centerfortransforminghealthcare.org/projects/detail.aspx?Project=1.

The Joint Commission. (2019). *2019 National Patient Safety Goals.* Retrieved from https://www.jointcommission.org/assets/1/6/2019_HAP_NPSGs_final2.pdf.

Virkstis, N. D., Westheim, J., & Boston-Fleischhauer, C. (2009). Safeguarding quality: Building the business case to prevent nursing-sensitive hospital-acquired conditions. *Journal of Nursing Administration, 39*(7–8), 350–355.

How Can I Determine the Strengths and Weaknesses of Team Members?

Often motivated by the fear that a delegate may make a mistake in an assigned task, nurses focus on the potential weaknesses of their team members. As nurses, we are educated to anticipate the worst so that we can prevent accidents, adverse drug reactions, and negative impacts from disease processes and treatments alike. As prudent as this approach may be for the safety of all concerned, it is worthwhile to discuss the advantages of recognizing the strengths of the team members as well.

Recall the last time you were given specific, positive feedback about your performance during your clinical experience as a nursing student. How did you feel? Most of us are energized and restored by the reinforcement that our hard work has been recognized. Recognition of strengths will begin to get us on the right track in our relationship.

Assigning tasks on the basis of the strengths of the person will allow the patient to experience the very best care—and allow the delegate to provide the very best care. As a supervising RN, you are in a new position with respect to the long-term performance of delegates. If assistive personnel are assigned only those tasks in which they perform well, they may not grow in their abilities and skills. This mistake is exemplified by a hospital that had created a new multi-skilled PCA role with CNAs. These CNAs had been trained to do phlebotomies as well, as authorized by the state board. Phlebotomists had been eliminated but were given the option of training for the new PCA role. When all of the PCAs worked together, those who had been phlebotomists, because they were more comfortable with that skill, drew the lab tests. When all the PCAs who were former phlebotomists were off on vacation and maternity leave, none of the other PCAs had become proficient at this skill. Recognize strengths and encourage the best patient care possible by using them, but also challenge delegates to grow.

Asking the right questions before delegating can often prevent dreaded performance gaps. Nurses can be reluctant to ask float personnel or agency replacement staff whether they feel comfortable in completing the assignment they have received. Ask if they have any questions, listen attentively, and answer all questions so that they can confidently and competently complete the task. Float and temporary personnel tell us that they would prefer being asked about their competency at the beginning of a shift or assignment, with the offer of help and clarification, rather than having to locate an RN later to request information. The ANA Code of Ethics states, "The nurse is responsible and accountable for individual nursing practice and determines the appropriate delegation of tasks consistent with the nurse's obligation to provide optimum patient care" (ANA, 2015). Be assured that although it is the responsibility of the RN to assess the competency of those they supervise, the delegate must be "accountable for accepting the delegation and for his/her own actions in carrying out the task" (NCSBN, 1995, p. 1). The RN who is familiar with the situation, however, must ask the correct questions to determine whether the person is competent.

For example, if an RN was planning to ask a nursing assistant to feed a baby with respiratory difficulties based on the team's plan that the baby would be able to ingest 12 ounces of formula this shift, what questions might the RN ask to determine the potential strengths and weaknesses? If the individual has not had experience in this procedure, how could the nurse ensure her or his future competency? In this situation, an RN would certainly ask questions about past experiences with feeding babies who had difficulty swallowing. If the delegate assures the RN that she or he is competent, the RN may go further in asking what the CNA would do if coughing or choking occurred. Depending on the situation, the RN would probably want to demonstrate feeding techniques and observe the skills to ensure the competency of the delegate. This situation is an example of a scenario where the delegate "may not know what she does not know" and you must determine if this particular baby's feeding can be assigned to this individual, whether or not "feeding infants" is listed on the skills checklist.

What Are the Causes of Performance Weaknesses?

Let us look at an example of a performance weakness and try to determine what the potential causes may be.

In this scenario, you are an RN working a night shift on a hematology-oncology unit, and an agency nursing assistant, Pam, comes to work with you this shift. Pam is excited about the possibilities of interviewing for a regular night-shift position and would love to work extra on holidays and weekends. As you begin to discuss her assignment for the night, she states, "Oh, I forgot to tell you, I never care for bloodborne pathogen–positive patients! Ever!"

There are some potential costs and benefits to your response to this statement. As the nurse, you could ignore it and continue with your work. You may decide that this person has problems, and you may elect to delay forwarding her request for an interview to your department supervisor. Or you may determine that there is something behind her refusal. How you respond may cost you a potentially valuable staff member and could upset the other members of your team and the patients. Avoiding the problem or accommodating Pam's refusal could become a terrible headache when you are making assignments and would be contrary to the mission of your organization.

Experience has shown that there are several potential causes of performance inadequacies (Critical Thinking Box 14.3). One of the most common is that employees are not aware of what is expected of them. Does Pam know that it is part of your policy at this facility for everyone to take care of all patients, whether or not they are known to be HIV- or hepatitis C–positive? Perhaps being aware of this expectation would help Pam in making her decision about whether to apply for work on this unit.

❓ CRITICAL THINKING BOX 14.3

Potential Sources of Performance Weakness

- Unclear expectations
- Lack of performance feedback
- Educational needs
- Need for additional supervision and direction
- Individual characteristics: past experiences, motivational or personal issues

Often, being clear about expectations is not enough. All of us have some blind spots in our own performance. Perhaps we think we are doing just fine, meeting performance competencies and beyond, but colleagues have noted that we are not performing procedures according to policy. So another common cause of performance difficulties is that others have not shared their perceptions of our performance with us. If these observations are not shared, we will blithely believe we are doing great. Pam may have adopted this attitude regarding bloodborne pathogens in other work settings, but because of the desperation for her help, no one had shared the fact that this behavior falls short of competencies in her current job description.

Another common origin of performance weakness is an educational need. Does Pam need more education about how bloodborne infection is transmitted and how it is prevented? Surely she had to complete some infection control content in her CNA certification course, but it seems that she did not internalize this content. Or is there a personal problem? She may have just witnessed the death of a loved one from hepatitis, AIDS, or Ebola and feels unable to cope with seeing others with this disease at this time.

The amount of supervision needed can be another source of performance problems. As an RN, you must determine the amount of "periodic inspection" needed for the delegate. Some people require additional direction but are still able to do the job competently. In the absence of that direction, they may be unable to create positive patient outcomes. Nurses tell us they wish that the assistive personnel on their staff would be self-directed and take the initiative without being told. This RN's hope that all will do their jobs without interaction or supervision on his or her part does not conform with the definition of supervision or the RN's accountability to protect the public's safety. Again, as a leader, the RN must determine how much supervision is needed for the individual delegate, just as we determine the degree of observation needed for each patient based on our assessment of the patient's needs. In Pam's case, her reluctance to work with patients infected with bloodborne pathogens may have nothing to do with supervision but may reflect a need for guidance, education, or a frank discussion of expectations.

As the RN who is supervising Pam this shift, what steps would you take to determine the cause of her performance weakness—her assertion that she refuses to care for particular patients? What questions would you ask? How would you respond so that you could continue to use Pam's services during this shift, maintain the integrity of your mission and preserve the potential for your manager being able to hire a new employee?

Matching the right person with the right task is the third step in the circular process of delegation. This process includes planning and articulating priority patient outcomes, assessing the competency of the delegate to perform the task, determining the potential strengths and weaknesses of the assistive personnel, and planning how much supervision is needed. To ensure that the right person will perform the right task, additional clarification of expectations, performance feedback, and planning for educational needs may be necessary; these steps will promote the long-term success of the team.

THE RIGHT PERSON

After you have determined that a task can be delegated, matching the task to the right person involves nurses selecting the right task for a competent person in each situation. We have already discussed how you would determine the correct task. But how do we select the right person in the right situation (Fig. 14.3)?

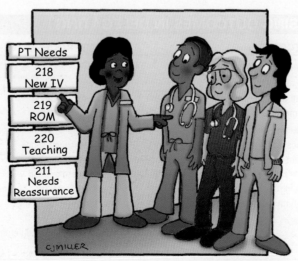

FIG. 14.3 It can be difficult to know who is the best person to handle a given situation.

How Can I Use Outcomes in Delegating?

In planning for the right person to handle a task, focusing on outcomes is essential (Critical Thinking Box 14.4). Alfaro-LeFevre's (2019) evidence-based critical thinking indicators are outcome-focused guides appropriate for delegation as well as critical thinking in nursing (p. 12).

❓ CRITICAL THINKING BOX 14.4

Talking About Outcomes: What's in It for Me?

- Provides a method to decide appropriate assignments: Who should be doing what task?
- Helps patients heal more quickly as we engage patient and family in the process of discussing their priorities and preferred goals/outcomes.
- Gives you a sense of purpose for the shift (short term and long term).
- Enhances your ability to motivate coworkers along a track to achieve the desired outcomes.
- Clarifies your role as leader of the team.
- Verifies and clarifies patient/family expectations and reduces anxiety and patient dissatisfaction when they are discussing and driving their own care plans.
- Promotes job satisfaction and collaboration for the whole team

For example, two patients are admitted to a hospital. Each will need hygienic care today (task), but who will give the baths is related to the outcome you are trying to achieve. For Mr. Peterson, who has been homeless and is in dire need of a bath so that you can perform a complete and accurate skin assessment, the priority outcome you and your patient desire is that Mr. Peterson will be clean. With Ms. Ibutu, who is a paraplegic, today is the day that her caregivers and she will demonstrate how they will assess her skin for areas of breakdown and how to perform range-of-motion exercises for her lower extremities. The RN's decision about who will do which task is dependent on the plan of care and the goals that the team has established in the discussion with the patient or family (Table 14.1).

This same logic applies when you have heard in report that a patient, Mr. Handelsky, is unstable. In your current care delivery system on your unit, the licensed practical (or vocational) nurse (LPN or

TABLE 14.1 USING OUTCOMES IN DELEGATING

PATIENT	OUTCOME	TASK/PROCESS	WHO WILL PERFORM IT?
Mr. Peterson	Patient will be clean.	Bath	Nursing assistant or other care associate
Ms. Ibutu	Patient and caregivers will know how to perform skin and range-of-motion assessment.	Bath with education regarding home care	RN: teaching plan; OT, PT, or rehabilitation aide may also assist
Mr. Handelsky	Patient will maintain cardiorespiratory homeostasis and continue on care path day 1. Patient will be free of pain and comfortable for this shift. Family members will be informed regarding his progress q2–3h. Long-term outcome: pain-free death.	Initial baseline vital signs and assessment, close monitoring Pain assessment and treatment, comfort measures (repositioning, skin care) Patient- and family-centered communication	RN: assessment and interpretation of data, communication and updating family members regarding progress LPN: data gathering and reporting RN: initial plan for comfort measures and pain assessment Assistant: comfort measures, report of progress

I PN, Licensed practical nurse; *OT,* occupational therapist; *PT,* physical therapist; *RN,* registered nurse

LVN) may handle the second set of vital sign data in your postoperative intensive care unit (PICU) after the initial bedside hand-off that you attend with the nurse in the postanesthesia recovery unit. Suppose, for example, that the report you received stated that there had been increasing cherry-red drainage from the chest tube and that the patient's cardiac monitor showed supraventricular tachycardia with an increasing respiratory rate. Based on the planned outcome for the shift, Mr. Handelsky will maintain cardiorespiratory homeostasis and continue on a critical path for the first day postthoracotomy, as had been discussed with him on his preoperative visit. Outcomes for the family would include them being informed every 2 to 3 hours about his stability and progress. Using your insight that his condition may be deteriorating, you may make a different decision regarding who will be there for the first several patient assessments. If the assistant working with you today is an experienced team member, you may choose to send him or her in to accompany you for subsequent patient evaluations, or send her to gather data on another patient. If the assistant is a "float" from an agency, known to you only by initial questioning, you may immediately make a visit to see Mr. Handelsky alone, assign her a less critical task, and begin to set up the plan for the data gathering and schedule for reporting that you will expect from your assistant later if the patient stabilizes. This would be a very different process if the outcome you wanted to achieve was pain relief and comfort for a terminal patient.

If you are working in an ambulatory care clinic or doctor's office setting, consider a situation in which you would use outcomes to change your delegation decision. Normally the MA may gather information and vital signs for all patients, obtaining their chief reason for coming in for their appointment today. However, the community health care worker told you that she had encouraged an anxious young teen to come in to obtain accurate pregnancy and sexually transmitted diseases (STDs) tests. You are aware that this teen may bolt at the slightest provocation. You tell the MA that you would like to be notified immediately when the patient arrives after school and that you will meet with her first to establish a trusting relationship. Intended outcomes would be to obtain definitive tests so that the "patient will understand her pregnancy status" and to create a plan for carefully relaying the news. Longer-term results would be that the patient would understand how to adopt safe sex and birth control practices. Your normal daily routines would be altered because of the patient's needs and would require the RN's interventions, teaching, and relationship-building rather than business as usual.

Take a moment to consider the outcomes for a particularly difficult patient you have been dealing with lately. Were you clear on outcomes? If so, have you shared them with colleagues? Focusing on outcomes takes time, but remember, "If you fail to plan, plan to fail." Why should an RN focus on outcomes? Discussion of the patient's goals and intended results of your interventions not only helps establish who should be doing what task but also allows RNs to motivate others. How many of us jump on a train if we do not know where it is going? A purpose and a destination allow all team members to function more effectively. When assistive personnel are given the same assignment daily, without variation, without any understanding of why they are doing what they are doing, it is similar to being an assembly line worker putting widgets in a machine. Satisfaction and motivation of coworkers generally come from the feeling that they are making a difference in the lives of their patients.

In a similar manner, you as the leader of the team would feel much better at the end of your shift or assignment if you could feel comfortable with the outcomes you have assisted the patient in achieving. You could actually verify the patient/family's priorities and plan with the patients, much as you were always told to do by the teachers in your nursing program! Streamlining the care to match the patient's expectations ultimately saves much time (Hansten, 2009; Hansten, 2014a, 2014b).

Again, the RN is accountable for the total nursing care of the patient, for determining the situation in which delegation will be used, and for the selection of the right person to do the right task in addition to the periodic inspection and follow-up of those they supervise. The right communication will begin that clarification process, bringing us to the next step in the five rights of delegation.

Remember that the building blocks of state practice regulations, job descriptions, skills records, and competency checklists in your organization and department, with clear communication with your delegate about their abilities, observation of their skills, and ongoing evaluation of the results of their work will allow you to be certain you have created a functioning team with the "right tasks" under the "right circumstances" being assigned to the "right person."

THE RIGHT DIRECTION AND COMMUNICATION

How Can I Get the Delegate to Understand What I Want?

How clear you make your initial direction will be the cornerstone in determining the success of your delegated task and, ultimately, the performance of your team. The bottom line, which is whether the patient outcome was achieved, hinges on your ability to provide initial direction that clearly defines your expectations of the delegate in performing the assigned task. It is not surprising that this is a step that is often done poorly or left out entirely, because the assumption is made that the individual "knows what the job is and should just do it."

The first component of supervision, according to its definition, is the provision of initial direction. Achieving a balance in which we provide enough information for the person to understand (and accept) the request without excessive repetition and risking confusion or condescension requires that we tread a fine line. The use of the "four C's" of initial direction will help you to plan your communication (Critical Thinking Box 14.5). Best practices include performing shift reports or handovers at the bedside, engaging the patients in the discussion of their priorities, the plan for care, and what each person will do for them during the shift (Hansten, 2008a, 2014a, 2014b).

? CRITICAL THINKING BOX 14.5

The Four Cs of Initial Direction

CLEAR: Does the team member understand what I am saying?
CONCISE: Have I confused the direction by giving too much unnecessary information?
CORRECT: Is the direction according to policy, procedure, job description, and the law?
COMPLETE: Does the delegate have all the information necessary to complete the task?

Data from Hansten, R., & Jackson, M. (2014). *Clinical delegation skills: A handbook for professional practice* (4th ed.). Sudbury, MA: Jones & Bartlett, pp. 287–288; LaCharity, L., Kumagai, C., & Bartz, B. (2019). *Prioritization, delegation, assignment* (4th ed.). St. Louis, MO: Elsevier, p. 6.

Let us assume that you are working in a home health agency and you are planning the care for a patient with heart failure (HF). You have made your initial visit, assessing the patient and planning the outcomes that you and the team will work toward in the next 3 weeks. Your patient is taking diuretics, antihypertensives, heart medications, and potassium supplements, in addition to being on a restricted diet. She is frequently short of breath and requires an assistant three times per week for hygienic care. In addition to providing hygienic care, you would like that assistant to monitor the blood pressure and check the patient's weight on the days you are not making a visit and to notify you if the blood pressure is outside of the range of 120 to 150 systolic and 50 to 90 diastolic or if there is any weight fluctuation. Using the four C's listed, you can evaluate your communication.

You tell your assistant the following:

Mrs. Jones has a heart condition and high blood pressure that requires medication and constant monitoring. One of our goals is to help Mrs. Jones have a stable blood pressure in a range that is normal for her. On the days that you are visiting and giving the patient her bath, I would also like you to take her blood pressure. If it is outside the range of 120 to 150 systolic and 50 to 90 diastolic, I would like you to let me know. We may need to adjust her medication, change her diet, and call her physician or the HF clinic for different orders. I would also like you to check her weight and let me know about any changes of more than 2 pounds from her home health admission weight of 185, so let me know if she weighs 187 or more. This will help us determine if she is retaining fluid.

Clear: Does the home health aide understand what is being asked of her? This direction is fairly straightforward—an easily understood instruction of taking the blood pressure. Is it clear that the aide is to determine and report the patient's weight? Does she know when to take it and where to record it?

Concise: Have you confused the assistant by giving too much information? Or is it enough information for her to complete the task? Only the assistant can help you with this determination. You will need to ask directly, "Am I confusing you?" or "Do you have enough information to do the job?" Every individual has different needs. However, you will want to make certain to check this out; some people will not be honest or accurate in their assessments of their understanding or abilities, leading to trouble later. Many of us are reluctant to ask questions, being afraid to admit our need for additional information. (We do not want to look like we do not know what we are doing!) This reluctance can ultimately result in harm to the patient, because assumptions are made that the direction was understood when, in fact, it was not.

Correct: Is a home health aide able and allowed to monitor blood pressures? Where would you look for additional information if you were not sure? Is the location of the scale identified? Does the time of day of the visit make any difference?

Complete: Does the assistant have enough information to fulfill your expectations? Once again, you will need to ask the delegate for clarification of his or her understanding of what you are asking. If you also expect this assistant to note the respirations and alert you to increased effort of breathing, have you shared that in your initial direction? Or did you assume she would naturally observe all vital signs because you alerted her to the patient's condition (and besides, she is a good assistant)? In our attempts not to appear condescending (I do not want to insult this assistant by reminding her to note the respirations—she might think I do not trust her to think!), we may often choose not to be as complete as we should be in communicating initial direction. What about lost weight? Is that significant to report? Asking her to repeat her instructions and explain what she plans to do at this patient's home would be useful. Be sure that she is able to read and understand the written details that are often required reading for home health aides.

Another common pitfall is the rationale that comes from working with someone over a period of time. A working relationship develops, and a routine or pattern of performance is established. When this happens, we start talking less and less to the other individual, believing that "she knows what I expect her to do." Consider the following situation:

You are working in an acute care behavioral health unit in partnership with Sam, a mental health technician (MHT); you have been working with him for the past several years. Your easygoing style has led to a comfortable reliance on each other and the feeling that each knows what the other expects. On this particular evening shift, the house supervisor is sending a direct admit of a patient who is intermittently paranoid and delusional and has a diagnosis of bipolar with substance abuse issues; you both know this patient well because of his periodic readmissions. "Well Sam, it's the same tune, different day. Mr. Dawkins is being readmitted again from his residential care home. You know the drill. He'll be here soon." Evaluate your initial direction.

Did you believe that Sam "just knew" that you wanted him to check on the patient, make sure the patient was safe, get the first set of vital signs, and report the patient's status to you as soon as possible until you could see the patient yourself?

An hour later, you see Sam at the portable computer in the hallway. You ask him, "Sam, how's Mr. Dawkins doing?" Expecting a brief report, you are surprised when Sam says, "I don't know. Is he here? I thought we were going to assess him together when he got here, especially considering our new suicide and ligature prevention process. Did the charge RN tell you about his arrival and get him settled?" What went wrong?

No matter how long you have been working with someone, the right communication is essential to ensure the success of teamwork. Sam did not accept the delegated task because he did not understand what you meant, nor did he think it was an appropriate assignment. Be sure that you check the person's understanding of what you are saying by maintaining clear communication patterns. Failing to do this may result in unmet expectations, which lead to anger and frustration. More important, the patient will not receive the optimal care that both you and your associate want to provide. In this case, a patient with psychiatric problems could have been left alone during a crucial period.

We have discussed how to carefully assess the patient, determine your plan on the basis of outcomes, and select the **right task** to delegate to the right person. We have learned about how to provide clear initial direction as part of the **right communication**. The final **right of delegation** is also a part of supervision: the periodic inspection of the actual act.

THE RIGHT SUPERVISION AND EVALUATION

How Can I Give and Receive Feedback Effectively?

The NCSBN reminds us that nurse must monitor the work that she has delegated or assigned, discovering the quality of the task completion and the patient results. Proper documentation should also be accomplished (NCSBN, 2017b, p. 8). Follow-up is crucial to complete the process and to keep patients safe. However, many nurses have shared their discomfort with giving and receiving feedback from coworkers. Few of us enjoy hearing about how we may have missed the mark; however, when you are supervising others, it is absolutely necessary to share feedback during your "periodic inspection." By following a formula for giving and receiving feedback and practicing it daily, RNs are assisted in the difficult job of correcting the performance of others." The reciprocal feedback process also permits you, as supervising RN, to hear how your own supervisory performance and communication affected the outcomes of the team (Critical Thinking Box 14.6).

❓ CRITICAL THINKING BOX 14.6

Feedback Formula

- Ask for the other individual's input first!
- Give credit for effort.
- Share your perceptions with each other.
- Explore differing points of view, focusing on shared outcomes.
- Ask for the other individual's input to determine what steps may be necessary to make certain desired outcomes are achieved.
- Agree on a plan for the future, including timeline for follow-up.
- Revisit the plan and results achieved.

Modified from Hansten, R., & Jackson, M. (2009). *Clinical delegation skills: A handbook for nurses* (4th ed.). Sudbury, MA: Jones & Bartlett.

Let's look at how this process can be used in a situation in which positive feedback is intended.

An RN (Pat) is working with a float RN (Julia) for the first time. Julia is new in the pool but is an experienced nurse. Pat is so pleased with Julia's experience and performance that she has gone off to have a nice long break and lunch with an old friend from the third floor. She has also taken time to meet with a colleague from the evening shift regarding a unit problem. Unfortunately she has not been present on the unit much today. When Pat is having lunch with her friend, she exclaims, "That new float Julia is just excellent! If it weren't for her, I couldn't be here having lunch with you. I hope that she knows how organized and valuable she is!" Her friend Alex states, "Well, you know you should tell her, not just me, about this." When Pat returns to the floor, flushed with good intentions of making Julia's day with effusive praise, she tells Julia about how lucky she has been to work with her today.

Because all of us crave positive feedback, and Julia is new to your organization, will Julia tell Pat that she's been trying to find Pat for hours? Probably not. But she *may* tell others, "Pat is one of those 'dump and run' nurses. I don't want to work on that floor again!" What if Pat asked *first*, "How have things been going for you today, Julia? I know this is your first day on the unit." Julia may have determined that it was possible (and expected) to give reciprocal feedback: "I've been trying to find you! I have completed everything, but it hasn't been easy. Where have you been?" The best intentions can be frustrated by not asking the other individual for input first. If you plan to give some negative feedback to an individual, you will also have to ask for her or his input first. For example: You have just noted that the night shift CNA did not record the intakes and outputs (I&Os) on three patients on your telemetry unit. You have called him and are thinking about how to discuss this with him in a positive manner; yet you know that he is not going to want to chat because it is about time for him to get some rest.

If you said, "Why didn't you record the I&Os in the electronic medical record (EMR)?!" the CNA would probably react defensively. If you state, "How was your night? (Wait for an answer.) I don't see the I&Os in the EMR, do you remember where they were recorded?" you have allowed the person to respond with what happened. If this CNA went home early with the flu or the unit experienced three codes or left the data somewhere else, it would not be an effective or popular action for you to pounce on the team member for missing data entry.

The next step in the process is giving credit for what has been accomplished. At this point, Julia's input has been received. Pat can state, "Well, I can see I didn't help you as much as I should have, and I forgot to give you my phone number. But I do want you to know that I've checked on all of our patients, and they are very happy with their care today." After hearing input and giving credit where it is due, exploration of the gaps in the relationship and their communication and initial direction at the beginning of the shift can now be undertaken with an open and frank discussion.

The discussion of differences will progress most smoothly if both parties recognize that they share common objectives: safe, effective care of the patients on their unit as reflected in the fulfillment of shared, planned outcomes or goals determined by collaborative discussion among patients and care team members. When difficulties or conflicts occur, remember the reason you are both there: the patients.

Julia and Pat may clarify what happened and what actions each may take to ensure that the missed communication does not happen in the future. Do not try to "fix" the situation for the other individual or prescribe what you will do for them. The other individual will know what he or she needs to do to achieve your shared goals. For example, Pat may have decided that it would fix it for Julia to convene with her an hour before shift tomorrow and go through the unit manuals and read the procedures. However, the most Julia may need is a phone number and some more discussion and planning about assignments at the beginning of the shift.

This process may seem to take too much time, because "Why wait for the others to come up with ideas when we can solve the problem for them?" RNs who lead teams throughout the nation tell us that their lives at work would be much better if everyone were behaving accountably. When we ask others for their step-by-step plan to prevent the problem in the future, it helps them determine that they are accountable for their own performance. In our scene with the missing I&O data, the RN will ask, "How can you make sure those I&Os are recorded before you leave in the future? What will work for you?" This type of statement confers the necessary respect for the assistant's ability to determine how to adapt his work performance to conditions.

Do not miss the final steps in the formula if you would like the positive changes to become embedded. Teams must agree on how they will proceed in the future and when they will revisit the problem or issue. Julia may determine that she'll remind Pat in the future when she arrives at the unit that she will need Pat's phone number and a plan for the day. When the next shift is completed, they will want to compare notes about how the shift has proceeded and whether their goals have been achieved. The CNA may decide to ask the RN the following week whether she has noted any missing I&Os. The pair will be able to evaluate whether the CNA's charting plan has been effective and can proceed to celebrate the success of the plan or to try other interventions. Although this formula seems like it might take a long time, these steps are often covered in 2 to 3 minutes and will save you both time in the future by avoiding other problems.

Practice using the feedback formula. Remember the following three most important points:
- Ask for the other person's input first.
- Give credit for accomplishments and efforts.
- Ask the other individual to come up with steps for resolving the issue.

How would you use this formula to tell a supervisor that you are concerned about how long it has been since you have heard about your intershift transfer, and you are becoming worried about whether it will take place? How would you provide positive feedback to an individual on your team who has been improving his ability to complete his shift on time? What about the person who is "missing in action"—the person you cannot seem to locate when you need her?

CONCLUSION

Nurses sometimes wish for an exact prescription for what to delegate and assign as well as when and how. Because nursing assessment and professional judgment are necessary for clinical delegation, each situation will be different. Whether you work in an ICU in a large tertiary hospital, a rural long-term care facility, home health, or ambulatory care, the template of the delegation process—*in the right circumstances, matching the right task with the right delegate, communicating instructions effectively, supervising and evaluating care, and offering and receiving feedback*—will be similar. In this fast-paced digital and robotic age, we suspect your leadership at the point of care will include new types of care providers and new delivery models. You will need to hone your abilities to assign care tasks effectively—and to supervise the work that is being done under your direction and supervision—to help your patients and their families achieve their preferred outcomes. The health of your community will be affected by your team and your leadership. To judge your comfort and assess your ability to integrate this process in your daily work life, complete the exercise in Critical Thinking Box 14.7. Good luck!

❓ CRITICAL THINKING BOX 14.7

Assessing Your Delegation Skills

Assemble these documents:
- Your state nurse practice act (includes statute, administrative codes, rules, policies, and advisory opinions)
- State statute, rules, codes related to your assistive personnel team members' roles
- Your job description and those of coworkers and delegates
- Skills checklists
- The patient list or assignment form from your unit
- A list of the usual staffing complement for your shift

1. Using these documents, determine the short-term outcomes for an average patient assignment based on the information you have been given in a report. What tasks could be delegated to the individuals you have on staff? Are these tasks OK to delegate or assign? When will you complete further assessment of the patient situations?
2. Based on the outcomes and job descriptions, how will you determine the competency of individuals to complete the tasks you have determined could be delegated?
3. How will you communicate the team's plan using outcomes in your discussion?
4. How often will you communicate with the delegates, based on their need for supervision and patient complexity and dynamics? Have you used the four Cs?
5. How will you evaluate the effectiveness of your plan? How will you provide positive feedback to the team?
6. A delegate made a mistake. You determined that the person was competent but the procedure was done improperly. For what are you accountable? How will you give feedback to the individual, encouraging his or her growth and accountability?
7. Have you implemented the five rights of delegation?

🌐 RELEVANT WEBSITES AND ONLINE RESOURCES

Alfaro-Lefevre, R. Promoting critical thinking in frontline nurses
Retrieved from www.AlfaroTeachSmart.com.

American Nurses Association (ANA)
http://nursingworld.org/. See: Unlicensed Personnel, Registered Nurses Utilization of Nursing Assistive Personnel in All Settings, Registered Nurse Education Relating to the Utilization of Unlicensed Assistive Personnel, Joint Statement on Delegation.

Duffy, M., & McCoy, S. F. (2014)
Delegation and you: When to delegate and to whom. Silver Spring, MD: American Nurses Association. ANA You Series: Skills for Success.

Hansten, R. (2008)
Relationship and results oriented healthcare™ planning and implementation manual. Port Ludlow, WA: Hansten Healthcare PLLC. www.RROHC.com, www.Hansten.com. Check for new delegation/supervision resources.

Hansten, R. (2014)
The master coach manual for the relationship & results oriented healthcare program. Port Ludlow, WA: Hansten Healthcare PLLC.

Hansten, R., & Jackson, M. (2009)
Clinical delegation skills: A handbook for professional practice (4th ed.). Sudbury, MA: Jones & Bartlett.

Continued

⊕ **RELEVANT WEBSITES AND ONLINE RESOURCES—CONT'D**

National Council of State Boards of Nursing

http://www.ncsbn.org, links to state boards and resources relating to delegation and supervision. Also download the ANA and NCSBN Joint Statement on Delegation.

Nursing Webinar Education for Delegation and Assignment: 3 part series

http://nursing.freecelms.education/by/ms-ruth-hansten-bsn-phd-mba-rn-fache

https://nurse.freecelms.education/by/ms-ruth-hansten-bsn-phd-mba-rn-fache/165678/leadership-at-the-point-of-care-part-1-delegation-supervision-and-teamwork

https://nurse.freecelms.education/by/ms-ruth-hansten-bsn-phd-mba-rn-fache/ms-ruth-hansten-bsn-phd-mba-rn-fache/165677/leadership-at-the-point-of-care-part-2-blueprint-for-successful-clinical-supervision-and-teamwork

https://nurse.freecelms.education/by/ms-ruth-hansten-bsn-phd-mba-rn-fache/ms-ruth-hansten-bsn-phd-mba-rn-fache/165676/leadership-at-the-point-of-care-part-3-effective-assignments-for-rns-and-assistive-personnel-acute-care

Website Resources

Books by Ruth Hansten Amazon Site: http://www.amazon.com/Ruth-l.-Hansten/e/B001IR3H1S

www.Hansten.com

www.RROHC.com

BIBLIOGRAPHY

Agency for Healthcare Research and Quality. (2018, June 5). *Decline in hospital-acquired conditions save 8,000 lives and $2.9 billion in acquired costs. In Retrieved from* https://www.ahrq.gov/news/newsroom/press-releases/declines-in-hacs.html.

Alfaro-LeFevre. (2019). *Critical thinking, clinical reasoning, and clinical judgment* (7th ed.). Philadelphia, PA: Elsevier Inc.

American Nurses Association. (2012). *ANA's principles for delegation by registered nurses to unlicensed assistive personnel.* Silver Spring, MD: ANA. Retrieved from http://www.nursingworld.org/MainMenuCategories/ThePracticeofProfessionalNursing/NursingStandards/ANAPrinciples/PrinciplesofDelegation.pdf.

American Nurses Association. (2015). *Code of ethics for nurses with interpretative statements.* Retrieved from http://www.nursingworld.org/MainMenuCategories/EthicsStandards/Tools-You-Need/Code-of-Ethics-For-Nurses.html.

Bittner, N., & Gravlin, G. (2009). Critical thinking, delegation, and missed care in nursing practice. *Journal of Orthopedic Nursing Association, 39*(3), 142–146.

Bittner, N., Gravlin, G., Hansten, R., & Kalisch, B. (2011). Unraveling care omissions. *Journal of Nursing Administration, 41*(12), 510–512.

Bobay, K., Fiorelli, K., & Anderson, A. (2008). Failure to rescue: A preliminary study of patient-level factors. *Journal of Nursing Care Quality, 23*(3), 211–215.

Brous, E. (2012). Professional licensure: Investigation and disciplinary action. *American Journal of Nursing, 112*(11), 53–60.

Garneau, A. M. (2012). The effect of human patient simulation on delegation performance among associate degree nursing students. (Doctoral dissertation). Retrieved from Proquest Dissertations and Theses. (Order Accession No: 3502633).

Gravlin, G., & Bittner, N. (2010). Nurses' and nursing assistants' reports of missed care and delegation. *Journal of Nursing Administration, 40*(7–8), 329–335.

Hansten, R. (2005). Relationship and results oriented healthcare: Evaluate the basics. *Journal of Nursing Administration, 35*(12), 522–525.

Hansten, R. (2008a). *Relationship & results oriented healthcare planning & implementation manual.* Port Ludlow, WA: Hansten Healthcare PLLC.

Hansten, R. (2008b). Why nurses still must learn to delegate. *AONE Nursing Leadership, 6*(5), 19–25.

Hansten, R. (2009). A bundle of best bedside practices. *Health Care Management, 28*(2), 111–116.

Hansten, R. (2014a). Coach as chief correlator of tasks to results through delegation skill and teamwork development, August/September. *Nurse Leader, 12*(4), 69–73.

Hansten, R. (2014b). *The master coach manual for the relationship & results oriented healthcare program.* Port Ludlow, WA: Hansten Healthcare PLLC.

Hansten, R., & Jackson, M. (2009). *Clinical delegation skills: A handbook for professional practice* (4th ed.). Sudbury, MA: Jones & Bartlett.

Hansten, R., Washburn, M., & Kenyon, V. (1999). *Home care nursing delegation skills: A handbook for practice.* Gaithersburg, MD: Aspen.

Institute of Medicine of the National Academies. (2013). In Mark Smith, Robert Saunders, Leigh Stuckhardt, & Michael McGinnism (Eds.), *Best care at lower cost: The path to continuously learning health care in America* (pp. 2–3). Washington, DC: The National Academies Press.

Institute of Medicine Report on the Future of Nursing. (2010). Retrieved from http://www.nationalacademies. org/hmd/~/media/Files/Report%20Files/2010/The-Future-of-Nursing/Nursing%20Education%202010% 20Brief.pdf.

Institute of Medicine. (2000). *To err is human: Building a safer health system.* Retrieved from http://www. nationalacademies.org/hmd/~/media/Files/Report%20Files/1999/To-Err-is-Human/To%20Err%20is% 20Human%201999%20%20report%20brief.pdf.

Kalisch, B. (2015). *Errors of omission: How missed nursing care imperils patients.* Silver Spring, MD: American Nurses Association.

Kalisch, B., & Schoville, R. (2012). It takes a team. *American Journal of Nursing, 112*(10), 50–54. https://doi.org/ 10.1097/01.NAJ.0000421024.08037.0d.

Kalisch, B., Landstrom, G., & Williams, R. (2009). Missed care: Errors of omission. *Nursing Outlook, 57,* 3–9.

Kalisch, B., Tschannen, D., & Hee Lee, K. (2011). Do staffing levels predict missed nursing care? *International Journal of Quality Health Care, 23*(3), 302–308. https://doi.org/10.1093/intqhc/mzr009.

Laws, L., & Hughes, C. (2018, April). Errors of omission in nursing care and its impact on patient care. *Texas Board of Nursing Bulletin, 49*(2), 4–5.

Mole, L. J., & McLafferty, I. H. (2004). Evaluating a simulated ward exercise for third year student nurses. *Nurse Education in Practice, 4*(2), 91–99. https://doi.org/10.1016/S1471–5953(03)00031-3 2004.

Mushta, J., Rush, K., & Andersen, E. (2017). Failure to rescue as a nurse sensitive indicator. *Nursing Forum, 53,* 84–92. https://doi.org/10.1111/n7f.122215.

National Council of State Boards of Nursing (NCSBN). (1990). *Concept paper on delegation.* Chicago, IL: NCSBN.

National Council of State Boards of Nursing (NCSBN). (1995). *Concepts and decision-making process. 1995 Annual Meeting Business Book.* Chicago, IL: NCSBN.

National Council of State Boards of Nursing (NCSBN). (2005). *Practical nurse scope of practice white paper.* Retrieved from https://www.ncsbn.org/Final_11_05_Practical_Nurse_Scope_Practice_White_Paper.pdf.

National Council of State Boards of Nursing (NCSBN). (2006). *Joint statement on delegation.* American Nurses Association (ANA) and the National Council of State Boards of Nursing (NCSBN). Retrieved from https:// www.nursingworld.org/practice-policy/nursing-excellence/official-position-statements/id/joint-statement-on-delegation-by-ANA-and-NCSBN/.

National Council of State Boards of Nursing. (2012). *NCSBN Model Act.* Chicago, IL: NCSBN.

National Council of State Boards of Nursing. (2016a). National guidelines for nursing delegation. *Journal of Nursing Regulation, 7*(1), 5–11. Retrieved from https://www.ncsbn.org/NCSBN_Delegation_Guidelines.pdf.

National Council State Boards of Nursing. (2016b). *2017 NCLEX-PN*®. *Test Plan.* Retrieved from https:// www.ncsbn.org/2017_PN_TestPlan.pdf.

National Council of State Boards of Nursing. (NCSBN) (2017a). *NCSBN Model Rules* (Updated from 2012). Chicago, IL: NCSBN. Retrieved from https://www.ncsbn.org/17_Model_Rules_0917.pdf.

National Council of State Boards of Nursing. (2017b). The 2017 environmental scan. *Journal of Nursing Regulation, 7*(4). Supplement, S1-S36. Retrieved from https://www.ncsbn.org/2017_Environmental_Scan.pdf.

National Council State Boards of Nursing. (2019a). *2019 NCLEX-RN® Test Plan.* Retrieved from https://www.ncsbn.org/2019_RN_TestPlan-English.pdf.

National Council of State Boards of Nursing. (2019b). *Nurse licensure compact (NLC).* Retrieved from https://www.ncsbn.org/compacts.htm.

Nhongo, D., Hendricks, J., Bradshaw, J., & Bail, K. (2018). Leadership and registered nurses (RNs) working after-hours in residential aged care facilities (RACFs): A structured online literature review. *Journal of Clinical Nursing.* https://doi.org/10.1111/jocn.14565.

Samuel, M. (2006). *Creating the accountable organization.* Katonah, NY: Xephor Press.

Scruth, E., & Pugh, D. (2018). Omission of nursing care: An international perspective. *Clinical Nurse Specialist, 32*(4), 172–174. https://doi.org/10.1097/NUR.0000000000000380.

Sheehan, J. P. (2001). UAP delegation: A step-by-step process. *Nursing Management, 32*(4), 22–24.

The Joint Commission. (2017). *Sentinel event alert: Inadequate hand-off communication.* Retrieved from https://www.jointcommission.org/assets/1/18/SEA_58_Hand_off_Comms_9_6_17_FINAL_(1).pdf.

Zhong, E. H. (2016). *NCSBN TERCAP Update: Analysis of 4,000 Cases of Practice Breakdown.* Retrieved from https://www.ncsbn.org/2016_TERCAP_PPT_BOD1130V2.pdf.

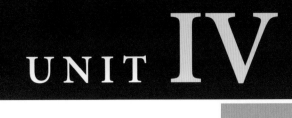

UNIT IV

Current Issues in Health Care

343

15

The Health Care Organization and Patterns of Nursing Care Delivery

Susan Sportsman, PhD, RN, ANEF, FAAN

ⓔhttp://evolve.elsevier.com/Zerwekh/nsgtoday/.

"The very essence of all good organization is that everybody should do her (or his) own work in such a way as to help and not hinder everyone else's work."

Florence Nightingale in her 1872 address to the nurses and students at St. Thomas Hospital. (Ulrich, 1992)

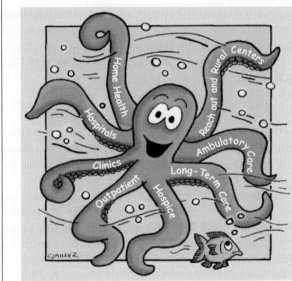

Health care should be within reach of everyone.

After completing this chapter, you should be able to:

- Describe challenges facing health care that affect the delivery of nursing care, including:
  - Changes to the Affordable Care Act since 2016
  - Reduction of health care costs
  - Evidence-based care
  - Shortage of health care professionals
  - Patient safety
  - Nurse staffing
- You should also be able to trace the history of the use of nursing care delivery models.
- Consider ways in which to structure nursing services to improve care while reducing costs in order to ensure that health care is within the reach of everyone.

The US health care delivery system has been changing dramatically over the past 40 years. Economic changes around the world and the passage of the Affordable Care Act of 2010, as well as the resulting political responses, focused the country's attention on the need to revise the US health care system to improve access and quality while reducing delivery costs. However, the results of the US national election in 2016 changed the dialogue around strategies to improve health care delivery. Nurses practicing in such an environment, regardless of their political leanings, must be comfortable with change and be willing to embrace the challenges that change brings.

345

A first step to ensuring that your nursing practice evolves in a positive direction is to be knowledgeable about current and potential future changes.

WHAT ARE SOME IMPORTANT CHALLENGES CURRENTLY FACING HEALTH CARE?

Cost of Health Care

High health care expenditures in the United States have long been a national problem. Total health spending is a function of both price paid to providers or for drugs and the volume of services used. These costs are measured by the percentage of health care costs relative to the gross national product (GNP). To illustrate the rise in the percentage of the cost of health care, in 1960, health care costs in the United States were 5% of the gross domestic product (GDP). In 2000, they were 13.3% (Sahadi, 2018). The costs of most health care services and prescription drugs are higher in the United States than in comparable countries. In contrast, the cost of using some services, including physician consultations and hospital stays, is lower than in other countries. However, the use of other services, such as C-sections and knee replacements, are higher than in other countries. Despite having fewer office visits and shorter average hospital stays, the United States overall spends twice as much per person on health care than do comparable countries (Kamal & Cox, 2018).

The continued growth in the cost of health care is a result of the greater use of prescription drugs and new medical technologies as well as higher administrative costs. The rise in the incidence of chronic disease, which accounts for a large portion of national health care expenditures, is also a major factor. For the past 30 years, various strategies have been instituted to halt this escalation in costs. One of the major approaches to reducing costs was **managed care**.

Managed Care

In the early 1900s, patients or their families paid the physician or the hospital directly for the care they received. As health care insurance became an employment benefit after the Second World War, third-party payers became more common. These third-party payers paid the provider an agreed-on fee for each service provided. The more the provider charged, the more the payer paid.

In the early 1980s, Medicare introduced the prospective payment system as a way of reimbursing hospitals. This marked the beginning of a movement to control health care costs. Under this system, which insurance companies soon adopted, a fixed fee was paid to the hospital according to a preset reimbursement rate for the diagnosis given at discharge. A hospital could treat a patient so that a shorter length of stay was necessary, thus reducing the consumption of resources. This allowed the hospital to show a greater profit or lower loss for caring for a patient if the care was more efficient than was the prearranged rate for the diagnosis. This practice began the trend of managed care in which health care is paid at a prearranged rate rather than as billed.

In the most extreme type of managed care, called *capitation*, employers pay a set fee each month to an insurance company for each covered employee and dependent. This amount does not vary based on the care given. Potential patients may never need any health care or they may require extensive hospitalizations. Regardless, the costs of care for all members of a particular employment group must be taken out of the set fee. Under this arrangement, there is incentive for the insurance company and the provider to work aggressively to keep patients healthy, because prevention or early intervention is likely to be less expensive than hospitalization. Conversely, if patients do not stay healthy or if they overuse hospitalization, the health care provider may actually lose money.

As a part of the managed care trend, health maintenance organization (HMO) plans became very popular as a form of insurance. In HMOs, an annual payment is made on behalf of the members to a group of providers who deliver all of the health services covered under the plan, including physician and hospital services. HMOs have grown because they provide a strong incentive to avoid hospitalization, which consequently reduces costs. HMO members often appreciate the ease of using health care with an HMO because there are fewer noncovered services and fewer forms to complete. However, the choice of providers is limited; members must use physicians who are part of the HMO network, and they may not see specialty physicians without a referral from their primary care provider.

The preferred provider organization (PPO) is another type of insurance plan designed to meet the goals of managed care. To avoid out-of-pocket expenses, members must use physicians who have agreed to provide services at a lower price to the insurer. However, members may use an "out-of-network" provider without a referral if they are willing to pay more for that service.

What Impact Has Managed Care Had on Costs?

Initially, managed care reduced the cost of health care. However, costs subsequently increased sharply in response to the backlash from restrictive managed care policies. Given the complexity of the issues surrounding the costs of health care, it is very difficult to say conclusively that managed care is effective, in part because the definition of "effective" may vary. Effectiveness can be measured by profit and loss, quality of care, and/or access to services. Improvement in one of these factors does not necessarily mean improvement in others. In addition, there are a number of stakeholders who must judge the effectiveness of care in any given situation, including the managed care organization, the employer, the Centers for Medicare and Medicaid Services (CMS), regulators, and providers, as well as individual patients, their significant others, and society as a whole. Since these groups often have different needs and agendas, one definition of *effective* is difficult to agree on.

AFFORDABLE CARE ACT

On March 23, 2010, Congress passed the Patient Protection and Affordable Care Act (ACA), which provided regulations to reduce health care costs as well as to improve access to care. On June 28, 2013, the US Supreme Court rendered a final decision to uphold this health care law. The goals of the ACA were to do the following:

- Make affordable health insurance available to people with family incomes between 100% and 400% of the federal poverty level (2017 FPL= $24,600) for a family of four
- Expand the Medicaid Program to cover all adults with income below 138% of the federal poverty level
- Support innovative medical care delivery methods designed to lower the cost of health care generally (HealthCare.gov, 2018b)

The ACA identified essential services that insurance companies must cover, including the following: ambulatory and emergency care; hospitalizations (surgery and overnight stays); pregnancy, maternity, and newborn care; mental health and substance use disorder treatment; prescription drugs; and birth control. Rehabilitative and habilitative services and devices, lab services, preventive and wellness services, chronic disease management, pediatric dental services, and breast feeding assistance were also included (HealthCare.gov, 2018b). These regulations expanded the availability of services required as a part of all insurance coverage.

In order to make insurance coverage under the ACA more affordable for individuals, the law required tax credits for eligible citizens. This refundable credit helped individuals and families cover the premiums for health insurance purchased through the federal or state health insurance marketplace. To qualify for this tax credit, taxpayers (1) had to indicate that they could not afford coverage through their employer; (2) could not be eligible for Medicaid, Medicare, CHIP, or Tricare; and (3) had to pay their share of the costs not covered by insurance (Internal Review Service [IRS], 2018).

For any health care insurance to be economically feasible, there must be sufficient numbers of healthy persons covered in order to support the reimbursement of care for those who require a great deal of care. In order to provide for this economic reality, the ACA requires individuals to buy insurance or pay a penalty at tax time unless they qualified for a limited number of exemptions.

The 2010 ACA regulations also included regulations to expand Medicaid coverage. In 2014, those under 65 years of age with incomes up to 133% of the federal poverty level, including individuals without children, were eligible for Medicaid. In addition, the State Children Health Insurance Plan (S-CHIP) was made simpler to access. Other requirements of the law included (1) free preventive benefits, such as wellness visits and cholesterol checks; (2) closing the prescription drug "donut hole" coverage gap; (3) investing more resources in efforts to fight health care fraud; and (4) tying payment to quality standards, investing in patient safety, and offering new incentives for providers who delivered high-quality care (HealthCare.gov, 2018a).

The ACA regulations let young adults stay on their parents' plan until age 26, a very popular regulation for many people of all political persuasions. In addition, insurance companies were no longer able to deny coverage, charge more based on health status, or drop coverage when the insured was sick. This meant that there were no more limitations of preexisting conditions. The policies could not discriminate based on gender or impose unjustified rate hikes or lifetime and annual dollar limits. The law also requires a rapid appeal of insurance company decisions. These regulations were to be fully funded by the federal government from 2014 to 2019. In 2019, the federal funding is to be dropped to 90% of the funding. States had the opportunity to opt out of this expansion; 19 states took this option. Most of these states were concerned about having to pick up the 10% of the cost after 2019 (HealthCare.gov, 2018a). The complete provisions of the law were to be implemented over a 5-year period.

In the intervening years since the implementation of the ACA, there have been some published evaluations to provide an understanding of the effectiveness of this legislation. That is, have these statistics changed as a result of the implementation of the ACA? In fact, the most measurable effects of the ACA have been the availability of health insurance to those who previously had no insurance and were often unable to access care. In January 2017, *Politifact* reported that roughly 28 million Americans were **uninsured,** down from 41.3 million in 2013, primarily because of the (1) expansion of Medicaid, (2) creation of online health insurance marketplaces, (3) ability of young people to stay on their parents' coverage through age 27, and (4) mandates of the law that require everyone to purchase a health insurance plan (Jacobson, 2017).

Unfortunately, the cost of health care in the United States has continued to rise since the implementation of the ACA. According to the Centers for Medicare and Medicaid Services (CMS, 2017), health care cost rose to 17.9% of GDP in 2016. CMS (2017) predicts that the health care share of the GDP will rise to 19.9% by 2025.

STRATEGIES TO CONTROL COSTS

In 2016, hospital care accounted for the largest share (32%) of health care expenditures; physician services were second, accounting for 20%. "Other spending"—including dental and other professional services, home health care, durable and nondurable medical equipment and products, government public health activities, and investments—accounted for 20%, and prescription drugs accounted for 10% (CDC, 2016). The reduction of costs in these areas would have the greatest impact on the reduction of total costs. Specific efforts to reduce hospital costs that affect the delivery of nursing care include case management, evidence-based practice (EBP), appropriate staffing, improving retention of staff, use of the electronic health record (EHR), and the reduction of patient care errors.

VALUE-BASED CARE, PAY FOR PERFORMANCE, AND ACCOUNTABLE CARE ORGANZATIONS

What Is Value-Based Care?

Value-based health care is a delivery model in which reimbursement to providers—such as hospitals, physicians, and other providers—is based on patient outcomes. In short, by using an evidence-based approach, providers are rewarded financially for helping patients to improve their health and thus to reduce chronic disease. This approach encourages patient safety and quality improvement through the elimination or reduction adverse events, adoption of evidence-based care standards, improved protocols, changes in hospital processes to create better patient care experiences and increasing care transparency for consumers. It is seen as the best method for lowering health care costs while also increasing quality, although moving from a fee-for-service to a fee-for-value system is difficult and will take time (NEJM Catalyst, 2017b).

What Is Pay for Performance?

Pay for performance (P4P), a value-based health care approach, is increasingly being used to reduce costs and improve the quality of health care. Although traditional fee-for-service reimbursement still represents a large percentage of income for hospitals, the shift toward payment for value-based health care programs is accelerating rapidly. In P4P programs, hospitals are required to address a large number of factors that they previously, in traditional fee-for-service systems, had no incentive to consider. Two basic types of P4P designs are used in hospital reimbursement. With the first, payers lower the fee-for-service payments and instead use funds to reward hospitals based on how well they perform across process, quality, and efficiency measures. In the second, hospitals are penalized financially for poor-quality performance (NEJM Catalyst, 2018).

Stimulated by the passage of the ACA, the CMS is leading the way in value-based care with a variety of P4P payment models. As the largest funder of health care at almost 40% of overall spending, CMS has developed various P4P models, including three programs that affect hospital reimbursement through Medicare (Medicare.gov, n.d.).

The first approach focuses on a pool of funds obtained by reducing all Medicare payments to acute-care hospitals by 2%. These funds are then redistributed to the hospitals based on their performance on measures related to (1) safety, (2) clinical care, (3) efficiency and cost reduction, and (4) patient- and caregiver-centered experience. Hospitals are scored on the various measures and their scores are compared over time with their own scores and the scores of other hospitals. CMS uses the higher of the two scores to determine financial awards (NEJM Catalyst, 2018).

In the second approach, hospitals are penalized if they had higher rates of readmissions compared with peer institutions. The program was established by the ACA and applies to specific episodes of care such as heart attack, heart failure, pneumonia, chronic obstructive pulmonary disease (COPD), hip or knee replacement, or coronary bypass surgery. Currently hospitals with poor performance in relation to other hospitals must accept up to a 3% reduction of their Medicare payments (NEJM Catalyst, 2018).

The third approach reduces payments by 1% to hospitals in the bottom quartile of performance based on risk-adjusted measures of hospital-acquired conditions, such as surgical site infections, hip fractures resulting from falls, or pressure sores. This reduction in payments to hospitals saves

TABLE 15.1 THE POSITIVE AND NEGATIVE ASPECTS OF PAY FOR PERFORMANCE

POSITIVE ASPECTS	NEGATIVE ASPECTS
Reduces costs	May harm and reduces access for socioeconomically disadvantaged population because they perform poorly on P4P surveys
Decreases bad outcomes	Lowered job satisfaction for providers
Stresses quality over quantity of care	Incentives to "game" the system
Encourages payers to redirect funds to encourage best practices and promote positive outcomes	Costly to implement and verify measurement systems
Transparency through the use of metrics	P4P processes may not always support individual care
Encourages accountability and competition	Difficult to accurately attribute performance outcomes given that patients receive care from multiple providers
Uses existing fee-for-service payment system to allow an incremental transition to value-based care	

P4P, Pay for Performance.
NEJM Catalyst. (2018). What is pay for performance healthcare? Retrieved from https://catalyst.nejm.org/pay-for-performance-in-healthcare/.

Medicare approximately $350 million per year and is based on six measures of patient safety and health care–acquired infections. Individual payers are also developing P4P processes. Table 15.1 outlines the positive and negative aspects of P4P.

What Are Accountable Care Organizations?

Accountable care organizations (ACOs) provide a pathway away from fee-for-service medicine and represent one of the first efforts to make value-based care a reality. ACOs are groups of doctors, hospitals, and other health care providers who come together voluntarily to give coordinated, high-quality care to the Medicare patients they serve. Coordinated care helps to ensure that patients, especially the chronically ill, get the right care at the right time, with the goal of avoiding unnecessary duplication of services and preventing medical errors. When an ACO succeeds in both delivering high-quality care and spending health care dollars more wisely, it shares in the savings it achieves for the Medicare program. Many providers view participating in an ACO as an opportunity to deliver better care in a coordinated fashion while also focusing on patient outcomes instead of processes (CMS, 2018a). Table 15.2 outlines the benefits and drawbacks of ACOs.

CASE MANAGEMENT

One of the defining characteristics of ACOs is coordination of care. This is not a new goal for health care; however, it is often difficult to achieve in the complex health care system. The Case Management Society of America (CMSA) notes that case (or care) managers are advocates who help patients understand their current health status, what they can do about it, and why those treatments are important. In this way, case managers guide patients through the health care delivery process and provide cohesion to other professionals on the health care delivery team. The purpose of case managers is to enable their clients to achieve goals effectively and efficiently. This role may take a variety of forms but generally includes coordination of care, communication, collaboration, and attention to the transition between levels of nursing care. Social workers and therapists may also be case managers, although how they perform their roles depends on the scope of practice within their discipline. All case managers must

TABLE 15.2 BENEFITS AND BARRIERS TO ACCOUNTABLE CARE ORGANIZATIONS

ADVANTAGES/DISADVANTAGES	EXAMPLES
Benefits	Improved population health
	Improved quality of patient care
	A focus on patients
	Physician leadership
	Reduced costs
	Shared savings
Barriers and drawbacks	Legal and regulatory barriers
	Anticipation of losing autonomy
	Population base is not large enough
	Inadequate capital for improvements in information technology
	Payment structure/financing

Adapted from Ortiz, J., Bushy, A., Zhou, Y., & Zhang, H. (2013). Accountable care organizations: Benefits and barriers as perceived by rural health clinic management. *Rural Remote Health, 13*(2), 2417. Retrieved from https://www.ncbi.nlm.nih.gov/pmc/articles/PMC3761377/.

be skilled at communication, critical thinking, negotiation, and collaboration. They must be knowledgeable about the resources available to patients. The case manager collaborates not only with individual patients but also with family and other of the patient's support systems.

Case management is effective in providing care, but all patients do not need this intensity of interaction. To provide case management services to all patients would be wastefully expensive. Patients should be assigned a case manager only if they

- Have complicated health care needs
- Are receiving care that is expensive as well as complicated
- Pose discharge planning problems
- Receive care from multiple providers
- Are likely to have significant physical or psychosocial problems

Case management may also be implemented in levels of care other than acute care hospitals, particularly in some outpatient and short-term rehabilitative settings. In many ways the roles and responsibilities of the case manager are the same regardless of the level of care at which they work. The differences in the emphasis of the role are often influenced by reimbursement.

Nurse Navigator Programs

Nurse navigator programs are a form of case management that is beginning to be more widely used to coordinate patient care. In 1990, Dr. Harold Freeman developed the first nurse navigator role at Harlem Hospital in New York in an effort to expedite diagnosis and treatment while also facilitating access to care for patients with abnormal breast screening results (Pedersen & Hack, 2010). Since that time nurse navigators have been used in a variety of settings.

In 2005, the Patient Navigator Outreach and Chronic Disease Prevention Act authorized federal grants to hire and train patient navigators; their role would be to help patients with cancer and other serious chronic diseases receive access to screening, diagnosis, treatment, and follow-up care. In 2006, the CMS funded six demonstration projects to help minority Medicare patients overcome barriers to screening, diagnosis, and treatment; in 2007, $2.9 million was allocated to this program (Wells et al.,

2008). To emphasize the growth of this role in cancer care, in 2013, the Oncology Nursing Society (ONS) published the *Oncology Nurse Navigator Core Competencies*, addressing the professional role, education, coordination of care, and communication of the nurse navigator (ONS, 2013).

Although a large number of nurse navigator programs target care of the cancer patient, there is also an opportunity to implement this role in caring for other chronic diseases (Case, 2011). For example, publications show that health care facilities carry out nurse navigator programs for conditions such as high-risk obstetric care, osteoarthritis, HIV (Horstmann et al., 2010), and asthma (Black et al., 2010).

The navigator role was conceived to reduce barriers to care faced by vulnerable patients who may be coping with delays in access, diagnosis, and treatment and/or with fragmented and uncoordinated care. An analysis of evaluations of nurse navigator programs from 2000 to 2010 identified improved patient satisfaction, positive changes in patients' attitudes and understanding of disease processes, and patients' perceptions of a timelier and more accessible treatment process (Case, 2011).

DISEASE MANAGEMENT

Disease management refers to multidisciplinary efforts to improve the quality and cost of care for patients suffering from chronic diseases. It involves interventions designed to improve adherence to appropriate scientific guidelines and treatments. The goal is similar to that of case management—to support patients with chronic diseases who may receive services from various levels of care (acute care to home-based care). However, it is a population health strategy as well as an approach to personal health.

Disease management programs are designed to target individuals with specific costly, chronic conditions such as asthma, diabetes, heart failure, coronary heart disease, end-stage renal disease, depression, high-risk pregnancy, hypertension, and arthritis. Disease management programs usually involve an interprofessional team, including physicians, nurses, pharmacists, dieticians, respiratory therapists, and psychologists. The goal of these programs is to educate individuals to manage and control their condition as a means of receiving better care thus leading to better outcomes and reduced costs. Counseling, home visits, 24-hour call centers, and appointment reminder systems can be used to support patients responsible for their chronic conditions (HPI, 2004). Although disease management shows considerable promise, significant additional attention is needed in testing and demonstrating best practices and sharing information on successful components across a variety of care settings.

Do Disease Management Programs Reduce the Cost of Health Care?

Disease management programs have been developed and implemented largely by managed health care plans. Almost all health care plans have implemented at least one type of disease management program, and many have multiple programs. The most common disease processes targeted include diabetes, asthma, and heart failure.

There is some evidence that these programs do reduce the expenditures for particular diseases. However, it is still unclear if disease management programs have the potential for long-term savings. This may be because studies that found substantial cost savings were usually of short duration and based on the experiences of a single plan or restricted to certain areas of the country. Disease management programs are still relatively new, and it is too early to determine whether they are cost-effective on a long-term basis (HPI, 2004).

What Tools Are Used to Support Care Coordination?

Clinical pathways and **disease management protocols** are similar strategies that support the work of the coordinator of care to reduce expensive variations in care.

> Clinical pathways, also known as *care maps*, are multidisciplinary plans of "best" clinical practice for groups of patients with a specific medical diagnosis.

These pathways support the coordination and delivery of high-quality care. A clinical pathway has the following four essential elements:

- A time line outlining when specific care will be given
- A statement of the categories of care or activities and their interventions
- A list of the intermediate- and long-term outcomes to be achieved
- A variance record

The variance record allows caregivers to document when and why the progress of individual patients varies from that outlined in the pathway. Clinical pathways differ from practice guidelines, protocols, and algorithms because they are used by the interprofessional disciplinary team and focus on the quality and coordination of care for individual patients. A sample of a clinical pathway can be found in the Evolve resources.

Clinical Guidelines

Both critical pathways and disease management protocols are generally based on clinical guidelines that incorporate nationally acceptable ways to care for a specific disease. These guidelines are typically developed by government agencies such as the Agency for Health Care Research and Quality (AHRQ, 2018a) or an organization devoted to health promotion and disease prevention, such as the American Public Health Association and the Centers for Disease Control and Prevention.

EVIDENCE-BASED PRACTICE

How Do We Know That Critical Pathways and Disease Management Protocols Reflect the Latest and Best Practice?

In 2000, the Institute of Medicine (IOM) released a landmark report titled "Crossing the Quality Chasm: A New Health System for the 21st Century" (IOM, 2000). It noted that it takes 17 years for findings of research in health care to be implemented consistently in practice.

> Evidence-based practice is one strategy to reduce the length of time required to integrate new health care findings into practice.

EBP is the use of the current best evidence to make decisions about patient care. It is intended to offer guidance as to the best way to deal with particular situations and, as an approach to clinical practice, it has been gaining ground since its formal introduction in 1992. Starting in medicine, it then spread to other fields, such as nursing, psychology, and education. Currently 55% of all nursing practice areas are estimated to be based on research findings. The ANA predicts that by 2020, some 90% of all nursing practice will be based on EBP research findings (Chrisman, Jordon, Davis, & Williams, 2014, p. 8).

There are some barriers to the effective use of EBP. Majid et al. (2011) found that more than 64% of the nurses they surveyed expressed a positive attitude toward EBP. However, the respondents indicated that heavy workloads often prevented them from keeping up with new evidence. The responding nurses also felt that EBP training, time availability, and mentoring by nurses with EBP experience would encourage them to implement EBP.

There are a number of evidence-based nursing centers around the world that provide the best available evidence to inform clinical decision making at the point of care. One of the largest is the Joanna Briggs Institute (JBI), an international not-for-profit research and development arm of the School of

Translational Science based within the Faculty of Health Sciences at the University of Adelaide, South Australia. It collaborates internationally with more than 70 entities across the world (http://joannabriggs.org/) (Critical Thinking Box 15.1). See Chapter 24 for more information on how EBP is utilized by nurses to provide safe patient care. Relevant websites and online resources are listed at the end of this chapter.

> **? CRITICAL THINKING BOX 15.1**
>
> What are the advantages of using evidence-based nursing care? What are the barriers? How might these barriers be overcome?

SHORTAGE OF NURSES

According to a 2018 ANA website, there will be more registered nurse (RN) jobs available through 2022 than in any other profession in the United States. The US Bureau of Labor Statistics (2018) projects that 1.1 million additional nurses will be needed to avoid a further shortage. Employment opportunities for nurses are projected to grow at a faster rate (15%) than in all other occupations from 2016 through 2026 (ANA, 2018c; US Bureau of Labor Statistics, 2018). This ongoing shortage of nurses is driven by the aging of the population, including currently practicing nurses, and work conditions in health care. This potential shortage is likely to continue to affect the cost and quality of health care provided in the United States for the foreseeable future.

How Can Health Care Organizations Retain Nurses?

Retention of nurses in their place of employment is as important as recruitment in suppling enough nurses to meet the demand.

To combat the need for staff to change jobs frequently, administrators and managers often emphasize attractive compensation packages, focusing on a culture of training that includes mentoring and constructive positive feedback as well recognition for excellence. Offering a variety of scheduling options to meet the needs of a variety of ages is also a popular retention strategy.

Currently there is particular interest in providing support for novice nurses in their first jobs. In *The Future of Nursing: Leading Change, Advancing Health*, a 2010 report from the IOM, a specific recommendation was that nurses should have the benefit of a residency program at the start of their careers and during career transitions. Bleich (2012) notes that the need for a residency program does not reflect failure on the part of nursing schools but rather the complexity of nursing. A detailed discussion on nurse residency programs can be found in Chapter 3.

The work environment is another critical component of maintaining a robust workforce, regardless of how long staff has been employed. One of the strategies to promote a positive workforce is for hospitals to aim for magnet status.

Magnet Hospitals

Recognition of the characteristics that influence a positive work environment on nurse retention is not new. In the early 1980s, during a previous nursing shortage, the American Academy of Nursing conducted research to identify the organizational attributes of hospitals that experienced success in recruiting and retaining nurses. The American Academy of Nursing Fellows nominated 165 hospitals throughout the nation that had reputations for attracting and retaining nurses and delivering high-quality nursing care. Ultimately, 41 hospitals were distinguished by high nurse satisfaction, low job turnover, and low nurse vacancy rates even when hospitals located in the same area were experiencing nursing shortages. These hospitals were called *magnet* hospitals because of their success in attracting and keeping nurses.

BOX 15.1 FORCES OF MAGNETISM

Force 1: Quality of nursing leadership
Force 2: Organizational structure
Force 3: Management style
Force 4: Personnel policies and programs
Force 5: Professional models of care
Force 6: Quality of care
Force 7: Quality improvement
Force 8: Consultation and resources
Force 9: Autonomy
Force 10: Relationships between the community and the health care organization
Force 11: Nurses as teachers
Force 12: Image of nursing
Force 13: Interdisciplinary relationships
Force 14: Professional development

Data from American Nurses Association. (2019). Forces of magnetism. Retrieved from https://www.nursingworld.org/organizational-programs/magnet/history/forces-of-magnetism/.

The Magnet Recognition Program identifies characteristics or outcomes, known as "forces of magnetism," that exemplify excellence in nursing (Box 15.1). Ten years after the identification of the original magnet hospitals, the American Nurses Credentialing Center (ANCC) established a new magnet hospital designation process, similar to accreditation by The Joint Commission (TJC). Recently the recognition program has been expanded to provide national recognition for excellence in long-term-care nursing facilities and smaller community hospitals. In the current competitive environment, receiving the magnet status may serve as a recruiting and marketing tool for hospitals, attesting to a professional work environment and high-quality nursing (Critical Thinking Box 15.2).

? CRITICAL THINKING BOX 15.2

What are the factors that *you* think result in a great working environment? What factors result in an unacceptable environment?

Drenkard (2010) suggests that magnet hospitals have higher percentages of satisfied RNs, lower RN turnover and vacancies, improved clinical outcomes, greater nurse autonomy, and greater patient satisfaction. Drenkard also notes that only 8% of the US hospitals have earned the magnet designation. Evidence suggests that preparing for magnet status ("Taking the Journey to Magnet Excellence") has an impact on quality, service, cost, and human resource measures.

THE IMPACT OF THE 2010 INSTITUTE FOR MEDICINE "FUTURE OF NURSING" REPORT

The convergence of the concerns about the challenges of the US health care system (high cost, primary care shortages, an aging and sicker population, health care disparities, and fragmentation of care) stimulated a national reaction regarding the need to transform the health care system. In response, the Robert Wood Johnson Foundation's Initiative on the Future of Nursing (INF) at the IOM was launched in 2009 (IOM, 2010).

As a part of this 2-year review process, the IOM brought together experts and thought leaders from multiple disciplines (nursing, business, law, medicine, and others) to develop a plan of action to transform the health care system. Since nurses compose the largest group of health care providers, the IOM believed that focusing on the challenges faced by the nursing profession would benefit the entire health care delivery system (IOM, 2010). The IOM and the Task Force held three national forums and numerous technical and policy-oriented workshops to gather insight into the challenges of nursing and develop a transformational report on the future of nursing. On October 5, 2010, the IOM released a landmark report titled *The Future of Nursing* (IOM, 2010).

The key messages of *The Future of Nursing* report (2010) include the following:

- Nurses should practice to the full extent of their education and training through an improved education system that promotes seamless academic progression.
- Nurses should be full partners with physicians and other health care professionals in redesigning health care in the United States.
- Effective workforce planning and policy making require better data collection and an improved information infrastructure.

The recommendations that were derived from these key messages were as follows:

1. Remove scope-of-practice barriers
2. Expand opportunities for nurses to lead and diffuse collaborative improvement efforts
3. Implement nurse residency programs
4. Increase the proportion of nurses with baccalaureate degrees to 80% by 2020
5. Double the number of nurses with doctorates by 2020
6. Ensure that nurses engage in lifelong learning
7. Prepare and enable nurses to lead change to advance health
8. Build an infrastructure for the collection and analysis of interprofessional health care workforce data (IOM, 2010)

The goals of this report were to be released in the year 2020. To what extent have the recommendations of the IOM been addressed? How has this important initiative affected nursing?

The website Campaign for Action Dashboard (2018) highlights the extent to which the *Future of Nursing* recommendations have been met as of July 27, 2018. Table 15.3 outlines these encouraging results.

QUALITY OF CARE AND PATIENT SAFETY

The IOM was a key player in the move toward high-quality health care. During the process of moving toward this goal, the IOM changed its name to the National Academy of Medicine (NAM, 2015). Despite the name change, the NAM has continued to emphasize health care quality, including patient safety.

The quality of care, including patient safety, remains an important issue in the current health care environment. In 1996, the IOM initiated a concerted, ongoing effort to assess and improve the quality of care in the United States. The first phase documented the seriousness of the quality problems. In the second phase (1999–2001), two reports were released. The first, "To Err Is Human: Building a Safer Health System," focused on how tens of thousands of Americans die each year because of medical errors (IOM, 2000). The second, "Crossing the Quality Chasm: A New Health System for the 21st Century" (IOM, 2001), defined six aims to improve health care quality, including care that is

1. Safe
2. Effective
3. Patient-centered
4. Timely
5. Efficient
6. Equitable

TABLE 15.3 RESULTS OF PROGRESS IN REACHING SELECTED INSTITUTE OF MEDICINE GOALS

INDICATOR	RESULTS (LATEST NATIONAL DATA AVAILABLE)
Increase the proportion of nurses in the United States with a baccalaureate degree to 80% by 2020.	2017—56%.
Double the number of nurses with a doctorate by 2020.	2017—a total of 28,004 nurses with doctoral degrees. 2009—a total of 8267 nurses with doctoral degrees. *This recommendation has been achieved.*
Advanced practice registered nurses should be able to practice to the full extent of their education and training.	Full access achieved *before* the campaign began—13 states. Full access achieved *since* the campaign began—9 states. Substantial improvement made—6 states. Incremental improvement made—9 states. Unchanged—13 states.
Make diversity in the nursing workforce a priority.	In the United States, the population is 50.8% female and 49.2% male. In 2017, prelicensure RN program graduates were 85.6% female and 14.1% male. Caucasian nurses represent a greater percentage in the US population overall.
Build infrastructure for the collection and analysis of interprofessional health care workforce data.	Desired: Databases on nurse education, nurse supply, and nurse demand • 25 states have all three databases. • 12 states have 2 databases (nurse education and supply). • 11 states have only 1 database (nurse supply). • 1 state has no database.

Campaign for Action. (2018). Dashboard. The Campaign is an initiative of AARP Foundation, AARP, and the Robert Wood Johnson Foundation. Retrieved from https://campaignforaction.org/resource/dashboardindicators/

The third phase, which is ongoing, focuses on ways the future health care delivery system described in earlier reports can be realized.

One of the IOM reports, "Keeping Patients Safe: Transforming the Work Environment of Nurses," suggests that the work environment of nurses must be changed to better protect patients. The report makes recommendations in the areas of (1) nursing management, (2) workforce deployment, and (3) work design and organizational culture (IOM, 2004). For example, restructuring of hospital organizations in response to managed care has often undermined the trust between nurses and administration. The report urged health care organizations to involve nurse leaders at all levels of management in decision making and to ask nursing staff their opinions about care design because nurses are very effective in detecting processes that contribute to errors.

In 2018, NAM published "Crossing the Global Quality Chasm: Improving Health Care World Wide." This report focused on improving the quality of health care across the world. The recommendations from this report can be read in full at https://www.nap.edu/resource/25152/Global%20Quality%20Chasm%20recommendations.pdf.

In 2008, the TJC published a report titled "Guiding Principles for the Development of the Hospital of the Future." This report outlines principles to (1) support economic viability, (2) guide technology adoption, (3) guide the achievement of patient-centered care, (4) guide the design of hospitals of the future, and (5) address staffing challenges.

The concern about patient safety extends to other areas within the TJC. In 2002, it established its "National Patient Safety Goals," which have been revised each year since then. The goals and related implementation expectations are identified by program: ambulatory care, assisted living, behavioral health care, critical access hospitals, disease-specific care, home care, hospital, laboratory, long-term care, networks, and office-based surgeries.

(See Box 22.1 for a complete list of the 2019 TJC Hospital National Patient Safety Goals.)

Institute for Health Care Improvement

The Institute for Health Care Improvement (IHI), a not-for-profit organization founded in 1991, is also focused on improving the quality of health care. The IHI's goal is to lead improvement of health care throughout the world based on the science of improvement, an applied science that emphasizes innovation, rapid-cycle testing in the field, and spread in order to generate learning. Currently, to advance its mission, IHI's work is focused in five key topic areas:

- Improvement capability: Ensuring that improvement science drives our work and that we extend the reach and impact of the improvement community
- Person- and family-centered care: Putting the patient and the family at the heart of every decision and empowering them to be genuine partners in their care
- Patient safety: Making care continually safer by reducing harm and preventable mortality
- Quality, cost, and value: Driving affordability and sustainability through quality improvement
- Triple aim for populations: Applying integrated approaches to simultaneously improve care, improve population health, and reduce costs per capita (IHI, 2018)

Another IHI effort to improve safety and quality in hospitals began in 2003, when IHI, in collaboration with the Robert Wood Johnson Foundation, developed a process for transforming care in hospital medical-surgical units. The initiative, known as "Transforming Care at the Bedside" (TCAB), involves a four-point framework design theme and six core values of work redesign. Front-line staff, with the full support of the executive team, creates, designs, tests, and implements patient care improvements (called "tests of change"). The improvement efforts are centered on a patient's or an employee's need. Small rapid tests of change provide a mechanism for avoiding delays, discussions, debates, meetings, and layers of administrative sign-offs that often occur in improvement efforts (Martin et al., 2007).

THE EFFECTS OF VARIOUS PATTERNS OF NURSING CARE DELIVERY

Through the years, nursing care has been delivered in many ways, including total patient care (the private-duty model); functional, team, and primary care; and relationship-based care (Fig. 15.1). These models were all designed to provide a framework for the organization of the care provided. As nursing has developed as a profession and its roles have expanded, the overarching name for all models became *the patient care delivery model* or *professional practice model*.

What Is the Total Patient Care or Private-Duty Model?

Historically nursing was organized around the *total patient care* or *private-duty model*. The RN was hired by the patient and provided care to that patient, typically in the patient's home. In the 1920s, 1930s, and again in the 1980s, this approach was used where one nurse assumed responsibility for the complete care of a group of patients on a one-on-one basis, providing total patient care during a shift.

The quality of care in the total patient care model is considered to be high, because all activities are carried out by RNs who can focus their complete attention on one patient. This model is efficient because it (1) decreases communication time between the staff caring for a patient, (2) reduces the need for supervision, and (3) allows one person to perform more than one task simultaneously. Some

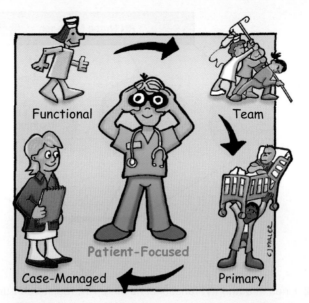

Functional

Team

Patient-Focused

Case-Managed

Primary

FIG. 15.1 Evolving patterns of nursing care delivery.

nurses prefer this model because they can focus on patients' needs without the work of supervising others; others feel that their skills and time are wasted doing patient care activities that could be done by others with less skill and education. Patient satisfaction tends to be high with this model if continuity of care and communication are maintained among nurses (Flagg, 2015).

What Is Functional Nursing?

The movement toward the use of RNs as employees of hospitals came with the outbreak of World War II. RNs took over the work in the hospital, and that, coupled with the war effort, stimulated the nursing shortage of that period. This forced hospitals to develop alternative models of nursing. The positions of aides and licensed vocational/practical nurses came into being, and in some states these individuals were allowed to perform functions such as the administration of medications and treatments. This functional kind of nursing, which broke nursing care into a series of tasks performed by many people, resulted in a fragmented, impersonal kind of care (Fig. 15.2). Fragmentation of care caused patient problems to be overlooked because the problems did not fit into a defined assignment.

This assembly-line approach provided little time for the nurse to address a patient's psychosocial or spiritual needs. Fragmentation of care and errors and omissions tended to occur or increase when functional nursing was used. This approach would seem to be cost-efficient because it can be implemented with fewer RNs. However, patients, nurses, and physicians have been critical of this approach because of the fragmentation and the lack of accountability for the patients' total care (Flagg, 2015).

What Is Team Nursing?

In the 1950s, *team nursing* evolved as a way to address the problems with the functional approach. In this type of nursing, groups of patients were assigned to a team headed by a *team leader*, usually an RN, who coordinated the care for a designated group of patients (Fig. 15.3). The team leader determines

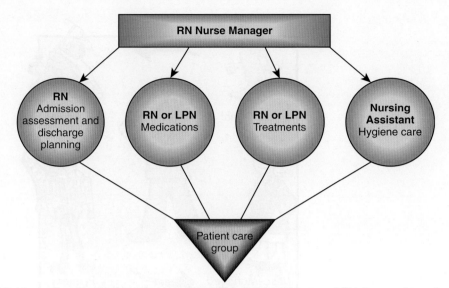

FIG. 15.2 Lines of authority: functional nursing. *RN,* registered nurse. *LPN,* licensed practical nurse.

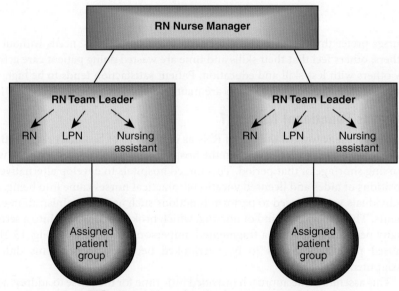

FIG. 15.3 Lines of authority: team nursing.

work assignments for the team on the basis of the acuity level of the group of patients and the ability of the individual team members. The following is an example of the components of a team:

■ An RN who is the team leader
■ Two licensed vocational nurses/practical nurses assigned to patient care
■ Two unlicensed assistive personnel (UAP)

The success of team nursing depends on good communication among the team members. It is imperative that the team leader continuously evaluate and communicate changes in the patient's condition to the team members. The team conference is a vital part of this approach, allowing team members to assess the needs of their patients and revise their individual plans of care on an ongoing basis. The team model allows the nurse to know patients well enough to make assignments that best match each patient's needs with staff strengths. Patients' needs are coordinated, and continuity of care may improve depending on the length of time each member stays on the team. However, care can be fragmented and the model ineffective when staff is limited. In addition, the amount of time required to communicate among team members may decrease productivity (Flagg, 2015).

What Is Primary Nursing?

In the 1960s and 1970s, *primary nursing* evolved. In this system, a nurse plans and directs the care of a patient during a 24-hour period. This approach is designed to reduce or eliminate the fragmentation of care between shifts and nurses, because one nurse is accountable for planning the care of the patient around the clock. Progress reports, referrals, and discharge planning are usually the responsibility of the primary nurse. When the primary nurse is off duty, an associate nurse continues the plan of care. An RN may be the primary caregiver for some of the assigned patients, whereas an associate nurse is the primary caregiver for others. Some forms of primary nursing evolved into an all-RN staff (Fig. 15.4). Primary nursing may also be mixed and modified with nurse extenders, such as paired partners or partners in care. Although team nursing took the RN away from bedside care, primary and modified primary nursing puts the nurse back in close contact with the patient.

Relationship-based practice is the new name for primary nursing. The RN—who may be called the care coordinator, the responsible nurse, the principal responsible nurse, the case manager, or the care manager—manages and coordinates a patient's care in the hospital and also coordinates the discharge plan. This nurse develops a relationship and can be identified by the patient, the patient's family, and the health care team as having the responsibility and authority for planning the patient's nursing care.

What Is Patient-Focused Care?

Patient-focused care is another delivery system that has evolved since the late 1990s. Because of earlier nursing shortages, some traditional nursing interventions such as phlebotomy and diet instruction have been assigned to members of departments that do not report to nursing. These ancillary workers

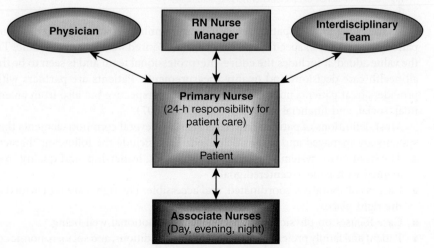

FIG. 15.4 Lines of authority: primary nursing.

spend a great deal of time in transit from one unit to another. Time is also lost when there is not enough work for such a single-function individual to do. These tasks can be centralized on the unit under the direction of the RN. UAPs are cross-trained to perform more than one function, thus increasing the level of productivity. In this system, the patient comes in contact with fewer people, and the RN, who is familiar with the patient's plan of care, supervises the delivery of care. This model also moves RNs to a higher level of functioning because they are now accountable for a fuller range of services to the patient. Tasks that do not require an RN can be delegated to a UAP under the supervision of the RN (Flagg, 2015).

There are also models of care associated with providing care during the patient's transition to home or to another less intense level of care. Such transitional care is particularly important in today's health care environment. Peikes et al. (2012) describe three such models. The first, the *transitional care model* (TCM), provides comprehensive in-hospital and follow-up care plans. The second model, *care transitions intervention* (CTI), teaches self-management and communication skills to patients and caregivers so they can coordinate care. There is also a follow-up component using a home visit and telephone call. The *reengineered discharge* (RED) model provides patient education, medication reconciliation and education, instruction about red flags to symptoms, teach-back learning processes, coordination of physician appointment and follow-up tests, and evidence-based written discharge plans (Peikes et al., 2012).

What Is the Most Effective Model of Nursing Care?

In the past, a great deal of literature about models of care delivery was published. However, there has been little systematic evaluation of the use of the various models, often because of the lack of similarity in staffing and patient populations on comparison units. It is therefore impossible to determine the impact that inpatient models of nursing care have on patient outcomes, costs, or job satisfaction. It may be that the model of nursing care delivery is less important than other factors—including nurse/patient ratios, the use of overtime, and the organizational culture in which the nurse works—in influencing outcomes (Critical Thinking Box 15.3). According to Peikes et al. (2012), there is rigorous evidence that at least some of the TCMs do improve outcomes. The impact on the reduction of cost is unclear.

? CRITICAL THINKING BOX 15.3

What factors influence the patterns of nursing care delivery?

As the name implies, patient-centered care, similar to patient-focused nursing care, focuses on the patient's (or family's) specific health needs and desired health care outcome. This approach is part of the value added; it includes the entire interprofessional team and is seen to be the driving force behind all health care decisions and quality measurements. Patients are partners with their providers, and providers treat patients not only from a clinical perspective but also from an emotional, mental, spiritual, social, and financial perspective (Shaller, 2007).

Most definitions of patient-centered care have several common elements that affect the way health systems are managed and care is delivered. This include the following characteristics:

- The health care system's mission, vision, values, leadership, and quality-improvement drivers are aligned with patient-centered goals.
- Care is collaborative, coordinated, and accessible. The right care is provided at the right time and in the right place.
- Care focuses on physical comfort as well as emotional well-being.
- Patient and family preferences, values, cultural traditions, and socioeconomic conditions are respected.
- Patients and their families are an expected part of the care team and play a role in decisions at the patient and system levels.

- The presence of family members in the care setting is encouraged and facilitated.
- Information is shared fully and in a timely manner so that patients and their family members can make informed decisions (NEJM Catalyst, 2017a).

Patient-centered care represents a shift in the traditional roles of patients and their families from one of passive order taker to one of active team member. Many providers are implementing patient satisfaction surveys, patient and family advisory councils, and focus groups, and they are using the resulting information to continuously improve the way health care facilities and provider practices are designed, managed, and maintained from both a physical and operational perspective so they become centered more on the individual person than on a checklist of services provided (Shaller, 2007). Table 15.4 outlines specific characteristics that are important in patient-centered care and Research for Best Practice Box 15.1 examines the patient experience and patient satisfaction.

TABLE 15.4 IMPORTANT CHARACTERISTICS OF PATIENT-CENTERED CARE

CHARACTERISTICS	EXAMPLES
Respect for patients' values, preferences and expressed needs	• Involve patients in decision making • Treat patients with dignity respect and sensitivity to their cultural values and autonomy
Coordination and integration of care	• Proper coordination of care to reduce feelings of vulnerability (coordination of clinical care, ancillary services support; and front-live patient care)
Information and education	• Information on clinical status, progress, and prognosis, processes of care, to facilitate autonomy, self-care and health promotion
Physical comfort	• Pain management • Assistance with activities and daily living needs • Hospital surroundings and environment

Emotional support and alleviation of fear and anxiety	• Anxiety over
	  • physical status, treatment and prognosis
	  • impact of illness on themselves and family
	  • financial impact of illness

Involvement of family and friends	• Providing accommodations for family and friends • Involving family and close friends in decision-making • Supporting family members as caregivers • Recognizing the needs of family and friends
Continuity and transition	• Understandable detailed information regarding medications, physical limitations, etc. • Coordinate and plan ongoing treatment and services after discharge • Provide information regarding access to clinical, social, physical and financial support on a continuing basis
Access to care	• Access to the location of hospitals, clinics and physician offices • Availability of transportation • Event of scheduling appointments • Accessibility to specialist or specialty services when a referral is made • Clear instructions provided on when and how to get referrals

Adapted from Shaller, D. (2007). Patient centered care: What does it take? The Commonwealth Fund. Retrieved from https://www.commonwealthfund.org/publications/fund-reports/2007/oct/patient-centered-care-what-does-it-take
Picker Institute. (2015). Picker Institute's eight principles of patient-centered care. Retrieved from https://nexusipe.org/informing/resource-center/picker-institute%E2%80%99s-eight-principles-patient-centered-care

RESEARCH FOR BEST PRACTICE BOX 15.1
The Patient Experience and Patient Satisfaction

Practice Issue

Patient's satisfaction with their experiences in health care is seen as a measure of the quality of care and is increasingly linked to reimbursement of hospitals and other providers. The author suggests that patient satisfaction is a complex dynamic that is poorly understood. This article discusses the factors related to patients' satisfaction with their experiences. She addresses the following questions: How does the patient's experience influence the patient's perception of satisfaction with this care? Is patient satisfaction accurately measured? What is the responsibility of nursing in assuring a satisfactory patient experience?

Implications for Nursing Practice

- Patient satisfaction is related to the patient's direct and indirect experiences in communicating with health care providers.
- The nurse's work environment can affect patient satisfaction in positive and negative ways.
- A patients' personal experiences may not directly relate to the quality of the care provided but rather is related to their expectations of what they believe should be provided or their expectations of their prognosis, treatment, family interaction, and environment.

Considering This Information

1. How would you explain the relationship between a positive work environment and patient satisfaction?
2. How does the organization where you have had clinical experiences measure the patient perspective of satisfaction?
3. Do you believe that patients and families can assess the quality or safety of the care they receive? Why or why not?
4. Do you believe that hospitals or providers should be rewarded financially for providing safe, high-quality care? What are the benefits of this approach? What are the limitations or liabilities?

Reference

Berkowitz, B. (2016). The patient experience and patient satisfaction: Measurement of a complex dynamic. *OJIN: The Online Journal of Issues in Nursing, 21*(1), E1–E8. https://doi.org/10.3912/OJIN.Vol21No01Man01.

Patient-centered care has become a central aim for the nation's health system, yet patient experience surveys indicate that the system is far from achieving its goals. Bokhour et al. (2018, p. 168) interviewed leaders of patient-centered organizations and initiatives and identified seven key factors for achieving patient-centered care at the organizational level: (1) top leadership engagement, (2) involvement of patients and families at multiple levels, (3) staff engagement, (4) focus on innovations, (5) alignment of staff roles and priorities, (6) organizational structures and processes, and (7) the environment of care.

The authors note that "Transforming healthcare systems to focus on patient-centered care and better serve the 'whole' patient is a complex endeavor influenced by completing priorities and regulations" (Bokhour et al., 2018, p. 168). However, they believe that implementing actions in each of the identified domains may help to transform the system to patient-driven care.

NURSE STAFFING

What Is the Impact of Staffing Patterns on the Quality of Care?

Regardless of the model of care used, nurse staffing must be addressed, particularly in hospitals in which 24-hour coverage is required. In 2004 and again in 2007, the AHRQ released landmark reports that summarized findings of AHRQ-funded research and other research on the relationship between nurse staffing levels and adverse patient outcomes. These reports included the following conclusions:

- Lower levels of hospital nurse staffing are associated with more adverse outcomes.
- Patients in hospitals today are more acutely ill than in the past, but the skill levels of the nursing staff have declined.

- Higher-acuity patients have added responsibilities that have increased the nurse workload.
- Avoidable adverse outcomes, such as pneumonia, can raise treatment costs by as much as $28,000.
- Hiring more RNs does not decrease profit.
- Higher levels of nurse staffing could have a positive impact on both quality of care and nurse satisfaction (AHRQ, 2004, 2007).

The 2004 studies showed significant associations between too few nurses on a unit and higher rates of pneumonia, upper gastrointestinal bleeding, shock/cardiac arrest, urinary tract infections, and failure to rescue. Other studies in the review showed associations between lower staffing levels and pneumonia, lung collapse, falls, pressure ulcers, thrombosis after major surgery, pulmonary compromise after surgery, longer hospital stays, and 30-day mortalities (AHRQ, 2004).

In 2007, the AHRQ funded research to review studies from 11 databases to assess how nurse/patient ratios and nurse work hours were associated with patient outcomes in acute care hospitals. These factors influence nurse staffing policies and strategies that improve patient outcomes. As a result, it was found that higher RN staffing was associated with less hospital-related mortality, failure to rescue, and other patient outcomes, but also that higher RN staffing might not be the cause of these outcomes because hospitals that invest in adequate nursing staff may also invest in other initiatives to improve quality. Researchers also found that the effect of increased RN staffing on patient safety was strong and consistent in intensive care units (ICUs) and in the care of surgical patients. A larger number of RN hours spent on direct patient care was associated with a lower risk of hospital-related death and also with shorter lengths of stay (AHRQ, 2007).

Martsolf et al. (2014) assessed the causal relationship between the level and skill mix of nurses, adverse events as measured by nurse-sensitive patient safety indicators, lengths of stay, and cost. Increases in hospital nurse staffing levels were associated with reductions in adverse events and lengths of stay and did not lead to increased costs. Increases in nurse staffing levels were associated with reductions in nursing-sensitive adverse events and lengths of stay but did not lead to increases in costs. Changing the skill mix by increasing the number of RNs as a proportion of licensed nursing staff, led to reductions in costs. This study further supports the value of inpatient nurse staffing as it contributes to improvements in inpatient care.

As the research suggests, identifying and maintaining the appropriate number and mix of nursing staff is critical to the delivery of high-quality patient care. A federal regulation, **42 Code of Federal Regulations (42CFR 482.23(b)**, requires hospitals certified to participate in Medicare to "have adequate numbers of licensed RNs, licensed practical nurses and other personnel to provide nursing care of all patients as needed" (ANA, 2015). In response to this regulation, various states have developed ways to ensure that hospitals maintain optimal nurse staffing.

State laws usually fall into one of three approaches to staffing regulation. They
1. Require hospitals to have nurse-driven staffing committees to develop staffing plans
2. Call for a legislative mandate for specific nurse/patient ratios
3. Include a regulatory requirement to disclose staffing levels to the public and/or a regulatory body (ANA, 2015)

The ANA has adopted the staffing committee approach to this issue, identifying the following as factors to consider in developing a staffing plan:
- Patient complexity, acuity, or stability
- Number of admissions, discharges, and transfers
- Professional nursing and other staff skill level and expertise
- Physical space and layout of the nursing unit
- Availability of technical support and other resources (ANA, 2015).

The ANA has worked with members of Congress to pass nursing staffing legislation for a number of years. Most recently, the Safe Staffing for Nurse and Patient Safety Act of 2018 was passed. This legislation considers not only the complexity and stability of patients but also nurse experience, available technology, resources, and unit workflow such as numbers of admission, discharges, and transfers (ANA, 2018a).

The ANA has also published the *Principles of Safe Staffing,* second edition, which addresses issues related to core components of nurse staffing, health care consumers, RNs and other staff, organization and workplace culture, and staffing evaluation (ANA, 2012).

How Are Nursing Work Assignments Determined?

After appropriate staffing levels for a unit have been determined, specific nurses must be scheduled. How work assignments are decided varies with individual organizations and is related to the model of care delivery, condition of the patient, architecture of the unit, and expertise of the staff.

> A major problem in scheduling nurses is the fact that patient acuity fluctuates dramatically from day to day and from season to season.

For example, during the Christmas holidays there is often a significant decrease in the number of elective surgeries. In response, some hospitals may close units or reduce the number of staff on any given unit. By contrast, in the middle of the influenza season, the hospital might be full and understaffed. See Critical Thinking Box 15.4 to consider how you might handle staffing issues.

❓ CRITICAL THINKING BOX 15.4

How might you handle a situation on your unit where staffing is a concern? What are the unit's census, acuity, and patient-classification systems?

- Does your organization have a float pool within the staff or an agency or outside staff available?
- Check whether your part-time staff can work an extra shift.
- Will another staff member cover the extra shift in exchange for a day off later in the schedule?
- Can you survive with partial-shift coverage during the "peak" shift hours?
- Ask a staff member to work a double shift—either stay late or come in early.
- Work the shift yourself.
- What other solutions can you think of?
- What are the advantages and disadvantages of each of these options?

In 2018, the ANA published, for public comment, *Principles of Staffing and Workforce Management: The Future of Nursing as Holistic Providers and Advocates of Care.* This document aligns the ANA's *Principles of Staffing* with the IHI's *Triple Aim* and notes that the staffing process involves the following four components:

- **Forecasting** budgeting and planning based on expected future patient volume and acuity
- **Scheduling** of adequate number of nurses and other nursing personnel to address current needs of patients
- **Assigning** staff based on needs of each patient and balanced workload across the scheduled nurses and nursing personnel
- **Improving** monitoring and analyzing, performance, quality and safety, and outcomes of nursing care (ANA, 2018b)

What About Scheduling Patterns?

Nursing has also been concerned about scheduling practices and options because in many health care environments nursing care must be provided 24 hours a day, 365 days per year. That is why there are numerous scheduling patterns other than the typical 8-hour shift 5 days a week. From working 10-hour days 4 days a week to the weekend alternative (known as the Baylor plan) of two 12-hour weekend shifts for 36 hours of pay, nurses have tried numerous patterns and combinations of shifts.

What About the Use of Overtime?

With the current shortage of health professionals, employees are also encouraged and sometimes required to work overtime. The landmark study of nurses by Rogers and associates (2004) was one of the first efforts to evaluate the effects of nurse work pattern on fatigue. It was found that that 14% of nurses in the study reported working shifts of 16 hours or longer in the previous 4 weeks and that 81% of shifts ran beyond their scheduled limits. This work pattern results in fatigue, which can produce a level of performance similar to that of someone who is drunk. Fatigue can also produce physical performance effects that inhibit critical cognitive functions, including lapses of attention, irritability, memory lapses, decreased ability to detect and react to subtle changes, slowed information processing, difficulties in handling unexpected situations, and communication difficulties.

Stimpfil and colleagues (2012) reported the results of a survey of nurses in four states; it showed that more than 80% of the nurses were satisfied with scheduling practices at their hospitals. However, as the proportion of hospital nurses working shifts of more than 13 hours increased, patients' dissatisfaction with care also increased. Nurses working shifts of 10 hours or more were up to two and a half times more likely than nurses working shorter shifts to experience burnout and job dissatisfaction and to plan to leave their jobs.

Kaliyaperumal et al. (2017), using the Epworth sleepiness scale (ESS) and the Montreal Cognitive Assessment (Mocha) questionnaire, studied sleep deprivation among 97 female and 3 male nurses between the ages of 20 and 50 years and all in good health. Mobile applications were used to test their vigilance, reaction times, photographic memory, and numerical cognition. These parameters were assessed at the end of a day shift and 3 to 4 days after the start of a night shift. Cognitive performance was found to be impaired among shift-working nurses due to poor sleep quality and decreased alertness during wake state. Thus shift work poses significant cognitive risks in the work performance of nurses (Critical Thinking Box 15.5).

? CRITICAL THINKING BOX 15.5

What Do You Think?

- How many hours are too long to work?
- Is there an increase in the number of errors made by nurses working 12 hours or longer?
- How would you handle it if your supervisor asked you to work 6 more hours after your 12-hour shift because the floor is short staffed?
- What is your responsibility as a professional nurse when it comes to overtime?

CONCLUSION

The emphasis on cost control and managed care has changed the way in which nursing care is delivered. New models of health care delivery are being developed in which we look at the desired outcome and "manage backward" to achieve that outcome at the lowest possible cost. Because of some of the unexpected negative consequences of managed care, there is now renewed emphasis on evidence-based care to enhance patient safety (see the Relevant Websites and Online Resources). We are continually challenged to develop more innovative and creative ways to ensure excellence in patient care with limited dollars. Nurses can meet this challenge.

🌐 RELEVANT WEBSITES AND ONLINE RESOURCES

The Academic Center for Evidence-Based Nursing (ACE) at the University of Texas Health Science Center at San Antonio
Retrieved from http://ebp.uthscsa.edu/

Agency for Health Care Research and Quality
Retrieved from http://www.ahrq.gov

American Association of Colleges of Nursing
Retrieved from http://www.aacn.nche.edu

American Nurses Association
Retrieved from http://www.nursingworld.org

Indiana Center for Evidence-Based Nursing Practice, in the Purdue University Calumet's School of Nursing
Retrieved from http://www.ebnp.org.

Institute for Health Care Improvement
Retrieved from http://www.ihi.org

Joanna Briggs Institute University of Adelaide, Australia
Retrieved from http://joannabriggs.org/

The Joint Commission
Retrieved from http://www.jointcommission.org

National Academy of Medicine (formerly the Institute of Medicine)
Retrieved from https://nam.edu/

The Sara Cole Hirsch Institute for Best Nursing Practice Based on Evidence at Case Western Reserve School of Nursing
Retrieved from https://case.edu/nursing/research/centers-of-excellence/sarah-cole-hirsh-institute

BIBLIOGRAPHY

Agency for Healthcare Research and Quality (AHRQ). (2004). Hospital nurse staffing and quality of care: Research in action. Retrieved from https://archive.ahrq.gov/research/findings/factsheets/services/nursestaffing/nursestaff.html.

Agency for Healthcare Research and Quality (AHRQ). (2018a). Clinical guidelines and recommendations. Retrieved from http://www.ahrq.gov/professionals/clinicians-providers/guidelines-recommendations/index.html.

Agency for Healthcare Research and Quality (AHRQ). (2018b). Evidence based practice center. Retrieved from https://www.ahrq.gov/research/findings/evidence-based-reports/centers/index.html.

American Nurses Association (ANA). (2012). ANA's Principles for nurse staffing (2nd ed.). Maryland: Silver Springs. Retrieved from https://www.nursingworld.org/~4af4f2/globalassets/docs/ana/ethics/principles-of-nurse–staffing–2nd-edition.pdf.

American Nurses Association (ANA). (2015). Nursing staffing. Retrieved from https://www.nursingworld.org/practice-policy/advocacy/state/nurse-staffing/.

American Nurses Association (ANA). (2018a). ANA applauds nurse staffing legislation. Retrieved from https://www.nursingworld.org/news/news-releases/2018/ana-applauds-nurse-staffing-legislation.

American Nurses Association (ANA). (2018b). Principles of staffing & workforce management: The future of nursing as holistic providers and advocates of care. Retrieved from https://www.nursingworld.org/~49fbb4/globalassets/practiceandpolicy/call-for-public-comment/principles-of-staffing_quadruple-aim_ew-edits_2018.06.19.pdf.

American Nurses Association (ANA). (2018c). Workforce. Retrieved from https://www.nursingworld.org/practice-policy/workforce

American Nurses Association. (2019). Forces of magnetism. Retrieved from https://www.nursingworld.org/organizational-programs/magnet/history/forces-of-magnetism/.

Black, H., Priolo, C., Akinyemi, D., et al. (2010). Clearing clinical barriers: Enhancing social support using a nurse navigator for asthma care. *Journal of Asthma, 47*(8), 913–919.

Bleich, M. (2012, May). In praise of nursing residency programs. *American Nurse Today, 7*, 5. Retrieved from https://www.americannursetoday.com/in-praise-of-nursing-residency-programs/.

Bokhour, B., Fix, G., Mueller, N., Barker, A., Lavela, S., Hill, J., et al. (2018). How can healthcare organizations implement patient-centered care? Examination of a large scale transformation. *BMC Health Service Research, 18*, 168. https://doi.org/10.1186/s12913-018-2949-5. Retrieved at https://www.ncbi.nlm.nih.gov/pmc/articles/PMC5842617/.

Campaign for Action. (2018). Dashboard. Retrieved https://campaignforaction.org/wp-content/uploads/2018/08/Dashboard-Indicator-Updates_July27.pdf.

Case, M. B. (2011). Oncology nurse navigator: Ensuring safe passage. *Journal of Oncology Nursing, 15*(1), 33–40.

Case Management Society of America. (2015). Retrieved from www.cmsa.org.

Collins, S., Gunja, M., Doty, M., & Bhupal, H. (2018). First look at health insurance coverage in 2018 finds ACA gains beginning to reverse. Retrieved from https://www.commonwealthfund.org/blog/2018/first-look-health-insurance-coverage-2018-finds-aca-gains-beginning-reverse?redirect_source=/.

Centers for Disease Control and Prevention (CDC). (2016). Health expenditures. Retrieved from https://www.cdc.gov/nchs/fastats/health-expenditures.htm.

Centers for Medicare & Medicaid Services (CMS). (2017). 2016–2025 projections of national health expenditures data released. Retrieved from https://www.cms.gov/newsroom/press-releases/2016-2025-projections-national-health-expenditures-data-released.

Centers for Medicare & Medicaid Services (CMS). (2018a). Accountable care organizations (ACOs): General information. Retrieved from https://innovation.cms.gov/initiatives/ACO/.

Centers for Medicare & Medicaid Services (CMS). (2018b). National health expenditure data. Retrieved from https://www.cms.gov/Research-Statistics-Data-and-Systems/Statistics-Trends-and-Reports/NationalHealthExpendData/index.html.

Christman, J., Jordan, R., Davis, C., & Williams, W. (2014). Exploring evidence-based practice research. *Nursing Made Incredibly Easy!, 12*(4), 8–12. https://doi.org/10.1097/01.NME.0000450295.93626.e7.

Drenkard, K. (2010). Going for the gold: The value of attaining Magnet recognition. *American Nurse Today, 5*, 3. Retrieved from https://www.americannursetoday.com/going-for-the-gold-the-value-of-attaining-magnet-recognition/.

Flagg, A. J. (2015). The role of patient-centered care in Nursing. *Nursing Clinics of North America, 50*(1), 75–86. https://doi.org/10.1016/j.cnur.2014.10.006.

HealthCare.gov. (2017). Key features of the Affordable Care Act, year by year. Retrieved from http://www.hhs.gov/healthcare/facts-and-features/key-features-of-aca-by-year/index.html.

HealthCare.gov. (2018a). Affordable Care Act (ACA). Retrieved from https://www.healthcare.gov/glossary/affordable-care-act/.

HealthCare.gov. (2018b). What marketplace health insurance plans cover. Retrieved from https://www.healthcare.gov/coverage/what-marketplace-plans-cover.

Health Policy Institute (HPI). (2004). Disease management programs: Improving health while reducing costs? In Georgetown University, Issue Brief, 4. Retrieved from https://hpi.georgetown.edu/agingsociety/pubhtml/management/management.html.

Horstmann, E., Brown, J., Islam, F., Brick, J., & Agins, B. D. (2010). Retaining HIV infection patients in care: Where are we? Where do we go from here? *Clinical Infectious Diseases, 50*(5), 752–761.

Institute for Healthcare Improvement (IHI). (2019). Topics. Retrieved from http://www.ihi.org

Institute of Medicine. (2004). Keeping patients safe: Transforming the work environment of nurses. Retrieved from https://www.ncbi.nlm.nih.gov/books/NBK216188/.

Institute of Medicine. (2010). Future of nursing. Retrieved from http://nationalacademies.org/hmd/Reports/2010/The-Future-of-Nursing-Leading-Change-Advancing-Health.aspx.

Joanna Briggs Institute. (2018). About JBI. Retrieved from http://joannabriggs.org/.

Kaiser Family Foundation (KFF). (2017). Summary of the American Health Care Act. Retrieved from http://files.kff.org/attachment/Proposals-to-Replace-the-Affordable-Care-Act-Summary-of-the-American-Health-Care-Act.

Kaiser Family Foundation (KFF). (2018). Health costs. Retrieved from https://www.kff.org/health-costs/.

Internal Review Service (IRS). (2018). The premium tax credit: The basics. Retrieved from https://www.irs.gov/affordable-care-act/individuals-and-families/the-premium-tax-credit-the-basics-0.

Jacobson, L. (2017). What would the impact be if the Affordable Care Act is repealed? In *PolitiFact*. Retrieved from http://www.politifact.com/truth-o-meter/article/2017/jan/05/what-would-be-impact-if-affordable-care-act-repeal/.

Kaliyaperumal, D., Elango, Y., Alagesan, M., & Santhanakrishanan, I. (2017). Effects of sleep deprivation on the cognitive performance of nurses working in shift. *Journal of Clinical Diagnostic Reasoning, 11*(8), CC01–CC03. https://doi.org/10.7860/JCDR/2017/26029.10324.

Kamal, R., & Cox, C. (2018). How do healthcare prices and use in the U.S. compare to other countries? *Kaiser Family Foundation*. Retrieved from https://www.healthsystemtracker.org/chart-collection/how-do-healthcare-prices-and-use-in-the-u-s-compare-to-other-countries/#item-on-average-other-wealthy-countries-spend-half-as-much-per-person-on-healthcare-than-the-u-s.

Martin, S., Greenhouse, P. K., Merryman, T., Shovel, J., Liberi, C. A., & Konzier, J. (2007). Transforming care at the bedside: Implementation and spread model of single-hospital and multihospital systems. *Journal of Nursing Administration, 37*(10), 444–451. https://doi.org/10.1097/01.NNA.0000285152.79988.f3.

Martsolf, G. R., Auerbach, D., Benevent, R., et al. (2014). Examining the value of inpatient nurse staffing: An assessment of quality and patient care cost. *Medical Care, 52*(11), 982–988. https://doi.org/10.1097/MLR.0000000000000248.

McDonald, A., & Ward-Smith, P. (2012). A review of evidence based practice to retain graduate nurses in the profession. *Journal for Nurses in Staff Development, 28*(1), E16–E20. https://doi.org/10.1097/NND.0b013e318240a740 January-February.

Medicare.gov. (n.d.). Hospital compare: Linking quality to payment. Retrieved from https://www.medicare.gov/hospitalcompare/linking-quality-to-payment.html

Melnyk, B. M., & Fineout-Overholt, E. (2015). *Evidence based practice in nursing and health care: A guide to best practice* (3rd ed.). Philadelphia: Lippincott Williams & Wilkins.

Majid, S., Foo, S., Luyt, B., Zang, X., Theng, Y., Chan, Y., et al. (2011). Adopting evidence-based practice in clinical decision making: nurses' perceptions, knowledge, and barriers. *Journal of Medical Library Association, 99*(3), 229–239. https://doi.org/10.3163/1536-5050.99.3.010.

National Academy of Medicine (NAM). (2015, April 28). Press release: Institute of Medicine to become National Academy of Medicine. Retrieved from http://www.nationalacademies.org/hmd/Global/News%20Announcements/IOM-to-become-NAM-Press-Release.aspx.

NEJM Catalyst. (2017a). What is patient-centered care? Retrieved from https://catalyst.nejm.org/what-is-patient-centered-care/.

NEJM Catalyst. (2017b). What is value-based healthcare? Retrieved from https://catalyst.nejm.org/what-is-value-based-healthcare/.

NEJM Catalyst. (2018). What is pay for performance healthcare? Retrieved from https://catalyst.nejm.org/pay-for-performance-in-healthcare/.

Oncology Nursing Society (ONS). (2013). Oncology Nurse Navigator Core Competencies. Retrieved from https://www.ons.org/sites/default/files/ONNCompetencies_rev.pdf.

Ortiz, J., Bushy, A., Zhou, Y., & Zhang, H. (2013). Accountable care organizations: Benefits and barriers as perceived by rural health clinic management. *Rural Remote Health, 13*(2), 2417. Retrieved from https://www.ncbi.nlm.nih.gov/pmc/articles/PMC3761377/.

Pedersen, A., & Hack, T. F. (2010). Pilots of oncology health care: A concept analysis of the patient navigator role. *Oncology Nursing Forum, 37*, 55–60.

Peikes, D., Zutshi, A., Genevro, J., Smith, K., Parchman, M., & Meyers, D. (February 2012). Early evidence on the patient-centered medical home. In Final report (Prepared by Mathematica Policy Research, under Contract Nos. HHSA290200900019I/HHSA29032002T and HHSA290200900019I/HHSA29032005T). AHRQ Publication No. 12-0020-EF. Rockville, MD: Agency for Healthcare Research and Quality. Retrieved from https://pcmh.ahrq.gov/sites/default/files/attachments/Early%20Evidence%20on%20the%20PCMH%202%2028%2012.pdf.

Picker Institute. (2015). Picker Institute's eight principles of patient-centered care. Retrieved from https://nexusipe.org/informing/resource-center/picker-institute%E2%80%99s-eight-principles-patient-centered-care.

Rogers, A. E., Hwang, W. T., Scott, L. D., Aiken, L. H., & Dinges, D. F. (2004). The working hours of hospital staff nurse and patient safety. *Health Affair, 23*, 202–212. https://doi.org/10.1377/hlthaff.23.4.202.

Sahadi, J. (2018). Warren Buffett is right. Health care costs are swallowing the economy. *@CCN Money,* January 30. Retrieved from https://money.cnn.com/2018/01/30/news/economy/health-care-costs-eating-the-economy/index.html.

Shaller, D. (2007). Patient centered care: What does it take? *The Commonweath Fund,* Retrieved from https://www.commonwealthfund.org/sites/default/files/documents/___media_files_publications_fund_report_2007_oct_patient_centered_care__what_does_it_take_shaller_patient_centeredcarewhatdoesittake_1067_pdf.pdf.

Stimpfil, A. W., Sloane, D. M., & Aiken, L. H. (2012). The longer the shift for hospital nurses, the higher the level of burnout and patient dissatisfaction. *Health Affairs, 3*(11), 2501–2509. https://doi.org/10.1377/hlthaff.2011.1377.

The Joint Commission. (2019). National patient safety goals. Retrieved from www.jointcommission.org/PatientSafety/NationalPatientSafetyGoals.

US Bureau of Labor Statistics. (2018). Occupational outlook handbook. Retrieved from https://www.bls.gov/ooh/healthcare/registered-nurses.htm#tab-6.

Wells, K. J., Bellagio, T. A., Dudley, D. J., et al. (2008). Patient navigation: State of the art or is it science? *Cancer, 113*(8), 1999–2010. https://doi.org/10.1002/cncr.23815.

16

Economics of the Health Care Delivery System

Julie V. Darmody, PhD, RN, ACNS-BC

ⓔhttp://evolve.elsevier.com/Zerwekh/nsgtoday/.

The registered nurse uses appropriate resources to plan, provide, and sustain evidence-based nursing services that are safe, effective, and fiscally responsible.
Standard 16, Resource Utilization, ANA Nursing Scope and Standards of Practice, 3rd ed. (2015b)

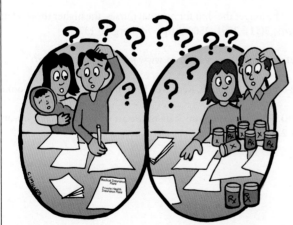

U.S. health care is a complex mix of public and private systems.

After completing this chapter, you should be able to:

- Define economics and health care economics.
- Compare the market for health care with a normal market for goods and services.
- Use a basic knowledge of health care economics to analyze trends in the health care delivery system.
- Describe what operating budget, personnel budget, and capital budget mean.
- Define economic research strategies.
- Describe what is meant by the term *fiscal responsibility* in clinical practice.
- Discuss strategies you will use to achieve fiscal responsibility in your clinical practice.

The rate of increase in U.S. national health care spending for 2016 was 4.3%, which was a deceleration from the faster growth in 2014 and 2015 due to coverage expansions under the Affordable Care Act (ACA) and increased prescription drug spending (Hartman et al., 2018). U.S. national health expenditures (NHEs) in 2016 were $3.3 trillion, or $10,348 per person, which comprises 17.9% of the gross domestic product (GDP) (Hartman et al., 2018). By the year 2026, those expenditures are projected to be $5.7 trillion and comprise 19.7% of GDP (Cuckler et al., 2018).

The outcome of this large investment of resources in health and health care in the United States is variable. Many Americans do not receive the care they need, receive care that causes harm, or receive care without consideration of their preferences and values. The distribution of services is often inefficient and uneven across populations. For the past 15 years, annual reports by the Agency for Healthcare Research and Quality (AHRQ) have summarized health care quality and disparities in the U.S. health care system and have identified strengths, weaknesses, and disparities (AHRQ, 2018). The most recent report for 2017 indicates that access has improved with a significant increase in the number of people who reported having health insurance (AHRQ, 2018). Overall quality has improved, but the pace of improvement varied depending on the priority area. More than two-thirds of care measures for person-centered care and patient safety improved and half of care measures for healthy living, effective treatment, and care coordination improved (AHRQ, 2018). A majority of care affordability measures did not change at all, and disparities of care continue, especially for poor and uninsured populations (AHRQ, 2018). Many challenges remain in improving access, quality, and reducing racial, ethnic, and income disparities. All of these clinical and financial measures of the health care system have implications for nursing practice.

WHAT ARE THE TRENDS AFFECTING THE RISING COSTS OF HEALTH CARE?

Both intrinsic and extrinsic factors contribute to the rising costs of health care. Intrinsic factors include characteristics of the population, the demand for health care, and health insurance coverage. Extrinsic factors include the availability of technology, prescription drug costs, and workforce costs (Fig. 16.1).

Intrinsic Factors

The 2010 Census reported that there were 308.7 million people in the United States, and population estimates for 2017 reported there were 325.7 million people, representing an estimated 5.5% change

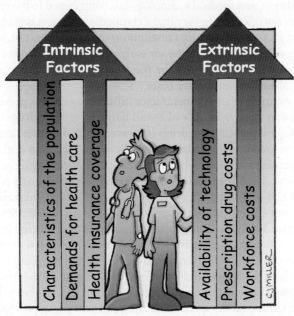

FIG. 16.1 Trends affecting the rising cost of health care.

from 2010 to 2017 (U.S. Census Bureau, 2017). According to projections for 2016 to 2050, the population age 65 years and older is expected to nearly double from 48 million to 88 million by 2050, accounting for 22.1% of the population. This increase in the aging population, an intrinsic factor, will influence health care costs and use of resources. Many persons 65 years and older on Medicare live with multiple health problems and chronic conditions, cognitive impairments, and limitations on activities of daily living (Kaiser Family Foundation, 2017a). In 2013, more than one-quarter of all Medicare beneficiaries (27%) reported being in fair or poor health (Kaiser Family Foundation, 2017a). In addition, nearly half of all people on Medicare had incomes less than $26,200 per person (Kaiser Family Foundation, 2017a). A critical challenge for the Medicare program will be to provide quality care for the increasingly aging population while keeping the program financially secure. The ACA of 2010 provided for the testing of new models, including accountable care organizations (ACOs), medical homes, and bundled payments (Kaiser Family Foundation, 2017a). Medicare spending growth is projected to be 4.5% between 2016 and 2026, an increase from 1.3% between 2010 and 2016 (Kaiser Family Foundation, 2017a). Demand, in the economic sense, is the amount of health care services that a consumer wishes to purchase. Demand for health care may be influenced by illness, cultural-demographic characteristics, and economic factors, including income and health insurance (Feldstein, 2012). Health insurance coverage is one of the most important factors that influences the quantity of health services demanded (Feldstein, 2012). With the 2014 implementation of the ACA Medicaid expansion and Health Insurance Marketplaces, the number of uninsured nonelderly Americans decreased from 44 million in 2013 to 28 million at the end of 2016 (Kaiser Family Foundation, 2017b). One of the first groups to gain expanded health insurance options under the ACA was young adults, age 19 to 25 years, who were allowed to remain as dependents on their parent's private insurance until age 26. The uninsured rate for these young adults dropped from more than 30% in 2009 to 19% in 2014 (McMorrow et al., 2015).

Extrinsic Factors

The availability of new medical technology has contributed to the rising costs of health care. If an organization does not offer technology that a competitor offers, it is likely that the market share (percentage of persons in an area selecting that institution) of the organization will decline. To attain a competitive edge, an organization needs to be an early adopter of expensive, new technology. Then, thinking sequentially, someone has to pay for the technology, and this cost will be passed on to consumers in the form of higher health care costs.

Another example of an extrinsic factor influencing costs is prescription drug spending, which may be influenced by the availability of brand name or generic drugs, new drugs, and consumer utilization. Spending for prescription drugs increased in 2014 (12.4%) and 2015 (8.9%), largely attributed to an increase in spending for hepatitis C medication (Hartman et al., 2018). In 2016, prescription drug spending decreased to 1.3%, which was more consistent with the rate of 1.2% during 2010 to 2013 (Hartman et al., 2018). Another factor driving health care costs is hospital care expenditures, which represented 32% of total health care spending during 2016, increasing by 4.7% (Hartman et al., 2018). Individuals' out-of-pocket spending for health care increased 3.9% in 2016, which was the fastest rate of growth since 2007. The increase is due to higher cost sharing in group health insurance plans and increased enrollment in consumer-directed health plans with high deductibles and copayments (Hartman et al., 2018). The Organization for Economic Cooperation and Development (OECD) compared health data for 36 industrialized countries in 2016 (OECD, 2018a). In 2016, health spending was 17.2% of GDP in the United States, which was well above the OECD average of 8.9% (OECD, 2018a). The United States spent more than $10,000 per capita (per person) on health care in 2016, which is also well above the OECD average health spending per capita in 2016 of $4069 (OECD,

2018a). In 2016, the United States continued to be number one in health care spending as a percent of GDP and also in per capita spending; however, the United States had an infant mortality rate of 5.9 deaths per 1000 live births, which is greater than the OECD average of 3.9, and a life expectancy of 78.6 years, which is 2.2 years less than the OECD average life expectancy of 80.8 years (OECD, 2018b).

> This has led some to question whether the United States has the best health care system in the world or just the most expensive.

WHAT IS THE EFFECT OF THE CHANGING ECONOMIC ENVIRONMENT ON CLINICAL PRACTICE?

Because nurses belong to the largest health care profession and are thus in a position to influence health care costs, it is essential that all nurses understand basic concepts of economics and fiscal (money) management. This knowledge was previously taught in graduate courses for nurse managers or nurse executives. However, the world has changed! Nurses at the point of care in all settings will be challenged to maintain caring values and practices in relationships with patients and families while maintaining financial responsibility within the economic reality of limited resources (Cara, Nyberg, & Brousseau, 2011).

> Currently all nurses need to couple their clinical skills with business skills that enable them to be full participants in designing and delivering health care.

HOW IS THE US HEALTH CARE SYSTEM FINANCED?

The U.S. health care system has a complex mix of public and private systems for providing health insurance and financing health care. Health insurance provides a means of financing health care expenses. In 2017, the most common ways to obtain health insurance were employer-based (56%), Medicaid (19.3%), Medicare (17.2%), individual direct purchase coverage (16%), or military coverage (4.8%) (Berchick et al., 2018). In addition, 8.8% of people, or 28.5 million, did not have health insurance during 2017 (Berchick et al., 2018). Medicaid, Medicare, and military coverage are all government or public funding. Medicaid is a public insurance program for low-income persons that is jointly administered by the federal and state governments (Kaiser Family Foundation, 2018b). Medicare is a public program administered by the federal government that is for persons 65 years and older, persons who are permanently disabled, and who have end-stage renal disease (ESRD) (Kaiser Family Foundation, 2017a).

The Affordable Care Act of 2010

The ACA of 2010 was the largest mandated health care change since Medicare and Medicaid were introduced in 1965. The timeline for implementing the ACA was from 2010 through 2015. The provisions of the law addressed issues of access, quality, and cost in the U.S. health care system (Kaiser Family Foundation, 2015) (Critical Thinking Box 16.1).

❓ CRITICAL THINKING BOX 16.1

What are the implications of the Affordable Care Act for nursing practice? Suggest strategies for nurses to assist individuals and families to understand their rights and choices under this law.

The ACA created a framework for increasing access to health coverage for Americans. Key features of the ACA include (Kaiser Family Foundation, 2015):

- Provides state and federal-based health insurance marketplaces where individuals can purchase private insurance with premium and cost-sharing assistance based on income level. Requires all health plans to provide a standardized, easy-to-read uniform Summary of Benefits and Coverage (SBC), which gives consumers consistent information and allows them to compare what health plans offer when making choices of coverage
- Prohibits denial of coverage for children with preexisting conditions beginning in 2010 and for adults with preexisting conditions beginning in 2014
- Allows young adults up to age 26 to stay on their parents' insurance policies
- Provides expanded Medicaid coverage for low-income children and adults
- Provides coverage for a range of preventive health services without any patient cost sharing (copayments, deductibles, or coinsurance)

Under the ACA, the number of uninsured Americans decreased from 44 million in 2013 to 28 million at the end of 2016 through Medicaid expansion and subsidies for low-income individuals on the Health Insurance Marketplace (Kaiser Family Foundation, 2017b).

Progress has been made to increase access and affordability of health coverage for many Americans. Challenges include that there are still 28.2 million people uninsured in 2016, and they cite high cost as the main reason for lack of insurance (Kaiser Family Foundation, 2017b). Other reasons include that they are not able to obtain insurance through a job or that they may be unaware of financial assistance available through the ACA (Kaiser Family Foundation, 2017b).

Employer-Sponsored Health Insurance

Employer-sponsored health insurance covers 152 million people, which is more than half of the nonelderly population in the United States (Kaiser Family Foundation, 2018a). The average annual premiums for employer-sponsored health insurance in 2018 were $6896 for single coverage and $19,616 for family coverage, which was an increase of 3% and 5%, respectively, over 2017. On average, most covered workers shared this cost by contributing 18% of the single premium and 29% of the family premium (Kaiser Family Foundation, 2018a).

Plan types offered by employers include preferred provider organizations (PPOs) at 49% of covered employees, high-deductible health plans with savings option (HDHPs/SO) at 29%, health maintenance organizations (HMO) at 16%, Point of Service (POS) Plan at 6%, and conventional or indemnity plan at less than 1% (Kaiser Family Foundation, 2018a). A PPO is a plan that creates a network of preferred providers, and use of the network providers is at a lower cost to plan participants than using out of network providers (Center for Medicare and Medicaid Services, 2018a). In contrast to a PPO, participants in an HMO are restricted to use of the network providers and will not be covered for out-of-network care except in an emergency (Center for Medicare and Medicaid Services, 2018a). In POS plans, participants will pay less if they use an in-network provider and, in addition, need to have a referral from their primary care provider to see a specialist (CMS, 2018a). The HDHP/SO is a high-deductible health plan with a lower premium combined with a savings account to allow participants to pay for health care expenses with money free from federal taxes (CMS, 2018a).

INTRODUCTION TO ECONOMICS

A simple definition of economics is the allocation of scarce resources. An analogy might be made to the income that an individual earns. The paycheck is a limited, finite amount of money, and choices must be made about how to spend, or allocate, the money. Such choices might include rent, a car payment, food, clothing, and health insurance payments. Individuals may not be able to pay for all of the goods or services that they wish to have, so decisions must be made and priorities established.

Similarly, health care is a limited resource, and choices have to be made. The choices about health care that concern economists are made at the national or government level. Every country must make three basic decisions that include how much the country wants to spend on health care, what services and methods the country will use to provide health care, and how health care will be distributed among the population. The first two choices are concerned with efficiency, whereas the third choice is concerned with equity. Different choices may be made by governments based on differing values and perspectives (Feldstein, 2012).

Just as governments make these choices, individuals also make choices about what they will spend and what health care services they will use. For example, health insurance coverage has a great impact on choosing to seek care. One in five uninsured adults in 2016 chose to go without needed health care due to cost (Kaiser Family Foundation, 2017b). The uninsured are less likely than those with health insurance to receive preventive care for major health problems and chronic illness. The uninsured may face unaffordable health care bills when they do seek care (Kaiser Family Foundation, 2017b).

The decisions about how health care is distributed or allocated involve the question of who gets what. The underlying question involves whether health care is a right or a commodity (like cars or clothing) to be allocated by the marketplace. The World Health Organization (WHO) states in its constitution that the enjoyment of the highest attainable standard of health is one of the fundamental rights of every human being (WHO, 2005). The American Nurses Association (ANA) Principles for Health System Transformation (ANA, 2016) also affirms that the health system must provide universal access to essential health care services for all citizens and residents. In another document, the ANA *Code of Ethics for Nurses* (ANA, 2015a) states that nurses should practice with respect for the dignity, worth, and unique characteristics of every person.

However, even if one believes that health care is a right, challenging questions remain. How much health care is a right? Who pays for the health care of people who cannot afford it? Let us assume that an instructor is teaching senior nursing students who all agree that health care is a right. The instructor then asks the students how much of their paycheck they would be willing to forfeit in taxes so that everyone could have this right to receive health care. It is rare that students are willing to subsidize others' health care at a cost of more than one-third of their own salaries.

> Think about your first paycheck as a registered nurse. How much would you be willing to give up?

Even beyond the costs of care is the question of allocation decisions—that is, who decides who receives what health care. Several responses are possible: the government, payers of health care, individuals, the marketplace, or rationing systems.

Government Allocation Decisions

Through its funding of Medicare, the government has made multiple allocation decisions. The U.S. government has decided it will pay for inpatient health care and some outpatient care for patients 65 years of age and older and for selected others. Unfortunately, many of the persons covered by Medicare have come to believe that Medicare covers "everything," and this is not so. It is particularly challenging to nurses when elderly patients assume that they "have Medicare" and thus "nursing home care is paid for." This is a frequent misinterpretation of Medicare coverage. There are many limitations to the services reimbursed by Medicare and many requirements that must be met before the government will make payment (Critical Thinking Box 16.2).

CRITICAL THINKING BOX 16.2

Hospice is reimbursed $75 per visit by Medicare Part B for home visits. For one particular group of patients, it costs hospice an average of $98 per day to provide care.
- What are the implications for hospice?
- What options should the hospice nurse manager and nurses consider?

Payer Allocation Decisions

The ACA of 2010 required all health plans to provide coverage for applicants regardless of health status, gender, or any other factors. In addition, the ACA requires plans to cover a range of preventive health services without any patient cost sharing (Kaiser Family Foundation, 2015). Within these overall guidelines, all insurance companies have rules about the services that will be covered or not covered and the requirements that must be met under their policies.

Most policies require preauthorization (preapproval) of services before the patient receives care, except in cases of emergency. For example, a physician's office will typically communicate the need for a surgical procedure to the insurance company and obtain this approval. However, if the patient is admitted to the hospital in an emergency, this requirement is normally waived, and the hospital has a limited amount of time to gain the payer approval or reimbursement for the care or the claim may be denied.

Another restriction on resource allocation involves the process of concurrent utilization review (UR). This is a strategy used by managed care companies to control both costs and quality. The process requires that hospital staff, typically registered nurses, communicate the plan of care for a hospitalized patient to the payer or their representative. The payer then determines whether the care is appropriate, is medically necessary, and is covered under the terms of the policy or the contract with the provider (Murray & Henriques, 2003). For example, if a patient is admitted to the hospital the day before elective surgery, that day's cost will almost certainly be denied reimbursement. Preoperative patient teaching and surgical preparation can be handled on an outpatient basis at a much lower cost than a day in the hospital.

Marketplace Allocation Decisions

A final alternative for the allocation of resources is the marketplace. This type of decision making implies that health care is a normal good, similar to a car or a piece of clothing, where an increase in income leads to an increase in demand for the good, and the rules of supply and demand apply. However, the market for health care includes some significant differences when compared with the market for normal goods.

Unpredictability of demand. The first difference in the market for health care is the unpredictability of demand. When a person is well, there is little demand for health care services. There is a great demand for health care when a person is ill, and the timing of illness is, of course, uncertain. For example, consider the case of a patient needing a heart transplant. A patient does not wait until the price comes down. Rather, the surgery is purchased at any price if a donor heart is available.

Consumer knowledge. Another difference in the health care market involves the knowledge of the consumer. If an individual is purchasing a coat or a car, the person usually knows a good deal about the item being purchased, or he or she consults *Consumer Reports* for further data. This is not the case in health care, about which patients tend to have limited knowledge and limited ability to interpret the available knowledge.

Barriers to entry to the market. Even if patients had sufficient knowledge to treat their own illnesses, the health care market is fraught with barriers. All providers must pass examinations and be licensed by appropriate boards. Prescriptive authority is heavily regulated and closely controlled.

Lack of price competition. The health care market, unlike the market for clothing and automobiles, does not engage in price competition. For example, when have you heard of a sale on appendectomies or "2 for the price of 1" hip replacements? Of course, it does not happen. More problematic is the fact that health care consumers frequently do not know the cost of their care—especially if an insurance provider is paying for it. In fact, many consumers indicate that they "never saw a bill" for their hospitalization. This is considered to be a measure of the quality of their insurance. Is there any other product that would be routinely purchased without knowledge of its price? The lack of this knowledge leads to predictable consumer health care purchasing behavior.

The classic Rand Health Insurance Experiment (Keeler & Rolph, 1983) was a controlled research study that examined the effect of different copayments on the use of health care. Participants in the study either received free care or paid copayments of 25%, 50%, or 95%. Economic theory would predict that as price increases, the purchase of goods or services would decline. That is exactly what happened. With a copayment of 25%, there was a decline in the use of health care of 19% compared with a free plan. There were even greater declines in the use of health care services at the higher rates of copayments. This consumer behavior is so predictable that health care economists have a term for it: *moral hazard*. It refers to a situation in which a person uses more health care services because the presence of insurance has lowered the price to the person.

A final method of allocating health care resources is some system of rationing. Rationing is a type of allocation decision that suggests a need-based system. One author defines rationing as a decision to "(1) withhold, withdraw, or fail to recommend an intervention; (2) informed by a judgment that the intervention has common sense value to the patient; (3) made with the belief that the limitation of health care resources is acute and seriously threatens some members of the economic community; and (4) motivated by a plan of promoting the health care needs of unidentified others in the economic community to which the patient belongs" (Sulmasy, 2007, p. 219). Americans find this inherently distasteful. One example of a rationing decision is to not perform heart transplants on patients older than 65 years, with the rationale that the money could be spent on, for example, well-child immunization programs. The major ethical questions (Sulmasy, 2007) involved in rationing decisions include (1) who makes the decision, and (2) using what criteria? However, most Americans find the concept of rationing inherently unacceptable. The counterargument to this position is that rationing occurs every day in the U.S. health care system, but the decision is currently made on the basis of the individual's ability to pay for care.

BUDGETS

A *budget* is a tool that helps to make allocation decisions and to plan for expenditures. It is important for staff nurses to understand budget processes, because these decisions directly impact their clinical practice. For example, staff nurses working on a patient-care unit may feel that there is not enough time to care for acutely ill patients on the unit. A clinical manager may respond that the "budget will not allow" additional staff. The reality is that the budget is a human-made planning tool and must be flexible to be useful. Savvy staff nurses will understand the budget process and be able to relate patient acuity to staffing needs. To engage in these discussions, all nurses need to understand basic concepts of budgets as well as different types of budgets: capital budgets, operating budgets, and personnel budgets (Fig. 16.2).

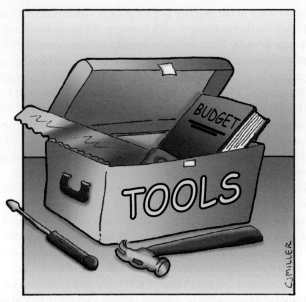

FIG. 16.2 Budget—a tool that helps make allocation decisions.

What Are the Basic Concepts of Budgets?

When preparing a budget, one must first consider the unit that the document or budget will serve. It could be an entire hospital, a department, or an individual patient-care unit. This discussion will focus on the budget of a patient-care unit, because that is the work environment of most registered nurses.

Here are the basic terms that nurses must know:

Revenue: All the money brought into the unit as payment for a good or a service. Some departments in the hospital are defined as revenue centers. Examples might include radiology or surgery. Typically, these departments generate a great deal of income for the larger organization.

Expense: All the costs of producing a product. Nursing care units are typically labeled as cost centers; that is, they do not directly generate revenue. Most hospitals have a fixed room rate that includes nursing care. Nurse leaders have questioned the appropriateness of nursing care being lumped into the room rate, but few have been able to effect a change. Some exceptions to this include nursing care to patients in the recovery room, intensive care unit, or labor and delivery area, where there is a separate charge for nursing care.

Margin (or profit): Revenue minus expenses equals margin or profit. Nurses may cringe at the thought of hospitals making a profit, but every hospital—whether it is defined as a *not-for-profit hospital* or a *for-profit hospital*—must make a profit. Profits are needed to replace equipment, purchase new technology, and, in some cases, provide care for indigent patients. In addition, for-profit hospitals must pay stockholders a return on their investment. The necessity of making a profit is so crucial to the continued existence of an organization that there is an old adage that states, "No margin, no mission." This means that if an organization does not make a profit, it is unable to fulfill the purpose or mission of the organization, no matter what it might be. The lay public will often describe hospitals as "for profit" or "not for profit." Often faith-based institutions are included in the latter category. In reality, all hospitals must make a profit. It is more significant how the profit is used.

What Are the Types of Budgets?

The budget process involves the development of three budget types that are combined to make an overall budget for the patient-care unit: the capital budget, operating budget, and personnel budget. The budget covers a 12-month period that may begin January 1, July 1, or October 1, depending on the organization.

Capital Budget

The beginning point of a budget cycle is usually the *capital budget*. Hospital administrators usually ask departments or patient-care units for a list of items that their area will need to purchase in the coming year. These items are usually restricted to equipment costing more than $5000 and lasting more than 1 year. Each manager must rank such requests for the unit and write a justification of the necessity for the item. For example, at a unit level, the nurse manager may request replacement beds, telemetry equipment, or computers. Most managers will discuss unit needs with staff nurses and seek their input. Staff nurses do the work of the organization and are in the best position to know what is needed for patient care. So be ready to make suggestions. Keep a running list of all the things you wish you had available to you to improve patient care, so when it is time to budget for the next year, and your manager asks for ideas, you will be ready to share. Next, all of the organization's needs are summarized and prioritized according to the funds available. Rarely is there sufficient capital to fund all the requests, and difficult allocation decisions and choices must be made.

Operating Budgets

This budget includes a statement of the expected expenses of the unit for a period, usually 1 year. The budget process begins with a statement of volume projections. The nurse manager projects how much patient care will be provided in the coming year. The volume that nurses are concerned with is measured in patient days, and thus the question is "How many patient days of care will be provided in the coming year?" The manager would first look at past data to examine how many days were given in the previous year. It is also helpful to look at monthly data, to determine whether there was a month that exceeded projections, perhaps a month in which there was a flu epidemic or one that had a very low number of patient days because of vacations of medical staff who admit patients. Knowledge of these trends helps the manager to project volume for the subsequent year. The manager would next consider any changes in the patient-care unit that might affect volume projections. For example, if two new surgeons were added to the staff, if the unit would begin to provide care for a new clinical population of patients, or if the unit would be newly designated as the overflow unit for same-day surgery patients, all of these factors would increase the volume projections.

In an outpatient setting, the nurse manager of a clinic considers the volume of patient-care visits. The manager carefully considers anything that might increase or decrease that volume in the coming year. This might include adding more clinic exam rooms, retirement or addition of professional providers, or events and changes within the provision of, and competition for, health care dollars in the geographic area.

In addition to projecting the patient day volume, nurse managers also examine the activity of the unit and the acuity (the intensity of care required) of patients. The activity is usually described as *admissions, discharges, and transfers* (ADTs). One measure of activity is the average daily census—that is, how many patients are occupying beds on the unit at midnight. However, this measure by itself results in an underestimation of the work of the unit. A more accurate picture is gained by the addition of the ADT data because even though these patients may not be counted in a midnight census, they require many hours of care by registered nurses (Critical Thinking Box 16.3).

❓ CRITICAL THINKING BOX 16.3

In most hospitals, nursing care is "lumped in" with the room charge, and thus nursing care is an expense in the budget and not a revenue center. Most patients (except intensive care unit, step-down, labor and delivery, recovery room) pay the same amount for nursing care.

What are the advantages/disadvantages of this situation for nursing?

Nurse managers must also consider the acuity of the patients on the unit. In an intensive care unit, patients are extremely ill and require many hours of care per day. The number of care hours decreases as patients are moved to general patient-care units. Each organization considers the acuity of patients but may use different methods of arriving at measurements. There are several computerized software packages available whereby nurses enter patient data and the software program produces estimates of the staffing needs of the unit. Programs are designed for each clinical population of patients (e.g., obstetrics, pediatrics, psychiatry). Nurses enter data concerning many factors, including numbers of patients, functional abilities, telemetry monitoring, and postoperative day. These factors help to define how much care patients need and thus can be used to project staffing needs. At the time the budget is created, the nurse manager can review the data to see whether the staffing planned for the unit was adequate to meet patient-care needs.

On a daily basis, there may be vacant beds on a patient-care unit. However, if there were not a sufficient number of registered nurses available to provide care for the patients who *could potentially* occupy these beds, the unit would not be able to accept additional admissions. Therefore the nurse manager frequently reports "available staffed beds" rather than "vacant beds." When there are no available staffed beds, it is a critical situation. The manager may be asked to work on increasing the supply of nurses by calling in additional staff. Another strategy might be to identify patients who could be safely discharged early if required. In the worst-case scenario, the emergency department may divert potential patients to another hospital, a situation that hospital administration executives deplore! The nurse manager must be prepared to advocate for safe patient care in these situations.

The *operating budget* also includes all of the items necessary for care on the unit. These are called *line items* in a budget and include such things as supplies, telephones, small equipment (e.g., wheelchairs, nurse pagers, fax machines), postage, and copying costs. Some of these are *variable costs* (i.e., costs that change with the volume of patients cared for in a year). Some institutions would include a factor for the variable costs of housekeeping or laundry. There may be a line item for travel for staff nurses to attend clinical conferences or to pay for specialty certification of nurses. These are expenses frequently paid by employing organizations. Other costs, such as heat and electricity, are considered *fixed costs* that do not change with the number of patients. A nurse manager considers all these things when planning an operating budget (Critical Thinking Box 16.4).

❓ CRITICAL THINKING BOX 16.4

As a staff nurse, you have been asked to serve on your unit's financial management committee. You have been told to reduce overall expenses by 3%—in any way you choose to do it.

Given the definitions of fixed and variable costs, where do you think you could begin to look for cost reductions? Develop some ideas of possible cost reductions. Remember that your commitment is to preserve the high quality of patient care.

Personnel Budget

The *personnel budget* for a nursing unit is the largest part of unit expenses, and nursing is the largest part of personnel expense. In most hospitals, nursing costs represent at least 50% of hospital expense budgets (Pappas, 2008). This has caused some hospital administrators, who need to reduce expenses, to state:

"Follow the dollars, and they will lead to nursing."

Staff nurses need to understand how a nurse manager determines the number of nurses required for patient care. As discussed, beginning considerations are acuity of patients and the volume or number of patients. The nurse manager must also consider the clinical expertise of the nursing staff. If a unit has a high percentage of new graduates, there will be a decreased ability to safely care for a higher volume of acutely ill patients on the unit. Next, the nurse manager engages in a series of calculations, all of which are easily understood by staff nurses.

Hours per patient day (HPPD). Each patient-care unit will have a designated number of hours of care per patient day. In an intensive care unit, this might be as high as 22 hours per day; on a general surgical unit, it might be 6 to 8 hours. However, nurses need to be aware that these hours must be spread over three shifts (if the organization uses 8-hour shifts) or two shifts (in the case of 12-hour shifts). Nurse managers typically derive *staffing patterns* (i.e., combinations of staff [RNs, LPNs, nursing assistants]) that are needed for each shift. These may vary for weekends, nights, and even days of the week. For example, if Monday is a day when many surgical procedures are performed, staffing must include higher numbers of registered nurses to assess and monitor postoperative patients.

Full-time equivalent. A full-time equivalent (FTE) represents the number of hours that a nurse employed full time is available to perform all of the employment activities. This is calculated to be 2080 hours (52 weeks times 40 hours), but it is usually split into productive and nonproductive time (Hunt, 2001).

Productive time. This figure reflects the amount of time the nurse is available to provide care to patients. For example, one work day (8 hours) is usually considered to be 7.5 productive hours.

Nonproductive time. This time reflects the amount of time that is not available for direct care. Some examples of nonproductive time include vacations, days off, holidays, time at educational seminars, time for committee work (e.g., quality improvement), breaks, and lunch. If these factors are not calculated into the budget, staffing needs may be seriously underestimated. Skilled nurse managers know their staff and can project nonproductive time. For example, if a unit has a very senior staff that accrues annual vacations of 4 to 6 weeks, this must be considered in the budgeting process.

What Are the Economics of Caring?

As clinicians, many nurses are reluctant to incorporate knowledge of health care economics into their clinical practice, feeling that it makes them somehow less compassionate or less caring. However, it can be argued that the reason nurses must understand health care economics is that they can bring the values of nursing to the decision-making process for patient care. They can become advocates for patients in the budget process. For example, an administrator with a masters of business administration degree may examine the budget of a nursing care unit and make a decision to decrease staffing. A nurse who understands the budgeting process and the research evidence about nurse staffing and patient outcomes can argue persuasively against reductions in nursing hours per patient day (HPPD).

It is also important for staff nurses to be able to evaluate the research that provides the evidence for clinical practice change. Many nurses report that their goal is to provide "cost-effective care." However, they use this term loosely and do not understand the economic analysis strategy of cost-effectiveness analysis (CEA). This strategy provides information about the cost of an intervention and the effectiveness of an intervention.

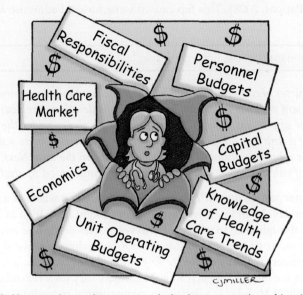

FIG. 16.3 Nurses play an important role in the economics of health care.

At the level of providing care for individual patients, staff nurses must understand fiscal responsibility for clinical practice. *Fiscal responsibility* concerns a threefold responsibility: first to the patient, second to the employing institution, and finally to the payer of health care. It is defined as the duty/obligation of the nurse to allocate (1) financial resources of the patient to maximize the patient's health benefit, (2) financial resources of the employer to maximize organizational cost-effectiveness, and (3) financial resources of the payer by using knowledge and efficiency (Fig. 16.3).

Fiscal Responsibility to the Patient

The primary fiscal responsibility of the nurse is always, most important, to the patient. This means that a nurse uses the most cost-efficient combination of resources to maximize the health benefit to the patient. Nurses need to understand the costs of care and different reimbursement systems, because this will affect the development of a care plan. It is important for nurses to assess the resources that patients have available to dedicate to health care. These may include not only insurance coverage but also the availability of family members or community resources to aid in care.

For example, many churches team up to provide transportation to treatment locations for patients receiving chemotherapy. Communities vary widely in the resources they offer to patients and families. There may be free support groups, online chat rooms, or Meals on Wheels services available. All of these are valuable community health care resources that are not monetary.

In another example, when creating a discharge plan for a patient, it is essential that a nurse understand the health care resources the patient requires and how they will be paid for. A physician may write orders for prescription medications that are not covered by the patient's insurance. Patients are often reluctant to admit that they cannot afford these medications, and they may either choose not to fill the prescription or may go without other necessities to purchase the medication. Sometimes patients even resort to cutting medications in half to make them "last longer," thereby receiving only a partial dose of the medication. If nurses understand patients' insurance coverage and include this in assessment data, they can make better plans of care. It is especially important that nurses understand Medicare coverage because in some hospitals, more than 50% of patients have this coverage. Table 16.1

TABLE 16.1 BASICS OF MEDICARE INSURANCE COVERAGE

WHICH PART OF MEDICARE	COST	DESCRIPTION OF COVERAGE	DOES NOT COVER
Medicare Part A	Usually no premium if the individual or the spouse paid Medicare taxes while working. Copayments, coinsurance, or deductibles may apply for some services.	Hospital care, hospice care, home health care, and inpatient care in a skilled nursing facility following a 3-day hospital stay	Custodial or long-term care in a skilled nursing facility
Medicare Part B	There is a monthly Part B premium. Most people will pay the standard premium amount, which was $134 in 2018. For covered services, enrollees must meet the yearly Part B deductible before Medicare begins to pay its share. Then, after the deductible is met, enrollees typically pay 20% of the Medicare-approved amount of the service if the health care provider accepts assignment.	Services from doctors and other health care providers, outpatient care, home health care, durable medical equipment, and many preventive services	Routine dental care, dentures, hearing aids, eye examinations for prescribing glasses, or cosmetic surgery
Medicare Part C	MA plans—a plan like an HMO or a PPO plan. Medicare will pay a fixed amount each month to the private insurance company providing the MA Plan.	Run by Medicare-approved private insurance plans. The MA Plan covers all of Part A and Part B and usually includes prescription drug coverage as part of the plan. May offer additional benefits such as hearing, vision, and dental coverage, as well as health and wellness programs for an additional cost.	Might not cover if an individual goes outside of the selected provider network. The individual must follow plan rules, such as obtaining a referral to see a specialist. The individual may only join a plan at certain times during the year and is expected to stay in the plan for a year.
Medicare Part D	Medicare drug coverage: Individual must have Part A and/or Part B. Most plans charge a monthly premium that varies depending on the plan chosen.	Prescriber must be enrolled in Medicare or have "opted-out" in order for prescriptions to be covered under Part D. There is a yearly deductible before the plan begins to pay. Copay—Amounts the individual pays at the pharmacy after the deductible. Coverage gap—After the individual and the plan have paid a certain amount for covered drugs, the "coverage gap" or "donut hole" is reached. In 2019, once you enter the coverage gap, you pay 25% of the plan's cost for brand name and 37% for generic drugs until you reach the end of the coverage gap. Not everyone will enter the coverage gap because their drug costs will not be high enough. After the yearly out-of-pocket limit is reached, the individual receives "catastrophic" insurance whereby the individual again pays only the copay for covered drugs the rest of the year.	Limits on how much medication the individual can obtain at one time Drugs not on the plan's list of approved drugs ("formulary") are not covered.

HMO, Health maintenance organization; *MA plans*, Medicare advantage plans; *PPO*, preferred provider organization.
(From Centers for Medicare & Medicaid Services [2018b]. *Medicare and you 2019*. Retrieved from https://www.medicare.gov/Pubs/pdf/10050-Medicare-and-You.pdf.)

summarizes the basics of Medicare insurance. Nurses need to be aware that the coverage for Medicare is very complex, and the complete documentation for coverage is available online.

It is also important that nurses engage in early discharge planning, beginning the process on admission or even before admission. For example, if a patient is to have a scheduled surgery for hip replacement, the nurse in the orthopedic surgery clinic may talk with the patient about convalescence and continued physical therapy in the rehabilitation unit of a skilled nursing facility. If this process is done before admission, the patient and the family will have the opportunity to visit several facilities and make a selection.

It is important to understand that this does not mean that patients will not receive care or medications if the patient cannot afford to pay for it. It does mean that the nurse will work to ensure that patients receive the care they need, regardless of their ability to pay. In the example of a patient who is to be discharged with a prescription that he or she cannot afford, there may be programs within the hospital that provide low-cost medications. Another alternative is to determine whether a generic drug is available at a lower cost. Some patients even choose to order their prescriptions by mail from Canada to obtain medication at lower costs. This practice is legal in some states and illegal in others. So, before you make this suggestion to a patient, make sure it is legal in your state.

It is also important that nurses understand that fiscal responsibility for clinical practice is a responsibility shared with all other health care disciplines. Nurse practitioners and physicians write orders requiring medications, diagnostic procedures, and laboratory tests. Therefore they share fiscal responsibility. Clinical social workers have a great knowledge of health care resources available to patients both in the hospital and in the community. All members of the interdisciplinary team share this responsibility and contribute to the goal of maximizing the benefit of health care resources for patients (Fig. 16.4).

Nurses also need to advocate for staffing levels that will permit them the time they need to monitor and assess their patients (i.e., time to exercise their clinical judgment). Research has demonstrated that nursing care makes a difference in preventing patient deaths and complications (Needleman et al., 2006). Using this evidence to support requests for additional nursing hours to care for acutely ill patients is a rational and respectful way to communicate.

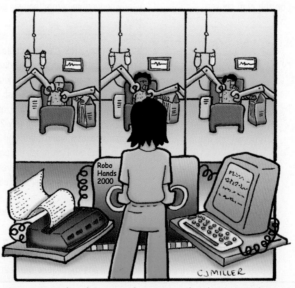

FIG. 16.4 Advances in computer technology continue to assist the nurse, but technology cannot replace the humanistic aspect of nursing care.

Fiscal Responsibility to the Employing Organization

Nurses also have a responsibility to the organization or agency where they are employed. The most important way for a nurse to demonstrate fiscal responsibility is by providing quality patient care. For example, thorough hand hygiene and the use of sanitizing gels prevent infections that may increase patient costs. Similarly, the prevention of falls and pressure ulcers is a clinical practice that has significant cost implications (Research for Best Practice Boxes 16.1 and 16.2).

> Nurses who continually improve their clinical practice by using evidence-based practice or "best practice" guidelines are also engaging in quality practice that is cost-effective.

🔍 RESEARCH FOR BEST PRACTICE BOX 16.1

Cost of Nurse-Sensitive Adverse Events

Practice Issue

In a time of increasing health care costs and an emphasis on providing safe, high-quality care to patients, nurses need to understand the cost of complications that are related to nursing care.

Implications for Nursing Practice

- Pappas (2008) studied five adverse events: medication errors, falls, urinary tract infections, pneumonia, and pressure ulcers.
- For patients with health failure, the cost of an adverse event was $1029.
- For surgical patients, the cost of an adverse event was $903.
- The odds of pneumonia occurring in surgical patients decreased with additional registered nurse hours per patient day.

Considering this Information

What is an argument grounded in best practice that you can make to ensure that quality care (remember this is the consideration of cost and quality) is provided to patients?

Reference

Pappas, S. H. (2008). The cost of nurse-sensitive adverse events. *Journal of Nursing Administration, 38,* 230–236.

🔍 RESEARCH FOR BEST PRACTICE BOX 16.2

Preventing Pressure Ulcers on the Heel: A Canadian Cost Study

Practice Issue

The heel is an area that is especially at risk for the development of pressure ulcers.

Implications for Nursing Practice

In a study conducted by Bou et al. (2009), two methods of preventing pressure ulcers on the heel were compared:

- Method A involved protective bandaging plus usual care.
- Method B provided a hydrocellular dressing for protection of the heel in addition to usual care.

  44% of patients in the Method A group developed pressure ulcers on the heel compared with 3.3% in the Method B group. The Method B group cost $11.67 more per patient to provide than the Method A group.

Considering this Information

Based on the research, what argument can you make for the more expensive treatment?

Reference

Bou, J. E., Rueda López, J., Camañes, G., Herrero Narváez, E., Blanco Blanco, J., Ballesté Torralba, J., et al. (2009). Preventing pressure ulcers on the heel: A Canadian cost study. *Journal of the Dermatology Nurses' Association, 21,* 268–272.

Nurses also have an obligation to use the resources of the institution wisely. The most costly health care resource that nurses allocate is their time. The nurse considers patient-care needs and prioritizes how professional nursing time shall be allocated. Although it would be ideal for nurses to have unlimited time with each patient, it is not possible. As a beginning point, the nurse knows that the most important reason that a patient is hospitalized is to receive assessment and monitoring by a registered nurse. If a patient does not need this assessment, it is likely that the patient can be safely treated in a less expensive health care setting, such as a skilled nursing facility. The care plans that nurses develop and implement include prioritizing the needs of unstable patients. At other times, it is decided that the patient and family require teaching from a professional nurse. It may also be that the patient and family require psychosocial support, a nursing intervention that requires a high level of nursing expertise.

Nurses also need to understand the *prospective payment system*. Under this system, the hospital is paid a set amount for the care of a patient with a certain condition or surgery. If the hospital engages in efficient clinical care practices, the organization makes a profit. If the hospital is not efficient, it may lose money. Medicare reimburses under this prospective system—called *diagnostic-related groups (DRGs)*—as do many private insurance companies.

This system has had a large impact on nursing practice. For example, if the nurse does not have a discharge plan in place on the day a discharge decision is made, perhaps because of the lack of planning for transportation for a patient, it may be that the patient will remain in the hospital for an additional day while arrangements are made. This incurs unnecessary costs for the hospital. From another perspective, an unnecessary hospital day is a quality issue. Patients in the hospital are subject to the possibility of infection, the hazards of immobility and bed rest, and even the potential for malnutrition. As mandated by the ACA, hospitals will not receive reimbursement for care related to "never events," such as pressure ulcers, falls, and hospital-acquired infections (Sherman & Bishop, 2012). In addition, hospitals will lose Medicare reimbursement if too many of their patients are being readmitted within 30 days of hospital discharge (Sherman & Bishop, 2012).

Another way that nurses practice fiscal responsibility is by accurately documenting the patient's condition. This must include the severity of the patient's illness, as well as the plan of care. If this is not documented, insurance companies may not reimburse for the care. For example, if the nurse documents "up and about with no complaints," it is very likely that the hospital day will not be covered by insurance. However, if the nurse documents the assessments and monitoring that are being done at frequent intervals, the care will likely be reimbursed.

There are other ways in which nurses recognize institutional fiscal responsibility. For example, the nurse should be aware of bringing only the needed supplies into a patient room because any unused supplies cannot be returned to stock. Some supplies are charged to patients when used. The fiscally responsible nurse makes this a part of practice, if required.

Another example involves breaks and meal times. The nurse takes breaks and meal times as scheduled, to remain healthy and fully functioning on the job. A shift may occasionally be hectic, and it may not be possible to take breaks, but if this is the norm, it is a situation that creates burnout and should be investigated and resolved.

Fiscal Responsibility to the Payer of Care

At present, the U.S. government is the largest single payer of health care. For government-funded care such as Medicare and Medicaid, the ultimate payer then is the taxpayer. For private insurance, the payer may be the insurance company selected by an employer or by an individual. In all cases, the nurse has the obligation to use resources efficiently and effectively. The nurse needs to provide documentation that the patient requires care in the appropriate setting. This includes communicating the severity of the patient's illness as well as the plan of care. Without this documentation, the payer may

---

BOX 16.1 STRATEGIES FOR FISCALLY RESPONSIBLE CLINICAL PRACTICE

The nurse:
- Provides quality nursing care that prevents complications
- Makes conscious decisions about the allocation of professional nursing time
- Understands Medicare and Medicaid insurance coverage
- Engages in evidence-based practice and follows best practice guidelines
- Shares information with patients and families about the costs of care and alternatives
- Assigns assistive personnel (nurse aides, certified medical assistants) appropriately to help with care and recognizes the nurse is ultimately responsible for the care provided
- Works with the members of other health care professions to promote fiscal responsibility for clinical practice
- Documents patient condition accurately
- Begins discharge planning on or before admission
- Completes charge slips for patient supplies, if required
- Avoids burnout by taking scheduled breaks, meal times, and vacations
- Engages in safe clinical practice that will avoid personal injuries

---

BOX 16.2 QUESTIONS FOR THE NEW GRADUATE TO CONSIDER ASKING DURING A JOB INTERVIEW

- How are financial concerns of patients handled? For example, if a patient is unable to afford needed medications on discharge, what resources are available to nurses to help the patient?
- How is acuity of patients assessed and factored into staffing?
- What are the budgeted hours per patient day for the unit?
- What is the turnover rate on this unit? Why do nurses stay on/leave this unit?
- How do staff nurses have input into capital budget requests for the unit?
- How are data about unit financial indicators communicated to the staff?
- What percentage of salary is used as an estimate of fringe benefits?
- What is the overtime rate on this unit?
- Can you tell me about the discharge planning process for patients on this unit?
- What is the staff development plan for professional nurses on this unit?

---

determine that a particular level of care is not necessary and may not reimburse for that care. It is also clear that the application of evidence-based practice guidelines will enable the nurse to select interventions that are cost-effective and that result in the best outcomes.

Box 16.1 summarizes some strategies to help achieve fiscally responsible clinical practice. Box 16.2 summarizes some questions that a new graduate of a nursing program might want to ask during a job interview to assess how a prospective employer views fiscal responsibility. See the end of the chapter for relevant websites and online resources regarding economics in nursing practice. These resources will be beneficial for you as you begin your profession.

CONCLUSION

Given the dire predictions about health care costs being forecast for the next 10 years, it is imperative that nurses consider the economics of clinical practice. Throughout most of nursing history, nurses have not wanted to learn about the costs of care, considering such concerns about as important or as appealing as unnecessary paperwork. Nurses proclaim that they want to be caregivers, not accountants. However, nurses humanize health care institutions. Not only do they bring the values of caring and compassion to the workplace, but they represent the largest health professional group. As representatives of the largest health professional group, nurses can contribute to controlling healthcare costs by incorporating fiscal responsibility into clinical practice.

🌐 RELEVANT WEBSITES AND ONLINE RESOURCES

Agency for Health Care Research and Quality (AHRQ)
www.ahrq.gov.

American Nurses Association: Health Care Reform
https://www.nursingworld.org/practice-policy/health-policy/health-system-reform/

Centers for Medicare & Medicaid Services (CMS)
www.cms.gov.

Health Care Reform: Affordable Care Act (ACA)
www.healthcare.gov.

Kaiser Family Foundation
http://kff.org/.

Medicare
http://www.medicare.gov/.

Medicaid
http://www.medicaid.gov/.

Organization for Economic Co-operation and Development (OECD)
http://www.oecd.org/.

World Health Organization
http://www.who.int.

BIBLIOGRAPHY

Agency for Healthcare Research and Quality (AHRQ). (2018). 2017 National healthcare quality and disparities report. Rockville, MD: AHRQ Publication. No. 18-0033-EF. Retrieved from www.ahrq.gov/research/findings/nhqrdr/index.html.

American Nurses Association. (2016). ANA's Principles for Health System Transformation. 2016. Retrieved from: https://www.nursingworld.org/~4afd6b/globalassets/practiceandpolicy/health-policy/principles-healthsystemtransformation.pdf.

American Nurses Association. (2015a). *Code of ethics for nurses with interpretative statements*. Silver Spring, MD: Publishing Program of ANA. Nursesbooks.org.

American Nurses Association. (2015b). Nursing: Scope and standards of practice. In *Silver Spring* (3rd ed.). MD: Publishing Program of ANANursesbooks.org.

Berchick, E. R., Hood, E., & Barnett, J. C. (2018). Health Insurance Coverage in the United States: 2017. Washington D.C.: US Government Printing Office. Retrieved from: https://www.census.gov/content/dam/Census/library/publications/2018/demo/p60-264.pdf.

Cara, C. M., Nyberg, J. J., & Brousseau, S. (2011). Fostering the coexistence of caring philosophy and economics in today's health care system. *Nursing Administration Quarterly, 35*(1), 6–14.

Feldstein, P. J. (2012). *Health care economics* (7th ed.). New York: Delmar.

Centers for Medicare and Medicaid Services (CMS). (2018a). HealthCare.gov glossary. Retrieved at: https://www.healthcare.gov/glossary/.

Centers for Medicare & Medicaid Services (CMS). (2018b). Medicare and You 2019. Retrieved from https://www.medicare.gov/Pubs/pdf/10050-Medicare-and-You.pdf.

Hartman, M., Martin, A. B., Espinosa, N., Catlin, A., & the National Health Expenditure Accounts Team. (2018). National health spending in 2016: Spending and enrollment growth slow after initial coverage expansions. *Health Affairs, 37*(1), 150–160. https://doi.org/10.1377/hlthaff.2017.129. Retrieved from https://www.healthaffairs.org/doi/pdf/10.1377/hlthaff.2017.1299.

Hunt, P. S. (2001). Speaking the language of finance. *Association of Perioperative Registered Nurses Journal, 73,* 774–787.

Kaiser Family Foundation. (2018a). 2018 Employer health benefits survey. Retrieved from https://www.kff.org/report-section/2018-employer-health-benefits-survey-abstract/.

Kaiser Family Foundation. (2018b). Issue brief: 10 things about Medicaid: Setting the facts straight. Retrieved at: http://files.kff.org/attachment/Issue-Brief-10-Things-to-Know-about-Medicaid-Setting-the-Facts-Straight.

Kaiser Family Foundation. (2017a). Issue brief: An overview of Medicare. Retrieved from https://www.kff.org/medicare/issue-brief/an-overview-of-medicare/.

Kaiser Family Foundation. (2017b). Fact sheet: Key facts about the uninsured population. Retrieved from https://www.kff.org/uninsured/fact-sheet/key-facts-about-the-uninsured-population/.

Kaiser Family Foundation. (2015). Issue brief: The coverage provisions in the Affordable Care Act: An update. Retrieved from http://kff.org/health-reform/issue-brief/the-coverage-provisions-in-the-affordable-care-act-an-update/.

Cuckler, G. A., Sisko, A. M., Poisal, J. A., Keehan, S. P., Smith, S. D., Madison, A. J., et al. (2018). National health expenditure projections, 2017-26: Despite uncertainty, fundamentals primarily drive spending growth. *Health Affairs, 37*(3), 482–492. https://doi.org/10.1377/hlthaff.2017.1655.

Keeler, E. B., & Rolph, J. E. (1983). How cost sharing reduced medical spending of participants in the health insurance experiment. *Journal of the American Medical Association, 249,* 2220–2222.

McMorrow, S., Kenney, G. M., Long, S. K., & Anderson, N. (2015). Uninsurance among young adults continues to decline, particularly in Medicaid expansion states. *Health Affairs, 34*(4), 616–620.

Murray, M. E., & Henriques, J. B. (2003). Denials of reimbursement under managed care. *Managed Care Interface, 16,* 22–27.

Needleman, J., Buerhaus, P. I., Steward, M., Zelevinsky, K., & Mattke, S. (2006). Nurse staffing in hospitals: Is there a business case for quality? *Health Affairs, 25,* 204–211.

Organization for Economic Co-operation and Development (OECD). (2018a). Spending on Health: Latest Trends. Retrieved from http://www.oecd.org/health/health-systems/Health-Spending-Latest-Trends-Brief.pdf.

Organization for Economic Co-operation and Development (OECD). (2018b). OECD Health Statistics 2018. Retrieved from http://www.oecd.org/els/health-systems/health-data.htm.

Pappas, S. H. (2008). The cost of nurse-sensitive adverse events. *Journal of Nursing Administration, 38,* 230–236.

Sherman, R., & Bishop, M. (2012). The business of caring: What every nurse should know about cutting costs. *American Nurse Today, 7*(11), 32–34.

Sulmasy, D. P. (2007). Cancer care, money, and the value of life: Whose justice? Which rationality? *Journal of Clinical Oncology, 25,* 217–222.

Census Bureau, U. S. (2017). Quick facts United States: Population estimates July, 1, 2017. Retrieved from https://www.census.gov/quickfacts/fact/table/US/PST045217.

U.S. Census Bureau. (March 28, 2016). U.S. population aging slower than other countries, Census bureau reports. Report Number CB16-54. Retrieved from https://www.census.gov/newsroom/press-releases/2016/cb16-54.html.

World Health Organization. (2005). Constitution of the World Health Organization. Retrieved from http://www.who.int/governance/eb/who_constitution_en.pdf.

17

Political Action in Nursing

Michael L. Evans, PhD, RN, NEA-BC, FACHE, FAAN

ⓔhttp://evolve.elsevier.com/Zerwekh/nsgtoday/.

One of the penalties for refusing to participate in politics is that you end up being governed by your inferiors.
Plato

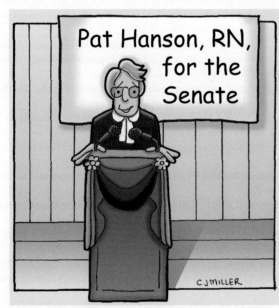

Nurses are playing a major role in the political process for planning the future of health care.

After completing this chapter, you should be able to:
- Define politics and political involvement.
- State the rationale for a nurse to become involved in the political process.
- List specific strategies needed to begin to affect the laws that govern the practice of nursing and the health care system.
- Discuss different types of power and how each is obtained.
- Describe the function of a political action committee.
- Discuss selected issues affecting nursing: multistate licensure, nursing and collective bargaining, and equal pay for work of comparable value.

Too often, nurses feel that the legislative process is associated with wheeling and dealing, smoke-filled rooms, and the exchange of money, favors, and influence. Many believe politics to be a world that excludes people with ethics and sincerity—especially given the controversies in presidential administrations and political party ideologies that so often result in gridlock. Others think only the wealthy, ruthless, or very brave play the game of politics. It seems that most nurses feel that the messy business of politicking should be left to others while they (nurses) do what they do best and enjoy most: taking care of patients.

However, nurses are currently coming to realize that politics is not a one-dimensional arena but a complex struggle with strict rules and serious outcomes. In a typical modern-day political struggle, a rural health care center may be pitted for funding against a major interstate highway. Certainly, both projects have merit, but in times of limited resources, not everyone can be victorious. Nurses are now aware that to influence the development of public policy in ways that affect how we are able to deliver care, we must be engaged in the political process.

A powerful asset that nurses have to build political influence is the public trust in nurses. The Gallup Organization has conducted an annual survey for years in which the honesty and ethical standards of 22 occupations is assessed. For well over a decade, nurses are rated at the top of the list each year; 84% of Americans describe nurses' ethical standards and honesty as "very high" or "high" (Gallup, 2018).

Leavitt and colleagues (2002) wrote that "the future of nursing and health care may well depend on nurses' skills in moving a vision. Without a vision, politics becomes an end in itself—a game that is often corrupt and empty" (p. 86). To demonstrate these skills, nurses must elect the decision makers, testify before legislative committee hearings, compromise, and get themselves elected to decision-making positions. Nurses realize that involvement in the political process is a vital tool that they must learn to use if they are to carry out their mission (providing quality patient care) with maximum impact.

Nurses' recognition of problems in the current health care system, and their commitment to the principle that health care is a *right* of all citizens, fuel their desire to become active in the political arena and to form a collective force to improve the health care system.

An example of the power of the nursing collective is evidenced in organized nursing's efforts to provide support and defense for a Texas nurse who was discharged from her hospital position for reporting a physician to the Texas Medical Board for medical patient care that the nurse believed was unsafe (ANA, 2010; Conde, 2010). The nurse, a member of the Texas Nurses Association and the American Nurses Association (ANA), also faced a third-degree felony charge for "misuse of official information."

The Texas Nurses Association became aware of the case and immediately offered to support the nurse involved in the case and enlisted the support from the ANA as well. The call went out from the ANA to all nurses, and more than $45,000 was donated both by individuals and organizations from across the United States to support the defense of this nurse. The ANA and the Texas Nurses Association strongly criticized the criminal charges and the fact that this case could have a long-term negative impact on nurses who are acting as whistle-blowers advocating for their patients.

The case went to trial, and a jury found the nurse not guilty. The ANA president at the time, Rebecca M. Patton, RN, MSN, CNOR, said of the outcome, "ANA is relieved and satisfied that Anne Mitchell (RN) was vindicated and found not guilty on these outrageous criminal charges—today's verdict is a resounding win on behalf of patient safety in the U.S. Nurses play a critical, duty-bound role in acting as patient safety watch guards in our nation's health care system. The message the jury sent is clear: the freedom for nurses to report a physician's unsafe medical practices is nonnegotiable. However, ANA remains shocked and deeply disappointed that this sort of blatant retaliation was allowed to take place and reach the trial stage—a different outcome could have endangered patient safety across the U.S., having a potential chilling effect that would make nurses think twice before reporting shoddy medical practice. Nurse whistle-blowers should never be fired and criminally charged for reporting questionable medical care" (ANA, 2010, para 5).

It is important for nurses to join and to support nursing organizations that advocate and lobby on behalf of nurses, nursing, and quality health care. Not all nursing organizations have a governmental affairs division for lobbying. The ANA has lobbyists in Washington, DC, to advocate for the concerns of the profession. In addition, most of the constituent state nurses associations have legislative activities at the state level. (Several nursing associations, including the ANA, are described in Chapter 9.) Before joining a nursing association, you should ask whether the association lobbies on behalf of the interests of its members. The future power of nurses depends on nurses joining and supporting such associations.

> Nursing will continue to lobby for new federal and state legislation that improves the quality and availability of nursing and health care.

The nursing profession will also continue to work with the national media to portray nurses in a positive, professional light. For nurses to be effective in promoting policy, the public needs a clear picture of what nurses bring to the American health care delivery system. For example, the ANA responded to an event dealing with a nurse who was competing in the Miss America contest and who was delivering a dramatic monologue about her experience as a nurse. A cohost of the television program "The View" mocked the monologue and the nurse for wearing a "doctor's stethoscope," as if the nurse were wearing a costume.

The ANA led a national outcry over this situation, with the message "nurses don't wear costumes; they save lives." As a result, there was so much public and advertiser backlash over this comment that the network, the television program, and the cohost issued an apology (ANA, 2015a).

WHAT EXACTLY IS POLITICS?

Politics, described by Mason et al. (2007, p. 4), is a vital tool that enables the nurse to "nurse smarter." Involvement in the political process offers an individual nurse a tool that augments his or her power, or clout, to improve the care provided to patients. Whether on the community, hospital, or nursing-unit level, political skills and the understanding of how laws are enacted enable the nurse to identify needed resources, gain access to those resources, work with legislative bodies to lobby for changes in the health care system, and overcome obstacles, thus facilitating the movement of the patient to higher levels of health or function (Fig. 17.1).

Let us look first at the nursing-unit level:

Your hospital is in the process of selecting a new supplier of intravenous (IV) pumps. You and the other nurses on your unit want to have input into that decision because IV pumps are essential to the care of your patients and you have a definite opinion about the type of IV pump that works best. However, the intensive care unit nurses have the only nurse position on the review committee (and therefore the director's ear!). You and the nurses on your unit strategize to secure input into this important decision.

Your plan might look like this:
- Gather data about IV pumps—cost, suppliers, possible substitutes, and so on.
- Communicate to the charge nurse and supervisor your concern about this issue and your plans to become involved in the decision (by using appropriate channels of communication).
- State clearly what you want—perhaps request a seat on the committee when the opportunity arises.
- Summarize in writing your request and the rationale, submitting it to the appropriate people.
- Establish a coalition with the intensive care unit nurses and other concerned individuals.
- Become involved with other hospital issues, and contribute in a credible fashion (i.e., do not be a single-issue person).

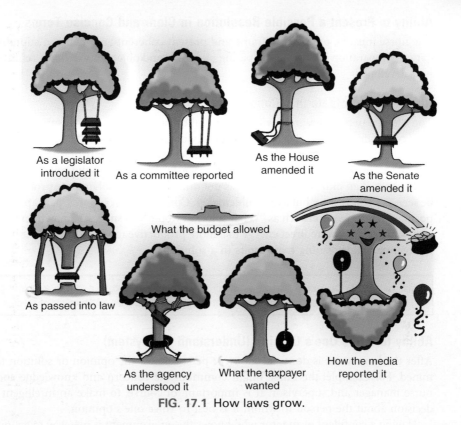

As a legislator introduced it

As a committee reported

As the House amended it

As the Senate amended it

What the budget allowed

As passed into law

As the agency understood it

What the taxpayer wanted

How the media reported it

FIG. 17.1 How laws grow.

What Other Strategies Would You Suggest?

The scenario described here illustrates what a politically astute nurse would do in this situation. Although the example applies to a hospital setting, the strategies are comparable to those necessary for becoming involved on a community, state, or even federal level. Practicing at the local level will provide good experience for larger issues—one has to start somewhere. Furthermore, a nurse involved on the local level will be able to hone her or his skills, thus gaining confidence in the ability to handle similar "exercises" in larger forums.

In the previous example, the nurse was able to formulate several "political" actions to influence the outcome of the IV pump decision (Critical Thinking Box 17.1).

🔘 CRITICAL THINKING BOX 17.1

What are some issues in your school or hospital that are examples of political issues or the result of politics?

What Are the Skills That Make Up a Nurse's Political Savvy?
Ability to Analyze an Issue (Those Assessment Skills Again!)
The individual who expects to "influence the allocation of scarce resources" must do the homework necessary to be well informed. She or he must know all the facts relevant to the issue, how the issue looks from all angles, and how it fits into the larger picture.

Ability to Present a Possible Resolution in Clear and Concise Terms

The nurse must be prepared to frame and present coherent arguments in support of the recommendation. Preparation includes anticipating questions and objections so that a rebuttal will be logical and well developed.

Ability to Participate in a Constructive Way

Too often, a person disagrees with a proposal being suggested to a hospital unit (or city council) but only complains about it. The displeased individual seldom takes the time to study the problem or to understand its connection with other hospital departments (or city programs in a broader issue). Most important, the displeased person seldom suggests an alternate solution.

In short, if an individual's concern is not directed toward solving the problem, that person will not be seen as a team player but as a troublemaker. Constructive responses, perhaps something as simple as posing a single question such as "What solution would you suggest?" may help those involved to think in positive terms and redirect energy to a more productive mode. Positive action can produce the kind of creative brainstorming that results in a solution.

> Simply complaining about something does not usually change anything. Proposing a solution, along with your rationale for choosing the solution, is a source of power because that solution may be chosen as the course of action.

Ability to Voice One's Opinion (Understand the System)

After the homework is done, let the *right* person know the opinion or solution that has been determined. For example, the nurse might communicate concern and knowledge about the issue to the nurse manager and supervisor. It is important, of course, to make an intelligent and well-informed decision about the person to whom it is best to voice one's opinion.

Having a confidant or mentor who knows the environment is one way to acquire this information, as he or she can provide you with insight regarding the appropriate person to whom you can express your opinion and suggestions. Another strategy is to use your listening skills. Simply standing back and listening are assets that will come in handy! Whatever the technique, studying the dynamics of the organization with all senses will help the nurse to decide on the best person and the most appropriate way to communicate the proposed solution and rationale.

Ability to Analyze and Use Power Bases

While discussing issues with colleagues and studying the organization, be alert to the various power brokers. In the previous IV pump vignette, the nurse notes the vice president (VP) of purchasing is an obvious source of power in the hospital. This VP will certainly concur with, if not make, the final decision. However, be aware that power does not always follow the lines on the organizational chart. The power of the nurse aide on the oncology unit who just happens to be the niece of the newly appointed member of the board of trustees may escape the notice of some. This person could be used to influence a decision if necessary. Similarly, the fact that the VP of purchasing's mother was on the unit should be filed in your memory for future use.

Understanding policy that has been promulgated by respected bodies can also be used as a power base. For example, the Institute of Medicine issued a report in 2011 called *The Future of Nursing*. One of the major tenets of this respected report is that nurses should be able to practice to the full extent of their education, licensure, and training (National Academies of Sciences, 2010).

If a nurse practitioner (NP) is trying to make a point about how the role of the NP in providing medication-assisted therapy (MAT) can address the opioid crisis in the rural area where he or she practices, using such information can reinforce the power behind the message. On a more global level, using such a power base can help to enact new laws to end the nation's opioid epidemic (i.e., "SUPPORT for Patients and Communities Act") and make the point that the expansion of the role of advanced practice nurses can help to alleviate the massive shortage of primary care physicians and can improve care processes (American Enterprise Institute, 2018; National Academies of Sciences, 2015).

Facts may be facts, but *where* one gets information can sometimes make a statement as powerful as the information itself. Having the ability to use many different channels of information will afford the nurse the power to choose among them.

WHAT IS POWER, AND WHERE DOES IT COME FROM?

Sanford (1979) describes five laws of power. She recommends that these laws be studied to identify strategies to develop power in nursing. The laws are as follows:

Law 1: Power Invariably Fills Any Vacuum

When a problem or issue arises, the prevailing desire is for peace and order. People are willing to yield power to someone interested in restoring order to situations of discomfort. Therefore someone will eventually step forward to handle the dilemma. It may be some time before the discomfort or unrest grows to heights sufficient for someone to take the lead.

Nonetheless, a person exerting power will step forward to offer a solution. In some situations, this person may be the previously identified leader, the nurse manager, or the department chair. More often there is an official power broker influencing the action. Know that there are opportunities to exert influence—for example, by taking the leadership role (i.e., stepping forward to fill the vacuum).

Law 2: Power Is Invariably Personal

In most instances, programs are attributed to an organization. For example, the state and national children's and health associations proposed a fictitious program called ImmunEYEs. However, if one investigated, it might be found that the program began with a small group of friends talking while eating a pizza one evening, lamenting the number of infants still not immunized. In the course of their conversation, one might have said, "If we were to create a media blitz that would get the need for immunizations into the consciousness of parents—get the need for immunizations in their face!" And the next person might have said, "In their *eyes!* Yea, ImmunEYEs. Let's do it!"

Initiatives such as this start with one person creating a new approach to a problem. That person exercises power by providing the leadership or spark to create the strategy to carry out such an initiative, thus inspiring and motivating people to contribute to the effort.

Law 3: Power Is Based on a System of Ideas and Philosophy

Behaviors demonstrated by an individual as she or he exerts power reflect a personal belief system or a philosophy of life. That philosophy or ideal must be one that attracts followers, gains their respect, and rallies them to join the effort. Nurses have the opportunity to ensure that a patient's right (versus privilege) to health care, access to preventive care, and similar values are reflected in policies and procedures.

Law 4: Power Is Exercised Through and Depends on Institutions

As an individual, one can easily feel powerless and unable to handle the complex problems facing a hospital, community, or state. However, through a nursing service organization, a state nurses association, or a similar organization, that individual can garner the resources needed to magnify her or his power. The person-to-person network, the communication vehicle (usually an organization's newsletter or journal), and the organizational structure are established for precisely this function— to support and foster changes in the health care system.

Law 5: Power Is Invariably Confronted With and Acts in the Presence of a Field of Responsibility

Actions taken create a ripple effect by speaking to the other nurses for whom nurses act and, most important, the patients for whom nurses advocate. The individual in the power position is acting on behalf of the group. Power is communicated to observers and is reinforced by positive responses. If the group thinks that its ideals are not being honored, the vacuum will be filled with the next candidate capable of the role and supported by the organization.

Another Way to Look at Power and Where to Get It

In a classic, much-referenced work, French and Raven (1959) describe five sources of power. They are (in order of importance) reward power, coercive power, legitimate power, referent or mentor power, and expert or informational power. These descriptions of power were presented in the discussion of nursing management in Chapter 10. The discussion there described the use of power within the ranks of nursing. Here, the use of power is presented as it applies to the political process, especially through political action in nursing.

The strongest source of power is the ability to *reward*. The best example of making use of the reward power base is the giving of money. For example, if someone gives a decision maker financial support for a future political campaign, the recipient will feel obligated to the donor and may, from time to time, "adjust opinions" to repay these obligations! Currently, because caps have been placed on campaign contributions, the misuse of this type of reward has been reduced.

An additional source of reward-based political power is the ability to commit voters to a candidate through endorsements. This illustrates the importance of having a large number of members in an organization—in other words, a large voting bloc. This reinforces the imperative for nurses to join and support nursing organizations that advocate on behalf of nurses, nursing, and quality health care.

Second in importance is the power to *coerce* or "punish" a decision maker for going against the wishes of an organization. The best example of this power, the opposite of *reward*, is the ability to remove the person from office at election time.

Third in importance is *legitimate* power, or the influence that comes with role and position. Influence derives from the status that society assigns individuals as a result of, for instance, inherited family money, membership in a respected profession, or a prominent position in the community. The dean in a school of nursing has a certain amount of influence just because of who he or she is. Right? A nurse's commitment to enhancing nursing's influence explains why nurses encourage and assist one another to achieve key decision-making positions—to build nursing's legitimate power base.

The fourth power base is that of *referent* or *mentor* power. This is the power that "rubs off" of influential people. When representatives of the student body talk with a faculty member about a problem they are having with a course, and they receive her or his support, the curriculum committee or dean is more likely to listen sympathetically than if the students were arguing only for themselves. The faculty member, joining with the students to solve their problem, adds to the students' power. The wish to build this type of power encourages nurses to join coalitions, especially those including organizations with greater power than their own.

The last and weakest of the power bases is that of *expert* or *informational* power. Nurses know about health and nursing care and are thus able to impart knowledge in this area with great confidence and style. Typically, nurses communicate this authority through letters written to legislators, testimonies presented in hearings, and through other contacts made on behalf of nursing and patients. In summary, power is derived from various sources. Nurses use, with the greatest frequency and ease, the weakest of the power bases—that deriving from their expertise. Although this is an important power base, nurses must develop and exercise the other types as well. Only then will nurses realize the full extent of their potential (Critical Thinking Box 17.2).

? CRITICAL THINKING BOX 17.2

Who are the people in positions that reflect the different power levels in your school, hospital, and community?

NETWORKING AMONG COLLEAGUES

It has been said that one should never be more than two telephone calls away from a needed resource, whether it be a piece of information, a contact in a hospital in another city, or input into a decision one is about to make. The key to successful networking is consciously building and nurturing a pool of associates whose skills and connections augment your own.

As a nursing graduate, one should begin the important task of networking by selecting an instructor from nursing school who is able to speak positively about your performance during nursing school. Ask this person if she or he would be willing to write a letter of reference for your first job. If the person agrees, nurture this contact from that time onward. Keep this individual apprised of your whereabouts, your successes, and your plans for the future. This person will be an important link not only to your school but also to your future educational and career undertakings. Then, at each future work site, find a charge nurse or supervisor willing to write a reference and with whom you can maintain contact. Keep building the network throughout your career.

Remember that this network must be nourished. Constant use of one's resources without reciprocation will exhaust them and make them unreliable sources of assistance in the future, but if properly cared for, this network will provide support for the rest of your career.

BUILDING COALITIONS

A *coalition* is a group of individuals or organizations who share a common interest in a single issue. Groups with whom nurses might form coalitions are as diverse as the topics about which nurses are concerned. For example, nurses are concerned about and lobby for adequate, safe child care, a safe environment, and women's issues. The numerous organizations interested in these diverse issues are potential candidates for a coalition with nursing organizations. However, it is not unusual for two organizations to be in a coalition on one issue but adversaries on another. Indeed, this is common in the political arena, where negotiations and compromises are the norm.

A warning: *the selection of coalition partners should strengthen your cause or organization.* Forming coalitions is a strategy to empower oneself. Therefore build coalitions with people more powerful than you, and build coalitions with organizations enjoying greater power than nursing, not less (Critical Thinking Box 17.3 and Fig. 17.2).

? CRITICAL THINKING BOX 17.3

What are examples of nursing coalitions in your community or state?

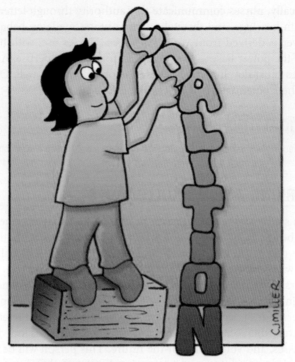

FIG. 17.2 How do we build a coalition?

What About Trade-Offs, Compromises, Negotiations, and Other Tricks of the Trade?

Politics is not a perfect art or science. In the heat of battle, nurses are often called on to compromise, but if they are unwilling to bend on some principle, they sacrifice all. To hold out for the ideal typically means that no progress toward the ideal will be realized. Often, changes in health care policies are achieved in incremental steps. However, the decision to compromise a value or principle must be carefully made with full realization of the implications—not an easy decision!

The political skills discussed so far apply to any situation, whether in a family, a hospital unit, or a community. The next part of the chapter is focused on skills that apply specifically to the governmental process.

How Do I Go About Participating in the Election Process?

One key to successful political activity is involvement in the election process. This is the stage where one can get to know the candidates; they also get to know you. In addition, it is a time when one makes important contacts for that network.

Getting involved in a candidate's campaign is simple. First, study the positions to be filled. Then, with the help of the local nurses' association, the local newspaper, or the county or state Democratic or Republican Party, select the candidate whose views on health care most closely match yours. Next, find the candidate's campaign headquarters. After this, contact the candidate's volunteer coordinator to see when volunteer help is needed. Most campaigns are crying for assistance with folding letters and stuffing envelopes, looking up addresses, and preparing bulk mailings. They will welcome you with great enthusiasm! Be sure to tell the campaign staff that you are a nurse and would be more than willing to contribute to the candidate's understanding of health care issues and to assist in drafting the candidate's positions on these issues (Critical Thinking Box 17.4).

? CRITICAL THINKING BOX 17.4

Who in your state government supports legislation that is pro nursing and pro health care?

Beware: Involvement in campaigns and party organizations can lead to catching the political "bug." Victims of the political bug are overcome by a powerful desire to make changes in the system, and they see a multitude of opportunities to educate people about the health needs of a county, state, and nation. An example of two nurses who caught the bug: During a past national presidential election, the nurses at a state caucus volunteered to write the resolution for the party's position on health care, which, if passed, would become a plank in the platform. After much work drafting the statement and bringing it before various committees, they were ecstatic when it passed and became the health statement for their party! (Review the case studies in the Evolve Resources for an example of the effectiveness of political action by nurses.)

What Is a Political Action Committee?

Another way that nurses can influence the elective process is through involvement in an organization's political action committee. Political action committees, or PACs, grew out of the Nixon/Watergate era, when Congress decided that candidates for public office were becoming too dependent on money supplied by special interests—individuals who give large political contributions and thereby exert undue influence over the elected official's decisions.

As a result, Congress limited the amount of money an individual may contribute to a candidate, established strict reporting requirements, and created a mechanism whereby individuals can pool their resources and collectively support a candidate.

The ANA National Political Action Committee is called ANA-PAC. Through this vehicle, nurses across the country organize to collectively endorse and support candidates for national offices. Likewise, state nurses associations have state-level PACs to influence statewide elections. There may be PACs in your area that endorse candidates in city elections. All PACs must comply with the state or federal election codes and report financial support given to candidates for public office.

Currently, PACs play an important role in the political process because they provide a mechanism whereby small contributors can act as a collective, participating in the electoral process when otherwise they would feel outmaneuvered by the bigger players.

The ANA's Endorsement Handbook stresses four points regarding PACs:

1. **Political focus.** The only purpose of any PAC is to endorse candidates for public office and then supply them with the political and financial support they need to win an election.
2. **No legislative activities.** A PAC does not lobby elected officials; that is the job of the ANA or the state nurses association and its government-relations arm. A PAC simply provides financial and campaign support for candidates whose views are generally consistent with those of its contributors.
3. **Not "dirty."** A PAC does not "buy" a candidate or a vote. However, the very nature of political life suggests that candidates who recognize an organization's ability to affect their electoral prospects will be inclined to listen to the group's views when considering specific pieces of legislation.

4. **Health concerns only.** Nursing PACs evaluate the candidates on nursing and health concerns only. In other words, ANA-PAC might solicit the candidates' ideas about how Congress might address the problem of older adult abuse in long-term care facilities or expanding health care insurance coverage for the uninsured. However, the organization as a nursing PAC should not include questions, for instance, about the source of funding for the new cabinet on foreign commerce. The organization speaks for members only on issues covered in its philosophical statements, resolutions, position statements, legislative platforms, or other documents that its members as an organization have accepted (Critical Thinking Box 17.5).

---

⑦ CRITICAL THINKING BOX 17.5

How has the American Nurses Association's Political Action Committee affected nursing on a national level? What have been the most recent activities of this organization? How does your state organization communicate or affect nursing and health care legislation in your state?

After Getting Them Elected, Then What?

Lobbying is the attempt to influence or sway a public official to take a desired action. Lobbying is also characterized as the education of the legislator about nursing and its issues. Educating officials, like educating patients, is an important part of the nurse's role.

As nurses, we can lobby in several different ways. The first and best opportunity to lobby comes when the nurse first meets the candidate and evaluates her or him as a potential officeholder. This is the time to assess the candidate's knowledge of health care issues. Take the time to teach and to learn.

A second opportunity comes when the official needs information to decide how to vote on an issue. Depending on time constraints, the issue, and other considerations, a nurse might decide to lobby the official in person or in writing. If time and financial resources permit, the most powerful type of contact is a face-to-face visit. The only way to ensure time with your senator or representative is to make an appointment. Even then, you may not be successful.

If you are making an unscheduled visit to the Capitol that precludes an appointment, the best time to catch your senator or representative is early in the day, before the legislative sessions or committee meetings start; they rarely start before 10 or 11 AM. Contact with the legislator's aid or assistant can be just as effective as time spent with the official. Busy federal and state officials depend heavily on their staff. Treat staff members with the respect they deserve! Be sure to leave a business card or your name and contact information in writing, including an e-mail address. Make sure that they know how to contact you if they should have any questions.

Finally, remember that contact should be made between legislative sessions and during holidays when the official is in her or his home district. The structure and content of the visit should be similar to that of a written contact. That is, know your issue, keep it short, identify the issue by its bill number and title, and communicate exactly what action you want the senator or representative to take. Box 17.1 is a list of specific "Dos and Don'ts When Lobbying." As you begin lobbying, add your recommendations to the list.

If you cannot visit your representative because of time or travel restrictions, a well-written letter, e-mail, or telephone call can communicate your message. Examine the sample letter in Box 17.2. Note that some pointers are listed at the foot of the page. Examples of the proper way to address a public official can be found in Box 17.3.

> ## BOX 17.1   DOS AND DON'TS WHEN LOBBYING
>
> ### Do
>
> - Make sure your legislator knows constituents who are affected by the bill; suggest visits to programs in his or her area.
> - Clearly identify the bill, using title and number if possible.
> - Be specific and know about the issue or bill before you write or talk.
> - Identify yourself (occupation, hometown, member of American Nurses Association).
> - Use your own words; if writing, use your own stationery. No form letters!
> - Send an e-mail and include your name.
> - Be courteous, brief, and to the point.
> - Provide pertinent reasons for your stand.
> - Show your legislator how the issue relates to his or her district.
> - Respect your legislator's right to form an opinion different from yours.
> - Present a united front. Keep your internal problems at home.
> - Write letters of appreciation or send an e-mail to your legislators when appropriate.
> - Write letters at appropriate times or send an e-mail; for example, when a bill is in committee, request action that is appropriate for that stage in the legislative process.
> - Establish an ongoing relationship with the public official.
> - Know issues or problems your legislator is concerned about, and express your interest in assisting him or her.
> - Attend functions sponsored by coalition members. Be seen!
> - Get involved in your legislator's campaign for reelection—or his or her opponent's, if necessary!
>
> ### Don't
>
> - Write a long letter or send a lengthy e-mail discussing multiple points; deal with a single bill or concern per letter, e-mail, or contact.
> - Use threats or promises.
> - Berate your legislator.
> - Be offended in the event of a canceled appointment. Things are unpredictable during a legislative session.
> - Demand a commitment before the legislator has had time to consider the measure.
> - Pretend to have vast influence in the political area.
> - Be vague.
> - Hesitate to admit you do not know all the facts, but indicate you will find out—and do!

Letters are common methods of communicating with elected officials; however, a telephone call, fax, or e-mail is often necessary to relay your opinion when time is limited before an important vote. The suggested format and content of the e-mail and telephone message are similar to that of a letter or face-to-face interview.

Deciding on the type of contact to make with the decision maker will vary depending on the situation. For example, if the bill is coming up for the first time in committee, the strategy may be that 10 to 15 people write letters or e-mails or call the members of the committee. At this point, the *number* of contacts with the office is important. The reason is that the legislator's assistant typically answers the telephone or opens the mail, tallies the subject of the contact, and puts a hash mark in the "Pro HB 23" or "Con HB 23" column for the bill. Therefore a greater impact will be realized if multiple contacts pertain to one bill. However, bags of form letters may have a negative impact on a lobbying effort. Make sure your callers/writers understand the issue and are able to individualize their contact with the elected official. People who contact the legislator's office with a script that they do not understand will not further the lobbying efforts of an organization.

The aforementioned efforts are sufficient early in the process; however, if a major controversial bill is coming up for a final vote in the Senate, activating a statewide network and bombarding the senators

BOX 17.2   EXAMPLE OF A LETTER TO A PUBLIC OFFICIAL

Ima Nurse, RN
123 Main Street
Any Town, USA 12345-6789
The Honorable U. R. Important, Jr.
United States Senate
Washington, DC 20510
Dear Senator Important:

I request your support of SB 101 regarding appropriations for nursing education and research. This bill is vital to the country's efforts to improve the number and quality of registered nurses. As you recall, the 2020 Very Important Nursing Study demonstrated the growing demand for Advanced Nurse Practitioners to work with the increasing numbers of people older than 65 years. This bill will provide funding to increase the number of faculty and student slots in the country's schools of nursing and to support nursing research in gerontological nursing. The expanding numbers of older people in our area of the country are not able to access the health care they deserve. During a trip home, I would like to take you to the Main Street Senior's Clinic. I know that you would be pleased with this service, as are the health care providers and the patients.

Will you support this bill? Do you have any questions about it? If so, please call me or call the State Nurses' Association Headquarters.

Thank you for your concern with this issue and your continuing support of health care issues.

Sincerely yours,
Ima Nurse, RN

Points to Note

Your letter or e-mail should

- Be neat, without typos or grammatical errors
- Be correctly addressed
- Be on professional letterhead, if written
- Cover only a single topic
- Refer to the bill by number and content
- State your request in the first sentence
- Include brief rationale for your request
- Use "RN" in your inside address and salutation

with letters, e-mails, telephone calls, faxes, and telegrams—as many as possible—is a typical strategy. The bigger the issue, the bigger the campaign should be.

At several points in a lobbying season, but certainly after contacting the elected official for a major vote, a follow-up thank you letter will strengthen your contact with the legislator and help to establish you in her or his political network. In addition to reinforcing the reason for your original contact, thank the official for her or his concern with the issue and the work in solving the problem by writing the bill, voting for it (or whatever), and for paying attention to your concern (Critical Thinking Box 17.6).

❓ CRITICAL THINKING BOX 17.6

When are the bills that affect nursing and health care going to be presented to your state legislature? Is safe staffing on the legislative agenda?

In summary, there are specific skills to learn for effective political involvement, but remember that many of the skills needed to be politically savvy are the very ones that will serve you well in everyday professional negotiations (Fig. 17.3).

BOX 17.3 HOW TO ADDRESS PUBLIC OFFICIALS

The President[1]
Writing
The Honorable (Full Name)
President of the United States
The White House
Washington, DC 20500
Dear Mr./Madam President:

Speaking
"Mr./Madam President"
"President (Last Name)"

The Vice President
Writing
The Honorable (Full Name)
Vice President of the United States
Executive Office Building
Washington, DC 20501
Dear Mr./Madam Vice President:

Speaking
"Mr./Madam Vice President"
"Vice President (Last Name)"

A Senator
Writing
The Honorable (Full Name)
United States Senate
(will have office building and room address)

Washington, DC 20510
Dear Senator (Full Name):

Speaking
"Senator (Last Name)"

A Representative
Writing
The Honorable (Full Name)
U.S. House of Representatives
(will have office building and room address)
Washington, DC 20515
Dear Mr./Ms. (Full Name):

Speaking
"Representative (Last Name)"
"Mr./Ms. (Last Name)"

A Member of the Cabinet
Writing
The Honorable (Full Name)
Secretary of (Cabinet Agency)
(will have office building and room address)
Washington, DC 20520
Dear Mr./Madam Secretary:

Speaking
"Mr./Madam Secretary"
"Secretary (Last Name)"

[1]The correct closing for a letter or e-mail to the president is "Very respectfully yours." The correct closing for all other federal officials noted here is "Sincerely yours."

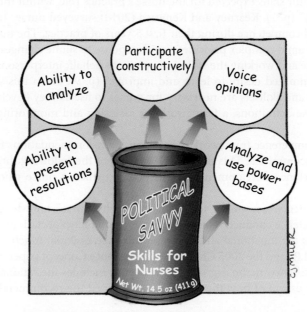

FIG. 17.3 Skills to make a nurse politically savvy.

As a recent graduate who is becoming oriented to your first job and is beginning to look around at what you and your colleagues need to improve, you will agree that political involvement is necessary to reach your goals.

> Don't wait to be "allowed" to make a difference, don't wait to be invited to join, and don't let someone else do the job. Please step forward! Act like the powerful, informed, influential nurse that you are. There is much that needs to be done; be a part of the action to achieve solutions!

Margaret Mead said, "Never doubt that a small group of thoughtful, committed citizens can change the world. Indeed, it's the only thing that ever has." The nursing profession has much to accomplish in addressing the problems with affordable, readily available health care for all. Make sure you are a part of the solutions that will be discovered in the future!

CONTROVERSIAL POLITICAL ISSUES AFFECTING NURSING

Uniform Core Licensure Requirements

What Is It?

The Nursing Practice and Education Committee, formed by the National Council of State Boards of Nursing (NCSBN), proposed the development of core licensure requirements. Now referred to as Uniform Licensure Requirements (ULRs), these requirements ensure that nurses practicing in one state have met the same requirements of nurses practicing across in other states (NCSBN, 2011). This was in response to an increasing concern regarding the mobility of nurses and the maintenance of licensure standards to protect the public's health, safety, and welfare. With the implementation of Mutual Recognition, it is important that health care consumers have access to nursing services that are provided by a nurse who meets consistent standards, regardless of where the consumer lives. NCSBN (2005) defined competence as "the application of knowledge and the interpersonal, decision-making, and psychomotor skills expected for the nurse's practice role, within the context of public health, welfare, and safety" (p. 1). Kearney and Kenward (2010) surveyed nurses to explore how nurses defined and developed competence during their first 5 years of practice. The nurses' defined competency as "efficient care amid complex priorities; rapid response to subtle changes in patients' conditions; seeing the big picture and working the system on patient's behalf; interpersonal warmth, respect, and authority; and a committed desire to learn and improve" (p. 9). From this study, it is apparent that essential functions and skillsets are necessary for nurses to use as they develop qualities of a competent nurse. From these definitions, a framework for assessing and monitoring competency in nursing practice is ideal.

The competence framework is based on the recommendations from the 1996 Continued Competence Subcommittee. This framework consists of the following three primary areas:

- Competence development: the method by which a nurse gains nursing knowledge, skills, and abilities
- Competence assessment: the means by which a nurse's knowledge, skills, and abilities are validated
- Competence conduct: refers to health and conduct expectations, including assurance that licensees possess the functional abilities to perform the essential functions of the nursing role

The ULRs and the 2005 Continued Competence Concept paper may be found at the NCSBN's website (https://www.ncsbn.org/index.htm), which includes the rationales for the proposed requirements and a discussion of how the committee developed the recommendations.

Agreements, known as *nurse licensure compacts (NLCs)*, began in 2000 and specify the rights and responsibilities of nurses who choose or who are required to work across state boundaries and the governing body responsible for protecting the recipients of nursing care. As of 2018, 31 states enacted NLCs.

States entering into NLC agree to recognize mutually a nursing license issued by any of the participating states. To join the compact, states must enact legislation adopting the compact. The nurse will hold a single license issued by the nurse's state of residence. This license will include a "multistate licensure privilege" to practice in any of the other compact states (both physical and electronic). Each state will continue to set its own licensing and practice standards. A nurse will have to comply only with the license and license renewal requirements of her or his state of residence (the one issuing the license), but the nurse must know and comply with the practice standards of each state in which she or he practices (NCSBN, 2018a) (Critical Thinking Box 17.7).

? CRITICAL THINKING BOX 17.7

How will the enhanced nurse licensure compact affect the licensure and practice of nursing in your state?

In 2018, the *enhanced nurse licensure compact* (eNLC) was started and was intended to be an improvement over the original NLC in terms of nurse screening requirements and addressing technology improvements in care provision.

There was resistance from some states regarding the requirements for licensure, such as the NLC not requiring that applicants undergo state and federal fingerprint based criminal background checks, whereas the new eNLC does mandate the participating states conduct the federal and state criminal background check (NCSBN, 2018b).

The program was begun in January 2018, with 29 member states and other states with pending legislation. The eNLC benefits nurses with the increased mobility to practice, and it also increases access to care for patients. In addition, there are new provision that address higher protections in patient safety.

The eNLC permits RNs and LPN/LVNs to have a single multistate license, and they are able to practice in person or via telehealth in the home state and other eNLC states.

Telehealth is growing rapidly, and nurses working with this type of technology-enhanced care have been required to have multiple state licenses. The eNLC addresses this requirement and covers nurses providing telehealth care across state boundaries.

Nursing and Collective Bargaining

March! There are no bunkers, no sidelines for nursing today. We find ourselves the center of attention. As the government and corporate America fight escalating health care costs, AIDS is wreaking havoc and technology swells unchecked. Underpaid, overworked, and overstressed nurses are in the midst of a conflagration. Nursing is in greater demand than ever before. Remember Scutari. We must organize, unite, go on the offensive.

Margretta Madden Styles, 1988, quoted in **Hansten and Washburn, 1990, p. 53.**

The National Labor Relations Act is a federal law regulating labor relations in the private business sector (extended to voluntary, nonprofit health care institutions in 1974). This law grants employees the right to form, to join, or to participate in a labor organization. Furthermore, the law gives employees the right to organize and bargain with their employers through a representative of their own choosing.

Collective bargaining continues to be a point of debate among nurses. Those supporting collective bargaining argue that it is a tool to force positive changes in the practice setting or a method of controlling the practice setting. Many positive changes in the clinical setting are attributed to advances made during contract negotiations.

Opponents feel that, as a profession, nurses should not use collective bargaining but instead should influence the practice setting by employee and employer working as a team and not as adversaries. They contend that a strike, the ultimate tool of any labor dispute, should not be used. Opponents further argue that practice standards are not negotiable. The points of disagreement between employer and employee are almost always economic: pay, vacation, sick leave, and similar issues. Chapter 18 presents a more detailed discussion of collective bargaining issues. Regardless of your opinion of collective bargaining, the process will involve political action.

What do you think? A paragraph in the ANA's publication *What You Need to Know About Today's Workplace: A Survival Guide for Nurses* summarizes the challenge for us, and the words are still accurate nowadays:

In a work environment that is constantly changing, it is imperative that nurses are able to assess the true merits of various labor-management structures, to evaluate the real value of proposals to upgrade compensation packages, to determine appropriate levels of participation in workplace decision-making bodies, and to distinguish between long-range solutions and "quick fixes" to workplace problems (Flanagan, 1995, p. 5).

Equal Pay for Work of Comparable Value or Comparable Worth?

The concept of comparable worth or pay equity holds that jobs that are equal in value to an organization ought to be equally compensated, whether or not the work content of those jobs is similar. Pay equity relates to the goal of equitable compensation as outlined in the Equal Pay Act of 1963, and "sex-based wage discrimination" is a phrase that refers to the basis of the problems defined by Title VII of the Civil Rights Act of 1964.

As long ago as World War II, the War Labor Board suggested that discrimination probably exists whenever jobs traditionally relegated to women are paid less than the rate of common-labor jobs such as janitor or floor sweeper. One of the first cases was that of the *International Union of Electrical Workers v. Westinghouse*. The union proved that male-female wage disparity existed and uncovered a policy in a manual that stated that women were to be paid less because they were women. Back pay and increased wages were given in an out-of-court settlement in an appellate-level decision.

It was nurses who initiated the action in *Lemons v. the City and County of Denver*. Nurses employed by the city of Denver claimed under the Civil Rights Act that they were the victims of salary discrimination because their jobs were of a value equal to various better-paid positions throughout the city's diverse workforce. The court ruled that the city was justified in the use of a market pricing system (a form of pay based on supply and demand) even though it acknowledged the general discrimination against women. The court said that the case (and the comparable-worth concept) had the potential to disrupt the entire economic system of the United States. Because of this judgment and the fact that the nurses were unable to prepare a job evaluation program to substantiate their claim, the judge dismissed the case.

Safe Nurse Staffing

The ANA (2015b) released a study called "Optimal Nurse Staffing to Improve Quality of Care and Patient Outcomes: Executive Summary." This study conducted a targeted review of published articles dealing with nurse staffing and patient outcomes. A panel was also convened consisting of experts in the field of nurse staffing. ANA believes that nurses themselves should be empowered to create staffing plans due to the complex nature of staffing and the large number of variables. ANA continues to stress that staffing is too complex to simply legislatively mandate staffing ratios. The study also stresses the evidence that appropriate staffing has a demonstrated effect on a variety of patient outcomes. Nurses can use the study to advocate for and implement sound evidence-based staffing plans.

In 2013, the Registered Nurse Safe Staffing Act (H.R. 2083/S. 1132) was endorsed by ANA. This would require Medicare-participating hospitals to establish RN staffing plans using a committee, comprised of a majority of direct-care nurses, to ensure patient safety, reduce readmissions, and improve nurse retention. As the act moved forward, it was introduced into the House of Representatives in April 2015, as the 2015 Registered Nurse Safe Staffing Act (H.R. 2083) and required amendments to title XVIII (Medicare) of the Social Security Act, requiring Medicare-participating hospitals to implement hospital-wide staffing plans for nursing services among other requirements. In 2018, the Safe Staffing for Nurse and Patient Safety Act was introduced into the U.S. Senate and House of Representatives, which requires Medicare participating facilities to ensure the formation of committees comprised of at least 55% of nurses to formulate and implement nurse-to-patient ratio staffing plans that are unit specific (ANA, 2018).

The Safe Staffing for Nurse and Patient Safety Act of 2018 considers not only nurse input but also availability of resources, technology, and unit workflow as key components of safe, staffing plans. ANA President Pamela F. Cipriano sums up the importance of nurse-driven initiatives guiding legislative change in the following statement, "Nursing care is like medication—we would never withhold a medication when we know its lifesaving effects. The Safe Staffing for Nurse and Patient Safety Act empowers direct care nurses to determine the unique and variable needs of their patients to ensure the safety and quality outcomes of care" (ANA, 2018, para 3). At the time of this publication, seven states have enacted safe staffing legislation using the committee approach: Oregon, Texas, Illinois, Connecticut, Ohio, Washington, and Nevada (ANA, 2018).

Much work still needs to be done in the area of safe staffing. Nurses are very concerned about staffing issues—mandatory overtime, increased numbers of assistive personnel replacing licensed personnel, and increased patient acuity are factors contributing to the problem. Changes will be achieved as we educate the public, as well as legislative representatives, and as nurses take the primary role to initiate changes in the workplace environment.

Nursing Workforce Development Programs

Nursing workforce development programs began in 1964 as Congress passed the Nurse Training Act of 1964, recognizing the vital role nurses play and the need for recruitment of additional people into the profession. This occurred during a time of a very serious nursing shortage.

Since that time, the programs, referred to as Title VIII programs, help to sustain a strong nursing workforce that is qualified to meet the country's needs. The programs include loan forgiveness and scholarship aid for nurses who agree to work in a critical shortage facility and communities in need. There are also provisions for increasing numbers of faculty (AONE, 2018).

Health Care Reform

Health care reform is a very broad, complex term that over the past decade has been focused on:
- Who is covered by health care insurance?
- Who pays for the coverage?
- How does the coverage address access?
- Is it mandated that each person has coverage, and what is the penalty for not having health care insurance?

The Patient Protection and Affordable Care Act of 2010 was passed to help insure coverage for all Americans. It has been changed as different political groups agreed or disagreed with the original provisions (ANA, 2017).

CONCLUSION

Politics, policy making, and advocating for patients are key processes for nurses to claim their "power" as a driving force in health care. Participating in ANA-PAC activities provides an opportunity to be at the grassroots level of lobbying (see the Relevant Websites and Online Resources later). Shaping policy and becoming active in the legislative area are practice roles for nurses. By having an understanding of the political process, nurses can and will make significant strides in promoting legislation that will positively affect the health of the nation.

🌐 RELEVANT WEBSITES AND ONLINE RESOURCES

American Nurses Association (ANA)
ANA official position statements. https://www.nursingworld.org/practice-policy/nursing-excellence/official-position-statements/
When nurses speak, Washington listens. https://ana.aristotle.com/sitepages/homepage.aspx

American Nurses Association-Political Action Committee (ANA-PAC)
https://ana.aristotle.com/SitePages/pac.aspx

American Nurses Credentialing Center (ANCC)
https://www.nursingworld.org/ancc/

The American Nurse: Official publication of the American Nurses Association
http://www.theamericannurse.org/

BIBLIOGRAPHY

American Enterprise Institute (AEI). (2018). *Nurse practitioners: A solution to America's primary care crisis.* Retrieved from https://www.aei.org/publication/nurse-practitioners-a-solution-to-americas-primary-care-crisis/.

American Nurses Association (ANA). (2010). *Not guilty—Texas jury acquits Winkler County nurse.* Retrieved from https://www.nursingworld.org/news/media-resources/legal-action/.

American Nurses Association (ANA). (2015a). *ANA President Pamela F. Cipriano, PhD, RN, NEA-BC, FAAN responds to comments on ABC's "The View" (9/16/15).* Retrieved from http://www.theamericannurse.org/2015/11/01/what-nurses-are-saying/.

American Nurses Association (ANA). (2015b). *Optimal nurse staffing to improve quality of care and patient outcomes: Executive summary.* Retrieved from http://info.nursingworld.org/staffingwp/.

American Nurses Association (ANA). (2017). *Health system reform resources.* Retrieved from https://www.nursingworld.org/practice-policy/health-policy/health-system-reform/resources/.

American Nurses Association (ANA). (2018). *ANA applauds nurse staffing legislation.* Retrieved from https://www.nursingworld.org/news/news-releases/2018/ana-applauds-nurse-staffing-legislation/.

American Organization of Nurse Executives (AONE). (2018). *Title VIII: Nursing workforce development programs.* Retrieved from http://advocacy.aone.org/title-viii-celebrating-50-years-nursing-workforce-development-programs-0.

Conde, C. (2010). Whistle-blower walks: Jury acquits nurse who reported physician to TMB. *Texas Medicine,* 106(5), 39–44. Retrieved from https://www.texmed.org/Template.aspx?id=16152.

Flanagan, L. (1995). *What you need to know about today's workplace: A survival guide for nurses.* Kansas City, MO: American Nurses Association.

French, J. R. P., & Raven, B. (1959). The bases of social power. In D. Cartwright (Ed.), *Studies in social power.* Ann Arbor: University of Michigan Press.

Gallup. (2018). *Nurses again outpace other professions for honesty, ethics.* Retrieved from https://news.gallup.com/poll/245597/nurses-again-outpace-professions-honesty-ethics.aspx.

Hansten, R. I., & Washburn, M. (1990). *I light the lamp.* Vancouver, WA: Applied Therapeutics.

Kearney, M., & Kenward, K. (2010). Nurses' competence development during the first 5 years of practice. *Journal of Nursing Regulation, 1*(1), 9–15. https://doi.org/10.1016/S2155-8256(15)30360-4.

Leavitt, J. K., Cohen, S. S., & Mason, D. J. (2002). Political analysis and strategies. In D. J. Mason, J. K. Leavitt, & M. W. Chaffee (Eds.), *Policy and politics in nursing and health care.* St. Louis, MO: Saunders.

Mason, D. J., Leavitt, J. K., & Chaffee, M. W. (2007). Policy and politics in nursing and health care. In D. J. Mason, J. K. Leavitt, & M. W. Chaffee (Eds.), *Policy and politics in nursing and health care.* St. Louis, MO: Saunders.

National Academies of Sciences. (2010). *The future of nursing: Leading change, advancing health.* Retrieved from http://nationalacademies.org/HMD/Reports/2010/The-Future-of-Nursing-Leading-Change-Advancing-Health.aspx.

National Academies of Sciences. (2015). *Assessing progress on the Institute of Medicine Report,* The Future of Nursing. Washington, DC: The National Academies Press. Retrieved from http://nationalacademies.org/hmd/reports/2015/assessing-progress-on-the-iom-report-the-future-of-nursing.aspx.

National Council of State Boards of Nursing. (2005). *Continued competence concept paper.* Retrieved from https://www.ncsbn.org/3947.htm.

National Council of State Boards of Nursing. (2011). *The 2011 uniform licensure requirements.* Retrieved from https://www.ncsbn.org/3884.htm.

National Council of State Boards of Nursing. (2018a). *Licensure compacts.* Retrieved from https://www.ncsbn.org/compacts.htm.

National Council of State Boards of Nursing. (2018b). *Enhanced nurse licensure compact (eNLC) implemented January 19, 2018.* Retrieved from https://www.ncsbn.org/11945.htm.

Sanford, N. D. (1979). *Identification and explanation of strategies to develop power for nursing in power: Nursing's challenge for change.* Kansas City, MO: American Nurses Association.

18

Collective Bargaining
Traditional (Union) and Nontraditional Approaches

Jennifer Wing, MSN, RN*

http://evolve.elsevier.com/Zerwekh/nsgtoday/.

It is time for a new generation of leadership to cope with new problems and new opportunities. For there is a new world to be won.
President John F. Kennedy

Difficulties are meant to rouse, not discourage. The human spirit is to grow strong by conflict.
William Ellery Channing

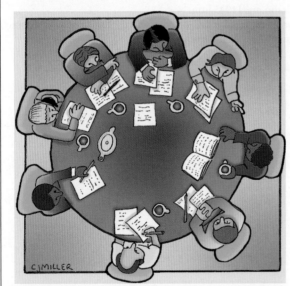

Is there a place for collective bargaining in nursing?

After completing this chapter, you should be able to:
- Identify the milestones in the history of collective bargaining.
- Compare traditional and nontraditional collective bargaining.
- Identify examples that indicate an employer's position on the role of professional nurses as it impacts practice.
- Identify conditions that may lead nurses to seek traditional or nontraditional collective bargaining.
- Identify the positive and negative aspects of traditional and nontraditional collective bargaining.
- Discuss the benefits of collective bargaining for professional groups.
- Discuss the impact of the silence of nurses in public communications and the public's perception of nurses.
- Identify barriers to the control of professional practice.
- Identify Advanced Practice Nurse role in advocating for the nursing profession.

*The authors would like to thank, **Joann Wilcox, RN, MSN, LNC,** for her previous contributions to this chapter.

Y ou will soon be accepting your first position as an RN. You will be adjusting not only to a new role but also to a new workplace. Even in these times of dramatic change in health care, many of you will start your career in a hospital. In fact, the demographics about nurses show that:

- Approximately 61% of nurses in practice are providing care in hospitals (Bureau of Labor Statistics, 2018). In addition, RNs are providing direct patient care in settings such as outpatient care settings, private practice, health maintenance organizations, primary care clinics, home health care, nursing homes, hospices, nursing centers, insurance and managed care companies, etc. (Bureau of Labor Statistics, 2018; Potter, Perry, Stockert, & Hall, 2017) in which care that was hospital-based in the past is now provided in these alternative settings.
- The hospital is also the most common employer of graduate nurses in their first year of practice; more than 82.2% of new graduates were working in a hospital in their first year of employment (National Council State Boards of Nursing [NCSBN], 2018a).
- Employment of RNs is projected to grow 16% from 2016 to 2026, faster than the average for all occupations. Growth will occur for a number of reasons, including an increased emphasis on preventative care; growing rates of chronic conditions, such as diabetes and obesity; and demand for health care services from the Baby Boomer population, as they live longer and more active lives (Bureau of Labor Statistics, 2018).

As you begin to interview for your first position in your career as a professional RN, there is no doubt you will find yourself both excited and anxious. Your prospective employer will assess your ability to think critically and to perform at a professional level in the health care setting. The potential employer will ask, "Is this applicant a person who will be able to contribute to the mission of the organization and to the quality of health care offered at this organization?"

While the employer assesses your potential to make a contribution, it is equally important that you remember that an interview is a *complex two-way* process. You will, of course, be eager to know about compensation, benefits, hours, and responsibilities. These are very tangible and immediate interests. However, these are not likely to be the best predictors of satisfaction with your practice over time, as the ability to practice your profession as defined by licensure and education will be the foundation leading to job satisfaction and professional fulfillment.

You should be prepared to assess the potential employer's mission and ability to support your professional practice and growth. It is extremely important that you gain essential information about the organization, its mission, and its culture. It is easy to overlook very significant organizational issues that will ultimately affect your everyday practice of nursing when your primary focus is on becoming employed and on wondering whether you will succeed in this first professional role. Lacey-Mabe (2016) identifies several questions to keep in mind: What is your supervisory style? What's your vision for this unit? In what ways are clinicians held accountable for high qualities of practice? Additionally, it is important to use the 2015 *Code of Ethics* for nursing to guide your questions about the role of the staff RN in decision making related to the practice of nursing in the facility. "Making decisions based on a sound foundation of ethics is an essential part of nursing practice in all specialties and settings…" (American Nurses Association [ANA], 2015).

Hospital structures and governance policies can have a dramatic influence on the effectiveness of a RN and how he or she can fulfill obligations to patients and families. RNs have defined the discipline of nursing as a profession, and, as members of this profession, they *must have a voice in and control over the practice of nursing*. When that voice and control are not supported in the work setting, conflicts most likely will arise. In some states, nurses have made a choice to gain that voice and assume control of their practice by using a traditional collective bargaining model, commonly known as a *labor union*. In other states, particularly those that function under the right-to-work regulations, nurses attempt to control practice through interest-based bargaining (IBB), which is a nontraditional approach to

BOX 18.1 TERMS

Traditional collective bargaining—A legally regulated collective bargaining unit or a union that assists members to gain control over practice, economics in the health care industry, and other health care issues that threaten the quality of patient care.

National Nurses United (NNU)—The new registered nurse super union formalized in December 2009.

Nontraditional collective bargaining—Shared governance, or interest-based bargaining (IBB); a collaborative-based, problem-solving approach to assist nurses to have a voice in the workplace and control over issues that affect their practice.

Center for American Nurses (CAN)—Organization that previously represented the interests of nurses who were not formally represented by a collective bargaining unit or union (Budd et al., 2004). It is now an integral part of the ANA.

American Nurses Association (ANA)—Provide support to advance the nursing profession. Advocating in Congress and setting the standards for nursing worldwide.

collective bargaining that is used to accomplish the provision of a voice and control over practice (Budd et al., 2004) (Box 18.1). In some states, nurses use both models to meet the needs of their diverse membership.

WHEN DID THE ISSUES LEADING TO COLLECTIVE BARGAINING BEGIN?

Since World War II, there have been phenomenal advances in medical research and the subsequent development of life-saving drugs and technologies. The introduction of Medicare and Medicaid programs in 1965 provided the driving force and the continued resources for this growth. This initiative opened access to health care for millions of Americans who were previously disenfranchised from the health care system.

The explosion in knowledge and technology, coupled with an expanded population able to access health care quickly, increased the demands on the health care system and many of the providers in that system. These advances required nursing to adapt as the complexity of health care and the number of patients accessing this care continued to increase. For example, at the time when the acuity of hospitalized patients increased because of shorter lengths of stay, organizations were responding to cost containment demands by downsizing the number of staff members. As more patients had access to all services in the health care system, the number of care hours available for each patient decreased, because fewer staff per patient were being hired. Overall, patients were sicker when they entered the system. Yet they were moved more quickly through the acute care setting because of such innovations as same-day admissions, same-day surgery, increased discharge to long-term care settings, and early discharge. Add to these changes the periodic shortages of nurses prepared for all levels of care, the increased use of unlicensed assistive personnel to provide defined, delegated nursing care, and growing financial pressures on the health care system, and tensions became understandably high.

The time between 2000 and 2013 also brought pressures on RNs, as the safety of hospitalization became a paramount concern among both patients and health care staff. The publication *To Err Is Human* (Institute of Medicine, 2000, p. 31) stated that, "Based on the results of the New York Study, the number of deaths due to medical error may be as high as 98,000 [yearly]." In an editorial review of the publication done in 2016, it was noted, in 2013 this number had risen to 400,000 (Palatnik, 2016). With RNs being at the bedside of acute care patients, their involvement in identifying and/or committing medical errors is high. Ensuring this staff has the appropriate resources to provide safe care is an issue that RNs need to address directly with the management of the facility and/or the collective bargaining agent for that hospital/organization. Enormous financial challenges confront health care institutions. As an RN working in the health care industry, you will encounter and use newly developed and very costly health care technologies. At the same time, you will experience firsthand the impact of public and private forces that are focused on placing restraints on cost and reimbursement for a patient's care.

Adding to these concerns regarding safe care, new technologies, and potential staff shortages was the implementation of the Patient Protection and Affordable Care Act (PPACA) of 2010 (commonly referred to as the Affordable Care Act [ACA] or Obamacare) (U.S. Department of Health & Human Services, 2017). A significant aspect of this act is the fact that it created the requirement for almost every person in this country to be covered by some form of health care insurance, thereby increasing the numbers of people who could/would present for care from the various health care facilities. It is unclear if PPACA will remain as it is in the future. There have been attempts, in Congress, to repeal and/or replace PPACA. For now, the number of people who are presenting for care remains increased.

As a professional RN, you are at the intersection of these potentially conflicting forces. For you, these forces will be less abstract; they are not just important concepts and issues facing a very large industry. As a nurse, these concepts and forces are patients with names, faces, and lives valued and loved within a family and a community. You are responsible for the care you provide and for advocating on behalf of these patients and—as you will soon discover—the health of the health care industry.

As an RN, you will become familiar with how, when, and why events occur that adversely or positively affect the patient and the health of the organization. This places you in a unique position to take an active lead in developing solutions. These solutions must be good for patients and for your organization. During your interview for potential employment, while you are busy assessing the potential employer's mission and support of your practice and growth, it is easy to overlook those significant organizational attributes that will ultimately affect your everyday practice of nursing. Therefore, during your interview it would be important for you to ask those questions identified in the beginning of this chapter, particularly those that address the ethical practice of RNs.

THE EVOLUTION OF COLLECTIVE BARGAINING IN NURSING

In the early 1940s, 75% of all hospital-employed RNs worked 50 to 60 hours a week and were subject to arbitrary schedules, uncompensated overtime, no health or pension benefits, and no sick days or personal time (Meier, 2000). In 1946, the ANA House of Delegates unanimously approved a resolution that formally initiated the journey of RNs down the road of collective bargaining. During the period between this resolution and 1999, the constituent organizations of ANA (state associations) were determined to be collective bargaining units for RN members who desired this representation in the workplace. Not all states provided collective bargaining services, so the debate over the acceptance of collective bargaining as appropriate for nurses became a divisive issue in the ANA for decades.

Legal Precedents for State Nursing Associations as Collective Bargaining Agents

The legal precedent that determined that state nursing associations are qualified under labor law to act as labor organizations is the 1979 Sierra Vista decision. The important consequence of this decision that affected nurses was that they were free to organize themselves and not to be organized by existing unions (Kimmel, 2007). Many RN leaders contend that these associations are not only proper and legal but are the preferred representatives for nurses in this country for purposes of collective bargaining. Ada Jacox (1980) suggested that collective bargaining through the professional organization was a way for RNs to achieve that collective professional responsibility that is a characteristic of a profession. It was thought by many that the state nursing association was the only safe ground that could be considered as neutral turf on which RNs from all educational backgrounds could meet and discuss issues of a generic nature and of importance to all RNs. However, as discussed in the section on the history of collective bargaining, it is beginning to appear that the preferred platform for meaningful collective bargaining for the profession is through a structure, such as the National Nurses United (NNU).

Many formally organized unions outside of the ANA have competed for the right to represent nurses. It was the opinion of many nurses that the state nurses associations were the proper and legal bargaining agents and were also the preferred representatives for nurses in this country for purposes of collective bargaining. During the late 1980s, the demand among nurses for representation continued to grow, yet efforts to organize nurses for collective bargaining were being stymied by a decision from the National Labor Relations Board (NLRB) that stopped approving the all-RN bargaining units. A legal battle then ensued, with the ANA and other labor unions against the American Hospital Association (AHA). The NLRB issued a ruling that reaffirmed the right of nurses to be represented in all-RN bargaining units.

Seeking a broader base of representation and greater support from the ANA for the collective bargaining program led activist nurses within the ANA to establish the United American Nurses (UAN) in 1999. They believed in the creation of a powerful, national, independent, and unified voice for union nurses. In 2000, the UAN held its first National Labor Assembly annual meeting. The participants in this meeting were staff nurse delegates. In February 2009, the UAN, the California Nurses Association, and the Massachusetts Nurses Association joined forces to form one new union that claims to represent 185,000 members. The new union, called the UAN–National Nurses Organizing Committee, would become a part of the labor movement as an AFL-CIO affiliate union. Shortly after this move, the union was renamed the National Nurses United (NNU, 2018).

As has been demonstrated, the representation of RNs for collective bargaining continues to change and grow to the point where affiliation with the ANA primarily for this purpose is no longer evident. Collective bargaining outside of ANA has become the route for RNs to gain the recognition many believe is essential for the growth of the profession. Others see this as the least effective way to gain recognition and benefits afforded to members of a profession.

Collective bargaining for professional groups (physicians, teachers, professors, scientists, entertainers, pilots, administrators) offers RNs another perspective regarding the process of collective bargaining. Identification with these professional groups can certainly help the nursing profession become accepted as a true profession with all the benefits of that identification.

Some of the differences noted between traditional collective bargaining and collective bargaining for professionals are agreeing to take lower wages in exchange for greater fringe benefits, setting a wage floor and then allowing individuals to negotiate for a salary based on individual performance, and/or negotiating for merit pay for outstanding performance (Department for Professional Employees [DPE], 2017). The opportunity to develop a variety of ways to earn wages begins the recognition that, even when bargaining collectively, there are opportunities to be compensated for significant differences in performance.

Collective bargaining for professionals also offers the opportunity to designate how a proposed increase in wages can be used to address other issues that might exist within the professional group.

WHO REPRESENTS NURSES FOR COLLECTIVE BARGAINING?

Traditional and Nontraditional Collective Bargaining

The national professional organization for nursing is the ANA, with its constituent units, the state, and territorial nursing associations. Through its economic security programs, the ANA recognized state nursing associations as the logical bargaining agents for professional nurses, and the states have been the premier representatives for nurses since 1946! These professional associations are indeed multipurpose; their activities include economic analyses, provision of related education, addressing nursing practice, conducting needed research, and providing traditional as well as nontraditional collective bargaining, lobbying, and political action.

The creation of the UAN by the ANA strengthened their collective bargaining capacity at a time when competition to represent nurses for collective bargaining was growing. The UAN was established in 1999 as the union arm of the ANA with the responsibility of representing the traditional collective bargaining needs of nurses. At the same time, a relatively new approach to collective bargaining was being developed and introduced into the labor market. This approach is a nontraditional process referred to as *interest-based bargaining* or *shared governance* (Brommer et al., 2003; Budd et al., 2004). This is a nontraditional style of bargaining that attempts to solve problems and differences between labor and management. Although this style of bargaining and mediation will not always eliminate the need for the more traditional and adversarial collective bargaining, many believe this nonadversarial approach to negotiation may be closer to the basic fabric of the discipline of nursing and its ethical code.

The organization that represented IBB, or the nontraditional collective voice in nursing, was the Center for American Nurses (Center). This was a professional association established in 2003, replacing the ANA's Commission on Workplace Advocacy that was created in 2000 to represent the needs of individual nurses in the workplace who were not represented by collective bargaining. The Center defined its role in workplace advocacy as providing a multitude of services designed to address the products and programs necessary to support the professional nurse in negotiating and dealing with the challenges of the workplace and in enhancing the quality of patient care (The American Nurse, 2010) (Critical Thinking Box 18.1).

? CRITICAL THINKING BOX 18.1

What is the status of your state nursing association in regard to workplace issues? Is your state a member of the National Nurses United? What is being done on a local basis that reflects the activities of your state association related to registered nurses' control over their practice?

In 2007, the ANA informed the UAN and Center that they would not be renewing their affiliation agreement (Hackman, 2008). Following this, in 2009, the largest union and professional organization of RNs was officially formalized. This organization is the NNU, and it is an outgrowth of the merger of three individual organizations—the California Nurses Association, the Massachusetts Nursing Association, and the UAN (the former UAN) (Gaus, 2009). This NNU union includes an estimated 185,000 members in every state and is the largest union and professional association of RNs in U.S. history (NNU, 2018).

In 2013, what remained of the Center was integrated into the structure of ANA and is now a part of the "products and services … and valuable resources that will directly assist nurses in their lives and careers" (The American Nurse, 2010, para 2).

Whether your state is a member of ANA or NNU, or both, it is necessary to recognize that workplace advocacy is a concern that directly affects every practicing nurse. It is critical that nurses support the organizational efforts to address the growing problems regarding the safety of the workplace, as well as safe and competent patient care, managed by RNs.

American Nurses Association and National Nurses United: What Are the Common Issues?

Staffing Issues

Staffing issues and policies related to nurse staffing are among the most prevalent topics discussed in any type of negotiation. There is much discussion in both the national and state legislatures regarding proposals aimed at addressing the way in which RNs should be staffed to be able to provide safe, as well as quality, patient care. There is also much objection to implementing mandated staffing plans rather than allowing nurses to maintain control over issues related to their professional practice. The Institute of Medicine (2004) completed a study entitled *Keeping Patients Safe: Transforming the Work Environment of Nurses*. The results of the study have led to significant recommendations that would begin to address the chronic shortage of RN staff without resorting to mandatory regulations from the legislatures. An assessment of progress was conducted in 2015, at the request of the Robert Woods Johnson foundation, after it was noted that even with the implementation of most of these recommendations, there was still a significant number of preventable errors, which caused harm. The conclusion of this assessment was that nurses need to continue to improve their skills in the areas of collaboration, leadership, and innovation (Fauteux, 2014; Institute of Medicine, 2015).

Staffing requirements are already mandated by various agencies. For example, Medicare, state health department licensing requirements, and The Joint Commission (TJC) each publish staffing standards that define the need to have sufficient, competent staff for safe and quality care. In 2018, the Safe Staffing for Nurse and Patient Safety Act was introduced to Congress. If passed, Medicare-participating hospitals would be required to develop safe staffing plans for each unit in the hospital. The staffing committee would be comprised of at least 55% RNs working in direct patient care (ANA, 2018). However, this legislation will need the factors that define safe, quality staffing as the basis for this legislation. It is also clear that staffing is more than numbers and any legislation or policy must include the fact that the RNs must demonstrate the competencies for the processes that are needed to provide safe care and to ensure the safety of patients. Refer to Chapters 17 and 25 for further discussion regarding staffing issues.

Objection to an Assignment

Professional duty implies an obligation to decline an assignment that one is not competent to complete. RNs cannot abandon their assigned patients, but they are obligated to inform their supervisor of any limitations they have in completing an assignment (Fig. 18.1). Not to inform and not to complete

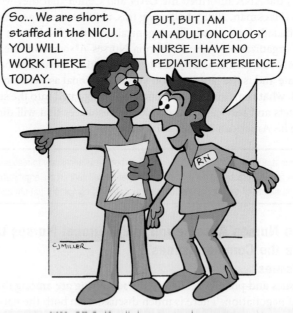

FIG. 18.1 Declining an assignment

the assignment, or not to inform and to attempt to complete the assignment, risks untoward patient outcomes and resultant disciplinary action up to and including some potential action taken by the board of nursing.

The right and the means for a nurse to register an objection to a work assignment are considered essential elements in a union contract that incorporates the values of a profession as the basis of the contract agreement. This same process must be provided to nurses not represented by a union because nurses are obligated *to only provide the care that they are competent to provide.* While they are participating in the interview process, RNs should ascertain the presence of a written policy regarding objections to an assignment.

Nurses are encouraged to submit reports indicating an objection to the assignment when the assignment is not appropriate. The report should follow the process defined in the contract or facility policy. These same problems should also initiate constructive follow-through by management or staff-management committees to improve the situations described in the reports. Inaction could serve as a basis for a grievance or negotiated change in a union contract or an incident or change in policy in a nonunion environment.

Concept of Shared Governance

Many facilities are implementing a variety of governance models called *shared governance, self-governance, participative decision making,* or *decentralization of management.* In its simplest form, shared governance is shared decision making based on the principles of partnership, equity, accountability, and ownership at the point of service (Swihart, 2006). The purpose of shared governance is to involve nurses in decision making related to control of their practice while the organization maintains the authority over traditional management decisions. The concept of shared governance can be a concern to unions representing nurses for purposes of collective bargaining, since collective bargaining is also thought to be a governance model that decentralizes aspects of management.

In general, shared governance focuses on clinical practice aspects of the RN staff while collective bargaining has a major focus on work rules/policies and so forth. While the line separating practice from work rules is minimal at times, it can be defined by those who are truly interested in achieving outcomes that are best for all parties. The discussion and understanding that must be reached address who or what controls the practice of professional nursing.

The concept of shared governance can be a concern to RNs who may feel that participating in shared governance can be a disadvantage to the practicing nurse if this participation is considered an alternative to collective bargaining. Whether greater latitude in decision making could be achieved through collective bargaining is the question to be considered. However, as more facilities are moving toward Magnet certification in which shared governance is a major function, it is recognized that some unionized facilities are also embracing the concepts of Magnet as recognition of the professional aspect of bargaining when representing the profession of nursing. Either way, it is essential that the practice of nursing be defined by nursing or the structure for implementing this practice is in place in each organization where nursing care is delivered.

Clinical or Career Ladder

The clinical ladder, or career ladder, has a place in both traditional and nontraditional styles of collective bargaining (Drenkard & Swartwout, 2005). The clinical ladder was designed to provide recognition of an RN who chooses to remain clinically oriented. The idea of rewarding the clinical nurse with pay and status along a specific track or ladder is the result of the contributions of a nurse researcher, Dr. Patricia Benner. Her descriptions of the growth and development of nursing knowledge and practice provided the basis for a ladder model that can be used to identify and reward the nurse along the steps from novice to expert (Benner, 2009).

Negotiations

While RNs in a facility have varied educational backgrounds and represent the multiple practice specialties available to nursing, there are common practice issues/processes that need to be addressed by the nursing negotiating team. Once the common issues are addressed, the differences in practice needs must then be addressed in ongoing negotiations.

Professional goals and practice needs are appropriate topics for contract negotiations. Because personnel directors, hospital administrators, and hospital lawyers may have difficulty relating to these discussions, the nurse negotiating team has to be able to provide sufficient information to help prepare these individuals to understand the inclusion of professional goals and practice needs into the collective bargaining process and as entries into the agreed-on contract. The resolution of disagreements about professional issues necessitates there be time for a thoughtful process by those who are appropriately prepared to reach agreements through the negotiating process. Perhaps the complex issues such as recruitment, retention, staffing, and health and safety are better addressed in the more collegial setting of the nontraditional model; however, many of these issues are paramount to the creation of a safe and effective work environment for nurses, and they need to be addressed in both types of negotiations (Institute of Medicine, 2004).

THE DEBATE OVER COLLECTIVE BARGAINING

Collective Bargaining: Perspectives of the Traditional Approach

Is There a Place for Collective Bargaining in Nursing?

Should RNs use collective bargaining if they are members of a profession? Is nursing a profession or an occupation? Those in the nursing profession have debated these questions since the late 1950s, and the discussion and debate continue today. Nurses often look for assistance outside of nursing to help resolve issues, but these two questions can and should be resolved by nurses if RNs are to be recognized as independent and in control of their practice.

According to the New York Department of Labor, "A registered professional nurse (RN) is a licensed health care professional who helps patients to achieve optimal health and prevent disease or injury. RNs provide compassionate care that is respectful of each patient's values and wishes. They coordinate and supervise care provided by other personnel, such as licensed practical nurses or home health aides. RNs provide health teaching to patients, families, other care providers and the public. They participate in health research and in making health care policies" (New York Department of Labor, 2016, para 1). Defining what each level of RN education best prepares one to practice can also be an issue discussed and agreed to through the process of collective bargaining. However, it must be recognized that these definitions are specific to each institution as the practice of professional nursing is defined at these individual facilities. Perhaps over time, the profession of nursing will reach consensus regarding practice and the level of education completed, and this will no longer have to be a negotiated item! Because of their expertise and the value of their service, members of a profession are granted a measure of autonomy in their work. This autonomy permits practitioners to make independent judgments and decisions on the basis of a theoretical framework that is learned through study and practice. Although there may still be some who do not agree with baccalaureate education being required for nursing to be designated as a profession, consider the fact that the absence of this professional designation continues to prevent nurses from the control over and definitions of their practice and of reaching their potential contributions to patient care and the health care system in which they are practicing.

In each state, registered nursing continues to be categorized as an *occupation* by the respective labor boards, and many decisions regarding the position of nursing in an organization are based on this classification as an occupation. However, for the purposes of the discussion on traditional and non-traditional collective bargaining, the role of nursing will be addressed as that of a profession.

RNs need to consider the power granted to them and to the profession when they earn their license to practice nursing. The legal authority to practice nursing is independent from any other licensed professional or regulatory organization. This power of independence includes taking the responsibility for one's practice and for the practice of others when that practice negatively impacts patients and/or the community. This power is also an important element when entering into collective bargaining, because the independently licensed RN must ensure the agreement supports this independence when addressing areas of clinical practice. Conflict arises as RN employees advocate for a professional role in patient care when they are not classified as a profession by labor definitions and by the hiring facilities. The health care institutions hire RNs as members of an occupation who are essentially managed and led by the organization's formal leaders who often focus on productivity and savings. However, the hiring organization may not put RNs in situations where their independent clinical responsibilities cannot be met.

This potential conflict is a factor leading RNs to consider unionization as the only way they can demonstrate control over their clinical practice, particularly if shared governance is not used at their place of practice.

> Nursing has used collective action to its benefit, achieving professional goals while protecting and promoting public interest through lobbying efforts in the political arena. Many registered nurses support collective bargaining in the workplace as a way to control their practice by redistributing power within the health care organization.

Registered Nurse Participation in Collective Bargaining

If the state nurses associations were considered to be logical bargaining agents for RNs, why do so few nurses join these associations, and why are even fewer associations pursuing collective bargaining? "ANA, a nursing organization … reportedly represents 163,111 RNs of the almost 3 million RNs that are active in this country" (Center for Union Facts, 2016). It is important to recognize that this low membership rate is not unique to nursing but is the same for most disciplines and for society in general. However, this low membership rate may also reflect the thinking of some that the professional organization for RNs may not be the best organization to represent the nursing population for collective bargaining. Perhaps the conflicts that would likely arise between a professional organization and a collective bargaining organization could be avoided by not combining these two distinct processes under one umbrella.

One of the problems with association memberships is that people tend to look at these associations and organizations for "what they can do for *me*"—for the work *I* do or the benefits *I* can receive. In reality, we need to look at these associations for what they can do for the profession and the population being served by the members of the profession/occupation. We then realize that the profession is only as strong as its members and the contributions they make to that occupation/profession. Perhaps looking at it in this way will encourage more to join and become members. The professional association can provide the standards and ethical platforms for a professional practice that would then be used as the basis for a collective bargaining contract.

> Collective bargaining for registered nurses occurs more frequently in states where there is significant union activity in other industries.

The current labor climate is very volatile across the country. Unions are trying to organize new categories of workers, with special emphasis on the growing health care sector in states that have not traditionally been active in the labor movement. Some state nursing associations stopped providing collective bargaining services because of external pressures, including challenges from competing unions, excessive resistance by employers, or state policies that make unionization difficult, such as right-to-work laws. In states with right-to-work laws, it is illegal to negotiate an agency shop requirement. Membership and dues collection can never be mandatory, even if the workers are covered by a collective bargaining agreement. The cost of negotiating and maintaining a collective bargaining agreement in these states is often more than the income received for providing these services. Philosophical differences regarding the benefits and risks of a professional association as the bargaining agent have also led RNs in some states to abandon or avoid union activities or to avoid joining the professional association.

There are 2.9 million employed RNs in the United States, but only a few hundred thousand are organized for collective bargaining, and only around 20% of RNs belong to a professional organization. Sixty-one percent of these RNs are employed by hospitals (Bureau of Labor Statistics, 2018).

How will collective professional goals be achieved if so many nurses depend on the time and finances of so few? Some believe that the profession's efforts to address workplace concerns from both the traditional and nontraditional perspectives will result in larger membership numbers in the near future. For now, there may be too few RNs involved in the nursing associations to make up the needed critical mass for the kinds of changes and support that need to take place. Perhaps learning that this is the case will motivate more RNs to join their professional organization to support the work that needs to be accomplished. The implementation of the NNU as the "RN Super Union" (Massachusetts Nurses Association, 2016) may supplant the state nurses associations as the primary provider of collective bargaining services for RNs.

Where Does Collective Bargaining Begin?

As stated in the National Labor Relations Act, RNs in the private sector are guaranteed legal protection if they seek to be represented by a collective bargaining agent. After a drive for such representation is under way and 30% of the employed RNs in an organization have signed cards signaling interest in representation, both the employer and the union are prohibited from engaging in any anti-labor action. Employers are prohibited from terminating the organizers for union activity, and they may not ignore the request for a vote for union representation. After the organizing campaign, a vote is taken; a majority, comprising 50% plus one of those voting, selects or rejects the collective bargaining agent.

The employer may choose to bargain in good faith on matters concerning working conditions by recognizing the bargaining agent before the vote. This approach usually occurs only if management believes a large majority of potential voters support the foundation of a union. In other cases, the employer may appeal requests for representation to the NLRB. Before and during the appeal, other unions may intervene and try to win a majority of votes for representation.

As a part of this appeal process, arguments are made before the NLRB regarding why, by whom, or how the nurses are to be represented. For example, the hospital may raise the question of unit determination. The original policy interpretation of the labor law simultaneously limited the number of individual units an employer or industry would have to recognize, yet allowed for distinct groups of employees, such as RNs, to receive separate representation. Nurses historically have been represented in all-RN bargaining units, and most bargaining units throughout the country reflect that pattern.

What Can a Union Contract Do?

Generally speaking, what can a union contract do in a hospital setting? Many believe that, today more than ever, RNs need a strong union such as the New York State Nurses Association (NYSNA, 2016). Nurse shortages and the rise of health care for profit have dramatically changed the environments in which RNs are practicing and the demands that are placed on them. Too many nurses are spending too much time on duties that can be completed by staff other than RNs. Too many nurses are enduring too much overtime and are working under conditions that are unsafe for them and their patients.

Members of the NNU believe a strong, unified workforce is the best solution to the problems facing RNs and their patients today. When RNs become members of NNU, for example, they gain the ability to negotiate enforceable contracts that spell out specific working conditions such as acceptable nurse–patient ratios, roles RNs will play in determining standards of care, circumstances under which RNs will agree to work overtime, pay scales, benefits, dependable procedures for scheduling vacations and other time off, and all other similar conditions important to nurses.

A contract can also include language related to clinical advancement, such as is measured by the use of a clinical ladder or a similar mechanism. This is one way to bring concepts that have traditionally been avoided in collective bargaining strategies into the contracts to address practice aspects of the profession. When actions such as this occur, it could be anticipated that more RNs will support collective bargaining.

Wages. Wages and benefits are the foundation of a contract. Wages are the remuneration one receives for providing a service and reflect the value put on the work performed. In an article on the history of nursing's efforts to receive adequate compensation, Brider (1990) reaffirmed the need to continue efforts to improve nursing salaries. The author correctly stated that, "from its beginnings, the nursing profession has grappled with its own ambivalence which is how to reconcile the ideal of selfless service with the necessity of making a living" (Brider, 1990, p. 77). The article confirmed the ambivalence of the nurses who recorded both their joy in productive careers and their disappointment with the way their work was valued. Registered nursing has certainly come a long way from the $8 to $12 monthly allowance in the early 1900s, but the challenge remains to bring nursing in line with comparable careers.

As we progress through the 21st century, it is clear periods of a shortage of nurses will occur. Like other occupations and professions, when the supply and demand favor the employee, wages are more critically evaluated. More recent shortages of RNs seem to be less responsive to some of the traditional solutions such as wage adjustments. This likely indicates that wages are not the only, or perhaps not even the primary, reason that individuals are not choosing registered nursing as a career or that many RNs are choosing to leave the field.

Another aspect of RN compensation involves the challenge of addressing the negative effects of wage compression. This economic concept means that RNs who have been in practice for 10 and 12 years may make less money than recent graduates in their first registered nursing jobs! Unfortunately, it is not uncommon during times of shortages to see hiring or relocation bonuses to attract RNs into new positions. It would be preferable to see those dollars redistributed for the purposes of maintaining the base that is formed by the retention of experienced RNs in the facility.

Job security versus career security. It is probably not news to any student enrolled in a registered nursing program that he or she has entered a field that is facing many challenges—both from within and from outside nursing. Challenges related to the need for more RNs will occur primarily because of technological advancements; an increased emphasis on primary and preventative care; and the large, aging Baby Boomer population who will demand more health care services as they live longer and more active lives (Bureau of Labor Statistics, 2018). Additionally, challenges related to the implementation of the Affordable Care Act of 2010 are to be expected, and planning for ways to address these challenges are under way.

> According to the Bureau of Labor Statistics' Employment Projections 2016 to 2026, registered nursing (RN) is listed among the top occupations in terms of job growth through 2026. The RN workforce is expected to grow from 2,955,200 in 2016 to 3,393,200 in 2026, an increase of 438,100 or 15% (Bureau of Labor Statistics, 2018).

The total number of licensed RNs in the United States in October 2018 was 4,693,937 (NCSBN, 2018b). The need for so many additional RNs, coupled with the anticipated growth in the profession, provides an opportunity to achieve some of the professional goals that have eluded nursing thus far, including full recognition as a profession and all that entails.

Seniority rights. RNs who remain on staff at an organization accrue seniority that is based on the length of time employed as an RN at that facility. Seniority provides specific rights, spelled out in the bargaining agreement, for those who have the highest number of years of service. These rights are derived from the idea that permanent employees should be viewed as assets to the organization and should therefore be rewarded for their service. In nurse employment contracts, there may be provisions (seniority language) that give senior nurses the right to accrue more vacation time and to be given preference when requesting time off, a change in position, or relief from shift rotation requirements. In the event of a staff layoff, the rule that states "the last hired becomes the first fired" protects senior nurses. Seniority rules may be applied to the registered nursing staff of the entire hospital or may be confined to a unit. However, transfers and promotions must reward the most senior qualified nurse in the organization.

Resolution of grievances. Methods to resolve grievances, which are sometimes explicitly spelled out in a contract, are an important element of any agreement. A grievance can arise when provisions in a contract are interpreted differently by management and an employee or employees. This difference often occurs when issues related to job security (a union priority), job performance, and discipline (a management priority) arise. *Grievance mechanisms* are used in an attempt to resolve the conflict with the parties involved. The employer, the employee, or the union may file a grievance. Nurses who are covered by contracts should be represented at any meeting or hearing they believe may lead to the application of disciplinary action. A co-worker, an elected nurse representative, or a member of the labor union's staff can provide such representation.

Arbitration. If the grievance mechanism does not lead to resolution of the issue, some contracts allow referral of the issue for arbitration. A knowledgeable—but neutral—arbitrator acceptable to both parties (union and hospital) will be asked to hear the facts of the case and issue a finding. In pre-agreed, binding arbitration, the parties must accept the decision of the arbitrator. For example, some contracts require that when management elects to discharge (suspend or terminate) a nurse, the case must be brought to arbitration. Based on the arbitrator's finding, the nurse may be reinstated, perhaps with back pay, may remain suspended, or may be terminated. If the contract states that the arbitrator's decision is final and binding, there is no further contractual or organizational avenue for either party to pursue.

Arbitration has also been used to resolve issues involving the integrity of the bargaining unit. Arbitrators have been asked to decide whether nurses remain eligible for bargaining unit coverage when jobs are changed and new practice models are implemented.

> Mediation, arbitration, and fact finding have all been used to resolve conflicts in union contracts.

There is strong support for the use of these three methods, but hospital management personnel often resist using them. Nurses usually fare well when contract enforcement issues are submitted to an arbitrator and facts, not power or public relations, determine the outcome.

Strikes and other labor disputes. What can nurses do in the face of a standoff during contract negotiations? The options that current RNs have are quite different from those before 1968, when nurses felt a greater sense of powerlessness. At that time, despite nurses' threats of "sickouts," walkouts, picketing, or mass resignations, the employer maintained an effective power base. Threats of group action attracted public attention, but nurses' threats had little effect on employers, because nurses who were represented through the ANA had a no-strike policy. As negotiations became more difficult, it was apparent that nurses were in a weaker bargaining position because of the no-strike policy. The ANA responded to the state nursing associations, and in 1968, it reversed its 18-year-old no-strike policy. The NNU does not have a no-strike policy.

Strikes remain rare among nursing units, but as mentioned previously, when the efficacy of patient care and patient and staff safety are at risk, RNs may believe they have to strike. Increased strikes were seen beginning in 2000 as facilities were imposing mandatory overtime to cover the staff shortages. Many nurses are uncomfortable with the idea of striking, believing that they are abandoning their patients. It is important for nurses who contemplate striking to discuss plans for patient care with nurses who have previously conducted strikes so that they will be assured that plans to care for patients are adequate.

When an impasse is reached in hospital negotiations, national labor law requires RNs to issue a 10-day notice of their intent to strike. In the public's interest, every effort must be made to prevent a strike. The NLRB mandates mediation, and a board of inquiry to examine the issue may be created before a work stoppage. The organization is supposed to use this time to reduce the patient census and to slow or halt elective admissions. In the meantime, the nurses' strike committee will develop schedules for coverage of emergency rooms, operating rooms, and intensive care areas. This coverage is to be used only in the case of real emergencies. Planning coverage for patient care should reassure nurses troubled by the possibility of a strike. Nurses who agree to work in emergencies or at other facilities during a strike often donate their wages to funds that are set up for striking nurses.

Business and labor are both in search of more positive ways to work together to be able to avoid the possibility of a work stoppage. Strikes are not easy for either side—one side is not able to provide services, and the other side is not able to earn its usual income. In the middle, when health care is involved, is the patient who loses trust in both the organization and in the body of employees who choose to strike, requiring the patient to seek care elsewhere. The Department of Labor and the Federal Mediation and Conciliation Service have sponsored national grants to undertake alternatives to traditional collective bargaining. At least two Midwestern nursing organizations have used win–win bargaining techniques and found them to be constructive methods for negotiation.

What Are the Elements of a Sound Contract?

Membership. The inclusion of union security provisions is an essential element of a sound contract (Fig. 18.2) and addresses one of the defined goals of collective bargaining (union integrity). *Security provisions* include measures such as enforcement of membership requirements (collection of dues and access by the union staff to the members). In a closed shop agreement, the employer agrees that they will only hire employees who are members of the union. Closed shops are generally illegal. Union shop agreements allow an employer to hire nonunion members but require the employee to join the union within a certain amount of time (usually after 30 days). In practice, though, employers are not allowed to fire employees who refuse to join the union, provided the employees pay dues and fees to the union. An *agency shop* agreement requires employees who do not join the union to pay dues and fees.

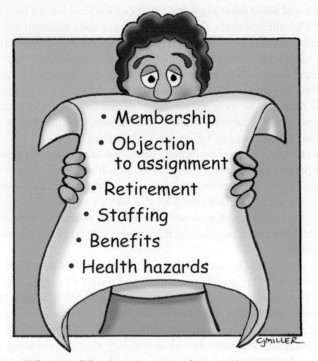

- Membership
- Objection to assignment
- Retirement
- Staffing
- Benefits
- Health hazards

FIG. 18.2 Effective elements of a sound contract.

Retirement. The usual pension or retirement programs for RNs have been either the social security system or a hospital pension plan. Because many employers are eliminating defined pension plans, individual retirement accounts, which are transferable from hospital to hospital in case of job changes, are becoming increasingly popular. The method of addressing issues related to financial support at the time of retirement should be a topic of negotiations. The ANA has entered an agreement with a national company to provide a truly portable national plan, unrestricted by geographic location or employment site. Although this plan could be complicated by conflicting state laws governing pension plans, a precedent was set as long ago as 1976, when California nursing contracts mandated employer contributions to individual retirement accounts for each nurse with immediate vesting (eligibility for access to the fund) and complete portability for the participants (meaning that the nurse could take the established retirement account to another hospital and could continue to add to this account either directly or by rolling it over into the new employer's individual retirement account).

One of registered nursing's most attractive benefits has been a nurse's mobility, which is the opportunity to change jobs at will. A drawback of this mobility is the loss of long-term retirement funds. With financial cutbacks in the hospital industry, retirement plans are in danger of being targeted as givebacks in negotiating rights or benefits to be traded away in lieu of another issue or benefit that may be more pressing at the time. One of the major benefits of individual retirement accounts is that they do belong to the employee, and the employee's contributions to the plan plus the employer's contributions to the plan can be taken with the employee when he or she leaves that employment, assuming all the defined rules of the plan are followed.

Health insurance coverage continues to be a key concern of employees and has been at the root of the majority of labor disputes in all industries in the past few years. It is not inconceivable that nurses may be asked to trade off long-term economic security (pensions) for short-term security (e.g., health benefits, wages). There is less chance this will occur if the organization has moved from the defined pension benefit. What is more likely to occur is that the employer will ask to contribute fewer dollars to health insurance premiums and/or retirement accounts and will ask employees to contribute an increased percentage of the cost of these benefits.

Other benefit issues. Other issues that have affected RNs as employees are family-leave policies, availability of daycare services, long-term disability insurance, and access to health insurance for retirees. These are the same issues that affect many workers in this country but may have a greater impact on employees such as RNs because of the 24-hour-a-day/7-day-a-week coverage that needs to be provided by this professional group.

An issue of special concern to RNs involves the scheduling of work hours. Although more men have joined the nursing occupation/profession, registered nursing remains a female occupation (Kaiser Family Foundation, 2016). This reality must be addressed by providing benefit packages that provide flexibility for women who assume multiple roles in today's society. Generally, it is women who provide ongoing care to both children and parents. The nurse in the family may be called on to do this more than the spouse or the siblings. RNs are asking nursing contract negotiators to secure leave policies that permit the use of sick time for family needs, which provide flexible scheduling that is flexible, and that allow part-time employment and work sharing.

An increasing number of men are entering the nursing field. According to the U.S. Census Bureau (2013), men comprise approximately 9% of the current RN workforce. It is also noted that males who are practicing in the nursing profession earned a median annual salary of $79,688, whereas the median annual salary for a female RN was $73,090 (Nurse.com, 2018). Would this difference exist in an organization in which there was a collective bargaining agreement? Staffing issues, such as objection to an assignment, inadequate staffing, poorly prepared staff, mandatory overtime, nurse fatigue, and health hazards, are all concerns that can be addressed in a union contract; however, these are also issues of ongoing concern for all RNs, regardless of the type of bargaining situation in their respective states or organizations. These issues are discussed further in Chapter 25.

How Can Nurses Control Their Own Practice?

The essence of the professional nurse contract is control of practice. For example, RN councils or professional performance committees provide the opportunity for RNs within the institution to meet regularly. These meetings are sanctioned by the contract. The elected registered staff nurse representatives may, for example, have specific objectives to

- Improve the professional practice of nurses and nursing assistants.
- Recommend ways and means to improve patient care.
- Recommend ways and means to address care issues when a critical nurse staffing shortage exists.
- Identify and recommend the elimination of hazards in the workplace.
- Identify and recommend processes that work to ensure the safety of patients.
- Implement peer review.
- Implement shared governance.

Nurse Practice Committees

RN practice committees should have a formal relationship with nursing administration. Regularly scheduled meetings with nursing and hospital administrators can provide a forum for the discussion of professional issues in a safe atmosphere. Many potential conflicts regarding contract language can be prevented by discussion before contract talks begin or before grievances arise. Ideally, all health care professionals should also be a part of these forums because they are an integral part of the care delivery system in a hospital and in other settings. Joint-practice language has been proposed in some contracts to facilitate these discussions.

Since the recognition of Magnet hospitals by the American Nurses Credentialing Center (ANCC) began in 1994, approximately 9.2% of all health care organizations in the United States have achieved ANCC Magnet recognition status (ANCC, 2018; Campaign for Action, 2017). Magnet status is not a prize or an award. Rather, it is a credential of organizational recognition of nursing excellence. Approximately 20% of the organizations awarded the recognition have a collective bargaining agreement with the nurses. This helps to validate the fact that control of nursing practice by RN staff members can be successfully achieved within the context of a collective bargaining agreement when both Magnet and collective bargaining have this as a common goal.

Collective Bargaining: Perspectives of the Nontraditional Approach

Effectively addressing the concerns of workplace advocacy, higher standards of practice, and economic security are not new issues. These concerns have caused nurses in some areas of the country to organize and to use unions and collective bargaining models to address practice and economic concerns. This section is designed to provide you with information and a rationale for a different approach to the position of the traditional collective bargaining. In the end, it will be up to you and your concept of the RN's role to grapple with this issue during your professional career.

Simultaneous Debates

Registered nursing today has acquired the majority of the generally recognized characteristics of a profession. One of these characteristics is a lengthy period of specialized education and practice preparation. The activities that are performed by professions are valued and recognized as important to society. In addition, a member of a profession has an acquired area of expertise that allows the person to make independent judgments, to act with autonomy, and to assume accountability. Nurses also have specialty organizations and are eligible to receive specialty credentialing in some defined areas of practice.

Another aspect of professional registered nursing is its strongly written ethical code. It is the obligation of every licensed RN to follow the tenets of the 2015 ANA Code of Ethics for Nurses (see Chapter 19). The Code articulates the values, goals, and responsibilities of the professional practice of nursing. The provisions of the Code that outline our duties to care for, advocate for, and be faithful to those people who entrust their health care to us are well integrated into the educational preparation of the RN. They are also widely recognized and respected by the public.

Collective Bargaining: The Debate That Continues

The debate about the appropriateness of collective bargaining continues. The combination of an explosion in knowledge and technology and an expanded population able to access health care quickly brought both public and private sector payers of health care to the inevitable quest to rein in the cost of health care. This gave birth and life to a growing collection of payment systems. There are now gatekeepers, specific practice protocols, contractual agreements between payers and providers, and provider and consumer incentives that govern the place, provider, type, and quantity of a patient's care. These developments have affected everyday care in a growing number of settings. Nurses are challenged daily in practice environments that have evolved to business models to survive financially while continuing to provide care to a defined population of patients. Many RNs feel these business and financial environments are not conducive to the patient-focused or family-centered models of care delivery or to the ethical values that have been an inherent part of the professional education and practice preparation of nurses. All too often, the intense clinical education of the RN practicing in today's health care environment has not prepared the individual to appreciate the financial and regulatory realities of a large industry. Perhaps even more disconcerting is the fact that as RNs enter the workforce, they may not see the magnitude of their potential for leadership and problem solving within an environment that continues to evolve so quickly while the environment continues to work hard to hold on to the traditional hierarchy of medicine and health care administration.

The history of the position of registered nursing during the first half of the 20th century may, in part, explain our slow journey toward leadership and control of nursing practice. In the last half of the 20th century, some RNs organized and relied on collective bargaining units to speak for them. Time and energy have been spent debating who can or should best represent professional nurses in the workplace. The transition of collective bargaining from the ANA, which established the foundation for acceptance of collective bargaining by RNs, to the growing NNU, may signal that the journey toward gaining control of nursing practice will move more quickly. These two strong organizations could take steps to gain acceptance of the concept that control of nursing practice by RNs is not congruent with "holding on to the traditional hierarchy of medicine and administration."

Traditional Collective Bargaining: Its Risks and Benefits

The goal of the traditional collective bargaining model is to win something that is controlled by another. There is an "us versus them" approach. The weapon is the power of numbers. Although a desired contract is achieved, long-lasting adversarial relationships may develop between the nurses and the employer (Budd et al., 2004) (Critical Thinking Box 18.2).

? CRITICAL THINKING BOX 18.2

With the soaring cost of health care, the changes in health care reimbursement, and the subsequent reining in of health care costs, where does that leave nursing in the collective bargaining process? Does this not further aggravate the already adversarial relationship of nurses and their employers?

Traditional collective bargaining held promise and assisted the professional nurse's evolution toward economic stability. These were important gains. However, the full power and potency of nursing as an industry leader has not emerged through traditional collective bargaining efforts. This may explain the dissatisfaction of the nurses with traditional collective bargaining or may also be an indication that the other basic debates within the body of RNs need to be resolved before nurses take the place in the industry they feel is appropriate for them.

Can nursing effectively step away from the adversarial process of traditional collective bargaining into an effective leadership role? IBB and/or processes such as shared governance may offer nurses a nonadversarial approach, but it will require nursing leaders to demonstrate an understanding of interests and outcomes that are important both to the nursing occupation/profession and to other members of the health care industry (Budd et al., 2004). As discussed earlier in this chapter, IBB is a nontraditional style of bargaining that attempts to solve problems and resolve differences between the workforce and the employer—or the nurse and the hospital. Although this style of bargaining and mediation will not always eliminate the need for the more traditional and adversarial collective bargaining, this nonadversarial approach of negotiation may be closer to the basic beliefs underlying professional nursing as well as the nursing code of ethics.

In considering nontraditional approaches, it is important to recognize state nurse associations that have made significant contributions to their local membership by offering IBB services to that membership. This has also resulted in contributions to the advancement of nontraditional, nonadversarial bargaining for the promotion of workplace advocacy on a national level (Box 18.2). Do these commitments sound familiar?

BOX 18.2   EIGHT COMMITMENTS TO WORKPLACE ADVOCACY

Workplace advocacy is a nurse-to-nurse strategy that can give registered nurses (RNs) a meaningful voice in their workplace. As a result of Texas Nurses Association (TNA) workplace advocacy efforts in the past, Texas now has one of the strongest nursing practice acts in the country. The following are eight commitments to workplace advocacy. The TNA will:

Work to secure mechanisms within health care systems that provide opportunities for registered nurses to affect institutional policies. Mechanisms include:

- Shared governance
- Participatory management models
- Magnet hospital identifications
- Statewide staffing regulations

Develop with stakeholders a conflict resolution process for nurse/nurse employers that addresses registered nurse concerns about patient care and delivery issues.

- Active participation with the Texas Hospital Association and the American Arbitration Association to develop a conflict resolution process that meets the needs of nurses in resolving patient care issues.

Provide legislative solutions to Texas registered nurses by reviewing issues of concern to nurses in employment settings and introducing appropriate legislation. Previous initiatives include:

- Whistle-blower
- Safe Harbor Peer Review
- Support for Board of Nurse Examiners rules outlining strong nursing practice standards

Explore the development of a legal center for nurses that could provide legal support and decision-making advice as a last recourse in cases of unresolved workplace issues. Its purpose would be to:

- Provide fast legal assistance
- Earmark precedent-setting cases that could impact case law and health care policy

Support the RN in practice with self-advocacy and patient advocacy information by providing products that increase knowledge about:

- Laws and regulations governing practice
- Use of applicable standards of nursing practice
- Conflict-resolution techniques
- Statewide reporting mechanisms that allow the nurse to report concerns about health care institutions and professionals
- Professional behaviors, core values, and conduct that support effective negotiation

Promote to RNs those health care institutions in Texas that demonstrate outstanding nurse/employer relations.

Work with Texas schools of nursing to develop materials that incorporate self-advocacy and patient advocacy information into the nursing curriculum.

Advocate for the elimination of physician abuse of RNs with the physician community and employers by:

- Working with physician professional organizations to develop a campaign to end physician abuse of RNs
- Working with health care facilities to establish zero tolerance for physician abuse of RNs
- Developing model policies against physician abuse of nurses
- Encouraging nurse-to-nurse advocacy to stop abusive situations

Reprinted with permission from Texas Nursing Association. (2006). *Eight commitments to workplace advocacy.* Austin, TX: tna@texasnurses.org.

FUTURE TRENDS

The public should be concerned about an inadequate supply of nurses. Based on that concern, along with the multiple other issues that are impacting the provision of health care now and in the future, there is increased interest by the press and policymakers to be sure RNs are prepared in adequate numbers and that their working environment supports quality nursing care. This attention is helping nurses achieve improvements in overall compensation and working conditions and may also lead to support for the preparation of sufficient numbers of RN faculty and methods of financial support for the education of RNs.

The nursing community should take a step back and try to identify those factors that appear to keep registered nursing from becoming a profession of choice, which should result in eliminating the continuous cycle of shortage/staff reduction/shortage. One of the classic issues is that nursing is still not considered a profession according to most definitions of a profession or according to the labor bureaus that classify employee groups. Until nurses accept the fact that we cannot just *say* we are a profession without meeting the minimum criteria for this designation, we will continue to be classified as an occupation only.

The movement to gain recognition as a profession is the next issue to be addressed in the next few years. Discussions regarding this requirement are found in Chapter 9. Another issue that must be addressed by organized nursing is the silence of nursing, as defined and discussed by Buresh and Gordon (2006). These authors completed extensive research to determine why nurses were rarely seen or heard in the various forms of media. They discovered that, for the most part, the media cannot find RNs who are willing to talk, to be interviewed, or to write editorials stating opinions or positions. The Worldwide Health Organization in collaboration with The International Council of Nurses has organized a global campaign, Nursing Now, to encourage nurses to be a strong voice in finding the solutions for the current health need issues (WHO, 2018).

As with many things in life, there is a tendency to look outside of the problem to define a cause for the problem and to look to others to find a solution. Nursing, as the largest group of health care providers and as the only group of providers entrusted to implement the majority of the medical plan of care, needs to look within to find how to communicate most effectively the vital role we take in the provision of health care.

Nurses throughout the country have felt firsthand the effects of cost containment. Those effects have often been detrimental to the quality of care that RNs are charged to provide. From a professional practice perspective, mandatory overtime and short staffing are some of the factors contributing to the preponderance of medical errors documented in the Institute of Medicine report, *To Err Is Human: Building a Safer Health System* (Institute of Medicine, 2000). The ANA was the initial voice in recognizing these as potential contributing factors and has led the way in encouraging research agendas that further quantify the number of work hours needed to provide safe care and further define how patient safety can be ensured. As with other major issues affecting the practice of RNs, the ANA and state nursing associations are in the lead in federal and state legislative efforts to address overtime and staffing in the context of safe patient care.

> What lies ahead for collective bargaining and all forms of collective action for nurses must be viewed within the context of the overall changes occurring in the health care system and in the financing mechanisms for that system.

As concerned nurses, we need to remain vigilant about our need to meet the basic obligation of licensure, which is to provide safe care to all patients. This issue of adequate access to health care services is one that will probably be with us for the rest of our professional careers. It is believed by many that one way to improve access to services is to deliver them in environments and by providers that have not traditionally been a part of our health care system. Each of these venues provides significant opportunities for RNs, because the essence of our work is the prevention of disease and the adaptability to chronic disease processes that will enable our patients to remain as active as possible in their own environment.

Advanced Practice Nurses Role in Advocating

In today's world the role of the Advanced Practice Nurse (APN) is expanding. Most people only consider nurse practitioners when they hear the term APN. In reality, this term is related to advanced education and not just one specific role. The two APN roles that can have a meaningful impact advocating for nurses are clinical nurse specialists and nurse practitioners. Their roles are twofold. They spend the majority of their time in direct patient care, but they do have a responsibility to be informal leaders in the areas in which they work. In a recent study, APNs were asked about their role as leaders in the clinical setting. This study found that although their leadership role lies mainly in the patient care area, they do have organizational leadership responsibilities, one of which is to "advocate for nursing—being a strong and supportive voice…" (Lamb, Martin-Misener, Bryant-Lukosius, & Latimer, 2018, p. 8).

By taking what they have learned as nurse leaders, APNs can encourage nurses to use their voices to advocate for themselves as well. APNs also have a unique position to be able to advocate for safer environments for both nurses and patients. This would include staffing numbers, work hours, and resources necessary to provide safe and effective care.

Besides being a voice for the nursing profession, APNs conduct research for best practice. This research provides evidence for nurses to present while negotiating for needed changes in the work environment. They also have a strong voice in the political world to advocate for legislature which can give nurses more power when negotiating for better work conditions and safer practices.

CONCLUSION

Nursing has a unique contract with society to promote effective health care and, as a natural outcome, promote the health and welfare of the nurse and the occupation/profession of nursing. The multipurpose nature of the professional nursing association will continue to work to preserve the future of nursing. This chapter cannot stand alone, nor can the nurses in the workplace stand alone if they are to offset the forces that negate the contributions of nurses. Political action and lobbying, research, and education are necessary to further the cause of nursing and to meet the health care needs of the public we serve. As nurses work to transform aspects of the health system and to improve access to care, they will continue to depend on collective action and a collective voice through the structures and functions initially established within the ANA to advocate for optimal working conditions and standards of practice. There are now multiple opportunities to continue to advance the collective voice of nursing to ensure that the profession of nursing will be available to provide the quality care and services to all those who are in need of this care and service (see the relevant websites and online resources below). Welcome to nursing! Join us in our efforts to unify our skills, knowledge, and voices as we ensure our vision is being met.

⊕ RELEVANT WEBSITES AND ONLINE RESOURCES

Back to the Future of Nursing: The Institute of Medicines 2013 Richard and Hinda Rosenthal Lecture
http://nationalacademies.org/hmd/activities/quality/rosenthallect/2013-dec-11.aspx.

IOM Report, The Future of Nursing
http://nationalacademies.org/HMD/Reports/2010/The-Future-of-Nursing-Leading-Change-Advancing-Health.aspx.

National Nurses United (NNU)
www.nationalnursesunited.org/.

Online Journal of Issues in Nursing
OJIN is a peer-reviewed, online publication that addresses current topics affecting nursing practice, research, education, and the wider health care sector. http://www.nursingworld.org/OJIN.

Patient Protection and Affordable Care Act
http://www.gpo.gov/fdsys/pkg/BILLS-111hr3590enr/pdf/BILLS-111hr3590enr.pdf.

BIBLIOGRAPHY

American Nurses Association (ANA). (2015). *Code of ethics for nurses with interpretive statements.* Retrieved from https://www.nursingworld.org/practice-policy/nursing-excellence/ethics/code-of-ethics-for-nurses/.

American Nurses Association (ANA). (2018). *ANA applauds safe staffing legislation.* Retrieved from https://www.nursingworld.org/news/news-releases/2018/ana-applauds-nurse-staffing-legislation/.

American Nurses Credentialing Center (ANCC). (2018). *ANCC magnet recognition program®.* Retrieved from https://www.nursingworld.org/organizational-programs/magnet/.

Benner, P. (2009). *Expertise in nursing practice* (2nd ed.). New York: Springer.

Brider, P. (1990). Professional status: The struggle for just compensation. *American Journal of Nursing, 90*(10), 77–80.

Brommer, C., Buckingham, G., & Loeffler, S. (2003). *Cooperative bargaining styles at federal mediation and conciliation services: A movement toward choices.* Retrieved from https://www.fmcs.gov/?categoryID=35&;itemID=15880.

Budd, K., Warino, L., & Patton, M. (2004). Traditional and non-traditional collective bargaining: Strategies to improve the patient care environment. *Online Journal of Issues in Nursing, 9*(1), 9.

Bureau of Labor Statistics. (2018). *U.S. department of labor, occupational outlook handbook, registered nurses.* Retrieved from http://www.bls.gov/ooh/healthcare/registered-nurses.htm.

Buresh, B., & Gordon, S. (2006). *From silence to voice.* New York: Cornell University Press.

Campaign for Action. (2017). *Number of hospitals in the United States with magnet status.* Retrieved from https://campaignforaction.org/resource/number-hospitals-united-states-magnet-status/.

Center for Union Facts. (2016). *2013 Union profiles: American Nurses Association.* Retrieved from https://www.unionfacts.com/union/American_Nurses_Association#basic-tab.

Census Bureau. (2013). *Men in nursing occupations.* Retrieved from https://www.census.gov/people/io/files/Men_in_Nursing_Occupations.pdf.

Department for Professional Employees (DPE) Research. (2017). *The benefits of collective bargaining for professionals.* Retrieved from http://dpeaflcio.org/programs-publications/issue-fact-sheets/the-benefits-of-collective-bargaining-for-professional-and-technical-workers/.

Drenkard, K., & Swartwout, E. (2005). Effectiveness of a clinical ladder program. *Journal of Nursing Administration, 35,* 502–506.

Fauteux, N. (2014). *Ten years after keeping patients safe. In Charting Nurse's Future.* Retrieved from https://www.rwjf.org/en/library/research/2014/03/cnf-ten-years-after-keeping-patients-safe.html.

Gaus, M. (December 4, 2009). *Nurses move toward a "superunion."* Retrieved from http://www.labornotes.org/2009/12/nurses-move-toward-superunion.

Hackman, D. (2008). ANA and UAN part ways. *Georgia Nursing, 68*(4), 1. Retrieved from http://nursingald.com/uploads/publication/pdf/561/GA11_08.pdf.

Institute of Medicine. (2000). To err is human: Building a safer health system. In L. Kohn, & J. Corrigan (Eds.), *IOM report.* Washington, DC: National Academies Press.

Institute of Medicine. (2004). Keeping patients safe: Transforming the work environment of nurses. In L. Kohn, & J. Corrigan (Eds.), *IOM report.* Washington, DC: National Academies Press.

Institute of Medicine. (2015). *Assessing progress on the institute of medicine report the future of nursing. In IOM report.* Retrieved from http://nationalacademies.org/hmd/~/media/Files/Report%20Files/2015/AssessingFON_releaseslides/Nursing-Report-in-brief.pdf.

Jacox, A. (1980). Collective action: The basis for professionalism. *Supervisor Nurse, 11,* 22–24.

Kaiser Family Foundation. (2016). *Total number of professionally active nurses.* Retrieved from http://kff.org/other/state-indicator/total-registered-nurses/#notes.

Kimmel, N. (2007). *Nurses and unions: Changing times.* Retrieved from http://ezinearticles.com/?Nurses-and-Unions--Changing-Times&id=584916.

Lacey-Mabe, C. (2016). 10 questions to ask the interviewer. *Advanced Healthcare Network.* Retrieved from http://nursing.advanceweb.com/10-questions-to-ask-the-interviewer/.

Lamb, A., Martin-Misener, R., Bryant-Lukosius, D., & Latimer, M. (2018). Describing the leadership capabilities of advanced practices nurses using a qualitative descriptive study. *NursingOpen, 5,* 400–413. https://doi.org/10.1002/nop2.150.

Massachusetts Nurses Association. (2016). *Building the RN super union*. Retrieved from http://www.massnurses .org/news-and-events/national.

Meier, E. (2000). Is unionization the answer for nurses and nursing? *Nursing Economic, 18*(1), 36–37.

National Council State Boards of Nursing (NCSBN). (2018a). 2017 RN practice analysis: Linking the NCLEX-RN examination to practice U.S. and Canada. *NCSBN Research Brief, 72.* Retrieved from www.ncsbn.org/17_RN_US_Canada_Practice_Analysis.pdf.

National Council State Boards of Nursing (NCSBN). (2018b). *Active RN licenses: A profile of nursing licensure in the U.S. The National Nursing Database.* Retrieved from https://www.ncsbn.org/6161.htm.

National Nurses United (NNU). (2018). *About NNU.* Retrieved from http://www.nationalnursesunited.org/pages/19.

New York Department of Labor. (2016). *Registered professional nurse.* Retrieved from http://www.labor.ny.gov/stats/olcny/registered-professional-nurse.shtm.

New York State Nurses Association (NYSNA). (2016). *What is a union?* Retrieved from http://www.nysna.org/strength-at-work/what-is-a-union#.VroVR_k4HNM.

Nurse.com. (2018). *2018 Nurse.com nursing salary research report.* Retrieved from http://mediakit.nurse.com/wp-content/uploads/2018/06/2018-Nurse.com-Salary-Research-Report.pdf.

Palatnik, A. (2016). To err is human. *Nursing Critical Nursing, 11*(5), 4. https://doi.org/10.1097/01.CCN.0000490961.44977.8d. Retrieved from https://journals.lww.com/nursingcriticalcare/Fulltext/2016/09000/To_err_IS_human.1.aspx.

Potter, P. A., Perry, A. G., Stockert, P. A., & Hall, A. M. (2017). *Fundamentals of nursing* (9th ed.). St. Louis, MO: Elsevier.

Swihart, D. (2006). *Shared governance: A practical approach to reshaping professional nursing practice.* Marblehead, MA: HCPro.

The American Nurse. (November–December, 2010). *Center for American nurses services to be integrated into ANA.* Retrieved from http://www.theamericannurse.org/index.php/2010/11/30/center-for-american-nurses-services-to-be-integrated-into-ana/.

U.S. Department of Health and Human Services. (2017). *The Affordable Care Act, section by section.* Retrieved from http://www.hhs.gov/healthcare/about-the-law/read-the-law/index.html.

World Health Organization (WHO). (2018). *Nursing now campaign. World Health Organization/Health Workforce.* Retrieved from http://www.who.int/hrh/news/2018/nursing_now_campaign/en/.

19

Ethical Issues

Karin J. Sherrill, RN, MSN, CNE, ANEF, FAADN*

ⓔ http://evolve.elsevier.com/Zerwekh/nsgtoday/.

Acting responsibly is not a matter of strengthening our reason but of deepening our feelings for the welfare of others.

Jostein Gaarder

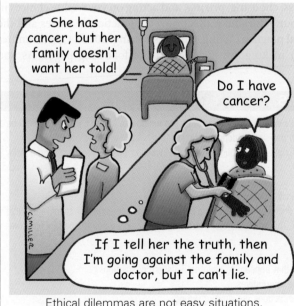

She has cancer, but her family doesn't want her told!

Do I have cancer?

If I tell her the truth, then I'm going against the family and doctor, but I can't lie.

Ethical dilemmas are not easy situations.

After completing this chapter, you should be able to:

- Define *the* terminology commonly used in discussions *of* ethical issues.
- Analyze personal values that influence approaches to ethical issues and decision making.
- Discuss the moral implications of the American Nurses Association and International Council of Nurses codes of ethics.
- Discuss the role of the nurse in ethical health care issues.
- Identify controversial health care issues that *affect* today's nurses.
- Recognize the ethical role of genetics and genomics in nursing practice.
- Recognize resources to assist in resolving an ethical dilemma.

I n developing the content for this chapter, a deliberate effort has been made to "simplify" the presentation of ethical issues and avoid complex philosophical debate. Many nurses shy away from formal ethical discussions because the terminology seems better suited to graduate school and a peer-reviewed journal. In reality, nurses deal with ethical issues every day in practice and must have the tools to advocate effectively for patients as well as for

*We would like to acknowledge Peter Melenovich, PhD, RN, CNE, for his previous contributions to this chapter.

themselves. The first step in equipping oneself for ethical debate is becoming comfortable with the language and issues. *Ethics* refers to principles of right and wrong behaviors, beliefs, and values. Thompson et al. (2007) add, "ethics is essentially concerned with our life as members of a community, and how we behave and function in society" (p. 36). Concern about ethical issues in health care has increased dramatically in the past three decades.

This interest has soared for a variety of reasons, including advances in medical technology; social and legal changes involving legalization of marijuana, the opioid epidemic, human papillomavirus (HPV) vaccine, and growing concern about the allocation of scarce resources, including a shortage of nurses. Nurses and the professional organizations that support them often speak out on these issues and have focused attention on the responsibilities and possible conflicts that they experience as a result of their unique relationship with patients and their families and their role within the health care team.

UNDERSTANDING ETHICS

Let us begin by defining commonly used terms (Box 19.1).

What Are Your Values?

Your values represent ideas and beliefs that you hold in high regard. Clarification of your values is suggested as a strategy to develop greater insight into yourself and what you believe to be important. Value clarification involves a three-step process: choosing, prizing, and acting on your value choices in real-life situations (Steele, 1983). Moreover, our values may affect how we practice as nurses and the decisions we make each day in our professional practice (Wang, Chou, & Huang, 2010). Opportunities to make choices and improve your decision making are included in the following pages. As you

---

BOX 19.1   DEFINITION OF TERMS

Advance directive: A written statement of a person's wishes about how he or she would like health care decisions to be made if he or she ever loses the ability to make such decisions independently.

Bioethical issues: Subjects that raise concerns of right and wrong in matters involving human life (e.g., euthanasia, abortion).

Bioethics: Ethics concerning life.

Confidentiality: The principle that one should not disclose information.

Durable power of attorney for health care: A document that allows a person to name someone else to make medical decisions for him or her if he or she is unable to do so. This spokesperson's authority begins only when the patient is incompetent to make those decisions.

Ethical dilemma

1. A situation involving competing rules or principles that appears to have no satisfactory solution.
2. A choice between two or more equally undesirable alternatives.

Ethics: Rules or principles that determine which human actions are right or wrong.

Living will: A document that allows a person to state in advance that life-sustaining treatment is not to be administered if the person later is terminally ill and incompetent.

Moral courage: The willingness to do what is right despite the fear of consequences.

Moral distress: Feeling of powerlessness to do what is right and ethical.

Moral or ethical principles: Fundamental values or assumptions about the way individuals should be treated and cared for. These include autonomy, beneficence, nonmaleficence, justice, fidelity, and veracity.

Moral reasoning: A process of considering and selecting approaches to resolve ethical issues.

Moral uncertainty: A situation that exists when the individual is unsure which moral principles or values apply in a given situation.

Values: Beliefs that are considered very important and frequently influence an individual's behavior.

consider your values, you will, I hope, gain more understanding about the underlying motives that influence them. This is not intended as a "right" or "wrong" activity but rather as a chance to examine the "what" and "why" of your actions. Do not be surprised if your peers or family hold different views on some topics. And remember, the values that are "correct" or "right" for you may not always be the "right" values for others, including patients and their families. Your values develop as a result of your culture, beliefs, and experiences; they may change through time as you encounter new life events.

Evaluate the critical thinking questions, write down your responses to them, and consider the possible reason or reasons for your choices. The critical thinking exercise in Critical Thinking Box 19.1 is suggested as a means of clarifying your values. Discuss your answers with peers and decide how comfortable you are in discussing and defending your values, especially if they differ from the values of your peers.

? CRITICAL THINKING BOX 19.1

Listing Values

List 10 values that guide your daily interactions.
Choose a partner (if available).
Discuss with a partner each of the values you listed and how they guide your interactions.
Compare your list of values with your partner's list, and discuss similarities and differences in the two lists.
Prioritize your list, and discuss why you feel some are more important than others.

From Steele, S., & Harmon, V. (1983). *Values clarification in nursing* (2nd ed., p. 90). East Norwalk, CT: Appleton-Century-Crofts; with permission.

Often, students are motivated to dive deeper into understanding their personal values and the reasons they make specific decisions. One opportunity to learn more about yourself is by taking the Ethical Lens Inventory (ELI). This evaluation tool is designed to help you understand the values that influence your choices. By making choices between 36 pairs of statements or words, the ELI provides a profile that explains what values are most important to you or how you would act in a specific ethical situation. Some sample statements and words can be found in Box 19.2 (https://www.ethicsgame.com/exec/site/eli.html)

BOX 19.2   ETHICAL LENS INVENTORY SAMPLE STATEMENTS

People should be rewarded more for
- Showing initiative and going the extra mile
- Cooperating with others to reach a mutual goal

When giving benefits for employees, companies should primarily consider:
- Family needs
- Individual needs

In choosing friends, it is more important to be with people
- With whom I agree
- That I find interesting

Mark the word that most accurately describes your personal values.
- Unselfish
- Self-disciplined
- Independent
- Committed
- Just
- Merciful

Reprinted with permission from Ethics Learning Inventory. For more information contact: info@ethicsgame.com.

Moral/Ethical Principles

What Is the Best Decision, and How Will I Know?

Despite different ideas regarding which moral or ethical principle is most important, ethicists agree that there are common principles or rules that should be taken into account when an ethical situation is being examined. As you read through each principle, consider instances in which you have acted on the principles or perhaps felt some conflict in trying to determine what was the best action to take (Fig. 19.1).

Autonomy: a patient's right to self-determination without outside control. Autonomy implies the freedom to make choices and decisions about one's own care without interference, even if those decisions are not in agreement with those of the health care team. This principle assumes rational thinking on the part of the individual and may be challenged when the individual infringes on the rights of others.

Consider this: What if a patient wants to do something that will cause harm to himself or herself? Under what circumstances can the health care team intervene?

Beneficence: duty to actively do good for patients. For example, you use this principle when you decide what nursing interventions should be provided for patients who are dying when some of those interventions may cause pain. In the course of prolonging life, harm sometimes occurs.

Consider this: Who decides what is good? Patient, family, nurse, or physician? How do you define *good*?

Nonmaleficence: duty to prevent or avoid doing harm, whether intentional or unintentional. Is it harmful to accept an assignment to "float" to an unfamiliar area that requires the administration of unfamiliar medications?

Consider this: Is it acceptable to refuse an assignment? When does an assignment become unsafe?

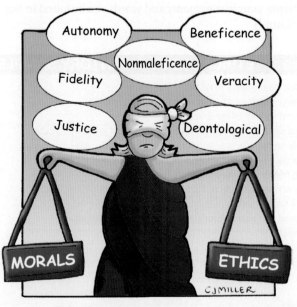

FIG. 19.1 Moral/ethical principles.

Fidelity: the duty to be faithful to commitments. Fidelity involves keeping information confidential and maintaining privacy and trust (e.g., maintaining patient confidentiality regarding illegal opioid use or "blowing the whistle" about unscrupulous billing practices).

Consider this: To whom do we owe our fidelity? Patient, family, physician, institution, or profession? Who has the right to access patient medical records? When should we "blow the whistle" about unsafe staffing patterns?

Justice: the duty to treat all patients fairly, without regard to age, socioeconomic status, immigration status, or other variables. This principle involves the allocation of scarce and expensive health care resources. Should uninsured patients be allowed to use the emergency department (ED) for nonemergency care—the most expensive route for delivering this type of care? Who should be paying for their care?

Consider this: What is fair, and who decides? Why are some patients labeled very important persons (VIPs)? Should they receive preferential care? Why or why not? What kind of access to health care should illegal immigrants receive: preventive or more costly ED care?

Veracity: the duty to tell the truth. The principle of veracity may become an issue when a patient who suspects that her diagnosis is cancer asks you, "Nurse, do I have cancer?" Her family has requested that she not be told the truth because their culture believes bad news takes away all hope for the patient.

Consider this: Is lying to a patient ever justified? If a patient finds out that you have lied, will that patient have any reason to trust you again?

Each of the aforementioned principles sounds so right; yet the "consider this" questions indicate that putting principles into practice is sometimes much easier said than done. Reality does not always offer textbook situations that allow flawless application of ethical principles. As Oscar Wilde, an Irish playwright, once said, "The truth is rarely pure and never simple." You will encounter clinical situations that challenge the way you apply an ethical principle or that cause two or more principles to be in conflict and to create moral distress; this is often referred to as an *ethical dilemma*.

Which Principle or Rule Is Most Important?

Current thinking on the part of ethicists favors autonomy and nonmaleficence as preeminent principles because they emphasize respect for the person and the avoidance of harm. However, there is no universal agreement, and many individuals rely on their spiritual beliefs as the cornerstone of ethical decision making.

Another possible approach to decision making is to consider the relative benefits and burdens of an ethical decision for the patient. If patients are capable of rational decision making, they may choose a different treatment approach than that of the care team. This fact is sometimes difficult for health care team members to accept, especially if it involves a decision to stop treatment. If patients are not capable of autonomous decision making, substituted judgment (decision making) by their designated family is then used. Problems frequently arise when family members disagree on a treatment choice or quality-of-life issue, as evidenced by the Terry Schiavo case in Florida (2003), when the husband's wishes to discontinue nutrition and hydration life support for his wife were granted after a prolonged court case that included attempted government intervention.

Traditional and contemporary models of ethical reasoning offer worldviews from which ethical principles, spiritual values, and the concepts of benefits and burdens can be derived, interpreted, and comparatively emphasized. Nevertheless, models of ethical reasoning are not without their critics, including nurses, who feel that abstract ideas about right and wrong are not helpful or "practical" at the bedside, especially in urgent situations.

In recent years, nursing ethicists have advanced a new approach to ethical issues, emphasizing an ethic of caring as the moral foundation for nursing. Nurses have been encouraged to consider all ethical issues from the central issue of caring. Because caring implies concern for preserving humanity and dignity and promoting well-being, the awareness of rules and principles alone does not adequately address the ethical issues that nurses confront, as in cases of suffering or powerlessness. Research regarding the application of caring to ethical issues is under way, but a practical model for applying this ethic of caring to clinical situations does not yet exist. Currently the most care-centered approach to ethical dilemmas is to consider the relative "benefits versus burdens" that any proposed solution offers to the patient. Health team members must try to consider benefits and burdens from the patient's perspective versus their own values on life, death, and the vast degrees of illness between the two. It is a difficult task to undertake.

So How Do I Make an Ethical Decision?

A number of approaches to ethical decision making are possible. The following is a brief overview of the three most commonly applied models of ethical reasoning. The first two types are considered normative because they have clearly defined parameters, or norms, to influence decision making. The third type is a combination of the other two models.

Deontological. Derived from Judeo-Christian origins, the deontological normative approach is duty-focused and centered on rules from which all action is derived. The rules represent beliefs about intrinsic good that are moral absolutes revealed by God. This approach reasons that all persons are worthy of respect and thus should be treated the same.

```
All life is worthy of respect.
```

As a result of the rules and duties that the deontological approach outlines, the individual may feel that he or she has clear direction about how to act in all situations. Right or wrong is determined based on one's duty or obligation to act, not on the consequences of one's actions. Therefore abortion and euthanasia are never acceptable actions because they violate the duty to respect the sanctity of all life, and lying is never acceptable because it violates the duty to tell the truth. The emphasis on absolute rules with this approach is sometimes seen as rigid and inflexible, but its strength is in its unbending approach to many issues, emphasizing the intent of actions.

Teleological. Derived from humanistic traditions, the teleological approach is outcome-focused and places emphasis on results. *Good* is defined in utilitarian terms: That which is useful is good. Human reason is the basis for authority in all situations, not absolutes from God. Morality is established by majority rule, and the results of actions determine the rules. Because results become the intrinsic good, the individual's actions are always based on the probable outcome.

```
That which causes a good outcome is a good action.
```

Simplistically, this view is sometimes interpreted as "the end justifies the means." Abortion may be acceptable because it results in fewer unwanted babies. Euthanasia is an acceptable choice for some patients because it results in less suffering. Giving preference for a heart transplant to a foreign national who can pay cash and donate money for a transplant program is acceptable because this will create a greater good for others. Using this approach, the rights of some individuals may be sacrificed for the majority.

Situational. Derived from humanistic and Judeo-Christian influences and most commonly credited to Joseph Fletcher (1966), an Episcopalian theologian, the situational view holds that there are no prescribed rules, norms, or majority-focused results that must be followed. Each situation creates its own set of rules and principles that should be considered in that particular set of circumstances. Emphasizing the uniqueness of the situation and respect for the person in that situation, Fletcher appeals to love as the only norm. Critics of this approach argue that this can lead to a "slippery slope" of moral decline.

> Decisions made in one situation cannot be generalized to another situation.

Chemically restraining a disruptive patient who has Alzheimer disease provides a calmer atmosphere for other patients in a long-term care facility. This approach is used after all other efforts to calm the patient have failed. "Pulling the plug" on a terminally ill patient who does not want any more extraordinary care can be considered an act of compassion. Withholding or withdrawing treatment is ethically correct from the individual patient's perspective if the burden of treatment outweighs the benefit of merely extending life. The definition of *burden* has to be approached from the patient's perspective, not from that of others who may feel burdened by the patient's need for care. Viewing a situation from the perspective of benefit versus burden can help patients and families make difficult decisions on the basis of the patient's clear or intended wishes discussed over a period of time. Nurses and other health care providers must be patient advocates, speaking out for those who are disadvantaged and cannot speak for themselves.

Table 19.1 compares the relative advantages and disadvantages of each approach. Remember that there is no perfect worldview. If there were, debate would stop and the need for continued ethical deliberation would cease. The ethical models presented here are not intended to be all-inclusive or exhaustive in depth. Rather, they should whet your appetite to learn more. Many journals and texts are

TABLE 19.1 THREE APPROACHES TO ETHICAL DECISION MAKING

Comparison of Advantages and Disadvantages

ETHICAL APPROACH	ADVANTAGES	DISADVANTAGES
Deontological	Clear direction for action.	Perceived as rigid.
	All individuals are treated the same. Does not consider possible negative consequences of action.	Does not consider possible negative consequences of actions.
Teleological	Interest of the majority is protected.	Rights of individual may be overlooked or denied.
	Results are evaluated for their good and actions may be modified.	What is a good result? Who determines good? Morality may be arbitrary.
Situational	This approach mirrors the way in which most individuals actually approach day-to-day decision making.	What is good? Who decides? Morality is possibly arbitrary.
	Merits of each situation are considered. The individual has more control/autonomy to make decisions in his or her own best interest.	Lack of rules of generalizability limits criticism of possible abuse.

devoted to clinical ethics, and you are encouraged to see how ethicists apply these and other models to issues that affect your area of practice. Surveys of nurses indicate an ongoing interest and an expressed need for ethical discussion and support in practice. Nurses experience ethical distress along with other health care team members, but the 24/7 experience of nursing is unique from the perspective of patient continuity and opportunities for advocacy. Nurses increasingly serve on hospital and religious ethics committees and are encouraged to contribute their perspectives to ethical debates.

How Do I Determine Who Owns the Problem?

The decision to choose a particular model of ethical reasoning is personal (see Table 19.1) and is based on your own values. Familiarize yourself with various models to decrease your own moral uncertainty and gain some understanding of the values of others. The following guidelines are suggested as a means of analyzing ethical issues that will confront you in nursing practice. You will not be a pivotal decision maker in all situations, but these guidelines can help you to make up your own mind as you listen to patients to voicing their wishes and asking questions.

First, determine the facts of the situation. Make sure you collect enough data to give yourself an accurate picture of the issue at hand. When the facts of a situation become known, you may or may not be dealing with an ethical issue.

For example, as an intensive care unit (ICU) nurse, you believe that the wishes of patients regarding extraordinary care are being disregarded. In other words, resuscitation is performed despite expressed patient wishes to the contrary. You must

1. Determine whether discussion about extraordinary care is taking place among patients, their families, and health care providers
2. Clarify the institution's policy regarding cardiopulmonary resuscitation (CPR) and do-not-resuscitate (DNR) orders
3. Determine what input the families have had in the decisions—that is, whether the families are aware of the patient's wishes
4. Explore the use of advance directive documentation at your institution and determine whether patients are familiar with the use and possible limitations of living wills
5. Share your concerns with health care providers to obtain their views of the situation. Discuss the situation with your clinical manager to clarify any misconceptions regarding policy and actual practice.

Second, identify the ethical issues in the situation. In the ICU scenario, if competent patients have expressed their wishes about resuscitation, this should be reflected in the chart. If a living will has been executed and is recognized as valid within your state, its presence in the chart lends considerable weight to the decision. The patient should be encouraged to discuss his or her decision with family to decrease the chances of disagreement if and when the patient can no longer speak for himself or herself. If immediate family members disagree with the living will, the physician may be reluctant to honor it, at least in part because of concern regarding possible liability. If a living will is executed without prior or subsequent discussion with the attending physician, there may be reluctance to honor the will because the physician was not informed of the patient's decision. The physician may feel that the patient did not make an informed decision. However, a durable power of attorney for health care combined with a living will completed before the patient's present state of incapacitation would stand as clear and convincing evidence of the patient's wishes, preventing such a problem. The example of extraordinary care in the ICU illustrates the existence of values and principles in conflict. When the care team, family, and patient have different views of the situation, the patient is likely to be burdened with less than the best outcome unless differences are resolved. The nurse can facilitate communication between the family and patient in resolving differences among all those involved. In this situation, the ethical components of this second step involve autonomy and fidelity versus beneficence.

Patient: Values autonomy, including the right to decide when intervention should stop.

Family: May value the patient's life at all costs and be unwilling to "let go" when a chance exists to prolong life regardless of life quality.

Physician: May feel that the patient has a fair chance to survive and that the living will was executed without the patient being "fully informed." The duty to care or cure may outweigh the physician's belief in the exercise of patient autonomy and fidelity.

Nurse: Values patient autonomy and the need to remain faithful to the patient's wishes. Concern for the needs of the family, in addition to respect for the physician–patient relationship, may cause some conflict.

Institution: Examination of institutional policy may show a conflict between stated policy (e.g., honoring living wills) and actual practice (e.g., performing CPR on all patients unless written physician orders indicate otherwise).

Third, consider possible courses of action and their related outcomes. Having collected data and after having attempted to discuss the issue with all involved parties, you are faced with the following three options:

1. Advocate for the patient with physicians and the family by facilitating communication.
2. Encourage the patient and family to share feelings with each other regarding desires for care.
3. Encourage the family, patient, and attending physicians to discuss the situation more openly.

If the advocacy role does not bring about some change in behavior, consider the possible input and assistance of an interdisciplinary ethics committee (IEC). Such committees have evolved in response to the growing number of ethical issues faced in clinical practice. Most hospitals now have an IEC, which is typically composed of physicians, clergy, social workers, lawyers, and, increasingly, nurses. Any health team member can access the committee with the assurance at least of receiving a helpful, listening ear. If necessary, the committee will convene to review a clinical case and will offer an unbiased opinion of the situation. Committee members may be helpful in clarifying issues or offering moral support; they may also be persuasive in suggesting that involved parties (i.e., family, physician, patient, and nurse) consider a suggested course of action. The authority of an IEC is usually limited because the majority of IECs are developed with the understanding that the advice and opinions offered are not binding to the individual. However, an IEC can serve as a potent form of moral authority and influence if used.

Taking the initiative to express your values and principles is not necessarily easy. As a recent graduate, you may think safer to "swallow hard," remain quiet, and invest your energies in other aspects of your role. You may risk ridicule, criticism, and disagreement when you speak out or have questions on an ethical issue, especially if your view is different or unpopular. However, you risk something far more important if you do not speak out and ask questions for clarification. Silence diminishes your own autonomy as a person and as a professional. Depending on the situation, you may raise eyebrows, but it is important to make your concerns known because some values may be imposed on the patient or on you in the clinical setting, and those values may not be morally correct. You may not agree with the values or believe that they are in the best interest of the patient. Evidence demonstrates that a nurse's intentions to leave or stay in a position are often determined from the level of experienced moral distress (Austin, 2017). Find your voice, ask questions, and speak up so that you will be able to control your practice more effectively.

Fourth, after a course of action has been taken, evaluate the outcome. In the ICU scenario, did improved communication occur among patients, families, and physicians? Were your efforts to advocate met with resistance or a rebuff? What could you try differently the next time? What values or principles were considered most important by the decision makers? What kind of assistance did you receive from the IEC? What role did you play in this situation, and was it appropriate?

What Other Resources Are Available to Help Resolve Ethical Dilemmas?

Nurses have several resources available to help them resolve ethical issues that may occur in professional settings. Nurses must first consider their personal views on any given issue and consider having an open and honest discussion with their peers and supervisors. After reflection and discussion, nurses may consider consulting the institution's ethics committee if the issue remains unresolved. Many professional resources are also available to provide direction about ethical issues and behavior. The first of these is the American Nurses Association (ANA) *Code of Ethics for Nurses* (2015, p. 196). The code is a statement to society that outlines the values, concerns, and goals of the profession. It should be compatible with the individual nurse's personal values and goals. The code provides direction for ethical decisions and behavior by repeatedly emphasizing the obligations and responsibilities that the nurse–patient relationship entails.

The provisions of the *Code of Ethics for Nurses* allude to the ethical principles mentioned earlier in this chapter and certainly imply that fidelity to the patient is foremost. A copy of the code with interpretive statements is available from the ANA. If you did not purchase a copy as a reference for school, consider buying it for your own use in practice. A copy of the code should be accessible within your place of employment.

Critics of the *Code of Ethics for Nurses* cite its lack of legal enforceability. This is a valid criticism, because the code is not a legal document, as licensure laws are. However, the code is a moral statement of accountability that can add weight to decisions involving legal censure. Many practicing nurses claim ignorance of the *Code of Ethics for Nurses* or believe that it is a document for students only. However, it is for all nurses and was developed by nurses. In 2001, the ANA published a *Bill of Rights for Registered Nurses*, a first-ever document of "rights" in contrast to the traditional focus on responsibilities. Awareness of these rights may provide nurses with a sense of comfort in voicing their advocacy for patients as well as for themselves. Take the opportunity to become familiar with its contents (ANA, 2001). Box 19.3 presents the *International Council of Nurses Code for Nurses*. This international code is valuable because it points out issues of universal importance to all nurses.

More recently, the ANA Center for Ethics and Human Rights (CEHR) was established to help nurses navigate ethical and value conflicts and life-and-death decisions, many of which are common to everyday practice. The CEHR is committed to the dissemination of information addressing professional, ethical, and human rights challenges at the bedside and throughout the community, nation, and world. In 2017, the CEHR published information on topics involving the conflicting roles of a correctional nurse, colleague impairment, and workplace violence, to name a few (ANA, n.d.).

In 1973, the American Hospital Association published a *Patient's Bill of Rights*. Now revised (Box 19.4) and called *The Patient Care Partnership*, this document reflects acknowledgment of patients' rights to participate in their health care and was developed as a response to consumer criticism of paternalistic provider care. The statements detail patient's rights with corresponding provider responsibilities. Read each statement and consider whether it seems reasonable. When first developed, many of the statements were considered radical. This document reflects the increasing emphasis on patient autonomy in health care and defines the limits of provider influence and control. Earlier beliefs that the hospital and physician know best (paternalism) have been challenged and modified. This document is likely to be refined further as joint responsibilities between patients and health care providers grow.

BOX 19.3 THE INTERNATIONAL COUNCIL OF NURSES CODE OF ETHICS FOR NURSES

The ICN Code of Ethics for Nurses has four principal elements that outline the standards of ethical conduct.

Elements of the Code

1. Nurses and People

- The nurse's primary professional responsibility is toward people requiring nursing care.
- In providing care, the nurse promotes an environment in which the human rights, values, customs and spiritual beliefs of the individual, family, and community are respected.
- The nurse ensures that the individual receives accurate, sufficient, and timely information in a culturally appropriate manner on which to base consent for care and related treatment.
- The nurse holds in confidence personal information and uses judgment in sharing this information.
- The nurse shares with society the responsibility for initiating and supporting action to meet the health and social needs of the public, in particular those of vulnerable populations.
- The nurse advocates for equity and social justice in resource allocation, access to health care, and other social and economic services.
- The nurse demonstrates professional values such as respectfulness, responsiveness, compassion, trustworthiness, and integrity.

2. Nurses and Practice

- The nurse carries personal responsibility and accountability for nursing practice, and for maintaining competence by continual learning.
- The nurse maintains a standard of personal health such that the ability to provide care is not compromised.
- The nurse uses judgment regarding individual competence when accepting and delegating responsibility.
- The nurse at all times maintains standards of personal conduct, which reflect well on the profession and enhance its image and public confidence.
- The nurse, in providing care, ensures that use of technology and scientific advances is compatible with the safety, dignity, and rights of people.
- The nurse strives to foster and maintain a practice culture promoting ethical behavior and open dialogue.

3. Nurses and the Profession

- The nurse assumes the major role in determining and implementing acceptable standards of clinical nursing practice, management, research, and education.
- The nurse is active in developing a core of research-based professional knowledge that supports evidence-based practice.
- The nurse is active in developing and sustaining a core of professional values.
- The nurse, acting through the professional organization, participates in creating a positive practice environment and maintaining safe, equitable social and economic working conditions in nursing.
- The nurse practices to sustain and protect the natural environment and is aware of its consequences on health.
- The nurse contributes to an ethical organizational environment and challenges unethical practices and settings.

4. Nurses and Coworkers

- The nurse sustains a collaborative and respectful relationship with co-workers in nursing and other fields.
- The nurse takes appropriate action to safeguard individuals, families, and communities when their health is endangered by a co-worker or any other person.
- The nurse takes appropriate action to support and guide coworkers to advance ethical conduct.

From International Council of Nurses. (2012). *ICN Code of ethics for nurses.* Geneva: Imprimerie Fornara; with permission.

BOX 19.4   PATIENT CARE PARTNERSHIP

Replacing the AHA's Patients' Bill of Rights, the Patient Care Partnership brochure informs patients about what they should expect during their hospital stay with regard to their rights and responsibilities. Here is a brief overview.

What to Expect During Your Hospital Stay
- High quality hospital care.
- A clean and safe environment.
- Involvement in your care.
- Protection of your privacy.
- Help when leaving the hospital.
- Help with your billing claims.
  The sections of the brochure explain some of the basics about how the patient can expect to be treated during a hospital stay. They also cover what the health care team will need from the patient to improve their care.

Note: You can download the full text Patient Care Partnership brochure at: https://www.aha.org/system/files/2018-01/aha-patient-care-partnership.pdf.
Reprinted with permission of the American Hospital Association, copyright 2003. All rights reserved.

Consider the settings in which you have had clinical experiences, and evaluate how well these rights have been acknowledged and supported. In your future practice, keep these rights in mind. Observing them is not only the right thing to do but also enforceable by law.

As a response to the rapidly growing home health care area of community nursing, the National Association for Home Care established a *Home Care Bill of Rights* for patients and families to inform them of the ethical conduct they can expect from home care agencies and their employees when they are in the home (National Association for Home Care & Hospice, n.d.). This document is widely used and addresses the rights of the patient and provider to be treated with dignity and respect; the right of the patient to participate actively in decision making; privacy of information; financial information regarding payment procedures from insurance, Medicare, and Medicaid; quality of care; and the patient's responsibility to follow the plan of care and notify the home health nurse of changes in his or her condition. Surprising as it may seem, there are instances of nurses who have lost their licenses as a result of unethical behavior toward patients in their homes. These abuses included financial and sexual exploitation—major violations of professional boundaries.

Home care nurses often face difficult ethical dilemmas about the delivery of care to patients. For example, a patient will require or desire more care or visits than Medicare or private insurance will pay for. All home care agencies have policies written to guide them through the decision-making process when they can no longer receive reimbursement for a patient's care. Often it is the responsibility of the home care nurse to find another community agency that can meet the patient's needs at a cost the patient can afford.

An additional document with which you should be familiar is the *Nuremberg Code* (Box 19.5). This code grew out of the blatant abuses perpetrated by Nazi war criminals during World War II in the name of science. Experiments were conducted by health care professionals without patient consent, resulting in horrific mutilations, disability, and death. The *Nuremberg Code* identifies the need for voluntary informed consent when medical experiments are conducted on human beings. It delineates the limits and restrictions that researchers must recognize and respect. Because of the preponderance of research in many clinical settings, nurses have a responsibility to understand the concept of voluntary informed consent and to support patients' rights throughout the research process. After reading this code, you should have a greater awareness of the patient's right to autonomy and the health care provider's responsibility to be faithful to that right.

BOX 19.5   THE NUREMBERG CODE

The great weight of the evidence before us is to the effect that certain types of medical experiments on human beings, when kept within reasonably well-defined bounds, conform to the ethics of the medical profession generally. The protagonists of the practice of human experimentation justify their views on the basis that such experiments yield results for the good of society that are unprocurable by other methods or means of study. All agree, however, that certain basic principles must be observed in order to satisfy moral, ethical, and legal concepts:

1. The voluntary consent of the human subject is absolutely essential. This means that the person involved should have legal capacity to give consent; should be so situated as to be able to exercise free power of choice, without the intervention of any element of force, fraud, deceit, duress, overreaching, or other ulterior form of constraint or coercion; and should have sufficient knowledge and comprehension of the elements of the subject matter involved as to enable him to make an understanding and enlightened decision. This latter element requires that before the acceptance of an affirmative decision by the experimental subject there should be made known to him the nature, duration, and purpose of the experiment; the method and means by which it is to be conducted; all inconveniences and hazards reasonably to be expected; and the effects upon his health or person which may possibly come from his participation in the experiment.
2. The duty and responsibility for ascertaining the quality of the consent rests upon each individual who initiates, directs, or engages in the experiment. It is a personal duty and responsibility that may not be delegated to another with impunity.
3. The experiment should be such as to yield fruitful results for the good of society, unprocurable by other methods or means of study, and not random and unnecessary in nature.
4. The experiment should be so designed and based on results of animal experimentation and a knowledge of the natural history of the disease or other problem under study that the anticipated results will justify the performance of the experiment.
5. The experiment should be so conducted as to avoid all unnecessary physical and mental suffering and injury.
6. No experiment should be so conducted where there is an a priori reason to believe that death or disabling injury will occur—except, perhaps, in those experiments where the experimental physicians also serve as subjects.
7. The degree of risk to be taken should never exceed that determined by the humanitarian importance of the problem to be solved by the experiment.
8. Proper preparations should be made and adequate facilities provided to protect the experimental subject against even remote possibilities of injury, disability, or death.
9. The experiment should be conducted only by scientifically qualified persons. The highest degree of skill and care should be required through all stages of the experiments of those who conduct or engage in the experiment.

Reprinted from *Trials of war criminals before the Nuremberg Military Tribunals under Control Council Law* (Vol. 2, no. 18, p. 181). (1949). Washington, DC: U.S. Government Printing Office.

Controversial Ethical Issues Confronting Nursing

Situations that raise ethical issues affect all areas of nursing practice. The following is a sampling of issues that consistently cause controversy.

Abortion

The debate over this issue has raged in the United States since the 1973 *Roe v. Wade* Supreme Court decision. The resolution of this case struck down laws against abortion but left the possibility of introducing restrictions under some conditions. Efforts toward that end continue today with mixed results for both the pro-choice and pro-life factions. Increasing efforts are focused on the need for parental notification/consent. The right to reproductive choice and access continues to be debated, and the argument affects nursing practice in both acute care and community settings.

Historic references to abortion can be found as far back as 4500 BC (Rosen, 1967). Abortion has been practiced in many societies as a means of population control and termination of unwanted pregnancies, yet sanctions against abortion are found in both ancient biblical and legal texts. It is interesting to note that the ancient sanctions against abortion generally related to fines payable to the husband if the pregnant woman was harmed. This form of sanction derived from the concept of the woman and fetus as male property. Greek philosophers, including Aristotle and Plato, made a distinction between an unformed fetus and a formed fetus. A fine was levied for aborting an unformed fetus, whereas the aborting of a formed fetus required "a life for a life." The number of gestational weeks that determine whether a fetus was formed was not stated, although the time of human "ensoulment" was understood: Aristotle believed that a male fetus was imbued with a soul at 40 days' gestation *(quickening)* versus 90 days for a female (Feldman, 1968). The subject of ensoulment became part of the ongoing debate regarding the time when the developing fetus becomes human. In other words,

---

When does life begin?

Judeo-Christian theologians generally came to identify the beginning of life as occurring at conception or at the time of implantation. However, even within this tradition, the Jewish Talmud and Roman law stated that life begins at birth, because the first breath represents the infusion of life. These varied views are still held today.

Social customs and private behavior regarding abortion have frequently differed from theological teaching. The first legal sanctions against abortion in the United States began in the late 19th century. Before that time, first-trimester abortions were not uncommon and, in fact, were advertised, supporting the idea that abortion before quickening was acceptable.

The ethical debate about abortion today is a continuing struggle to answer the question of when life begins and to determine an answer to the following questions:

1. Does the fetus have rights?
2. Do the rights of the fetus (for life) take precedence over the right of the mother to control her reproductive functions?
3. When is abortion morally justified?
4. Should minors have the right to abortion without parental consent or awareness?
5. Should fetal stem cells be used for research, helping to end the suffering of patients with chronic disorders such as Parkinson disease?

The struggle to answer these questions has polarized individuals into pro-life and pro-choice camps. Yet opinion polls on the subject have shown that very few people are against abortion in all circumstances or favor abortion as a mandatory solution for some pregnancies. Most Americans express views somewhere between these extremes, and the legal battle to maintain or restrict abortion access continues. The controversy has escalated into violence in some areas of the country, with abortion clinics and personnel subjected to attack; some abortion providers have been killed. This violence has resulted in the decreased availability of abortion services in many areas. In recent years, some pharmacists have refused to fill prescriptions for birth control pills and the "morning after" pill, claiming that this violates their moral beliefs, exacerbating the pro-life/pro-choice debate.

The Roman Catholic Church has been the religious group most frequently identified with the pro-life movement, but there are other groups—religious and otherwise—that support a ban on abortion. Pro-life proponents generally condone abortion only to save the life of the mother. These antiabortion groups are often criticized by pro-choice as extremist, against women, and repressive.

The pro-choice movement is vocal in championing the woman's right to choose and promoting the safety of legalized abortion. They cite the tragedy of past "back alley" abortions and compare restrictions on abortion to infringements on the civil liberties of women. Within the pro-choice movement are many individuals who favor restrictions on abortions after the first trimester and oppose the use of abortion as a means of birth control. Pro-life proponents often view pro-choice supporters as antifamily extremists who do not represent the views of the majority of Americans.

How does the abortion issue affect nursing? Nurses are involved as both individuals and professionals. The following are some general guidelines to consider.

Evaluate your values and beliefs in relation to abortion and how you can best apply these values to your work and to possible political action.

If you choose to work in a setting in which abortions are performed, review Provision 1 of the ANA *Code of Ethics for Nurses*: "The nurse practices with compassion and respect for the inherent dignity, worth, and uniqueness attributes of every person" (ANA, 2017, p. 1). This statement outlines your responsibility to care for all patients. If you do not agree with an institution's policy or procedure regarding abortion, the patient still merits your care. If that care (e.g., assisting with abortions) violates your principles, you should consider changing your job or developing an agreement with your employer regarding your job responsibilities. If you cannot provide the care that the patient requires, plan for someone else to do so.

You do not have to sacrifice your own values and principles, but you are barred by the ANA *Code of Ethics for Nurses* from abandoning patients or forcing your values on them. Such abandonment would also constitute legal abandonment, and you would be subject to legal action.

Some hospitals have developed conscience clauses that provide protection to the hospital and nurses against participation in abortions. Find out if your institution has such a clause.

Consider your response and the possible conflict in the following situations:

- You are a labor and delivery nurse working on a unit that performs second-trimester saline abortions in a nearby area. You are not a part of the staff for the abortion area, but today, because of short staffing, you are asked to care for a 16-year-old who is undergoing the procedure.
- You work in a family-planning clinic that serves low-income women. Because of escalating violence against abortion providers, the nearest abortion clinic is 100 miles away. You are restricted from providing information regarding abortion services because of federal guidelines.
- A 41-year-old mother of five has expressed interest in terminating her pregnancy of 6 weeks' gestation. She confides that her husband would beat her if he knew she was pregnant and contemplating abortion.
- You are teaching a class on sexuality and contraception to a group of high school sophomores. Two of the girls state that they have just had abortions. In response to your information regarding available methods of contraception, one of the girls states, "I'm not interested in birth control. If I get pregnant again, I'll just get an abortion. It's a lot easier."
- You have a history of infertility and work in the neonatal ICU. You are presently caring for a 24-week-old baby born to a mother who admits to having taken "crack" as a means of inducing labor and "getting rid of the baby." The mother has just arrived in the unit and wants to visit the baby.

These sample scenarios are meant to illustrate the conflicts that personal values, institutional settings, and patients may create for the recent graduate. In your responses, consider how you might lobby or participate in the political process to change or support existing policies regarding abortion and access to such services.

Euthanasia

Euthanasia is commonly referred to as "mercy killing." It is a Greek word that means "good death" and implies painless actions to end the life of someone suffering from an incurable or terminal disease. Euthanasia has been closely tied to a "right to die" argument, which has gained a good deal of attention in the past decade. Euthanasia is classified as *active, passive,* or *voluntary. Active euthanasia* involves the administration of a lethal drug or another measure to end life and alleviate suffering. Regardless of the motivation and beliefs of the individuals involved, active euthanasia is illegal in the United States and can result in criminal charges of murder if performed. In recent years, incidents of active euthanasia have become periodic news events, as spouses or parents have used measures to end the suffering of their mates or children from, for example, advanced Alzheimer disease or a persistent vegetative state. *Passive euthanasia* involves the withdrawal of extraordinary means of life support (e.g., ventilator, feeding tube) and is a fairly common practice in health care, especially when advanced medical directives are in place that indicate the patient's preferences. *Voluntary euthanasia* or physician-assisted suicide involves situations when the dying individual expresses his or her desires regarding the management and time of death to a physician who then provides the means for the patient to obtain a lethal dose of medication.

Today, advanced technology routinely keeps alive patients who would never have survived a few short years ago. Concerns regarding prolonging life and suffering for those individuals have resulted in a movement to have right-to-die statutes and living wills accepted. In those states that have such statutes and recognize living wills, termination of treatment in such cases has become easier. Right-to-die statutes release health care personnel from possible liability for honoring a person's wishes that life be not unduly prolonged (Rudy, 1985). Many years ago, the state of Oregon enacted the Death with Dignity Act (2011), which allows terminally ill Oregonians to obtain and use prescriptions from their physicians for self-administered lethal doses of medications. Since that time, other states have adopted similar legislation.

Another legal document, the Durable Power of Attorney for Healthcare Decisions (DPAHC), helps to ensure that a living will is carried out. The DPAHC identifies the individual who will carry out the patient's wishes in the event that he or she is incapacitated and also informs health care providers about the specific wishes of the patient regarding life-support measures.

A major impact on the availability of living wills and the DPAHC (which are referred to as *advance medical directives*) resulted from the introduction of the Patient Self-Determination Act in December 1991. Advance directives are federally mandated for all institutions receiving Medicare or Medicaid funds. On admission to a health care facility, information about advance directives must be offered to all competent adults. This means that all adults are told about the purpose and availability of living wills *(treatment directive)* and DPAHCs *(appointment directive)*. They are then helped to complete these documents if desired. After years of having advance directive information available to patients, the impact of this document on decision making has been varied. It certainly has influenced the communication that many patients have with their families, physicians, and other health care providers regarding their wishes at the time of signing, but patients often change their minds when their health care status changes, frequently opting for the prolongation of life. A problem has surfaced regarding the timing of information to patients regarding advance directives. If patients first hear about advance directives on admission to an acute care setting, anxiety about their admission and the separate concept of advance directives may seriously affect informed decision making at that time. Advance directives should ideally be discussed *before* serious illness occurs, and at the very least in a therapeutic environment to encourage well-informed and thoughtful decision making. It is important to consider individual cultural and religious beliefs and to clearly document these preferences so that the health care team has proper guidance and direction. Patients and families need reassurance that declining extraordinary care does not mean the abandonment of caring and palliative care when needed. Both patients and families must be reassured that palliative comfort care will never stop, even when aggressive curative efforts are withdrawn.

Decisions to withdraw or withhold nutrition and hydration from patients are complex and are the subject of ongoing debate by ethicists, health care personnel, and the legal system. In response to the issues of hydration and nutrition, the Ethics Committee of the ANA developed guidelines in 1988 and revised them in 1992. These guidelines state that there are instances when withholding or withdrawing nutrition and hydration are morally permissible. Although intended only as a guideline, this document provides direction for nurses who face such issues. Its wording has been both praised for its clarity and criticized for possible ambiguity. The primary exception to the withdrawal of hydration and nutrition is when harm from these measures can be demonstrated. This document is available from the ANA.

Futile Care and Physician-Assisted Suicide

Futile care (futility) and physician-assisted suicide (PAS) are two ethical and human rights issues that have drawn a great deal of attention and debate. Several studies over the last decade have shown the relationship between futile care and its impact on a nurse's moral distress, burnout, turnover, and lack of professional autonomy (Rostami & Jafari, 2016). Additionally, it has been found that moral distress associated with clinical situations representing futile care increased with time spent in the ICU (Mobley et al., 2007).

What is futility? *Medical futility* refers to the use of medical intervention (beyond comfort care) without any realistic hope of benefit to the patient. *Benefit* is defined as improvement of outcome. A concrete example of futility would be the continuation of ICU care for a patient in a persistent vegetative state who would, on discharge from the hospital, return to a nursing home incapable of interacting with the environment. The futility debate concerns the very nature of the definition of *benefit* in addition to who defines it. The economic pressure to control health care costs also leads to a focus on ways to eliminate "unnecessary" intervention.

On paper, futility can be defined, but its application to diverse clinical situations remains a challenge. The debate involves multiple parties whose interests and values are not always compatible. For example, patients and families have argued both for the right to refuse care that they believe is futile and the right to receive all possible care in the face of a medical opinion of futility. This argument raises two related questions:

1. Do patients or families have the right to demand and receive treatment that health care providers believe is futile?
2. Do physicians have the right to refuse to provide treatments that they believe are futile despite patient or family desire to initiate or continue such treatment?

Ethics committees have struggled to agree on a working definition of futility to provide support for clinicians, patients, and families who are faced with difficult decisions regarding care. Many institutions have developed guidelines for the withdrawal of treatment (except for comfort care). These guidelines emphasize the importance of clear, ongoing communication among all health care team members and with the patient and family. Accurate, compassionate discussion is essential to convey a unified approach to the realities and limitations of possible medical care. The guidelines should never be used as a threat or to imply abandonment of care. They are, as their name implies, guidelines. Lack of agreement among the patient, family, and health care team is likely to delay or prevent withdrawal of treatment primarily because of the fear of liability, even in cases of brain death. Supporting the patient or family decision may be difficult because of personal values and professional opinions. It is crucial to clarify where professional loyalties should lie and to keep the discussion patient-centered.

Pressures to eliminate unnecessary costs also influence the futility debate. Insurers, clinicians, and health care institutions increasingly question medical expenditures that produce futile outcomes and prolong the inevitability of impending death. Insurance reimbursement payments are likely to be further limited or denied for treatment judged to be of no benefit to the patient. A possible risk is that beneficial treatment may be eliminated or denied solely because of economic concern in cases having an uncertain outcome. Nurses must stay informed about institutional guidelines regarding medical futility; they must communicate clearly with patients, families, and physicians regarding expected goals and likely outcomes of care. The patient's welfare—and not economic concerns—should be the primary driving force for the withdrawal of treatment.

Physician-assisted suicide. PAS gained national attention years ago because of Dr. Jack Kevorkian's persistent efforts to publicize and bring legitimacy to a formerly taboo topic. Kevorkian assisted or attended in the deaths of more than 130 terminally and chronically ill patients (Schneider, 2011). His work caused the state of Michigan to pass legislation barring PAS, which led to Dr. Kevorkian's imprisonment. In 1994, Oregon approved PAS legislation. It was immediately challenged in the Oregon court by right-to-life advocates, but the Death with Dignity Act went into effect October 27, 1997. Currently, California, Washington, Montana, Vermont, Hawaii, Colorado, Oregon, and Washington, DC have similar legislation (Pro Con, 2018). For right-to-life advocates, even one of these deaths is too many and is a step down the path of state-approved murder. Quality-of-life advocates support PAS as an example of personal autonomy and control; however, the debate continues.

PAS has been debated for years, and opinions on both sides among physicians and the public are very strong. The American Medical Association opposes PAS because it violates the most basic ethical principle, which is "First, do no harm." Physicians have traditionally taken care of the living patient, and support for PAS threatens to destroy this fundamental relationship. Many individual physicians have, however, changed their minds in recent years because of their work with terminally ill patients. More than a few of these clinicians have come to believe that the only option for the relief of some patients' intractable pain and suffering is death.

Although the legalization of PAS continues to be debated in the courts, the practice goes on—generally in private and without headlines. Both critics and supporters of PAS state that the secrecy goes on because of the fear of arrest for homicide. There have been some court rulings supporting the right to PAS by terminally ill patients on the basis of the 14th Amendment's guarantee of personal liberty. These decisions have been assailed by right-to-life groups as an antilife philosophy that dishonors the intrinsic value of life.

PAS affects nursing practice because a decision to perform PAS may involve the nurse. The term *PAS* implies that the physician is the active agent, but a lethal dose may be ordered by the physician for the nurse to administer. Nurses must be aware of the legal and ethical implications of such an order. The administration of a lethal dose for the explicit purpose of ending a patient's life is an illegal act that can be prosecuted as homicide. From an ethical point of view, many would consider this the ultimate act of mercy, yet it is an illegal act in the United States except in the states mentioned earlier. Clinicians, ethicists, the public, and the courts continue to struggle with how best to respect the life and wishes of terminally ill patients without "doing harm." In 2013, the ANA issued a position statement prohibiting nurses from participating in any form of assisted death (ANA, 2013).

Ethicists generally agree that although the prolongation of life by extraordinary means is not always indicated, clarifying the circumstances when such care may be stopped (withdrawn) or possibly never begun (withheld) frequently creates controversy, particularly when the quality of life (coma, persistent vegetative state) is likely to be questionable.

Opponents of the right-to-die movement believe that it represents an erosion of the value of human life and may encourage a movement toward the acceptance of suicide as part of a "culture of death." They caution that the lives of the weak and disabled may come to be devalued as society concentrates on the pursuit of "quality of life." If passive euthanasia achieves societal acceptance, who will speak out in favor of protecting incompetent or dependent individuals who are not living what society views as a high-quality life? The well-publicized Schiavo controversy demonstrates the political polarization that this topic can cause (Caplan, 2015).

Proponents of the right-to-die movement believe that it provides a more natural course of living and dying for the individual and family by avoiding the artificial prolongation of life through technology. The availability of technology to prolong life often raises the question, "We can, but should we?"

Surveys of medical and nursing school curricula in the United States continue to show minimal content involving end-of-life care. Schools continue to focus curricula more on the curative approach to illness and disease, neglecting to address the palliative, comfort-directed needs of individuals who require care in the last months and days of their lives. This fact, combined with the aging of our population, points to the need for improvements in educating both current clinicians and students in health care institutions on ethical issues surrounding end-of-life care. A growing number of proactive clinicians and educators concerned with the quality of care provided to dying patients and their families are supporting an educational movement called *End-of-Life Care*. The specific program targeted for nursing is called the *End-of-Life Nursing Education Consortium Project*, targeting nursing faculty and nursing leadership in many specialty organizations. This consortium project has educated hundreds of nurses in the past few years, slowly influencing a change in both education and clinical practice. It will be interesting to see the impact of these efforts on patient care during the next decade. As nurses, we are challenged to make this last event of life a better experience for all. The growing popularity of the palliative care movement in the United States is a significant paradigm change, acknowledging the value and complexity of supportive, noncurative care for many conditions. Supporting the broader picture of palliative interventions—which may continue for months or years—will increase our understanding of the needs of patients who do not have a cure awaiting them but who want to embrace the time they have left with our support.

Consider your response and possible conflict in the following critical thinking situations (use the terms defined in Box 19.1 to guide your consideration or discussion with others):

A 22-year-old quadriplegic repeatedly asks you to disconnect him from the ventilator. His family rarely visits, and he believes that he has nothing left to live for.

The spouse of a patient with advanced Alzheimer disease states that he can no longer watch his wife of 43 years suffer. "She would not have wanted to live this way." His wife is being treated for dehydration, malnutrition, and a urinary tract infection. She is confused and is frequently sedated to manage her combativeness. The use of a feeding tube is being contemplated because of her refusal to eat.

The attending physician for a patient with terminal AIDS refuses to order increasing doses of pain medication because of her concern that it may cause a repeat episode of respiratory depression. The patient's pain is unrelieved, and he begs you for medication. "Please help me. I know I'm dying."

A patient on long-term dialysis wants to discontinue treatment, citing the side effects of dialysis and her medications. She feels that the quality of her life has disappeared. Her life partner died a year earlier, and she sees no reason to continue suffering. She has been on the transplant list for 6 years. She has indicated that her last appointment will be in 1 month and would like to know what kind of supportive care will be available.

For each of these scenarios, consider what your reaction would be and the possible resources you would use to resolve the conflicts.

What Are the Ethical Issues Regarding Transplantation?

There are more than 115,000 people on transplant lists in the United States today, and the majority of these individuals will die without a transplant because of the shortage of available organs (American Transplant Foundation, 2018). On what basis should someone receive an organ? Should the severity of illness serve as the primary criterion, or what other factors should be taken into consideration? Should economic status be used as a contributing factor in the process? How are donors solicited? What are the religious and cultural issues that influence someone's decision to be considered as a potential donor? Should the government intervene to enlarge the donor pool by deciding that victims of accidents imply donor consent if their driver's license does not have a statement specifically refusing donation? What protections need to be put into place to prevent coercion for organ donation? This is a reality in many countries where organs are paid for or condemned prisoners are sources for donation.

All of the aforementioned questions offer a window into the complexity of issues surrounding organ transplantation. The technology exists with ever-increasing precision, but there is a tremendous scarcity of organs. On what basis do we as a society attempt to create a process of organ access that is just and equitable? Who decides?

What Is the Ethical Issue Regarding the Use of Fetal Tissue?

Fetal tissue from elective abortions has been identified as potentially beneficial in the treatment of Parkinson disease and other degenerative disorders because of its unique embryonic qualities. Proponents argue that it is available tissue that can be put to beneficial use in patients who do not have any other hope of significant improvement or cure. They further argue that the availability of fetal tissue from elective abortions is a separate issue from the later use of the tissue for stem cell research. The abortion would have occurred regardless. Later use of the stem cell derives some good from the discarded tissue.

Critics who assail the use of fetal tissue for stem cell research as a further erosion of respect for the unborn were successful in spurring a federal ban on the use of fetal tissue for research in the United States during the 1980s. They believe that the limited research that has already been done regarding fetal tissue has created the mentality that pregnancy can be used as a means of providing parts and tissues for others. The ban was removed in early 1993 after President Clinton took office, and in 2001, the use of stem cells received narrowly defined approval by the Bush administration for genetic research. Individual states have the authority to pass laws to permit human embryonic stem cell research using state funding. This right has not been overridden by congressional ban (NIH, 2016), but funding contracts have been revoked by the US Department of Health and Human Services in response to the controversy (National Public Radio, 2018). As the largest group of health care providers, nurses must keep themselves informed regarding the issues. Consider your own viewpoint and how it can affect your nursing care. Does the good (beneficence) achieved from the use of fetal tissue for patients with spinal cord injuries, type 1 diabetes, Parkinson disease, Alzheimer disease, heart disease, stroke, burns, cancer, and osteoarthritis outweigh the harm inflicted by viewing a fetus as a source of parts?

What Are the Ethical Issues Regarding In Vitro Fertilization?

This procedure involves the fertilization of a mother's ovum with the father's sperm in a laboratory followed by implantation of the embryo in the mother's uterus. Since the birth of the first successful in vitro fertilization baby in the late 1970s, the procedure has gained popularity as a method for some infertile couples to have a child. The availability of the technique has created a new subspecialty practice in obstetrics and has raised ethical issues for consideration. Opponents of the procedure argue that it is an unnatural act and removes the biological act of procreation from the intimacy of marriage. The cost of the procedure is also a source of criticism, calling into question whether it should be covered by insurance and whether the procedure should be available to all couples regardless of their ability to pay. Many couples are now able to select the sex of their baby, choosing the desired embryo for implantation and destroying the undesired embryos. If technology can be made to meet our desires for a "designer baby" with a particular hair or eye color, does that make it a morally correct course of action?

Questions concerning informed consent for the procedure merit attention as well. Some infertility clinics offer this service but have not been up-front about their success rates or qualifications.

Standardized methods for reporting this information have just recently been established. To be ethical, all such clinics should define success in the same way; for example, success equals pregnancy or success equals live birth. The two definitions are very different. Information about the qualifications of the staff should be available to patients, and the subspecialty should lobby for standards of practice that are enforceable and available to the public. Possible side effects from the drugs used to induce hyperovulation, from anesthesia, or from surgical injury during the laparoscopy should also be a part of the discussion.

Should anyone who desires the in vitro procedure have access, or should the procedure be limited to those in a heterosexual marriage? Some clinics have limited their services to heterosexual couples to avoid adverse publicity, but this policy is starting to change as single and lesbian women seek out avenues to become biological parents. Most important: to whom does the embryo belong and what are the embryo's rights? There have been court cases involving marital disputes regarding the custody of frozen embryos. What are the rights of the embryos in such instances? Can a parent choose to destroy the embryos over the objection of the estranged spouse, or should one parent be able to obtain custody of the embryos when his or her spouse wants them to be thawed out and destroyed? What responsibility does the staff have for maintaining parental ownership of the embryos?

What Are Genetics and Genomics?

The study of genetics and genomics has led to the increased ability of health care professionals to help patients improve their health outcomes and the treatment of their disease processes. Genetic research has led to the improved diagnosis and treatment of diseases with the creation of new types of drugs based on what we know about genes. These newer drugs target certain sites in the body, causing better effectiveness with fewer side effects (NIH, 2018).

"Genetics is a term that refers to the study of genes and their role in inheritance—the way certain traits or conditions are passed down from one generation to another.
Genomics is a relatively new term that describes the study of all of a person's genes including interactions of those genes with each other and the person's environment" (Lea, 2009, p. 2).

But what is the role of nursing in this emerging area? Nurses will provide education to patients about genetic and genomic testing, research, and treatment. As research-based improvements in the recognition of familial disease traits are identified and emerging disease treatments are discovered, nurses will play an increasingly important role in the study and application of genetic findings and the role of genetics and genomics in the health of the patients they serve. Genetics and genomics will undoubtedly play a significant role in current and future patient care. Nurses at all levels have the opportunity to engage in this opportunity and provide needed education, support, and treatment based in the most current research, even though ethical challenges may arise as a result of this emerging research and treatment (see the relevant websites and online resources at the end of this chapter). Kirk et al. (2011) purported that the study of genetics and genomics is one of the fastest growing areas of health care research. The authors contended that nurses must have a sound understanding of the impact of this area of health care research to provide comprehensive and effective care to their patients.

How should we use the ability to diagnose genetic defects prenatally? Genetic disorders such as Tay-Sachs disease, cystic fibrosis, Huntington chorea, and retinoblastoma can be diagnosed early in pregnancy. As this detection technology advances, how should it be used? Should screening remain voluntary or, as some have suggested, should it be mandatory to detect fetal disorders, with a view to possible abortion or treatment? Should the results of such genetic screening be made available to insurance companies? Critics argue that this information could be used as a means of coercion for couples over reproductive decisions if future insurance coverage is then limited. As this technology advances, safeguards must be applied to prevent invasions of privacy and any societal movement toward eugenics. As the human genome project allows us to become capable of knowing our genetic code and possibilities for developing disease, it raises the question of who should have access to that information. And for what reason or reasons? If a family with a known genetic disorder chooses to have more children with that disorder, is it the obligation of society to pay for their care? Is there any reason for insurance or the government to become involved with genetic counseling, or is this a private family affair?

Allocation of Scarce Resources

When the subject of scarce resource allocation is mentioned, justice is the core issue. What is fair and equal treatment when health care financing decisions are made? Who should make such decisions and on what basis? Critics argue that health care is not a scarce resource in this country but that the *access* to such care is scarce for many. They believe that this scarcity of access could be eliminated if our priorities in governmental spending were altered. Managed care put a temporary brake on runaway costs in the 1990s, but that brake has failed in the past few years. The solution to this issue remains unclear and is highly politicized. In the meantime, managed care of one form or another is influencing a larger and larger share of the insured population, raising related issues of restricted access to specialized care and loss of patient and physician autonomy.

Allocation also raises a number of questions. For example, do all individuals merit the same care? If your answer is an immediate yes, would you change your mind if the patient were indigent and not able to pay the bill? If you still say yes, should this same indigent patient receive a liver transplant as readily as someone who has insurance or cash to pay for it? Should taxpayers be obliged to pay for organ transplants, cardiac bypass surgery, or joint replacements for incarcerated felons? These and other questions continue to be asked by individuals, government bureaucrats, and ethicists in addition to health care providers. Perhaps at the core of this subject is a more fundamental question: Is health care a right or a privilege that comes with the ability to pay? If access to health care is a right that should be provided to all citizens, are we as a society prepared to pay the bill? And is there a level of health care that is essential for all, beyond which financing becomes a private matter?

The type of care that is provided and supported is another aspect of the debate. For example, should health promotion and prevention be emphasized as much as or more than illness-oriented and rehabilitative care? It is widely acknowledged that each dollar spent on preventive care (e.g., prenatal care) saves $3 or more in later intervention (e.g., neonatal ICU), yet our national and state health care expenditures (Medicare and Medicaid) are traditionally weighted in favor of an illness model for reimbursement. Managed care is an effort to control health care costs, but it is increasingly criticized as prioritizing the financial bottom line over the quality of care.

What Are Some of the Possible Solutions Being Debated?

Some individuals see a central point of controversy being whether the potential benefit is large enough or likely enough to occur in order to justify the expense (Scheunemann, 2011). Proponents of health care rationing argue that high-tech "11th-hour expenditures" are unwanted by some older adults and consume disproportionate amounts of health care resources. Proponents of rationing stress the need to acknowledge the finite resources of society. As our society continues to age, younger workers will increasingly be asked to pay the costs of Medicare, Medicaid, and Social Security. Disparities between generations will increasingly become part of the conversation regarding health care financing.

Many believe that more vulnerable groups, such as uninsured children, should be given a more equitable portion of health care services (e.g., well-baby clinics, universal health insurance for children). Others argue that health care is already being rationed and that we should recognize this fact and articulate our priorities. Few would disagree that our present health care financing needs a comprehensive overhaul before we experience a chaotic breakdown.

Health care rationing. You may already have experienced situations of health care rationing or limited access. As a nurse you may, on one hand, feel powerless and frustrated when patients do not receive care because they cannot afford it or, on the other hand, feel angry because indigent patients are placing heavy burdens on both private and public facilities. Consider your values and professional responsibilities as you think through this issue. Efforts to address it include the passage of the 1986 Emergency Medical Treatment and Active Labor Act (EMTALA), which requires hospitals to provide care to anyone needing emergency health care treatment regardless of citizenship, legal status, or ability to pay. As an individual and a nurse, you must take a stand regarding health resource allocation and support efforts to improve access while also determining what type of health care you believe to be ethically justifiable.

What Are the Ethical Issues Around Involuntary Commitment?

As we have discussed in previous sections, sometime legal statues and ethical decisions clash. One example of this is with the process of involuntary commitment. In certain situations, people with a mental illness or irrational behavior will be court-ordered to enter an outpatient or inpatient psychiatric treatment center against their will for treatment. This process of involuntary commitment is guided by the laws of each state and is most commonly limited to patients who are a threat to themselves or others.

Those supporting involuntary commitment feel that these individuals are a safety threat to the community. This teleological stance ensures that the rights of the majority (the public at large) are protected regardless of the fact that the rights of the individual are being denied. From a civil rights perspective, involuntary commitment creates a class of people who feel victimized at the hands of the legal and health care systems. Consider, for example, how the process of involuntary commitment violates the *Patient Care Partnership* discussed earlier in this chapter.

Professional Boundaries

According to the annual Gallup poll on honesty and ethical standards, nurses were ranked the most trusted profession in 2017, having topped the list of 22 professions for the past 16 years. Some 82% of Americans described nurses' ethical standards as high or very high (AHA, 2018). The public we serve expects nurses to act in their best interest, respect their dignity, and avoid personal gain. We have an ethical duty to our patients to establish and maintain well-defined professional boundaries when in the nurse-patient relationship (Benbow, 2013).

The National Council of State Boards of Nursing (NCSBN) believes that there is a continuum of professional behavior that ranges from underinvolvement to overinvolvement, with a therapeutic relationship being at the center. In Box 19.6 you will see the perspective for professional boundaries of our regulatory organization and, in Fig 19.2, a couple examples.

What Is the Impact of Social Media and Social Networking on Nursing Practice?

The use of social media and social networking sites has made it easy and convenient for nurses to stay connected to current events as well as to keep up to date on emerging clinical guidelines and evidence-based practice measures in the provision of patient care. However, with the increased use of technology

BOX 19.6   BOUNDARIES AND THE CONTINUUM OF PROFESSIONAL NURSING BEHAVIOR

- The nurse's responsibility is to delineate and maintain boundaries.
- The nurse should work within the therapeutic relationship.
- The nurse should examine any boundary crossing, be aware of its potential implications, and avoid repeated crossings.
- Variables such as the care setting, community influences, patient needs and the nature of therapy affect the delineation of boundaries.
- Actions that overstep established boundaries to meet the needs of the nurse are boundary violations.
- The nurse should avoid situations where he or she has a personal, professional, or business relationship with the patient.
- Posttermination relationships are complex because the patient may need additional services. It may be difficult to determine when the nurse-patient relationship is completely terminated.
- Be careful about personal relationships with patients who might continue to need nursing services (such as those with mental health issues or oncology patients).

Reprinted with permission from the National Council of State Boards of Nursing (NCSBN). (2018). *A nurse's guide to professional boundaries*, p. 6. Retrieved from https://www.ncsbn.org/ProfessionalBoundaries_Complete.pdf.

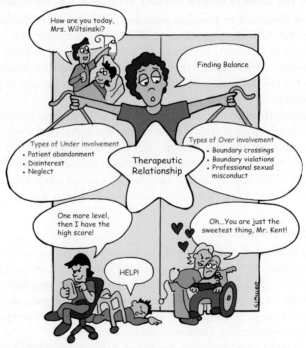

FIG. 19.2 Continuum of professional boundaries.

and social media, nurses must be aware of the legal limitations for using social media in both their professional and personal lives. The National Council of State Boards of Nursing (2011) and other professional nursing organizations have developed guidelines for nurses and students to follow in an effort to avoid any potential legal conflicts (Box 19.7).

BOX 19.7 GUIDELINES FOR USING SOCIAL MEDIA

Nurses must be aware of potential patient confidentiality and privacy breaches that may occur as a result of sharing private and confidential patient information via social networking sites and on the internet.

Here are a few points to consider:

- Any type of information, document, image, video, or material that you post on a social networking site or internet is subject to being shared with others.
- There is no such thing as permanently deleting information from a site. Even if deleted, the information may still be accessible by others.
- It is a breach of confidentiality to discuss a patient's condition or identify the patient by another name, room number, agency location, or diagnosis, even if you do not disclose the patient's legal name.

When using social media, consider the following:

- Recall that you have an ethical obligation to maintain and protect patient privacy and confidentiality.
- Never share or post patient images, videos, or any information pertaining to a patient on any form of electronic media; this includes the use of cell phones, smart phones, cameras, and other electronic devices in the clinical setting.
- Follow the institution's policies and procedures for taking photos or videos of patients for treatment purposes on electronic devices provided by the employer.
- Do not disclose any information that may identify the patient; this includes but is not limited to biographical data (name, age, occupation), medical diagnosis, room number, implantable medical devices, and diagnostic reports.
- Do not write or verbalize negative or rude comments about a patient, family member, or health care team member.
- Do not make harassing, profane, uncivil, hostile, sexually explicit, racially derogatory, homophobic, threatening, or other offensive comments about coworkers, the employing institution, patient, or patient's family.
- Recognize that professional boundaries between you, your patient, and the patient's family exist and must be carried out in both the practice setting as well as in the online environment.
- You have an ethical duty to report any type of breach of confidentiality or privacy.
- Know your employing institution's policies and procedures regarding the use of electronic media and personal devices in the workplace.
- Never speak on behalf of your employer or a co-worker unless you have been authorized to do so; also be sure to you follow the employer's policies and procedures.

Data from National Council of State Boards of Nursing (NCSBN). (August 2011). *White paper: A nurse's guide to the use of social media.* Retrieved from https://www.ncsbn.org/Social_Media.pdf.

Emerging Ethical Issues in Health Care

Rarely does a month pass that the media do not identify a new ethical issue in health care. As we soon enter the third decade of this century, the following issues are likely be the most debated ethical dilemmas that nurses will face:

- Health care for illegal residents
- Safe consumption spaces for people who use drugs under the supervision of trained nurses
- Lateral, patient, and family violence toward nurses
- The opioid epidemic and untreated pain
- Care of patients with illnesses that threatens the life of the nurse (i.e. Ebola virus, chemical/biological warfare, etc.)
- Legalized use of medical and recreational marijuana
- Providing inclusive services and care for individuals of all races, ethnicities, religions, ages, sexual identities, and social backgrounds

CONCLUSION

As technology advances, ethical issues and concerns will play an ever-increasing role in your nursing practice. The public, health care professions, spiritual traditions, increasing cultural diversity, and the legal system will all influence the ethical issues affecting health care in the future. It will be difficult to keep an open mind regarding these controversial dilemmas, but it is hoped that you will examine your personal values and continue to make decisions that are based on the welfare of your patients.

🌐 RELEVANT WEBSITES AND ONLINE RESOURCES

American Nurses Association (ANA)
Center for Ethics and Human Rights. https://www.nursingworld.org/practice-policy/nursing-excellence/ethics/
Center for Ethics and Human Rights 2017 Annual Report. https://www.nursingworld.org/~496198/globalassets/practiceandpolicy/nursing-excellence/center-for-ethics-and-human-rights-2017-annual-report-5.compressed.pdf
Code of ethics for nurses with interpretive statements. http://www.nursingworld.org/DocumentVault/Ethics_1/Code-of-Ethics-for-Nurses.html
Position statement on ethics and human rights. https://www.nursingworld.org/~4af078/globalassets/docs/ana/ethics/ethics-and-human-rights-protecting-and-promoting-final-formatted-20161130.pdf
Social media. https://www.nursingworld.org/social/
Social networking privacy toolkit. https://www.nursingworld.org/practice-policy/nursing-excellence/social-networking-Principles/

Centers for Disease Control and Prevention
Public health genomics. http://www.cdc.gov/genomics/.

Ethics Game
Ethical Lens Inventory (ELI). https://www.ethicsgame.com/exec/site/eli.html

International Council of Nurses
The ICN code of ethics for nurses. https://www.icn.ch/sites/default/files/inline-files/2012_ICN_Codeofethicsfornurses_%20eng.pdf

National Council of State Boards of Nursing
A Nurse's Guide to Professional Boundaries. https://www.ncsbn.org/ProfessionalBoundaries_Complete.pdf
A Nurse's Guide to the Use of Social Media. https://www.ncsbn.org/NCSBN_SocialMedia.pdf
Social Media Guidelines for Nurses. https://www.ncsbn.org/347.htm

National Human Genome Research Institute
Policy, legal and ethical issues in genetic research. http://www.genome.gov/Issues/.

White paper: A nurse's guide to the use of social media (2011, August)
https://www.ncsbn.org/11_NCSBN_Nurses_Guide_Social_Media.pdf.

BIBLIOGRAPHY

American Hospital Association. (2018). *Nurse watch: Nurses again top Gallup poll of trusted professions and other nurse news.* Retrieved from https://www.aha.org/news/insights-and-analysis/2018-01-10-nurse-watch-nurses-again-top-gallup-poll-trusted-professions.

American Nurses Association. (2013). *Euthanasia, assisted suicide, and aid in dying.* Retrieved from https://www.nursingworld.org/~4af287/globalassets/docs/ana/ethics/euthanasia-assisted-suicideaid-in-dying_ps042513.pdf.

American Nurses Association. (2001). *Nurses' Bill of Rights.* Retrieved from https://www.nursingworld.org/practice-policy/work-environment/health-safety/bill-of-rights-faqs/.

American Nurses Association. (2017). *Code of ethics for nurses.* Kansas City, MO: ANA. https://www.nursingworld.org/practice-policy/nursing-excellence/ethics/code-of-ethics-for-nurses/.

American Nurses Association. (n.d.). The ANA Center for Ethics and Human Rights. Retrieved from https://www.nursingworld.org/practice-policy/nursing-excellence/ethics/

American Transplant Foundation. (2018). *Facts: Did you know?* Retrieved from https://www.americantransplantfoundation.org/about-transplant/facts-and-myths/.

Austin, C., Saylor, R., & Finley, P. (2017). Moral distress in physicians and nurses: Impact on professional quality of life and turnover. *Psychological Trauma: Theory, Research, Practice, and Policy, 9*(4), 399–406. https://doi.org/10.1037/tra0000201.

Benbow, D. (2013). Professional boundaries: When does the nurse-patient relationship end? *Journal of Nursing Regulation, 4*(2), 30–33. https://doi.org/10.1016/S2155-8256(15)30154-X.

Caplan, A. (March 31, 2015). Ten years after Terri Schiavo, death debates still divide us: Bioethicist. *NBC Health News.* Retrieved from http://www.nbcnews.com/health/health-news/bioethicist-tk-n333536.

Centers for Medicare and Medicaid Services. (2012). *Emergency medical treatment and active labor act (EMTALA).* Retrieved from http://www.cms.gov/Regulations-and-Guidance/Legislation/EMTALA/index.html?redirect=/emtala/.

Feldman, D. M. (1968). *Marital relations, birth control and abortion in Jewish law.* New York: Schocker.

Fletcher, J. F. (1966). *Situation ethics.* Philadelphia: Westminster.

Kirk, M., Calzone, K., Arimori, N., & Tonkin, E. (2011). Genetics-genomics competencies and nursing regulation. *Journal of Nursing Scholarship, 43*(2), 107–116.

Lea, D. (2009). Basic genetics and genomics: A primer for nurses. *OJIN: The Online Journal of Issues in Nursing, 14*(2), 1–11.

Mobly, M., Rady, M., Verheijde, J., Patel, B., & Larson, J. (2007). The relationship between moral distress and perception of futile care in the critical care unit. *Intensive and Critical Care Nursing, 23*(5), 256–263. https://doi.org/10.1016/j.iccn.2007.03.011.

National Association for Home Care & Hospice. (n.d.). What are my rights as a patient? Retrieved from https://www.nahc.org/consumers-information/home-care-hospice-basics/hoime-health-and-hospice-patient-rights/

National Council of State Boards of Nursing. (2018). *A nurse's guide to professional boundaries.* Retrieved from https://www.ncsbn.org/ProfessionalBoundaries_Complete.pdf.

National Council of State Boards of Nursing. (2011). *White paper: A nurse's guide to the use of social media.* Retrieved from https://www.ncsbn.org/11_NCSBN_Nurses_Guide_Social_Media.pdf.

National Institutes of Health (NIH). (2016). Stem cell information. Retrieved from https://stemcells.nih.gov/info.htm

National Institutes of Health (NIH) National Human Genome Research Institute. (2018). *Frequently asked questions about genetic research.* Retrieved from https://www.genome.gov/19516792/faq-about-genetic-research/.

National Public Radio (NPR). (Sept. 26, 2018). *Health and human services says it's reviewing use of fetal tissue for research.* Retrieved from https://www.npr.org/2018/09/26/651838889/health-and-human-services-says-its-reviewing-use-of-fetal-tissue-for-research.

Oregon's Death with Dignity Act. (2011). Thirteen years. CD Summary. *Oregon Public Health Division, 60*(6).

Pro Con. (2018). *State-by-state guide to physician-assisted suicide.* Retrieved from: https://euthanasia.procon.org/view.resource.php?resourceID=000132.

Rosen, H. (1967). *In Abortion in America.* Boston: Beacon Press.

Rostami, S., & Jafari, H. (2016). Nurses perceptions of futile medical care. *Journal of the Academy of Medical Sciences, 28*(2), 151–155. https://doi.org/10.5455/msm.2016.28.151-155.

Rudy, E. B. (1985). The living will: Are you informed? *Focus on Critical Care, 12*, 51.

Scheunemann, L., & White, D. (2011). The ethics and reality of rationing in medicine. *Chest, 140*(6), 1625–1632.

Schneider, K. (2011, June 3). Dr. Jack Kevorkian dies at 83: A doctor who helped end lives. *New York Times.* Retrieved from https://www.nytimes.com/2011/06/04/us/04kevorkian.html.

Steele, S. M. (1983). *Values clarification in nursing* (2nd ed.). East Norwalk, CT: Appleton & Lange.

Thompson, I. E., et al. (2007). *Nursing ethics* (5th ed.). St Louis, MO: Churchill Livingstone/Elsevier.

Wang, K., Chou, C., & Huang, J. (2010). A study of work values, professional commitment, turnover intention and related factors among clinical nurses. *Journal of Nursing, 57*(1), 22–34.

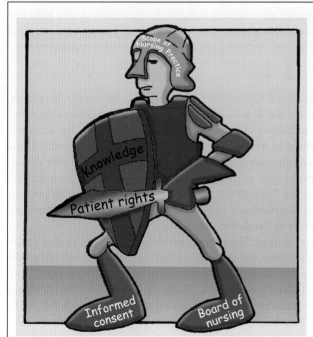

20

Legal Issues

Alice E. Dupler, MSN, JD, ANP-BC, Esq.*

ⓔhttp://evolve.elsevier.com/Zerwekh/nsgtoday/.

I attribute my success to this; I never gave nor took any excuse.
Florence Nightingale

It is not how much you do, but how much love you put in the doing.
Mother Teresa

Evidence-based knowledge is the best way to prevent poor patient and professional outcomes. Thus, knowledge is the best offense as well as the best defense.

After completing this chapter, you should be able to:
• Discuss sources and types of laws.

• Relate the Nurse Practice Act to the governance of your profession.
• Recognize the functions of a state board of nursing.
• Describe your responsibilities for obtaining and maintaining your license.
• Research and discuss scope of practice limitations on your license.
• Identify the elements of nursing negligence and how each element is proven in a negligence claim.
• Incorporate an understanding of legal risks into your nursing practice and recognize how to minimize these risks.
• Discuss the concerns surrounding criminal charges in nursing practice.
• Identify legal issues involved in the medical record and your documentation, including the use of electronic medical records.
• Understand legal concepts such as informed consent and advance directives.
• Improve the quality of health care as required by legal standards.
• Utilize professionalism when dealing with nurses who are impaired or functioning dangerously in the work setting.
• Discuss the concerns surrounding two or more legal issues in nursing practice.

*We would like to acknowledge, Nikki Austin, JD, RN, for her past contributions to this chapter.

L aws are rules of human conduct designed to keep civilized societies from falling into anarchy. A law is a prescriptive or proscriptive rule of action or conduct promulgated by a controlling authority such as government. Because laws have binding legal force and are meant to be obeyed, failure to follow the law may subject you to a wide variety of legal consequences. The Latin phrase *ignorantia legis neminem excusat* means "ignorance of law excuses no one." It is important for all persons, including nurses, to know, understand, and follow the law as it relates to their personal and professional lives.

There are many laws from a variety of sources that directly and indirectly impact the practice of nursing. Understanding these laws can have a profound effect on the way you practice nursing and may help ensure safe nursing practice. This chapter is an important start in becoming a legally educated nursing professional. Your journey does not stop here, however, because the law is always evolving and under constant scrutiny and challenge. Nursing professionals must assume ongoing responsibility for keeping up with relevant changes in the federal, state, and local laws that govern nursing practice.

SOURCES OF LAW

Where Does Law Come From?

Have you ever wondered where the law comes from? Laws can be created by regulatory, legislative, and litigation processes involving different branches of government (executive, legislative, and/or judicial). There are several primary and secondary sources of law that directly and indirectly impact the practice of nursing, including constitutional law, statutory law, common law, and administrative regulatory law.

What Is Constitutional Law?

The U.S. Constitution is the supreme law of the land. *Constitutional law* refers to the power, privileges, and responsibilities stated in, or inferred from, the U.S. Constitution as well as state constitutions. Constitutions prescribe the power and responsibilities of federal and state governments. For example, the powers of the federal government are defined in Article I, Section 8 of the U.S. Constitution. These powers include such things as the power to coin money, the power to establish a uniform rule of naturalization, the power to declare war, the power to tax and spend, and the power to regulate interstate commerce. Medicare and Medicaid were enacted through the spending powers of the federal government. Taxes are collected and then spent as distributions to the states to subsidize their Medicaid programs or directly to hospitals and providers as Medicare payments.

The Tenth Amendment to the Constitution states, "The powers not delegated to the United States by the Constitution, nor prohibited by it to the States, are reserved to the States respectively, or to the people." This means the powers of the state government include anything and everything that is not specifically described as being a power of the federal government. These powers, referred to as "police powers," include the power to license professionals, including nurses, and generally provide for public health and safety of the community (Ramanathan, 2014). States may not pass laws or institute rules that conflict with constitutionally granted rights or powers. Thus, federal and state constitutions are the most powerful statements of law in the nation and cannot be changed without approval of the citizenry.

What Is Statutory Law?

Statutory law is an important source of law. Statutes are created by federal, state, and local legislatures, which are comprised of elected officials who have been granted the power to create laws. It would be an impossible feat for governments to anticipate all possible scenarios in which a statute might be needed to regulate human conduct. Therefore, statutes are often written broadly enough to be applicable in a variety of situations. Courts must apply statutes, if available, to the facts of a case. If no statute exists, courts defer to *common law* (see below).

Statutory definitions are one of the most important parts of a statute. There you can find what the authors of the statute mean when they use a certain word. Because we all use words differently, a more precise understanding is necessary when reading and understanding statutory laws. Box 20.1 lists definitions of common legal terms. When a statute is vague or unclear, courts must engage in statutory interpretation to determine the legislature's intent.

BOX 20.1   COMMON LEGAL TERMS

Advance directive: A document made by an individual to establish desired health care for the future or to give someone else the right to make health care decisions if the individual becomes incapacitated; examples include living wills and durable powers of attorney for health care.

Defamation: A civil wrong in which an individual's reputation in the community, including the professional community, has been damaged.

Defendant: The person who is being accused of wrongdoing. The person then must defend himself or herself against the charges. In a negligence claim, this is the nurse or other health care provider.

Deposition: Out-of-court oral testimony given under oath before a court reporter. The purpose is to enable attorneys to ask questions and receive answers related to a case. The deposition process may involve expert witnesses, fact witnesses, defendants, or plaintiffs.

Diversion program: Voluntary, confidential monitoring programs for nurses whose practice may be impaired due to substance use disorder.

Expert witness: A person who has specific knowledge, skills, and experience regarding a specific area and whose testimony will be allowed in court to prove the standard of care.

Good Samaritan law: A law that provides civil immunity to professionals who stop and render care in an emergency. Care rendered cannot be done so in a grossly negligent manner.

Interrogatory: A process of discovering the facts regarding a case through a set of written questions exchanged through the attorneys representing the parties involved in the case.

Jurisdiction: The court's authority to accept and decide cases. May be based on location or subject matter of the case.

Malpractice: Improper performance of professional duties; a failure to meet the standards of care, resulting in harm to another person.

Negligence: Failure to act as an ordinary prudent person when such failure results in harm to another.

Plaintiff: The person who files the lawsuit and is seeking damages for a perceived wrongdoing. In malpractice, this is the patient and/or the patient's family.

Reasonable care: The level of care or skill that is customarily rendered by a competent health care worker of similar education and experience in providing services to an individual in the community or state in which the person is practicing.

Standard of care: A set of guidelines describing behaviors of what a reasonable and prudent health care professional would do in the same or similar circumstances.

Statutes of limitations: Laws that set time limits for when a case may be filed. These limitations differ from state to state.

Telemedicine: Using telecommunication technology, usually interactive, to provide health care information and services remotely.

Torts: Civil (not criminal) wrongs committed by one person against another person or their property. Includes the legal principle of assault and battery.

Whistleblower: Individual "on the inside" who reports incorrect or illegal activities to an agency with the authority to monitor or control those activities.

Whistleblower statute: Law that protects a whistleblower from retaliation. Usually involves specific criteria about how whistle was blown.

What Is Administrative Regulatory Law?

As agents for the executive branch of federal and state government, administrative agencies protect the public health and welfare. *Administrative law* is made by administrative agencies that have been granted the authority to pass rules and regulations and render opinions, which usually explain in more detail the statutes on a particular subject.

The administrative agency that is generally most familiar to nursing professionals is the state board of nursing, sometimes called the nursing commission. Nursing boards accomplish their mission through licensing competent and qualified individuals and then regulating licensees' safeness and scope of practice as outlined in each state's Nurse Practice Act.

What Are Nurse Practice Acts?

Each state has enacted important legislation known as a Nurse Practice Act. The Nurse Practice Act in each state defines the qualifications for nursing licensure and establishes how the practice of nursing will be regulated and monitored within that state's jurisdiction. Nurse Practice Acts generally describe nursing scope of practice boundaries, unprofessional conduct, and disciplinary action. In most states, the Nurse Practice Act and the regulations that interpret it do the following:

- Describe how to obtain licensure and enter practice within that state.
- Describe how and when to renew a nursing license.
- Define the educational requirements for entry into practice.
- Provide definitions and scope of practice for each level of nursing practice.
- Describe the process by which individual members of the board of nursing are selected and describe the categories of membership.
- Identify situations that are grounds for discipline or circumstances in which a nursing license can be revoked or suspended.
- Identify the process for disciplinary actions, including diversionary techniques.
- Outline the appeal steps if the nurse feels the disciplinary actions taken by the board of nursing are not fair or valid.

It is required to keep your state board of nursing informed of your current residence so that you are informed of events that can affect the safe delivery of patient care and thus your license and practice. Never ignore or take lightly any document received from your state board of nursing. Even if you think you have received a notice in error, contact the board of nursing immediately (Box 20.2). You also need to be informed of Nurse Practice Act requirements in a new state of residence before you begin to practice there. All Nurse Practice Acts are readily accessible online and/or easily obtained from any state board of nursing (see Appendix A on the Evolve website). Read the Nursing Practice Act and the regulations related to it for your state of licensure and/or state of practice.

BOX 20.2 PROTECT YOUR LICENSE

- Provide current evidence-based care reflecting current knowledge, your clinical judgment, and your patient's preferences, values, and beliefs.
- Be direct, respectful, honest, and timely when communicating with patients and families.
- Assure that information about you is current and accurate with your state board.
- Know the Nurse Practice Act and its related regulations in your state(s).
- Practice nursing according to the scope and standards of practice in your state(s).
- Know the self-reporting laws and self-report when required.
- Have professional licensure defense insurance.

What Is Criminal Law?

Statutory laws and their related regulations are either criminal or civil. Negligent conduct can be criminal acts or they may be considered civil actions. Civil actions concern private interests and rights between individuals and/or businesses. *Criminal law* involves prosecution and punishment for conduct deemed to be a crime. Most complaints against nurses are civil actions.

Criminal negligence is based on a criminally culpable state of mind in addition to a deviation from the standard of care. The lapse in standard of care can be intentional or unintentional. For example, in November 2006, a Wisconsin nurse made an unintentional medication error that resulted in a patient's death during childbirth. The nurse was criminally charged with patient abuse and neglect causing great bodily harm, a felony that carried a penalty of imprisonment and a significant monetary fine. The nurse eventually received probation after pleading no contest to two criminal misdemeanors. Additionally, the Wisconsin Board of Nursing suspended the nurse's license for 9 months to be followed by a 2-year practice limitation (ASQ, 2007).

■ *Case study 1*

You are working in a hospital where a very well-known actor is admitted with a diagnosis of *Pneumocystis jiroveci* pneumonia. During the patient's stay, you are asked by a physician to administer an intravenous medication for purposes of conscious sedation to the patient while the physician performs a procedure. During the procedure, the patient has a respiratory arrest secondary to oversedation and dies. You are devastated and realize that you may have administered too much medication. You decide to confide in your best friend, who is also a nurse, about the incident. While speaking to your best friend, you mention the actor's name and diagnosis. Your friend says that it was "illegal" for you to administer intravenous conscious sedation and expresses concern that your actions and possible medication error might land you in trouble (Critical Thinking Box 20.1).

❓ CRITICAL THINKING BOX 20.1

In Case Study 1, where might you be able to search to determine whether this is true? What type of legal trouble might you have?

What Is Case Law?

The role of the judiciary (court) is to apply and interpret the law. In our judicial system, two opposing parties present evidence before a judge and/or a jury who applies the law to the facts to determine the outcome of the case. When the court's interpretation of the law leads to law itself, it is known as case law. *Case law* and *common law* are often used interchangeably to describe law that is developed by courts when deciding a case as opposed to law created through a legislative enactment or a regulation promulgated by an administrative agency.

Civil Actions—Torts

Tort law, as described by Pozgar (2016), is a civil wrong committed against a person entitling the injured party to file a lawsuit to receive compensation for damages he or she suffered as a result of the alleged wrongdoing. The purpose of tort law is to determine culpability, deter future violations, and award compensation to the plaintiff if applicable. There are two categories of tort actions: unintentional and intentional. Medical negligence or professional negligence is an example of an unintentional tort and is discussed in more detail in the following (Jacoby & Scruth, 2017).

What Are Intentional Torts?

Intentional torts are civil "wrongs" that are done on purpose to cause harm to another person. Instead of seeking to put the *tortfeasor* (the wrongdoer) in jail, however, an intentional tort claim attempts to right the wrong by compensating the plaintiff. These types of claims are less common than negligence claims, which are not purposeful acts and can be asserted against a nurse in some circumstances.

There are several types of intentional torts. *Assault and battery* and false imprisonment are two examples of intentional torts. *Assault and battery* are the legal terms that are applied to nonconsensual threat of touch (assault) or the actual touching (battery). The practice of nursing involves a great deal of touching. Permission to do this touching is usually implied when the patient seeks medical care. All patients have the right, however, to withdraw their implied consent to medical care and refuse the procedure or treatment or medication being offered. So long as a patient has the capacity to make decisions, their refusal to consent or withdrawal of consent must be respected by the health care team or there could be legal implications. For instance, the Louisiana Supreme Court awarded $25,000 to a patient's family in a lawsuit wherein the nurses had ignored the patient's refusal of a Foley catheter. The patient was ultimately injured in the process of removing the catheter, and the court determined that the nurses had committed battery by performing an invasive procedure against the patient's wishes (*Robertson v. Provident House,* 1991). Also, a patient may wish to leave an institution against medical advice (AMA). If nurses use physical restraint or touching to keep this patient from leaving, these actions can lead to a civil claim of assault and battery.

False imprisonment means making someone wrongfully feel that he or she cannot leave a place. It is often associated with assault and battery claims. This can happen in a health care setting through the use of physical or chemical restraints or the threat of physical or emotional harm if a patient leaves an institution. Threats such as "If you don't stay in your bed, I'll have to sedate you" may constitute false imprisonment. This tort might also involve telling a patient that he or she may not leave the emergency department until the bill is paid. Another example is using restraints or threatening to use them on patients to make them do what you want them to do against their wishes. Unless you are very clearly protecting the safety of others, you may not restrain a competent adult (Critical Thinking Box 20.2) (Guido, 2013).

> **? CRITICAL THINKING BOX 20.2**
>
> In what situations would it be acceptable to restrain a patient?

In psychiatric patient populations in which patients may pose a danger to themselves or others, there are many very specific state and federal laws to follow as well as institutional policies. The challenge, of course, is in preventing patients from self-harm while also maintaining the patients' constitutional rights to liberty. This is not always an easy balance. There are many restrictions on the appropriate use of both hard and soft restraints and elevated scrutiny on their use in both hospital and long-term care facilities (Tolson & Morley, 2012). Claims of elder abuse have been filed for the misuse of restraints. You must be aware of the policies in your institution as well as any applicable statutory requirements.

Defamation (libel and slander) refers to causing damage to someone else's reputation. If the means of transmitting the damaging information is written, it is called *libel*; if it is oral or spoken, it is called *slander*. The damaging information must be intentionally communicated to a third person. The actions likely to result in a defamation charge are situations in which inaccurate information from the medical record is reported, such as in Case Study 1, or when speaking negatively about your co-workers (supervisors, doctors, other nurses).

Two defenses to defamation accusations are *truth* and *privilege*. If the statement is true, it is not actionable under this doctrine. However, it is often difficult to define truth, because it may be a matter of perspective. It is better to avoid that issue by not making negative statements about other people unnecessarily. An example of privilege would be required for good-faith reporting to child protective services of possible child abuse or statements made during a peer-review process. If statements made during these processes are without malice, state statutes often protect the reporter from any civil liability for defamation.

Recovery in defamation claims usually requires that the plaintiff submit proof of injury—for instance, loss of money or job. Some categories, such as fitness to practice one's profession, do not require such proof, as they are considered sufficiently damaging without it. Comments about the quality of a nurse's work or a health care provider's skills in diagnosing illness would fit in this category. You can avoid this claim by steering clear of gossip and by not writing negative documents about others in the heat of the moment and without adequate facts (Smith, Morin, Wallace, & Lake, 2017).

Invasion of Privacy and Breaches of Privacy and Confidentiality

A good general rule involving the sharing of patient information is always to ask yourself, "Do I have the patient's consent to share this information, or is it necessary to deliver health care services to this patient?" If the answer to either is "no," then the information should not be communicated.

Privacy regulations under the Health Insurance Portability and Accountability Act of 1996 (HIPAA) remain as a central focus for the public. There are specific privacy regulations under HIPAA that became effective in April 2003 and include an elaborate system for ensuring privacy for individually identifiable health information. Information used to render treatment, payment, or health care operations does not require the patient's specific consent for its use. This includes processes such as quality assurance activities, legal activities, risk management, billing, and utilization review (Whitehurst, 2017). However, the rules require that the disclosure be the "minimum necessary," and a clear understanding of what information can be shared under this exception is necessary (Furrow et al., 2018). Notice must be given to the patient regarding how the information will be used. All nurses working in health care must be aware of this law and how their institutions specifically comply with it.

Another aspect of HIPAA involves electronic information and the security measures necessary to ensure that protected patient information is not accessed by those without the right or need to know. These rules came into effect in April 2005. Each institution must have data security policies and technologies in place based on their own "risk assessment." Many institutions require that any health information transmitted under open networks, such as the Internet, telephones, and wireless communication networks, be encrypted (coded).

The Health Information Technology for Economic and Clinical Health Act (HITECH Act, 2009) was passed in conjunction with HIPPA. HITECH focuses on social media and newer technologies where disclosure of personal health information could occur. Nurses are especially vulnerable under HITECH when inadvertently disclosing health information without permission of the patient.

Many states have physician–patient privilege laws that protect communications between physicians and their patients. This enables information to pass freely between physician and patient without concern that it will be shared with those who do not need to know it. This includes law enforcement organizations. The privilege usually extends to information about a patient in the medical record or obtained while providing care. Most states extend physician–patient privilege to nurses and sometimes to other health care providers as well. This privilege generally belongs to the patient and not the health care professional, which means that only the patient can decide whether to relinquish it.

As a professional, it is important to observe *confidentiality* when talking about patients at home and at work (Fig. 20.1). Nurses must be very careful to keep information about the patient confidential and

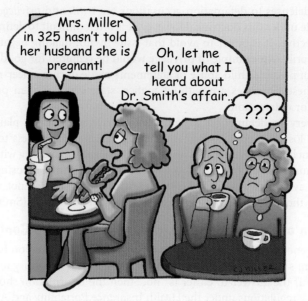

FIG. 20.1 Maintaining confidentiality is both an ethical and a legal consideration in nursing.

to share information only with health care workers who must know the information to plan or to give proper care to the patient. This is sometimes difficult to do, as seen in Case Study 1.

EHRs and national clearinghouses for health information present significant confidentiality concerns. Such technologies offer many advantages, including easier and broader access to needed information and more legible documentation. These same advantages also create issues because they make it more difficult to ensure confidentiality. Most hospitals and agencies have policies and procedures in place, such as access codes, limited screen time, and computers placed in locations that promote privacy (Malfait, Van Hecke, Van Biesen, & Eeckloo, 2018). The nurse is still responsible for the protection of confidentiality when computers, e-mail, voice paging systems, mobile devices, or other rapid communication techniques are used.

Privacy violations can result in a legal cause of action for the tort of *invasion of privacy*. This cause of action can apply to several behaviors, such as photographing a procedure and showing it without the patient's consent, going through a patient's belongings without consent, or talking publicly about a patient.

Miscellaneous Intentional Torts and Employment Civil Rights Claims

The aforementioned torts and others can be relevant to nurses in relation to their employment. These intentional torts can be brought personally against the nurse. *Tortious interference with contract* is a claim alleging that someone maliciously interfered with a person's contractual (often employment) rights. This can occur, for instance, if a nurse attempts to get another nurse fired through giving false or misleading facts to a supervisor. *Intentional infliction of emotional distress* is described by its name, and it can also be attached to malicious acts in the employment setting. These and certain civil rights claims such as *sexual harassment* and *discrimination* are both rights and potential liabilities for every person in the work force. Although beyond the scope of this text, policies and information regarding these issues demand further investigation by each health care employee to ensure that their rights and the rights of others are not violated.

What Are Unintentional Torts?

The most common type of *unintentional tort* is called *negligence*. A person is considered to have acted negligently when he or she unintentionally causes personal injury or harm to property where the person should have acted reasonably to avoid such harm. Because professional negligence (also referred to as malpractice) can potentially affect every nurse, it is important to explore what this means. Before we delve into negligence, let's examine classifications of legal actions and nursing licensure.

> The most common unintentional tort action brought against nurses is a negligence claim.

COURT ACTIONS BASED ON LEGAL PRINCIPLES

There are two major classifications of legal actions that can occur as a result of either deliberate or unintentional violations of legal rules or statutes. In the first category are *criminal actions*. These occur when you have done something that is considered harmful to society as a whole. The trial will involve a prosecuting attorney, who represents the interests of the state or the United States (the public), and a defense attorney, who represents the interests of the person accused of a crime (defendant). These actions can usually be identified by their title, which will read "*State v. [the name of the defendant]*" or "*U.S. v. [the name of the defendant].*" Examples include murder, theft, drug violations, criminal mistreatment of vulnerable adults, and some violations of the Nursing Practice Acts, such as misuse of narcotics. Serious crimes that can cause the perpetrator to be imprisoned are called *felonies*. Less serious crimes typically resulting in fines are *misdemeanors*. The victim, if there is one, may or may not be involved in a decision to prosecute a case and is considered only a witness in the criminal trial. Laws differ in states as to victim rights and/or if the person or the state will receive any of the money from fines. In Case Study 1, your actions would not likely result in a criminal action. Recently, however, there have been instances in which a nurse was thought to have recklessly caused a patient's death, and a case was brought in criminal court for negligent homicide. The issues involved in such criminal actions will be discussed later in this chapter.

The second category of legal claims includes *civil actions*. These actions concern private interests and rights between the individuals involved in the cases. Private attorneys handle these claims, and the remedy is usually some type of compensation that attempts to restore injured parties to their earlier positions. Examples of civil actions include malpractice, negligence, and informed consent issues. The victim (patient) or victim's family (patient's family) brings the lawsuit as the *plaintiff* against the *defendant*, who may be the individual (nurse) or company (hospital) that is believed to have caused harm. In the situation presented, you might be sued for malpractice by the actor's spouse if it is felt that you acted below a standard of care and caused the actor's death.

Sometimes an event can include both criminal and civil consequences. When that happens, two trials are held with different goals. The amount of evidence required to support a guilty verdict is different for each type of trial. The criminal case requires that the evidence show that the defendant was guilty beyond a shadow of a doubt. The civil case requires only that the evidence show that the defendant was more likely guilty than not guilty. This is what makes it possible for someone to be found "not guilty" in a criminal trial but "guilty" or negligent in a civil trial.

NURSING LICENSURE

All states prohibit the practice of nursing without a license. Many other professional occupations require a license. Have you ever asked yourself what is the purpose of licensure and why some occupations require a license while others do not? When specialized knowledge and skill are required to perform often complex professional activities, particularly activities involving potential harm to the public, licensure is usually required. Licensure protects the public health and welfare by establishing entry-level qualifications and ongoing competencies to maintain and ensure safe practice.

A license to practice nursing is a privilege, not a right. According to the National Council of State Boards of Nursing (NCSBN, 2018c), licensure is "the process by which boards of nursing grant permission to an individual to engage in nursing practice after determining that the applicant has attained the competency necessary to perform a unique scope of practice." Each state Board of Nursing follows licensing statutes and rules designed to determine if potential applicants possess the competency and necessary skills to practice safely in their chosen field.

Even the successful completion of an educational program in nursing and/or passing the National Council Licensure Examination for Registered Nurses (NCLEX-RN) does not guarantee that a state board of nursing will grant you a license to practice nursing. A license is granted by a state after a candidate has successfully met *all* the requirements in that state. Examples of these requirements may include criminal background checks and successful completion of a board-approved nursing education program.

When you graduate from nursing school and successfully complete the state licensing process to become a practical or registered nurse, you achieve professional licensure status under the law. Having a license to practice nursing brings you into close contact with laws and government agencies. Professional licensure is governed by Nurse Practice Acts that you must follow in the state(s) in which you are licensed and/or practicing nursing. Once you are licensed, the state continues to monitor your practice and has the authority to investigate complaints against your license. If you are found to have violated the Nurse Practice Act, a state board of nursing can take disciplinary action against your license.

Disciplinary Actions

Several levels of disciplinary actions can occur based on the severity of the practice act violation and the ongoing risk to the public. For instance, state boards of nursing have disciplinary power ranging from censure to probation, suspension, revocation, and denial of licensure. One of the most common reasons for state board action against nurses involves substance misuse and the diversion of prescription medications for personal use (Guido, 2013). Boards of nursing are increasingly concerned about this issue, because it has significant impact on rendering safe, effective patient care (NCSBN, 2018a).

Final disciplinary actions are a matter of public record and can be accessed by contacting a state board of nursing. Additionally, final disciplinary actions are reported to governmental and nongovernmental authorities for public protection. For example, NURSYS is a nongovernmental electronic information system that includes the collection and warehousing of nurse licensing information and disciplinary actions (NCSBN, 2018e). The Healthcare Integrity and Protection Data Bank (HIPDB) and the National Practitioner Data Bank (NPDB) are two federal data banks of information about health care providers in the United States. Adverse actions taken against a health care professional's license are required by federal law to be reported to the HIPDB and NPDB. However, the general public may not access information included in the NPDB and HIPDB, as the information is limited by law to entities such as hospitals, health plans, and government agencies.

Scope of Practice

The scope of practice for professional nursing is the range of permissible activity as defined by the law; in essence it defines what nurses can and, sometimes more important, cannot do. Because the scope of nursing practice is defined by state legislation, there is great variation from state to state both in specificity and in the range of activities that are legally authorized. Many state legislatures have enacted very specific scope of practice statements whereas others have drafted very vague and broad scope of practice statements and have left the job of describing the specific activities to the state board of nursing. Some state scope of practice statements are very restrictive, whereas others allow a much broader range of activities. It is very important that a nurse become very familiar with the practice act and the scope of practice as defined by the legislature or the state board of nursing in the state where he or she intends to practice.

There is significant variability for the scope of practice of licensed practical or vocational nurses (LPN/LVN) and even more variability for the scope of practice for advanced practice nurses (nurse practitioners, midwives, anesthetists, collectively called APRN) (NPDB, 2018). Because of the restrictive nature of the scope of practice statements of many states, all APRNs are not able to practice to the full extent of their education and training.

■ *Case study 2*
Recalling your incident Case Study 1, where you administered IV medication for conscious sedation to an actor who subsequently died from respiratory arrest as a result of oversedation, you decide to leave the state. You have to answer detailed questions on your licensure application for the new state about any previous malpractice claims. You had heard something about a claim being filed against your former hospital but had left shortly after that. Now you have received a notice from the state board of nursing of your previous residence inquiring about the incident with the actor and asking for a response within 2 weeks. The letter has taken a long time to be forwarded to you, and the 2-week deadline has passed. What should you do?

Multistate Licensure

The enhanced Nurse Licensure Compact (eNLC) is a "mutual recognition agreement" between states that have adopted the Compact legislation. The enhanced Nurse Licensure Compact allows both registered and practical nurses with a license in good standing in their "home state" to practice nursing in any of the other Compact states ("member states") without going through the process of obtaining additional licensure. According to the National Council of State Boards of Nursing (NCSBN), many states have enacted the enhanced Nurse Licensure Compact (NCSBN, 2018d).

An enhanced compact license is also known as a "multistate license." It is important to note that only nurses who declare a Compact state as their primary state of residence are eligible for a multistate license. This means that if you obtain a license in a state that is not participating in the Nurse Licensure Compact, you do not have a multistate license and cannot practice nursing outside of your primary state of residency without obtaining additional licensure in a new state. It is also very important to note that when you permanently relocate to another Compact or non-Compact state, all licensure laws including the Nurse Licensure Compact require you to obtain licensure in the new state.

The APRN Compact, approved by the NCSBN on May 4, 2015, allows an advanced practice registered nurse to hold one multistate license with a privilege to practice in other Compact states. The APRN Compact is under consideration in several states.

What About Substance Use Disorder in Nursing?

Substance use disorder describes a pattern of substance use behavior that encompasses substance misuse to dependency or addiction (NCSBN, 2018a, 2018b). Substances can be alcohol, prescription drugs, or illegal drugs. Substance use disorder can affect nurses and anyone regardless of their age, gender, or economic circumstances. Boards of nursing are increasingly concerned about this issue, because it has significant impact on rendering safe, effective patient care.

Nurse Practice Acts and their related statutes have mandatory reporting obligations regarding impairment. Many nurses say they are "afraid to get them in trouble" when they have reasonable suspicion that a colleague may have a substance use disorder. Allowing an impaired nurse to practice puts the patient at risk and negatively impacts the facility's reputation and the nursing profession. Concern for your colleagues is admirable; however, allowing them to continue to practice at the risk of patient harm is unacceptable. It is important that you know what the reporting requirements are for your state board of nursing and your facility.

One of the most common reasons for state board action against nurses involves the diversion of prescription medications for personal use (NCSBN, 2018a, 2018b). Do not ever assume that you or your colleagues are immune from substance misuse, abuse, or addiction. High stress and easy access to drugs contribute to the problem for health care providers.

If you do find yourself misusing drugs or alcohol, it is advisable to voluntarily report your substance misuse or abuse to your state board of nursing and seek immediate treatment. The boards of nursing in most states, including the District of Columbia and the Virgin Islands, have alternative monitoring programs to assist nurses with substance use disorders, which may prevent their licenses from being suspended or revoked. The non-disciplinary rehabilitative approach to substance use disorders recognizes the importance of returning a sober abstinent nurse to the work force (NCSBN, 2018a, 2018b).

States with alternative monitoring programs allow enrolled nurses to meet specific behavioral criteria, such as blood or urine testing, ordered evaluations, and attendance at rehabilitation programs, either while disciplinary action is being undertaken or instead of bringing formal disciplinary proceedings. The primary concern is to ensure safe nursing practice. If a nurse is in a voluntary rehabilitation program through a contract with a state board and has additional problems, the board may bring formal disciplinary action against the nurse that may negatively affect licensure for the rest of his or her life.

NEGLIGENCE

■ *Case study 3*

You are a nurse working in a hospital. The physician tells you that you need to administer an injection of Vistaril (hydroxyzine pamoate). You make sure that the order is documented in the medical record. The medication comes up from the pharmacy, and you check it against the physician's order and find that it is correct. You walk into the patient's room and use at least two patient identifiers to make sure you have the right patient. You give the injection in the patient's right dorsogluteal muscle and document this in the medical record.

The patient leaves the hospital. A year later, you are told that a lawsuit has been filed against the hospital by the patient. It seems the patient is claiming that the injection you gave him caused sciatic nerve damage and his whole leg is numb (Critical Thinking Box 20.3).

? CRITICAL THINKING BOX 20.3

Who may have negligence liability in this situation and why? You? The physician? The hospital? What defenses may be available to you?

Many nurses worry about being sued for something when, in the eyes of the law, no negligence has occurred. Not all poor outcomes are a result of negligence or are a violation of the Nurse Practice Act

(Jacoby & Scruth, 2017). A nurse also may legitimately make an error in judgment. Therefore, it is important for a nurse to know the basic elements that must be proved before negligence can occur. Then the nurse can evaluate incidents realistically.

Basic Elements of Negligence

What are the basic elements of negligence?
1. You must have a duty. In other words, there must be a professional nurse–patient relationship.
2. You must have breached that duty. In other words, you must have fallen below the standard of care for a nurse.
3. Your breach of duty must have been a foreseeable cause of the injury.
4. Damages or injury must have occurred.

There are four basic elements of negligence, all of which must be proven by the plaintiff in a negligence lawsuit in order for the plaintiff to be awarded compensation.

The job of the patient's (plaintiff's) attorney is to prove to a jury that each element of negligence has occurred. This is not always a simple straightforward process, and it can be frustrating and confusing for all involved parties. It is important for the nurse to understand the elements of negligence and how each element may be proved in a court of law (Jacoby & Scruth, 2017).

Do You Have a Professional Duty?

Generally, all persons owe a duty of "due care" to others in our daily activities and lives. This means that you must conduct yourself in a reasonable and prudent manner to avoid causing harm to another person or his or her property. The duty of due care also applies to nursing professionals who have a professional duty to act as a reasonable nurse would act in the same or similar circumstances to avoid causing foreseeable harm to patients.

To prevail in a negligence action, the plaintiff must establish that there was a nurse–patient relationship in which a professional duty was owed by the nurse to the patient. If you are working as a nurse in a hospital, the nurse–patient relationship is usually implied, and you owe a professional duty of care to your patients. What if you are giving advice in your home informally to a friend, relative, or neighbor? In this setting, it may not be implied that you are acting as a nurse, particularly in the absence of payment, institution, or formal contract.

What if you stop at an accident to assist someone who is injured? Good Samaritan statutes provide immunity from malpractice to those professionals who attempt to give assistance at the scene of an accident. You do not have any professional duty to stop, although you may feel an ethical duty to do so. However, a nurse may be sued in some states for rendering Good Samaritan aid if the nurse is found to have acted in a grossly negligent manner. If you do stop at the scene of an accident to provide aid, know that in most—if not all—states you cannot be sued for malpractice for what you might or might not do, unless the aid you provide is grossly negligent. That is, you do not have a professional standard of care to adhere to unless you are a professional at the scene as part of your employment. All persons, of course, are expected not to leave a victim in a position that is more dangerous than when found. After you stop to help the injured person, stay with him or her until you are given clearance by emergency responders.

Sometimes nurses volunteer to provide nursing assistance at sporting events or other activities where it is foreseen that professional services may be needed. In thinking about this, you may see that such a situation is not quite as clear as other situations. If you are at a first-aid station or if you are wearing a badge indicating you are a nurse, then you have the appearance of a professional, and people may rely on that appearance when seeking advice or assistance.

It is important to know your status under these various circumstances in your state. You should know whether you have immunity and whether you are covered by malpractice insurance.

Falling Below the Standard of Care: Was There a Breach of the Professional Duty?

After establishing that a professional duty is owed, the question becomes, "What is that duty?" The duty owed by a nurse to a patient is different from the duty owed to the patient by another health care discipline such as a physician or physical therapist. The duty of a nurse will be to act as a reasonable nurse would act under the same or similar circumstances. This is known as the standard of care and is a very important factor in most negligence cases. You may be asking yourself, "How will my attorney prove that I acted as a reasonable nurse and within the standard of care?"

The following aspects may be considered when attempting to establish through evidence what the standard of care for the nurse might be.

What About the Nurse Practice Act?

Perhaps the most important guideline for nurses will be the Nurse Practice Act in the state in which you are practicing. Most acts describe in general terms what a nurse may or may not do. Prohibitions, or things that are unprofessional conduct, are usually more specific. A Nurse Practice Act violation means that you have fallen below a standard of care set by the state for nurses. It also may mean that you risk an action against your license. If you do not know what these prohibitions are, you are putting yourself in jeopardy. As stated previously, and as applied here to the standard of care, it is important that you obtain a copy of the Nurse Practice Act for the state(s) in which you are or will be licensed to practice and be sure to stay current with your licensing standards. For instance, Texas now requires that all applicants for licensure pass a nursing jurisprudence examination, which is based on the Texas Nursing Practice Act and the Texas Board of Nursing Rules and Regulations (Texas BON, 2013).

What Is an Expert Witness?

The most common way to establish the duty owed by a nurse is by the testimony of a registered nurse who usually, but not always, has training and a background like yours. This expert witness will then testify regarding what a reasonable nurse in the same or similar circumstances would be expected to do—and, in the case of an expert witness for the plaintiff, will argue that you did not do it. If a plaintiff's attorney cannot find an expert nurse to testify that you did not act reasonably, then in most instances the case cannot go forward. In general, a patient cannot simply claim professional malpractice without having a professional witness to corroborate this.

In the same manner, if the plaintiff has an expert witness to prove you fell below the standard of care, you will need an expert witness to testify that you did not. Some nurses appreciate this role to use their expertise either for the defense of a nurse or as part of the plaintiff's claim against a nurse. Either role requires both integrity and professionalism to be effective and credible in front of a jury (Pozgar, 2016).

There is a type of malpractice case in which an expert is not required. This type of claim is called *res ipsa loquitur*, or "the thing speaks for itself." This claim is very difficult to prove, because the patient must have enough evidence to show that (1) the injury would ordinarily not occur unless someone were negligent; (2) the instrumentality causing the injury was within the exclusive control of the defendant; and (3) the incident was not a result of any voluntary action on the part of the plaintiff. If a patient can prove that all of these conditions exist, the burden then shifts to the defendant nurse to prove that malpractice did not take place. Incidents such as operating on the wrong body part or leaving a surgical sponge in a patient fall into this category of claim.

What Are Established Policies and Procedures?

Policies and procedures established by the institution in which you work are crucial pieces of evidence for establishing a standard of care (Edwards & Twomey, 2015). Attorneys who represent plaintiffs will request a set of hospital policies as soon as a lawsuit is filed. For instance, in Case Studies 1 and 3, a lawyer might ask for the hospital's policies on documentation and administration of medications. If you did not follow that policy, then you fell below a standard of care set by your institution.

You can see why you need to know and read the policies within your health care facility or corporation. These policies should also be a resource when you have questions about how to perform certain procedures or what your rights are in certain situations. Policies are the processes under which you must live. It is also important for you as a professional to participate in making or changing policies so that they accurately reflect what nurses are doing in your institution. In addition, the policies set standards for providing high-quality and consistent patient care. If you have followed a current evidence-based policy, it can be used proactively to prove that you followed the standard of care set by your institution.

What About Accreditation and Facility Licensing Standards?

Most health care facilities and other health care organizations must go through a process whereby they become licensed and/or accredited. The Joint Commission (TJC) and the National Committee of Quality Assurance (NCQA) are two such organizations that set accreditation standards for health care organizations. For instance, TJC has issued National Patient Safety Goals (NPSGs) every year since 2003 that include standards to improve safe identification of patients and their medications, prevent infections using proven guidelines, and improve communication among care providers (TJC, 2019). A state facility-licensing requirement would be that the facility develops policies and procedures to optimize patient safety when administering medications.

What About Textbooks and Journals?

Articles, textbooks, or portions of such publications may be used as evidence of the standard of care for nurses to follow. For instance, if a nursing journal has published a recent article on correct administration of intramuscular injections, that may be used to demonstrate what you should have done.

What Are Professional Standards for Nursing Organizations?

Professional nursing organizations, such as the American Nurses Association (ANA) or the Association of periOperative Registered Nurses (AORN), publish certain standards or practice guidelines. These may be used as evidence for what a reasonable nurse should do under certain circumstances.

In summary, there are many types of evidence used by plaintiff attorneys to demonstrate an expected standard of care. The nurse needs to remember that these same documents can be used to demonstrate that you did follow the standard of care. Let us see how.

Applying the Standard of Care to the Case Study

In Case Study 3, the plaintiff must find a nurse who will testify about the correct method for administering intramuscular injections. If you did not give the injection in such a manner, then the jury can infer that you did not act reasonably. However, if the correct method is to give the injection intramuscularly in the right dorsogluteal site, and you have documented that you did this, the plaintiff may not be able to establish a breach of the standard of care. Also, if you can show that you followed evidence-based hospital policies in the administration of the medication, again, there will be no proof of falling below the standard of care.

What if the patient attempts to claim a case using the theory of *res ipsa loquitur*? Again, the patient's lawyer must prove that the claimed injury could not have happened unless there was negligence. As demonstrated earlier, you would be able to prove through your documentation that you were not negligent. In addition, your attorney would also demonstrate your lack of liability through the third element of malpractice. Do you remember what that is?

Did the Breach of Duty Cause an Injury?

Causation is an important element that must be demonstrated in a negligence action. The plaintiff must prove that the nurse's action actually caused the injury and that the injury was a foreseeable consequence of the nurse's actions. Did the difficult birth cause the child to have cerebral palsy, or did a genetic birth defect cause the baby to experience a difficult delivery? Was the injury caused by the auto accident or by the medical care? Did the patient have the physical problem before the medical care or after? Was the injury caused subsequently by the patient's lack of compliance with the treatment plan, or did the patient subsequently injure herself after the medical care was rendered?

Applying "Causation" to Case Study 3

Returning to Case Study 3, the patient will have to prove that your injection caused the numbness in his leg. There are many intervening factors that could have caused this numbness. You do not have to prove anything because you, as a defendant, do not have the burden of proof. The plaintiff may have a very difficult time, especially if there are no documented complaints by the patient of problems at the time of the injection or shortly thereafter.

Just remember that a patient's claim that you or another provider caused some particular injury or problem should not automatically be assumed to be true. Although you do not have to argue the point with the patient, you also do not have to agree. Injuries have many causes and many stories behind them:

- Document the facts.
- Document what you see and do.
- Your role is to render nursing services, not to judge or give your opinion.
- Your actions and factual documentation will be your best defense.

Did the Patient Suffer Damages or Injury?

The last element that must be proved is that your breach of duty caused injury (damages) to the patient. This last element of negligence can also be overlooked when the nurse becomes distracted by the fact that he or she fell below the standard of care in making a mistake in patient care. Many practice errors do not cause injury or damages but are the result of multiple factors (Park, Hanchett, & Ma, 2018). For instance, if a nurse administers a one-time dose of 650 mg of Tylenol instead of 350 mg of Tylenol, the medication error is not likely to cause permanent injury or damages. This does not mean, however, that any medication error should be ignored or taken lightly or that some medications cannot cause death or serious injury with a single mistake. Medication errors are serious breaches of the standard of care (Harkanen, Tiainen, & Haatainen, 2017; Khalil & Lee, 2018; Rutledge, Retrosi, & Ostrowski, 2018). It is very unlikely though that a malpractice claim will be brought for a medication error that does not cause injury or damages. You may still suffer an employment-related consequence such as disciplinary action for errors that do not result in patient harm.

Damages can be viewed as the sum of money a court or jury awards as compensation for a tort action. *General damages* are those given for intangibles such as pain and suffering, disfigurement, interference with ordinary enjoyment of life, and loss of consortium (marital services) that are inherent in the injury itself (Furrow et al., 2018; Pozgar, 2016). *Special damages* are the patient's out-of-pocket expenses such as medical care, lost wages, and rehabilitation costs. *Punitive damages* are those damages that seek to punish those whose conduct goes beyond normal malpractice. Claims in which this might occur are rare, but they involve issues such as changed medical records, lies being told to patients, or intentional misconduct while under the influence of alcohol or drugs. Such punitive awards can add millions of dollars to an otherwise low-damage claim. Some states have limited the amount for specific types of damages that a plaintiff can receive (Critical Thinking Box 20.4).

> ### ? CRITICAL THINKING BOX 20.4
> Does your state limit the amount of damages a plaintiff can receive?

Damages Applied to the Case Study

In Case Study 3, numbness of a limb may be difficult to prove. Nerve conduction studies may be performed in an independent medical examination to demonstrate that the injection could not have caused the neurologic injury about which the patient complains. Numbness also does not mean lack of function and may not usually prevent any activity of daily living. The age and status of the plaintiff would have an important role, as would your documentation of the patient's lack of complaints and ability to ambulate.

> Your actions and documentation are the best defense.

WHO MIGHT HAVE LIABILITY (RESPONSIBILITY) IN A CLAIM?

■ Case study 4

You are a nurse working on a surgical unit in a hospital. One evening you are asked to float to pediatrics. The only experience you have had with children was when you were a student. A physician asks you to give digoxin to an infant and writes an order for 2 mg. This seems like a lot of medication to you, so you ask the charge nurse on the unit about the dose. The charge nurse assumes you are speaking about an oral dose of the medication and states this is normal. You give the medication by injection and shortly thereafter the child's heart stops beating, and he is coded. When you attempt to use an Ambu bag, it is not on the crash cart. The child eventually recovers; however, 21 years later, you receive notice that a young man is suing you for giving him the wrong dose of digoxin when he was an infant.

Personal Liability

Who can be held accountable for your actions as a nurse? You may hear things such as, "Don't worry, I'll take responsibility for this." There is no defense called "She made me do it." For many years, physicians were seen as the "Captain of the Ship" and thus ultimately responsible for everything that happened to the patient. This doctrine is no longer true. In the eyes of the law, each individual is accountable for his or her own actions. Even if you are not personally named in a lawsuit, you will be asked to provide evidence regarding your involvement and will be expected to defend your nursing care under oath. "I was just following orders" does not explain why you, as a professional nurse, made a medication error. You are held to a professional standard of care to know about the medications you are administering, including the correct dose.

There are 5,657,831 licensed RNs and PNs in the United States (CMS, 2018). A professional nurse includes registered nurses, licensed practical nurses, licensed vocational nurses, nurse practitioners, nurse anesthetists, nurse midwives, clinical nurse specialists, advanced nurse practitioners, and doctors of nursing practice. Clinical analysis of complaints and closed claims are rare. Of 10,639 reported adverse events that included 549 closed claims, 88.5% were complaints regarding care provided by registered nurses. Of those, the average settlement was $165,491; the average cost incurred to defend the nurse was $36,424 (NSO, 2015). The largest settlements were paid to patients who incurred harm in neurology or obstetrical units; this is due to anticipated harm over extended lengths of time. However, more claims were filed when patients were harmed on medical units (NSO, 2015). In particular patients were inaccurately assessed resulting in harm such as worsening pressure injuries or decreased abilities to move either when walking or turning in bed without assistance. Typically, malpractice insurance purchased by the workplace will be triggered when patients are harmed; however, this insurance does not include coverage to defend the nurses' license to practice. Thus, it is essential that every nurse maintain their individual professional licensure defense coverage to assure that when these instances occur, they can act to present their version of the circumstances to the state boards of nursing. In Case Study 4, who is likely to be named in a lawsuit? Who might share liability for the patient's injury? Although nurses do have a duty to follow physician's orders under most circumstances, this is never true if the nurse believes or has reason to believe that the provider's order is unsafe for the patient or not within the nurse's scope of practice. In Case Study 4, if the nurse did not know the correct dose of IV digoxin, the nurse had an independent duty to verify the correct dose.

In Case Study 1, receiving an order to give IV conscious sedation does not relieve the nurse of a duty to determine whether this is within his or her scope of nursing practice. If an order falls outside of the nurse's scope of practice, the nurse must notify the provider and refrain from carrying out the order. When accepting orders from health care providers, remember that you should only accept duties and orders that you are competent to perform and that are within your scope of practice.

Supervisory Liability

Questions often arise regarding the nurse's responsibility for the actions of others. The standard of care for a supervisor is to act as a reasonable supervisor under the same or similar circumstances. A supervisor can be expected to ensure the following:

- The task was properly assigned to someone competent to perform it safely.
- Adequate supervision was provided as needed.
- The nurse provided appropriate follow-up and evaluation of the delegated task.

As in Case Study 4, a supervisor could be expected to supervise more closely a float nurse or a recent graduate than someone who is an experienced nurse on a pediatric unit. It is also incumbent on a person being supervised to ask for assistance if that person is faced with a problem that he or she lacks the necessary skills to resolve. In Case Study 4, this was done, but the nurse administering the medication and the supervisor miscommunicated regarding the method or route of administration. How often do you think this happens in health care?

Delegation of nursing duties to unlicensed health care workers presents supervisory nurses with some special risks. Changes in health care delivery systems and financing are resulting in some unfamiliar categories of unlicensed caregivers with a wide variety of skills and expertise. Some boards of nursing have informed their licensees that each nurse remains personally liable for any task delegated to an unlicensed worker on the theory that the delegated task is considered the nurse's responsibility rather than being within the scope of practice of the unlicensed worker. Other boards of nursing have stated that they will apply to delegation the traditional standards for supervising any health care worker, as described earlier.

Certain nursing responsibilities, such as nursing diagnosis, assessment, teaching, and some portions of planning, evaluation, and documentation, should not be delegated to unlicensed staff. Contact the board of nursing in your state to understand better your responsibilities in the delegation of nursing duties.

Institutional Liability

Health care institutions such as hospitals are usually sued under a theory of *respondeat superior* for the actions of their employees. Almost all health care institutions carry insurance to cover the acts and omissions of their employees. Although institutions are often named as defendants in a lawsuit, this does not relieve the nurse from having to answer formally to the court for his or her own actions or inaction.

An institution's policies or lack thereof is also a common claim in a lawsuit. For instance, there can be a claim in Case Study 4 that the institution should have had a policy on nurses floating to other units in the hospital and that such persons should never be given the responsibility of transcribing physicians' orders. Additionally, in this case, there may be institutional liability through the pharmacy. If the pharmacy filled the wrong medication dose, and there are systems in place to check dosages, the pharmacist and/or technician may also be brought into the claim through the institution. There are certainly more systems than ever before in place in most hospitals to prevent medication errors. When they all fail, many persons can be involved in the liability.

Student Liability

Nursing students have responsibility for their own actions and can be held liable (Pozgar, 2016). The adage that "students practice under their instructor's license" is not true. Student nurses will be held to the standard of care for the tasks they perform (Pozgar, 2016). It is therefore important that students never accept assignments beyond their preparation and that they communicate frequently with their instructors to obtain assistance and guidance.

Instructors and preceptors are responsible for reasonable and prudent clinical supervision. An instructor could be held liable for inadequate supervision in erroneously determining that a student was competent to perform a skill, when he or she was not competent (Pozgar, 2016).

It is important to know your status under these various circumstances in your state and/or if you have immunity and/or are covered by malpractice insurance.

Instructors and preceptors need to remember that the level of expertise may vary for individual students, and the standard used to evaluate the students' performance usually involves more supervision than the standard used for some other, more experienced workers.

WHAT DEFENSES MIGHT BE AVAILABLE IN MALPRACTICE CLAIMS?

If the plaintiff in a malpractice claim does not prove each of the elements previously discussed, the defense can ask for a dismissal of the claim by making various motions (formal requests) to the court. There are several other issues that may influence the outcome of a malpractice claim.

A *statute of limitations* is a law that sets a time period during which a lawsuit must be filed after an event. States have different statutes and case law surrounding this time limit. Usually, the limit is measured from the time of the event or incident, last date of treatment, or time the event was discovered (or should have been discovered). For minors, some states allow the time to be counted from the time they reach majority (usually 18 years old), unless a suit has already been brought on their behalf by parents or others. Therefore, in Case Study 4, a suit could be brought 2 or 3 years after a person reaches 18 years (majority) for an injury occurring as an infant. Other states do not permit this delay. Lack of mental competence will also delay the time requirements in some states.

Failure to file the lawsuit within the statute of limitations time results in the loss of the right to sue. This can be considered a defense, because filing after the date allows the defendants to have the case dismissed. It is important to know, however, that in most states, the statute starts running when the patient knows of the injury. If there is any type of cover-up regarding an incident, the statute will not run.

Proving that the patient assumed the risk of harm or that the patient contributed to the harm by his or her actions provides another type of defense. *Assumption of the risk* defense states that plaintiffs are partially responsible for consequences if they understood the risks involved when they proceeded with the action (Furrow et al., 2018). An example would be a patient who has the capacity to make their own decisions and who has been warned to use a call light but instead crawls out of bed and thus injures herself.

Contributory negligence is an older doctrine that was at one time an "all or nothing" rule. Plaintiffs who had any part in the adverse outcome were barred from compensation. Today, most jurisdictions use a comparative negligence theory and reduce the money award by the injured party's responsibility for the ultimate harm done (Furrow et al., 2018). The results of one case indicated that a patient could be negligent and thus be at least partially responsible by (1) refusing to follow advice or instructions; (2) causing a delay in treatment or not returning for follow-up; (3) furnishing false, misleading, or incomplete information to a health care provider; or (4) causing the injury that results in the need for medical care (*Harvey v. Mid-Coast Hospital*, 1999).

COMMON CATEGORIES OF NEGLIGENCE

There are common categories of negligence and certain situations that involve a high risk for a lawsuit against nurses. These situations most often relate to patient safety, improper treatment, problems with monitoring and reporting, medication errors, failing to follow proper procedures and policies, and failure to document (Azuero, 2018; Bragadóttir, Kalisch, & Tryggvadóttir, 2017; Duffy, Culp, & Padrutt, 2018).

Medication Errors

A study by the Institute of Medicine (IOM) reported that medication errors harm 1.5 million people every year. The additional medical cost of treating drug-related injuries in the hospital was at least $3.5 billion per year. The study did not indicate whether the sources of the errors were nurses, physicians, or pharmacists. The reporting committee found that medication errors are common at every stage, from the writing of the prescription, to the filling of the prescription, to the administration of a drug and the monitoring of the patient's response (IOM, 2006). While the number of medication errors have significantly decreased, those that do occur appear to be causing much more significant harm (NSO, 2015). Claims involving medication errors are augmented when the nurse fails to record the medication administration properly, fails to recognize side effects or contraindications, or fails to ascertain a patient's allergies. Any initiative that improves patient safety also lowers the chance of someone being sued. At the same time, it sets a benchmark on which the standard of care may rest and thus becomes important for every nurse to know and follow.

The nurse's ability to listen to a patient or family member who notices that a medication is new or recheck when anything such as color or amount seems unusual may prevent a serious error. Many nurses feel rushed by the amount of work they are expected to accomplish, and they do not want to take extra time for anything. Making this check a priority will prove to be time well spent

BOX 20.3 TIPS FOR BEING AT YOUR BEST WHEN ADMINISTERING MEDICATIONS

- Minimize distractions. It is important to avoid interruptions when administering medications to reduce the risk of making a medication error.
- Utilize a bar coding medication administration scanning system when available.
- Recognize fatigue. If you are fatigued, you are more likely to make mistakes. Twelve-hour shifts, double shifts, and long shifts put patients at risk.
- Listen to your patients. Stop. Often, they will tell you if what you are planning to do is different or unusual. The patient is always the decision maker, not you.
- Double check high-alert medications. Take the time to do a second check, and you may save yourself and your patient from a medication error. Do not bypass black box warnings.
- Ensure competence. Never do a procedure you do not know how to do at the appropriate standard of performance. It is better to admit you need help or supervision than to risk hurting someone.
- Be accountable. Never be afraid to admit you made a mistake. Prompt corrective action may stop or at least reduce patient harm.
- Take your time. Do not rush when you are especially busy because being hasty can result in errors. Set realistic priorities and ask for help.
- Keep current and up to date in your practice knowledge base. An article in a professional journal may keep patients safe and avoid a lawsuit.

(Box 20.3). Dealing with an error and the consequences to the patient will take longer and will be more painful.

Although many medication errors do not cause permanent or serious damage to patients, there are certain medications that can. TJC standards require each institution to identify high-alert medications used in the institution and to initiate safety procedures for managing these medications (TJC, 2019).

Whenever a medication error occurs, the source of the error and the system failure should be carefully investigated. TJC also requires that health care organizations have a plan for responding to adverse drug events and medication errors, for example, sending reports to the Medication Error Reporting Program operated cooperatively by U.S. Pharmacopeia (USP) and the Institute for Safe Medication Practices (IOM, 2006; TJC, 2015).

Provide a Safe Environment

Patient safety is more and more recognized as a duty of the health care team and health care institutions. Providing a safe environment and implementing a fall reduction program were originally included in TJC's 2010 NPSGs. When a NPSG becomes a standard, the goal number is retired and is not used again. In 2010, TJC moved the goal to a standard for hospitals but kept it as a goal for long-term care facilities and home care. Ensuring patient safety includes many aspects. Nurses sometimes do not recognize the multiple roles they have in this area. They are responsible for knowing how equipment should work and not using it if it is not functioning correctly; removing obvious hazards such as chemicals, which might be mistaken for medications; and making the environment free of hazards such as inappropriately placed furniture or equipment and spills on the floor. An additional preventive measure is knowing how to document correctly if an incident occurs, so that there cannot be a doubt regarding the facts of what happened and everything you did to protect the patient.

Patient Falls

Falls are not inevitable as we age, but 25% of adults 65 and older fall every year (CMS, 2018). Falls that cause serious patient injury are routinely among the Top 10 sentinel events voluntarily reported to

TJC's Sentinel Event database. The most common factors contributing to falls with injury are inadequate assessment, failure to communicate, failure to adhere to facility protocols and safety practices, inadequate staff supervision or staffing, lack of leadership, and physical environment deficiencies (TJC, 2018b). Being proactive in response to a fall is essential, as those who do fall will repeatedly fall until they are significantly injured and unable to move without maximum assistance of staff. Much time and effort have been spent attempting to change patient care so that falls do not occur. Elimination of restraints, individualized comprehensive patient care plans, and decreasing the number of certain types of medications have been effective and have become evidence-based interventions when attempting to reduce significant injury falls (TJC, 2018b). TJC has specific tools targeted toward preventing harm to patients as a result of falls (TJC, 2018b). It is important to assure that your actions are evidence-based to prevent patient harm (Critical Thinking Box 20.5).

❓ CRITICAL THINKING BOX 20.5

What fall guidelines have you observed in your clinical settings? How are they the same, and how are they different from each other? How are fall guidelines in acute-care hospital settings different from long-term care settings?

Nurses are best able to defend themselves in these cases when their institution has a policy regarding protecting patients against falls, sometimes called an evidence-based guideline to prevent falls. These policies establish levels of risk in patients, such as age, confusion, sedation, and steps the nurse must take to protect the patient. If the nurse follows the guideline, it is difficult for a plaintiff to prove that the nurse fell below a standard of care. In developing policies and procedures, it is important to know the laws in your state, federal CMS guidelines, and TJC standards regarding falls (TJC, 2018b). Documentation is extremely important when a patient falls. Here are a few suggestions for documenting a patient fall situation; however, it is vital you follow the agency policy and procedural documentation guidelines where you are employed.

- Document the facts regarding how the fall was discovered, where the patient was found, and any other facts surrounding the fall. An example is to document that the patient was found beside the bed, with the side rails up, and the bed in the low position.
- Document the nursing assessment data, any obvious injuries, and nursing actions to maintain patient safety.
- Document what the patient says regarding the fall. A statement such as "I know you told me to put on the call light, but you all seemed so busy that I didn't want to bother you," can be of great benefit to the nurse. Of course, a patient's statement "I put on the call light, but nobody came" can have the opposite effect.
- Document whom you notified, such as the physician or the family.
- Document what was done for the patient, such as an examination, radiographs, orientation to surroundings, monitoring after the incident, bedside sitter, and assistance with further ambulation.
- Document your adherence to any policies of the hospital regarding vulnerable patients or those at risk for falls.

In *Shaw v. Plantation Management*, a nurse found a patient on the floor with a puddle of liquid next to him. The patient stated that the liquid was urine from another patient and that this caused him to fall. The nurse assessed the patient and got him the medical attention that he needed. The patient later died after surgery for a broken hip. The nurse did not know what the liquid was, and she did not know whether the patient had actually urinated after he fell. The nurse only charted what she had actually seen and what she did. Her clear documentation later prevented the patient's family from being able to prove that the incident was caused by any negligence on behalf of the facility (*Shaw v. Plantation Management*, 2009).

Equipment Failure

Today many nurses feel they spend more time nursing equipment than they do patients. This can be true. There is a certain standard of care connected with equipment. It must be used as directed by the manufacturer, and the nurse has a duty to know what that use is and to follow such directions. There is also a duty to make sure that the equipment is properly maintained and that records are kept of this maintenance. The equipment needs to be working properly and should not be used when a known defective condition exists. Additionally, the device must be available for use. For instance, in Case Study 4, the fact that the Ambu bag was not available can be viewed as a liability for either the nurse responsible for checking crash carts or the institution for not seeing that the carts are checked.

When there is a failure of a device or piece of equipment and a patient is injured, the focus should of course initially be on helping the patient. After that, it is extremely important that the device (e.g., catheter, pump, instrument) be sequestered and a clear record of its handling (chain of custody) be maintained. In a lawsuit, the nurse will need to prove that equipment failure, rather than human error, caused the injury. Part of the proof will rest in the piece of equipment itself. Therefore, one of the most important aspects of the defense will be not to lose or let go of the equipment or device before it is thoroughly evaluated by a neutral party after an incident. Often the manufacturer will ask for the equipment, but their interests might be adverse to yours: to prove user error rather than equipment failure. Information regarding the failure can be shared, but never let the device or equipment out of the custody of the institution. In addition, the nurse should adhere to any institutional policies regarding incidents involving equipment failure.

Nurses may also have a duty to be sure their institution complies with the Safe Medical Device Act of 1990. This federal law requires that all medical device–related adverse incidents be reported to manufacturers and, in the case of death, to the U.S. Food and Drug Administration (FDA), within 10 days. The purpose of this act is to protect the public from devices that may be defective (Furrow et al., 2018).

■ *Case study 5*

A 67-year-old woman with chronic obstructive pulmonary disease is having increasingly difficult respirations, increased cyanosis, and increased anxiety. She tells you she just cannot breathe. You have done all the measures for which you currently have orders, without her obtaining relief. It is 2 AM. You call the physician. She orders Valium 10 mg intramuscularly now. Even as a recent graduate, you know that Valium is contraindicated in a patient with this respiratory status. You call your supervisor, who tells you that Dr. Jones is a good physician and must know what she is doing. What should you do?

Failure to Assess Adequately, Monitor, and Obtain Assistance

Most often, the nurse should not delegate to another the responsibility for assessing and evaluating patient care and progress. If some portions of this duty are handled by others (e.g., another RN, LPN/LVN, unlicensed personnel), the nurse who is primarily responsible for the care of the patient must still be aware of the findings and confirm them when they indicate a change in patient condition or progress. Documentation of the changes and events surrounding the changes is critical. Accreditation standards and licensure requirements specifically address improving the effectiveness of communication between caregivers when reporting changes in a patient's condition. Effective communication includes clear documentation of critical events.

In Case Study 5, there may also be liability for failure to challenge an inappropriate order. These areas are uncomfortable for many experienced nurses, not just for the recent graduate. Frequently, these situations involve challenging a physician or other health care professional. They require that the nurse have current, accurate, and evidence-based information. They also require the nurse to be assertive and advocate for the patient, regardless of who the health care professional may be.

> It is not enough to identify problems. The nurse must identify the problems and contact the responsible health care provider to obtain appropriate care. And, the nurse must contact the nursing supervisor, medical director, and/or the chief executive officer as deemed necessary.

Most helpful in situations such as Case Study 5 is a policy that clearly delineates who to contact for the institution. With a policy in place, the nurse can be clear about who must be notified about a potentially problematic order, and it can be documented appropriately. It is important the nurse be protected from retaliation in such instances by the institution that stands to lose if the patient's safety is not put first.

Accurate documentation of the nursing assessment and of frequent monitoring will be required to demonstrate what you have done. Flow charts and forms can be timesaving devices in this area. Electronic communications now make such time-consuming documentation more readily available. Assure that you have reviewed prior entries by other nurses; explain differences in your assessments. Otherwise, they may reflect a change in condition that you may have missed and that should have been reported to the provider.

Failure to Communicate Adequately

Perhaps the most important role of everyone on the health care team is to communicate adequately. The patient's total care rests on this communication, whether it is verbal or written in the medical record.

> One of the most frequent claims against nurses in this area is the failure to communicate changes in the patient's condition to a professional who has a need to know.

Good communication is especially needed during the night hours, as in Case Study 5. Communication is not always welcomed in the middle of the night and can be impaired because it is not face to face and because the receiver may not be fully awake and alert. Best practice requires verification "read back" of all verbal and telephone orders (not limited to medication orders) by the person taking the order and the use of a standardized set of abbreviations, acronyms, and symbols throughout the organization. Thorough documentation of the communication will provide valuable information, but it should not be done defensively or thought of as a substitute for proper care. Defensive documentation is readily noticed by a reader, including a juror. And while you think it may "cover you," it does not; it highlights and points out to the reader that you knew or should have known to get assistance for the patient and did not.

Communication with hearing- and speech-impaired patients and with ethnically and culturally diverse patients may impact nursing care. The Americans with Disabilities Act is a federal statute that has requirements for institutions rendering health care to have translators available for key health care interactions. Failure to do so may put the institution at risk for fines and penalties (*Freydel v. New York Hospital*, 2000).

Failure to Report

States have many statutes that require health care providers to report certain incidences or occurrences. If the provider fails to report as required, and a person is injured, there can be negligence per se, and no expert testimony will be needed to prove the case. In addition, both institutional and professional licensure can be affected. It is important that nurses be aware of the reporting statutes in the state in which they are practicing. In some states, it is not only a duty but also the law to report certain incidences. The following are examples of such statutes involving a duty to report.

- A duty to self-report a criminal charge or conviction
- A duty to report other health care professionals whose behaviors are unprofessional and/or could cause harm to the public; this includes drug and alcohol abuse
- A duty to report evidence of child or adult or elder abuse and neglect, including any acts of a sexual nature against vulnerable (i.e., anesthetized) patients
- A duty to report certain communicable diseases
- A duty to report certain deaths under suspicious circumstances, including deaths during surgery
- A duty to report certain types of injuries that are or could be caused by violence
- A duty to report evidence of Medicare fraud
- Emergency Medical Treatment and Active Labor Act (EMTALA) violations

Nurses should know what to report, who should report, how the report should be accomplished, and to whom a report should be made. Institutional policies and Nurse Practice Acts on these topics are valuable. In *State v. Brown*, criminal charges were brought against an emergency room nurse who failed to report suspected child abuse to an agency when a 2-year-old boy was brought in with suspicious bruises. The trial court dismissed the charges claiming the Missouri statute was unconstitutionally vague as to the term "reasonable cause to suspect"; however, the Missouri Supreme Court later reversed that decision, reinstating criminal charges against the nurse (*State v. Brown*, 2004).

Many nurses are hesitant to report their employers, other professionals, or other agencies because of the possibility of retaliatory action against them. Many mandatory reporting statutes provide immunity to those who report in good faith. Some states have specific whistleblower statutes that not only protect nurses from retaliatory action but also may reward them. The content of the whistleblower statutes differs from state to state, so the nurse must find out whether one exists in his or her state of practice and learn what protection is provided. A federal statute, the False Claims Act, provides protection under certain situations for reporting Medicare fraud. Additionally, federal compliance standards require that institutions maintain a mechanism to report unlawful activities, such as a "hotline" where problems can be reported anonymously. In response to such reports, institutions must demonstrate that they responded appropriately and that they disciplined all individuals engaged in the illegal activities (Furrow et al., 2018; Pozgar, 2016) (Critical Thinking Box 20.6).

? CRITICAL THINKING BOX 20.6

Which states have "whistleblower" protection?

Failure to Document

Documentation is one of the best ways to protect your patient, yourself, and your license. Failure to document jeopardizes patient safety and puts you at risk should there be an adverse outcome. It is important to document all the patient's responses to treatment as well as the patient's progress or lack of progress. Nursing assessments must be documented in the medical record in a timely manner, and any contact with any provider should be promptly and accurately noted in the medical record. Other important areas to document include time and date of nursing care provided in addition to all procedures, medications, monitoring, and interactions with the patient or his or her family.

In many instances, you can become a nurse hero or be in deep trouble based on the accuracy and timeliness of your documentation in the medical record. One of the most important tools for all providers in a malpractice claim or licensure complaint is the medical record. The medical record is the first piece of evidence closely examined in any allegation of negligence. Accurate, timely, and thorough documentation is critically important. By recording the care administered, the specific time it was administered, the patient's response, and the overall status of the patient's condition, the nurse can demonstrate that the standard of care was met (Fig. 20.2).

Your defense attorney will use the medical record extensively and will make a timeline of events that surrounded the incident. Documentation regarding an incident should be thoroughly and factually done in the medical record and not in personal records or a diary (Fig. 20.3).

There is an adage that states, "If it is not documented, it wasn't done." It is simply difficult to prove something was done if there is no documentation and the plaintiff claims it was not done. It is then a "he said/she said" type of argument. A more accurate statement might be: "If it is documented, it was done." When an incident is documented at the time of the event, there is a strong presumption that the documentation is accurate and whatever a patient says to the contrary is simply self-serving. That is why it is so important to document extensively, accurately, and factually in the medical record (Box 20.4). This is especially true when there is an adverse event.

Forms often provide a difficult problem for defense attorneys when they are not completed properly. A blank space on the form or a box that is not checked, when it appears that the space or box was there to indicate the performance of a needed therapy, can be very detrimental to the nurse involved.

Most institutions are utilizing or in the process of implementing the electronic medical record (EMR) or electronic health record (EHR). The rules of documentation still apply, but additional safeguards will have to be considered. This is especially true when some of the health records are paper and

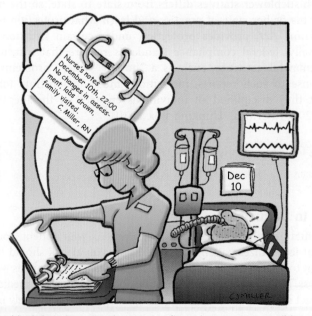

FIG. 20.2 It is critical that the nurse's notes reflect the current condition of the patient.

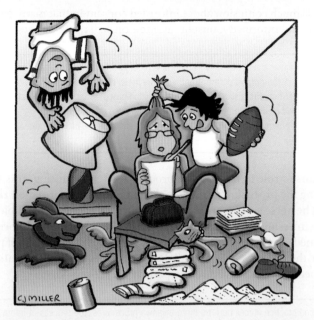

FIG. 20.3 Charting in the home setting can be challenging.

BOX 20.4 DOCUMENTATION GUIDELINES

- All entries should be timely, accurate, factual, and grammatically correct (objective).
- Documentation should be legible, including your name and your credentials.
- Make late entries and corrections appropriately and according to agency or hospital policies. Do not ever obliterate or destroy any information that is or has been in the chart.
- All assessments, monitoring data, medications administered, plans of care, and provider orders, whether verbal or written, must be noted in the medical record.
- Document all patient refusals of care and your communication with the patient's provider regarding the patient's refusal.
- Any communication with the patient's provider must be documented in the medical record including the time and date of the communication. Particularly note when the physician or health care provider visited the patient or if you contacted the provider for a problem. Record the information you communicated to the patient's provider and their response, your nursing actions, and the patient's response.

---

some electronic. Both records will have to be accessed, coordinated, and made complete to manage and safeguard the patient. It is believed that the EHR will promote more accurate and safe record keeping (Whitehurst, 2017).

RELATED LEGAL CONCEPTS

Informed Consent

Consent is usually a defense to all the intentional torts. You cannot have a claim for assault and battery if the patient has given consent for the procedure. Likewise, there can be no invasion of privacy if the patient has given consent to share confidential information with someone else, such as his or her lawyer.

There is much confusion about informed consent in that many people believe that it must be a piece of paper with "Informed Consent" written on it. This is not always true.

> Informed consent in the health care setting is a process whereby a patient is informed of:
> 1. The nature of the proposed care, treatment, services, medications, interventions, or procedures.
> 2. The potential benefits, risks, or side effects, including potential problems including death, related to recuperation.
> 3. The likelihood of achieving care, treatment, and service goals.
> 4. Reasonable alternatives and their respective risks and benefits including the alternative of refusing all interventions (AHRQ-PSNet, 2018).

The nurse's role in the consent process is often confusing. It is the responsibility of the provider performing the procedure to provide the patient with information regarding risks, benefits, and alternatives. The nurse's signature attests that the patient appears capable of making decisions and that the nurse is witnessing the patient's voluntary signature signifying informed consent before the procedure is performed. The form must be signed before the administration of preprocedural medications, which may alter the patient's judgment. Additionally, never witness a patient's consent to a procedure that has not been fully explained to the patient by the provider.

> As advanced practice nurses perform more invasive procedures, the process of informing the patient of what is to occur is the advanced practice nurse's responsibility.

Consent forms must be signed when a patient is considered capable to make informed decisions and before the procedure is performed. The patient is the only person who may give consent if he or she is capable of making decisions. Capacity is defined differently from state to state, and the nurse should be aware of how it is defined in his or her state of practice. Capacity is presumed, and therefore any claim of incapacity must be proved in court. When a motion has been entered into court indicating that a patient is no longer capable of making decisions on their own behalf, the court must consider the evidence. If the court agrees, the person is then declared incompetent and a guardian is appointed who then makes all decisions on behalf of the patient (Furrow et al., 2018; Pozgar, 2016).

Some situations may require special consideration. An example would be a patient suffering from "sundowning" syndrome, who shows no signs of cognitive impairment during the day but is quite confused and/or agitated throughout the night. Although the patient may verbalize understanding of an upcoming procedure, and you believe that he is currently capable of signing a consent form, his capacity could possibly be brought into question in a malpractice case if the record reflects periods of confusion.

Patients may always decline to give informed consent for a procedure, even if doing so may have serious consequences for their health status. This legal standard respects the fundamental liberty interest in personal autonomy protected by American jurisprudence (Furrow et al., 2018; Pozgar, 2016). Consent may be withdrawn at any time before the procedure.

> Informed consent is not required if the procedure is necessary to save a life and is done during an emergency.

Advance Directives

All states have laws guiding the execution and enforcement of health care directives including living wills and medical powers of attorney. It is important to allow patients to direct the course of their care and treatment whenever possible; however, they must be protected from making harmful decisions when their cognitive status is impaired or fluctuates. States differ about how consent can be given if the patient is incompetent or lacks capacity to make medical decisions. Advance directives such as a medical power of attorney or a living will may provide information about the patient's wishes. These documents allow individuals to prepare in advance for possible incapacity by formalizing their wishes in writing about their further health care decisions. The living will allows an adult to direct what he or she wishes regarding health care upon becoming incapacitated.

Often used in conjunction with the living will is the durable power of attorney for health care. This document allows the adult to appoint a specific person to authorize care if he or she becomes incapacitated. The durable power of attorney for health care does not usually become effective until a person is incapacitated. This document may be used in conjunction with or without a living will (see Chapter 19 for more information on advance directives). Congress passed the Patient Self-Determination Act of 1990 requiring hospitals to inform their patients of the availability of advance directives. State law defines the required wording for these documents and any other formalities necessary in their preparation. Because patients must be educated on these laws and documents, so should nurses. If not, you could be caught in a violation of the law at a crucial moment of life and death.

If a family challenges a living will or a medical power of attorney, a nurse will need to go through the administrative chain of command. A general rule is for nurses to follow the advance directives unless or until there is a court order to do otherwise. This means that families need to obtain legal services and go to court to overturn or challenge these documents. All persons, no matter what their ages, should complete advance directives. The Terri Schiavo case is a sad demonstration of the difficulties faced by families when there are no documented advance directives and family members differ in beliefs about what should or should not be done. Questions then arise as to whether acts or omissions of health care providers prolong life or prolong the dying process. Judges are certainly not the preferred ultimate decision makers.

When a patient does not have an advance directive and is incapacitated, there are state laws that give guidance regarding who can act as a *surrogate decision maker*. Parents must usually sign for minor children. Spouses or immediate family members may sign for unconscious adults. In other instances, if no one is available or designated, a court can appoint in a very short time someone to make health care decisions. A special consent under stricter standards applies to research studies, and often surrogates may not be able to make such decisions (Pozgar, 2016).

Documentation of informed refusal should be accurate, complete, and in accordance with the policies and procedures for your facility. It should include the results of a mental status assessment to show that the patient was neurologically and psychologically capable of refusing treatment. Clearly document the information that was provided to the patient, quoting the patient's reason(s) for refusing treatment, any questions he or she may have had, and your responses (Furrow et al., 2018; Pozgar, 2016).

CRIMINAL ACTIONS

Nurses who violate specific criminal statutes (such as those having to do with illegal drug use, negligent homicide, and assault and battery) risk criminal prosecution. Conviction of certain types of crimes must be reported to the state board of nursing and will usually result in a review of licensure status. You must be aware of the rules in the state in which you practice.

What Criminal Acts Pose a Risk to the Nurse?
Theft and Misappropriation of Property
- Protect the patient's property by thoroughly documenting and locking up all valuables when the patient is admitted to the facility.

■ Keep all items and property owned by the facility at the facility. This includes tape, bandages, and pens, to name a few.

Sometimes, nurses fail to protect a patient's property adequately and thus open themselves up to claims of theft. Many patients bring valuables to health care facilities or think that they do. It is helpful to give clear notice to the patients before admittance to leave valuables at home. A thorough and documented list of property on admission is imperative to prevent such claims, as is the locking up of valuables. When dentures and other property have not been adequately stored or monitored, the nurse may be held responsible.

Another aspect of this problem is stealing from the employer. Because of the extensive and costly nature of this problem, many employers have developed elaborate systems to discourage theft. With an ever-increasing focus on lowering health care costs, those costs related to employee theft will not be tolerated. Occasionally, nurses accidentally leave the job with tape, bandages, or other supplies in their pockets. These should be returned. Better yet, establishing a routine of checking your pockets before leaving for home will help reduce this risk. A nurse should never intentionally take property belonging to an employer.

Nursing Practice Violations

Scope-of-practice violations that result in the death of a patient may be the result of nurses performing tasks or procedures that the state board of nursing has not accepted as being within the appropriate scope for nurses, or these violations could be a result of doing actions that have been approved for advanced practice nurses only. In some states these violations and other possible violations of the Nurse Practice Act are misdemeanors, but in other states they may be felonies.

In rare cases, charges of murder or negligent homicide may be filed against the nurse (Furrow et al., 2018). In November 2000, the State of Hawaii convicted an individual of manslaughter in the death of a nursing home patient for permitting the progression of pressure ulcers without seeking appropriate medical help (Di Maio & Di Maio, 2002). In November 2006, the Wisconsin State Attorney General's Office charged a nurse with "neglect of a patient causing great bodily harm" when she accidentally connected an epidural infusion bag instead of an antibiotic to an IV, resulting in the death of the teenage mother during childbirth. The felony charge was later reduced to two misdemeanors through a plea bargain (ASQ, 2007).

This should be of concern to all nurses, because mistakes will always occur in health care. To err is human. Kohn and colleagues (2000) stated, "It may be part of human nature to err, but it is also part of human nature to create solutions, find better alternatives, and meet the challenges ahead" (p. 15). If fear of criminal prosecution and prison is added to these personal responses, how can we believe thoughtful, caring people will continue in the profession? As Curtin (1997) asks, "What conceivable social good will be achieved by putting these nurses in jail?" (Kowalski & Horner, 1998, p. 127).

Violations of the Food and Drugs Act

Participating in any activity with illegal drugs or the misappropriation or improper use of legal drugs may result in criminal action against the nurse. Conviction for a crime in this area will almost always result in action against a nurse's license. As described earlier, there is a high incidence of substance abuse in health care professions, so nurses need to be aware of the risks and avoid them. Writing prescriptions for drugs without the authority to do so is a criminal activity. Obtaining drugs illegally for friends and/or family needs, even if they seem legitimate, will still have criminal consequences.

RISK MANAGEMENT AND QUALITY IMPROVEMENT

How Do I Protect Myself and My Patient From Risks?

The safety of patients often involves many different formalized processes in institutions. One involves quality and goes by many names, such as "quality assurance" (QA), "continuous quality management" (CQM), or "continuous quality improvement" (CQI). In relationship to nursing practices, *peer review* is the process of using nurses to evaluate the quality of nursing care. This means that you, as a professional nurse, will be continuously involved in evaluating the care that you and other nurses provide. In the past, this was only done through retroactive review of care using techniques such as nursing audits to evaluate care already given. The current focus is on looking for ways to do better all the time. Examples of activities that may be involved in this process include the following:

- Evaluation of what nurses are doing for patients
- Policy and procedure development
- Staff preparation, competency, and skill documentation
- Continuing education and certification
- Employee evaluations
- Ongoing monitoring, such as infection control and risk management systems

TJC requires quality measures that meet four criteria identified to produce the greatest positive impact on patient outcomes when hospital agencies demonstrate improvement: (1) research—evidence-based care process improves outcomes; (2) proximity—performing the care process is closely connected to patient outcomes; (3) accuracy—measure assesses whether or not the care process has actually been provided; and (4) adverse effects—implementing the measure has little or no chance of causing unintended adverse effects (TJC, 2018a).

Risk management is a formal process to investigate incidents or untoward events that may pose a financial risk or risk of lawsuit to the institution. A designated department, through a risk manager, will often take the first step, which is to gather evidence surrounding the event in anticipation of litigation. Such evidence will include interviews with those involved and physical evidence, including relevant documents. If you are being interviewed, understand that a truthful accounting is the most important aspect of this process and will best serve the institution and you.

Risk managers, many of whom are registered nurses, will often then evaluate how to prevent a recurrence by changing systems to prevent reoccurrence. This might mean setting a new standard that can then be evaluated and vetted through a quality assurance process (Whitehurst, 2017).

One tool used by a risk management team is the *incident or occurrence report*. Incident reports generate many legal concerns, because in most states they must be produced in a lawsuit and can be used as evidence against individuals and the institution (Furrow et al., 2018). Caution should be used when completing an incident report, and only the person directly involved should objectively document the facts. Conclusions, opinions, defensiveness, and judgment or blame of others have absolutely no place in this document or process. In addition, the form should never be used for punitive reasons, because this will almost certainly increase the possibility that the report will not be completed honestly if at all (Furrow et al., 2018; Pozgar, 2016).

Although you would not mention in the medical record that you filled out an incident report, the person involved in the incident should make the same objective, factual documentation of an incident in the medical record. Information entered in the record should mirror information written on an incident report. Lack of documentation in the face of a known occurrence will always be considered a cover-up and will thus be extremely detrimental to any subsequent legal action. Never speculate about who or what caused an incident, because this may inadvertently give the plaintiff "causation" proof, which may not be true.

Cloud computing has also impacted nursing and should be considered when entering data electronically. Medical records can be obtained from data entered on any designated day and time. When making corrections to the record, it is especially important to follow the facility's procedure regarding late entries. When compared from day to day without explanation, it may appear that a record has been purposefully altered. Never delete and then reenter different language representative of the same date and time as had been previously erased. Regardless of intent, the record subsequently may be considered altered to protect the agency and hide information from the court regarding care received or not received by the patient.

Risk managers manage risk; quality assurance managers mitigate (lessen) the possibility of risk. Many times, they are the same registered nurse. An example of risk management and quality assurance working together would be the following:

A fire breaks out in the operating room, and a patient is burned. Immediately after this event, a risk manager might be notified through a telephone call and then later in an incident report. The risk manager would come immediately to the scene and collect all items and/or equipment involved in the fire (evidence) to determine the cause of the fire. He or she would also interview those who saw the fire (witnesses) to determine and record relevant facts. The risk manager may take specific actions to assist the patient and/or family, and to advise others working in the surgical area.

Sometimes financial settlements are made very early to avoid the costly process of a lawsuit. Risk management might identify ways to prevent another occurrence, such as removal of all alcohol-based skin preparations from the operating room. The quality-assurance department may then periodically evaluate this standard to ensure the continued safety of patients.

Risk managers usually work very closely with insurance companies that cover institutions and their employees for all types of financial risk, including malpractice and general liability. The defense and prevention of many claims start with good risk management. Yet every individual on the health care team who identifies a risk to patient safety and does something constructive to correct it must also make such efforts. Several simple risk management actions by nurses can often prevent a lawsuit. These include the following:

- Approaching angry patients with an apology and an offer to help (Gutheil et al., 1984). Moving toward the patient who has experienced an unexpected outcome rather than away is always the best policy. Isolation and a feeling of abandonment in the face of an untoward event can only augment the feeling that a wrong was done.
- Sharing uncertainties and bringing patients' expectations to a realistic level during the informed consent process can also prevent claims based on disappointment that an outcome is not perfect (Gutheil et al., 1984).
- Refusing to participate in hospital gossip, to document disparaging comments about a health care provider in the medical record, or to judge others on the health care team will contribute to an atmosphere of teamwork and compassion rather than competition, blame, and retaliation. The latter can ultimately contribute to unsafe patient care. An inadvertent negative remark documented in the medical record or verbalized to patients and families about a physician, the pharmacy, the laboratory, or other nurses is very frequently the genesis of a lawsuit. Such remarks are often based on limited knowledge and personal bias. Making such remarks could cause you to be a witness in a malpractice claim against your peers and/or other medical team members. This is seldom a desirable position for anyone.

Malpractice Insurance

One of the more controversial topics for nurses involves the question whether to purchase individual malpractice insurance policies. There is often misinformation about what these individual policies will do or cover, and there is little substantiation for what most authors say. In addition, insurance companies sometimes use scare tactics to induce nurses to purchase their products.

As the nurse's role continues to expand, so does the amount of liability exposure in a malpractice claim. Careful consideration should be given to a decision about whether to carry an individual malpractice insurance policy. An informed nurse should at least know what questions to ask.

What About Individual Malpractice Insurance?

Some individual nurse policies claim that you can prevent settlement of a claim if you wish to do so (have a consent clause). However, a close reading of the policy might demonstrate that if the case is then lost at trial or settled for more than the insurance company wished to offer, the company has the right to collect that difference and the cost of defense from you. Therefore, the consent you have a right to withhold may have very little meaning.

The cost for a nurse to purchase an individual malpractice policy is based on the area of nursing and the state of practice. Check your professional journals and your professional associations for insurance companies that offer malpractice insurance for nurses.

What Is Institutional Coverage?

Almost all health care corporations or institutions carry insurance policies that specifically cover acts or omissions of their employed nurses. This includes cases in which only the institution is named under the previously described *respondeat superior* doctrine or when an individual nurse employee is named. Most individual personal nursing malpractice policies are secondary to this policy. This means that they cannot be used in any manner if the institutional policy is used to cover the claim. It is not correct to assume that you can have your personal attorney present to represent your personal interests in addition to the institutional attorney. Even if you could, having two attorneys will often divide the defense.

The attorney selected by the health care institution to represent the institution is ethically required to represent both your interests and those of the institution. In addition, the institution's interests are rarely, if ever, adverse to yours.

The claim that an institution will insure you but then turn around and sue you is belied by the fact that one cannot find statistics to verify this common assumption. Institutions spend millions of dollars on insurance specifically to cover the acts of nurses. In addition, if institutions sued the nurses working for them, they would not retain many nurses.

It is true that if an employee commits a criminal act that by its nature is outside the scope of the employment, such as forced sexual intimacies with a patient, an institution may not defend the employee or cover costs. In this regard, however, criminal acts are not insurable under laws in most states and therefore are not covered by any policy (Simpson, 1998).

What Should I Ask About Institutional Coverage?

There are certain things that a prudent nurse concerned about coverage should do. All nurses should request and have a right to receive a document that provides the following information regarding their employer's insurance coverage for them:

- The name of the institution's insurance carrier, the limits of the policy, and the rating of the insurance company (Best Rating A+++ is the highest)
- Whether they are covered for all acts occurring within the scope of their employment and during the time they are employed
- The acts for which they do not have coverage
- Whether the hospital will cover them if they need to appear before the state board of nursing in relation to a malpractice claim. If not, an individual insurance policy that clearly does cover them may be valuable.

- How the nurse is covered by the institutional employer. This is particularly important if the nurse is an independent practitioner and/or in an extended practice role.

What Is Professional Licensure Defense Insurance?

Professional licensure defense insurance is a policy intended to reimburse costs incurred by you should a complaint be entered against you with the state board of nursing. Malpractice insurance is different and does not cover these expenses (Brous, 2012a, 2012b; Dowie, 2017). When it is alleged that you have harmed a patient, even though it is not yet established, a mandatory reporter is required to notify your licensing agency. Remember, the reporting standard is if that person has a reasonable suspicion that you may or may not have done something that resulted in possible harm to a patient. This is a very low burden placed on the reporter. Under this standard, almost all allegations must be reported. Professional licensure defense attorneys are required to help you retain your license when an investigation is triggered by a complaint. Your licensure is your livelihood; be confident that you will have the financial assistance necessary to keep it.

What Happens When I Go to Court?

Sometimes, despite all your efforts, you find yourself in litigation as a defendant. Know that very few claims go to trial. You do not need to picture yourself in a setting from *Law and Order* with a prosecutor tearing you apart. Most personal injury lawsuits are either dismissed or settled out of court, usually after an investigatory process called discovery (Furrow et al., 2018). This involves exchanging information about the case in the form of written questions called *interrogatories,* as well as a recorded oral questioning process called a *deposition.*

Depositions are oral statements given under oath and are extremely important in any negligence claim (Furrow et al., 2018; Miller, 2018). Depositions are used to evaluate the merits of the case, the credibility of the witnesses, and the strength of the defendants. Cases are sometimes won or lost in this process; thus, with the help of your attorney, you must be prepared. If you have not been offered the chance to meet with your attorney before your deposition, request the time to do so. Being prepared ahead of time can have a significant effect on your performance under stress.

Depositions occur in a less formal setting than the courtroom. Attorneys for both sides will be present. The attorney questioning you will be the attorney for either the plaintiff or for the other defendants, or both, and their interests may be adversarial to yours. Your attorney can object to certain questions, but generally speaking you will be expected to answer the questions to the best of your recollection because in the deposition there is no judge to rule on the objections.

> Remember, in a deposition you are there to answer questions in a truthful manner to the best of your recollection.

A lawsuit can be a very disconcerting and disheartening process. Your ability to realize this and not to feel alone in the process is extremely important. Often institutions mandate that persons involved in litigation receive counseling to help them resolve the anger and depression that almost inevitably occurs. Be sure to use the resources available to you, including your lawyer. Your risk management team is often a good resource as well and can usually answer questions or help resolve problems you might have in relation to the case. Remember the truth of the old adage that "this too will pass."

LEGAL ISSUES AFFECTING NURSING

Because developments and advances in medical and nursing care occur constantly, many areas of practice do not have firm rules to follow when making decisions. Changes in health care delivery and society's values have sparked controversy about a variety of issues.

Health Care Costs and Payment Issues

One example of a controversial issue is third-party reimbursement, or the right of an individual nurse, usually a nurse practitioner, to be paid directly by insurance companies for care given. Medicare has passed rules that allow nurse practitioners to bill independently under their own provider number. This is a very important step in the field of independent practice for nurses, because many health care insurers follow the lead of Medicare as related to billing issues.

In relation to the right to bill, all nurses need to understand billing and reimbursement rules so that they cannot be accused of participating in fraudulent billing schemes. For instance, although a bill can be generated for certain follow-up care performed by nurses in the outpatient clinic, as services rendered "incident to" what the physician does, there are strict requirements of physician involvement that nurses must understand. Nurse practitioners need to be careful that physicians with whom they collaborate are not also illegally billing for the nurse's services.

The most frequent areas where nurses can inadvertently become involved in fraud and abuse claims are the following:
1. Questionable accuracy and monitoring of provider visit coding
2. Improper use of diagnosis codes
3. Failure to provide patient care or providing poor patient care
4. Anesthesia services
5. Unneeded critical or acute-care services
6. Billing for physician assistant services
7. Improper billing of nursing or provider services

To avoid these areas, it is important to know about and understand your institution's compliance plan and to report suspected abuses through the required hotline or directly to nursing administration (Furrow et al., 2018).

From another perspective, the high cost of health care is also resulting in the proliferation of health care workers with less training and education than nurses, who can be hired for less money. Often these unlicensed workers have no laws circumscribing their practice and are doing tasks that have traditionally been done by RNs or LPN/LVNs, such as administering medications and giving injections. This is an important issue for nurses, especially when asked to supervise such workers and/or compete for positions in the health care market.

Controversial legislative changes have been made to address some of these problems. In response to concerns about whether increased acuity of patients, increased caregiver workload, and declining levels of training among patient-care personnel have threatened the quality of patient care, California passed Assembly Bill 394. This bill set a minimum nurse–patient ratio in acute-care general, special, and psychiatric hospitals (Lang et al., 2004). A year after it went into effect, nurses were battling Governor Arnold Schwarzenegger to keep what they fought so hard to obtain—an RN-to-patient ratio of 6 to 1 in 2004 and 5 to 1 in 2005. The controversy seems to stem from the difficulty of maintaining ratios "at all times" and in finding enough nurses to fulfill the ratios.

Related topics involve practice models and case management. Practice models involve attempts by institutions to answer what types and ratios of health care providers should constitute a patient-care team. Case management looks at how patient-care teams can best derive better outcomes and continuity for patients while effectively managing the variable costs of care delivery. Institutional decisions on these matters become policies and thus the "laws" under which you must deliver patient care.

Your knowledge of the issues, participation in the processes, and support for legislation and policies that are favorable for your profession and for patient care will be important when your state and/or institution decides such issues. Professional behavior includes concern with and participation in the direction that health care, and particularly nursing care, will take in the future.

Health Care Delivery Issues

Changes made in the types of systems used to deliver health care and in the techniques used by the systems have created many concerns for nurses. Hospitals and other expensive acute-care settings are giving way to outpatient clinics and same-day surgery centers. This means that people are being sent home while still acutely ill to take care of themselves or to be cared for by relatives without the benefit of hospital nursing services. This makes the nurse's role in discharge planning and patient education extremely important to prevent deterioration of certain health or surgical conditions in the home. In addition, it means that home health care nurses are routinely organizing care that formerly was rendered only in hospitals. For example, respirators in the home are not unusual. With this change, however, come more independent responsibilities for nurses. Responsibility can translate into liability.

Telephone nursing triage and telehealth nursing care present new and unusual legal concerns because of the difficulties of providing accurate long-distance care and the independent nature of these tasks (ASHRM, 2018). Although these nurses bring nursing care to many areas that have not had access to this care in the past, selecting appropriately prepared individuals to provide the care and educating them to function effectively when they cannot see the patient are challenging tasks.

HMOs and other forms of prepaid health care have helped reduce the rapidly growing costs of health care through a process called *utilization review*. Nurses hired to do this review are often asked to make judgments regarding whether a patient should be discharged. Early discharge of patients and limits on insurance reimbursements for certain allowable medications, equipment, and external services have sometimes caused ethical and legal problems for health care professionals.

Past laws protecting the HMOs from malpractice claims when patients were harmed because of flawed utilization review practices are now being challenged. There is a growing public concern that managed care organizations are making large profits while patients covered under their programs are not receiving adequate care.

The many changes occurring in the workplace often create levels of confusion and frustration, which make it more difficult to focus on the quality of the care being given on a day-to-day basis. These issues are examples of how legal issues interweave with all the other events in your professional life. Nurses must remain involved in these matters to stay aware of how their legal responsibilities are influenced by them.

Issues About Life-and-Death Decisions

Controversial ethical issues surrounding life and death also, of course, present controversial legal issues. Scientific research and new technologies can blur the line between life and death. As a nurse, you can often find yourself in the center of such controversies, so you need to be very aware of your state's laws at least on the following subjects.

Termination of Pregnancy

Where can pregnancies be terminated? Who can terminate a pregnancy? When can a pregnancy be terminated? Under what conditions? Under what, if any, conditions can teenagers terminate a pregnancy without parental consent?

Fetal Rights

When does a fetus become a person? If a fetus is born alive, what rights does the infant have? What rights do the parents have? What rights do health care workers have? What are the laws surrounding fetal death and/or the cessation of life-preserving treatments?

Human Experimentation or Research

Who owns tissue or organs removed from a patient's body? What can be done with the products of conception? What types of consent are necessary to enroll a patient in research studies? What types of boards and oversight must be involved to approve and monitor human research studies? What is the role of a nurse who administers research protocols to patients?

Patient Rights

What rights do patients in your state have in relationship to medical records, medical information, giving consent, participating in their care, suing providers, dictating issues surrounding their death, donating organs, being protected from abuse, receiving emergency treatment, being protected from the practice of unlicensed providers, transplantation of organs, accessibility of the disabled to health care, privacy, and confidentiality? What is your role to assure that they can exercise each of these rights?

CONCLUSION

As time goes on, laws will change, and new areas will arise that nursing will have to address. Continuing education, critical thinking, and an open mind will help you to learn about, and deal with, the legal issues that will touch your professional life daily. Get involved whenever possible with patient safety, quality, and risk management processes in your institutions, and become familiar with your state's Nurse Practice Act and advisory opinions. Be someone who has an educated opinion about conflicts inherent in health care and nursing (see the relevant websites and online resources at the end of this chapter). Take the opportunity to visit the hearings conducted by your state's board of nursing and by the state legislature. By becoming involved with the legal and disciplinary process, you will be much more aware of how you can protect yourself and your patients, and influence the direction of health care issues. After concluding this chapter, it is hoped that you also feel more confident when faced with "the law."

🌐 RELEVANT WEBSITE AND ONLINE RESOURCES

American Nurses Association
www.nursingworld.org.

Centers for Disease Control and Prevention
www.cdc.gov.

Centers for Medicare & Medicaid Services
www.cms.gov.

Institute for Healthcare Improvement
www.ihi.org.

National Academies of Sciences, Engineering, and Medicine
https://www.nationalacademies.org/hmd/.

National Center for Biotechnology Information
http://www.ncbi.nlm.nih.gov/.

Continued

🌐 RELEVANT WEBSITE AND ONLINE RESOURCES—CONT'D

National Council of State Boards of Nursing
www.ncsbn.org.

National Network of Libraries of Medicine
Resources for members of the National Network of Libraries of Medicine. www.nnlm.gov.

National Patient Safety Foundation
www.npsf.org.

Nursys Online Verification
www.nursys.com.

The Joint Commission
www.jointcommission.org.

U.S. Department of Health and Human Services
Agency for Healthcare Research and Quality. http://www.ahrq.gov/clinic/epcix.htm.

U.S. Department of Health and Human Services
www.hhs.gov.

U.S. Department of Health and Human Services
The Data Bank: National practitioner healthcare integrity and protection. http://www.npdb-hipdb.hrsa.gov.

U.S. Department of Veterans Affairs
VA National Center for Patient Safety. www.patientsafety.va.gov.

U.S. National Library of Medicine
www.pubmed.gov.

BIBLIOGRAPHY

Agency for Healthcare Research and Quality (AHRQ) and PSNet. (2018). *Glossary: Definition of informed consent.* Retrieved from https://psnet.ahrq.gov/glossary/I.

American Society of Healthcare Risk Management (ASHRM). (2018). *Telemedicine: Risk management considerations.* Retrieved from http://www.ashrm.org/pubs/files/TELEMEDICINE-WHITE-PAPER.pdf?pdf=telemedicine1.

American Society for Quality (ASQ). (2007). *Nurse charged with felony in fatal medical error.* Retrieved from http://asq.org/qualitynews/qnt/execute/displaySetup?newsID=1056.

Azuero, A. (2018). Likelihood of nursing care being missed is influenced by several work-based factors. *Evidence Based Nursing.* https://doi.org/10.1136/eb-2018-102933.

Bragadóttir, H., Kalisch, B. J., & Tryggvadóttir, G. B. (2017). Correlates and predictors of missed nursing care in hospitals. *Journal of Clinical Nursing.* https://doi.org/10.1111/jocn.13449.

Brous, E. (2012a). Professional licensure: Investigation and disciplinary action. *American Journal of Nursing, 112*(11), 53–60. https://doi.org/10.1097/01.NAJ.0000422256.95706.9b.

Brous, E. (2012b). Professional licensure protection strategies. *American Journal of Nursing, 112*(12), 43–47. https://doi.org/10.1097/01.NAJ.0000423512.68887.8d.

Dowie, I. (2017). Legal, ethical and professional aspects of duty of care for nurses. *Nursing Standard, 32*(16-19), 47–52. https://doi.org/10.7748/ns.2017.e10959.

Drach-Zahavy, A., & Srulovici, E. (2018). The personality profile of the accountable nurse and missed nursing care. *Journal of Advance Nursing.* https://doi.org/10.1111/jan.13849.

Duffy, J. R., Culp, S., & Padrutt, T. (2018). Description and factors associated with missed nursing care in an acute care community hospital. *Journal of Nursing Administration.* https://doi.org/10.1097/NNA.0000000000000630.

Edwards, N., & Twomey, M. (2015). Policies and procedures as a basis for liability. In *Carlock Copeland Civil Litigation.* www.CarlockCopeland.com.

Freydel v. New York Hospital, No. 97 Civ. 7926 (SHS), January 4, 2000.

Furrow, B. R., Greaney, T. L., Johnson, S. H., Jost, T. S., Schwartz, R. L., Brown, E. C., et al. (2018). *Health law: Cases, materials and problems* (8th ed.). Academic West Publishing.

Guido, G. (2013). *Legal and ethical issues in nursing* (6th ed.). Upper Saddle River, NJ: Prentice Hall.

Harkanen, M., Tiainen, M., & Haatainen, K. (2017). Wrong-patient incidents during medication administrations. *Journal of Clinical Nursing, 27*(3-4), 715–724. https://doi.org/10.1111/jocn.14021.

Harvey v. Mid-coast Hospital, 36 F.Supp. 2d 32 (D. Maine 1999).

Institute of Medicine. (2006). *Preventing medication errors.* Retrieved from http://www.nationalacademies.org/hmd/Reports/2006/Preventing-Medication-Errors-Quality-Chasm-Series.aspx.

Jacoby, S. R., & Scruth, E. A. (2017). Negligence and the nurse: The value of the Code of Ethics for Nurses. *Clinical Nurse Specialist.* https://doi.org/10.1097/NUR.0000000000000301.

Khalil, H., & Lee, S. (2018). Medication safety challenges in primary care: Nurses' perspective. *Journal of Clinical Nursing.* https://doi.org/10.1111/jocn.14353.

Kohn, L. T., Corrigan, J. M., & Donaldson, M. S. (2000). *To err is human: Building a safer health system.* Washington, DC: National Academies Press.

Lang, T. A., et al. (2004). Nurse–patient ratios: A systematic review on the effects of nurse staffing on patient, nurse, employee and hospital outcomes. *Journal of Nursing Administration, 34,* 326–327.

Malfait, S., Van Hecke, A., Van Biesen, W., & Eeckloo, K. (2018). Is privacy a problem during bedside handovers? A practice-oriented discussion paper. *Nursing Ethics.* https://doi.org/10.1177/09697330/879/348.

Miller, L. A. (2018). Litigation in perinatal care: The deposition process. *Journal of Perinatal Neonatal Nursing.* https://doi.org/10.1097/JPN.0000000000000304.

National Council of State Boards of Nursing. (2018a). *A nurse guide to substance use disorder in nursing.* Retrieved from https://www.ncsbn.org/SUD_Brochure_2014.pdf.

National Council of State Boards of Nursing. (2018b). *A nurse manager's guide to substance use disorder in nursing.* Retrieved from https://www.ncsbn.org/3692.htm.

National Council of State Boards of Nursing. (2018c). *Licensure.* Retrieved from https://www.ncsbn.org/licensure.htm.

National Council of State Boards of Nursing. (2018d). *Nurse Licensure Compact.* Retrieved from https://www.ncsbn.org/nlc.htm.

National Council of State Boards of Nursing. (2018e). *NURSYS.com—e-verify.* Retrieved from https://www.nursys.com/.

National Practitioner Data Bank. (NPDB). (2018). *Public use data file.* Retrieved from https://www.npdb.hrsa.gov/resources/publicData.jsp.

Nurses Service Organization (NSO). (2015). *Nurse professional liability exposures: 2015 claim report update.* Retrieved from https://www.nso.com/Learning/Artifacts/Claim-Reports/Nurse-Professional-Liability-Exposures-2015-Claim.

Park, S. H., Hanchett, M., & Ma, C. (2018). Practice environment characteristics associated with missed nursing care. *Journal of Nursing Scholarship.* https://doi.org/10.1111/jnu.12434.

Pozgar, G. D. (2016). *Legal aspects of health care administration* (12th ed.). Sudbury, MA: Jones and Bartlett.

Ramanathan, T. (2014). Law as a tool to promote healthcare safety. *Clinical Governance, 19*(2), 172–180. Retrieved from https://www.cdc.gov/phlp/docs/article-healthcaresafety.pdf.

Russell, D. (2018). Disclosure and apology: Nursing and risk management working together. *Nursing Management.* https://doi.org/10.1097/01.NUMA.0000533773.14544.e2.

Rutledge, D. N., Retrosi, T., & Ostrowski, G. (2018). Barriers to medication error reporting among hospital nurses. *Journal of Clinical Nursing, 7*(9-10), 1941–1949. https://doi.org/10.1111/jocn.14335.

Robertson v. Provident House, 576 So. 2d 992 (La. 1991).

Shaw v. Plantation Management, 2009 WL 838680 (La. App., March 27, 2009), cited in Patient's Fall: Solid Nursing Documentation Afterward, Negligence Lawsuit Dismissed. *Legal State v. Brown,* 140 S.W.3d 51 (Mo. 2004) No. SC85582. Retrieved from http://law.justia.com/cases/missouri/supreme-court/2004/sc-85582-1.html.

Smith, J. G., Morin, K. H., Wallace, L. E., & Lake, E. T. (2017). Association of the nurse work environment, collective efficacy, and missed care. *Western Journal of Nursing Research, 40*(6), 779–798. https://doi.org/10.1177/0193945917734159.

Texas Board of Nursing (Texas BON). (2013). *Examination information.* Retrieved from www.bon.state.tx.us/olv/examination.html.

The Joint Commission. (2019). *2019 National Patient Safety Goals.* Retrieved from http://www.jointcommission.org/standards_information/npsgs.aspx.

The Joint Commission. (2015). *Sentinel event alert.* Retrieved from http://www.jointcommission.org/assets/1/18/SEA_55.pdf.

The Joint Commission. (2018a). *Facts about accountability measures.* Retrieved from http://www.jointcommission.org/facts_about_accountability_measures/.

The Joint Commission. (2018b). *Targeted solutions tool for preventing falls.* Retrieved from http://www.centerfortransforminghealthcare.org/tst_pfi.aspx.

Whitehurst, K. (2017). Minimizing litigation risks in skilled nursing care. Accountable clinical processes aligned with EHR workflow can boost risk management efforts. *Provider: Long Term & Post-Acute Care.* Retrieved from http://www.providermagazine.com/archives/2017_Archives/Pages/0517/Minimizing-Litigation-Risks-In-Skilled-Nursing-Care.aspx.

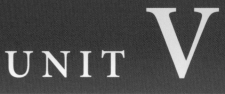

UNIT V

Contemporary Nursing Practice

21

Cultural and Spiritual Awareness

*Ashley Zerwekh Garneau, PhD, RN**

ⓔ http://evolve.elsevier.com/Zerwekh/nsgtoday/.

A nation's culture resides in the hearts and in the soul of its people.
Mahatma Gandhi

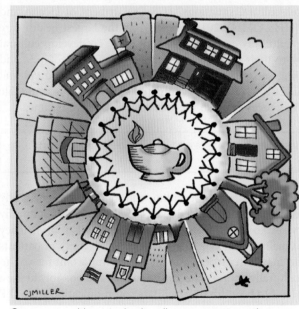

Our communities need culturally competent nursing care.

After completing this chapter, you should be able to:
- Define cultural and linguistic competence.
- List practice issues related to cultural and linguistic competence.
- List nursing measures for providing culturally and linguistically competent care.
- Identify challenges in defining spirituality.
- Determine the cultural and spiritual beliefs of patients in the health care setting.
- Assess the spiritual needs of patients in the health care setting.

*We would like to thank Peter Melenovich, PhD, RN, CNE, for his previous contributions of this chapter.

CULTURE AND SPIRITUALITY

What Is Meant by Cultural and Linguistic Competence?

In today's global society, cultural competence is a necessary component of excellence in nursing care. People can travel as never before. Nurses are connecting to patients remotely through the internet and other virtual modalities. Medical "tourism" is now a reality. Individualizing the care nurses provide to patients is dependent on a thorough understanding of each patient's cultural identification. These factors demonstrate the need for nurses to understand cultural and spiritual differences between themselves and others.

The American Nurses Association (ANA) affirms in its *Code of Ethics* the need for the nurse to be sensitive to individuals' needs: "The need for and right to health care is universal, transcending all individual differences. Nurses consider the needs and respect the values of each person in every professional relationships and setting" (ANA, 2015).

Leininger, considered a top authority on culture care and diversity, proposed that cultural understanding would allow for peaceful relations among groups of people (Leininger, 2007). Some considered this philosophy so important that Leininger was nominated for the Nobel Peace Prize. Cultural competence is essential for nurses.

But what exactly is cultural competence? The Office of Minority Health (OMH) defines it as "a set of congruent behaviors, attitudes, and policies that come together in a system, agency or among professionals that enables effective work in cross-cultural situations" (US Department of Health and Human Services Office of Minority Health [HHS OMH], 2016, para. 1). As the largest health care group, nurses are at the center of providing culturally competent patient care. To develop cultural competence, it is essential for nurses to explore their own personal views, beliefs, stereotypes, and assumptions about different cultures. By doing so, nurses acquire cultural sensitivity and cultural knowledge of different cultural groups (Cai, 2016). Culturally competent nurses are accountable for assessing and recognizing not only the differences but also the variation of being the same.

> The culturally competent nurse has an enhanced ability to provide high-quality care, which fosters better patient understanding and involvement in the plan of care.

Additionally, communicating with patients is essential for providing culturally and linguistically competent nursing care. Linguistic competence can further be defined as the inclusion of culturally appropriate oral and written language services to individuals with limited English proficiency (LEP) (Agency for Healthcare Research and Quality [AHRQ], 2013). Given the diversity of patients you will encounter whose cultural background may differ from yours, it will be important for you to ensure that written and printed materials are culturally appropriate for the patient and possibly to use a trained medical interpreter or translator may have to be utilized to facilitate communication with LEP patients.

The mnemonic CULTURE, developed by Zerwekh (2016), can help nurses to assess and improve their level of cultural competence (Box 21.1). In addition, nurses must use effective cultural interviewing questions, which are best if left semistructured and open-ended. Salvin and colleagues (2016) have developed a mnemonic for enhancing communication when gathering cultural assessment data by asking the patient the right questions (Box 21.2).

BOX 21.1   CULTURE—A NURSING APPROACH

Consider your own cultural biases and how these affect your nursing care.
Understand the need to recognize cultural implications in planning and implementing nursing care.
Learn how to use cultural assessment tools.
Treat patients with dignity and respect.
Use sensitivity in providing culturally competent care.
Recognize opportunities to provide specific culturally based nursing care.
Evaluate your own previous encounters with patients from other cultures and backgrounds.

From Zerwekh, J. (2016). *CULTURE: A mnemonic for assessing and improving cultural competence.* Chandler, AZ: Nursing Education Consultants, Inc.

BOX 21.2   THE 4C'S OF CULTURALLY SENSITIVE CARE: A MNEMONIC FOR HEALTH CARE PROFESSIONALS

1. What do you *call* your problem. (Remember to ask, "What do you think is wrong?" as a way of getting at the patient's perception of the problem. Don't ask, "What do you call your problem?"
2. What do you think *caused* your problem? (This gets at the patient's beliefs regarding the source of the problem.)
3. How do you *cope* with your condition? (This reminds the practitioner to ask, "What have you done to try to make it better? Who else have you seen for treatment?" Also, "How have you been coping with your illness?" "What effect has it had on your life/daily routine?"
4. What *concerns* do you have regarding your condition? (This should address questions such as "How serious do you think this is?" "What potential complications do you fear?" "How does it interfere with your life, or your ability to function?" It is important to understand the patient's perception of the course of the illness and the fears that he or she may have regarding it so that you can address his or her concerns and correct any misconceptions.)

Courtesy of Geri-Ann Galanti, PhD, Stuart Slavin, MD, and Alice Kuo, MD. Retrieved from www.ggalanti.org.

What Practice Issues Are Related to Cultural and Linguistic Competence?
Barriers to Cultural and Linguistic Competence

There are two categories of barriers to cultural competence: provider barriers and system barriers (Mazanec & Tyler, 2003). Provider barriers are those that a nurse may have, including lack of information about a culture's customs regarding health care. System barriers are those that exist in an agency because the agency's structure and policies are not designed to support cultural diversity (McGibbon et al., 2008).

Scenario: An American Indian family may wish to spend the night in the intensive care unit room with a critically ill family member. However, the room does not have cots on which they could sleep, and the waiting room is not large enough to accommodate all the family and extended family members who have come to support the patient. The community in which the hospital is located has a large American Indian population.

The nurse, as an advocate for patients and their families, can intervene through activities such as joining a hospital committee focused on hospital redesign. The nurse can point out the need for space for family members to stay overnight near their loved ones. In this way the nurse supports the needs of the culturally diverse community.

Lack of awareness of the National Standards for Culturally and Linguistically Appropriate Service (CLAS), cultural competency training, and limited resources regarding cultural competency are additional barriers to implementing culturally and linguistically competent nursing care (Ogbolu, Scrandis, & Fitzpatrick, 2018). Another example of a system barrier would be nurses' limited access to language services when they are communicating with LEP patients. Look at the following case:

You are attempting to teach your patient, who has a surgical incision, how to perform daily wound care and dressing changes. Your patient speaks only German. The only medical interpreter at your hospital who is trained in German is sick today. As a last resort, you ask the patient's spouse to help in communicating the needed instructions to the patient. The family member agrees, but during the interview, the spouse becomes confused about the frequency of dressing changes and misinterprets your instructions as saying to change the surgical dressing once a week, not once daily.

Considering this, what additional services could be used in this scenario? Review Box 21.3 for additional language assistance services that may be of use in communicating with LEP patients. Another barrier to cultural competence in the nursing profession is the need for a more diverse nursing workforce. It makes sense that the more diverse the nursing profession, the more diverse the delivery of care, resulting in improved patient outcomes.

Health and Health Care Disparities

One of the goals of *Healthy People 2020* is to achieve health equity, eliminate health disparities, and improve health in all groups (*Healthy People 2020,* 2018a). Health disparities are inequalities in disease morbidity and mortality in segments of the population. These disparities may be a result of differences in socioeconomic status, race, or ethnicity. They are believed to be the result of the interaction among genetic variations, environmental factors, and health behaviors. Limited access to health care and health-related services is a social determinant of health that contributes to health disparities. Findings from the *2017 National Healthcare Quality and Disparities Report* showed that individuals at or below 100% of the federal poverty level experienced the worse access to care compared with high-income groups (AHRQ, 2018).

Inequalities in income and education are at the root of many health disparities. In general, those populations that have the worst health status are those that have the highest poverty rates and the least education. Low income and low education levels are associated with differences in rates of illness and death, including heart disease, diabetes, and obesity. Higher incomes may allow better access to

---

BOX 21.3   TYPES OF LANGUAGE ASSISTANCE SERVICES

- Full-time trained and certified medical interpreters
- Part-time or contracted certified medical interpreters
- Dual-role interpreters (i.e., a staff nurse who is bilingual and has received training as a medical interpreter; serves as a medical interpreter on a limited basis)
- Ad hoc interpreters (i.e., any person who does not have formal training as a certified medical interpreter. The use of ad hoc interpreters is discouraged and may be illegal in some situations.)
- Telephonic and video interpretation (i.e., remote interpretation services where interpreter, patient, and staff, communicate via telephone or video camera and TV monitor; communication is sent and received through a speakerphone or headset device)
- Written materials available in the patient's preferred language

Adopted from Center for Medicare and Medicaid Services. (n.d.). Providing language services to diverse populations: Lessons from the field. Retrieved from https://www.cms.gov/About-CMS/Agency-Information/OMH/Downloads/Lessons-from-the-Field-508.pdf.

medical care, enable people to afford better housing and live in safer neighborhoods, and increase the opportunity to engage in health-promoting behaviors. Ongoing initiatives focus on adolescent health, genomics, global health, national security preparedness, sleep, social and environmental factors that promote optimal health; they also address the health needs of the lesbian, gay, bisexual, and transgender (LGBT) community (Healthy People, 2020, 2018b).

According to the Institute of Medicine (IOM) report *Unequal Treatment*, conscious (explicit) bias and unconscious (implicit) bias from health care professionals affect the quality of care and hence lead to health disparities. Explicit bias is an individual's preconceived judgment or belief for or against something or someone. Implicit bias is an unintentional judgment or belief for or against something or someone; a person may not even be aware of such an attitude or have control over it (Dovidio & Fiske, 2012; Project Implicit, 2018). Some of the causes of health care disparities include provider variables and patient variables.

Provider variables are provider–patient relationships, lack of minority providers, as well as health care provider bias and discrimination. Studies have clearly demonstrated that providers will often suggest different treatment options for different patients when the only difference is cultural background or skin tone (van Ryn, Burgess, Malat, & Griffin, 2006; White-Means et al., 2009). In an effort to eliminate health care disparities, the Institute for Healthcare Improvement (2018) recommends assessing and evaluating your own implicit biases so that you can implement measures for removing this type of bias when you interact with others. Project Implicit (2018) offers a test that assesses and determines your implicit biases. If you're interested in learning about your own implicit biases, you can take a virtual test via Project Implicit at https://implicit.harvard.edu/implicit/takeatest.html/.

Patient variables are mistrust of the health care system and refusal of treatment (Greer, Brondolo, & Brown, 2014). Often this mistrust comes from barriers in communication. For example, what types of interviewing questions would you include during an initial nursing history of a transgender patient? When you are obtaining a patient's sexual history, how would you address these questions to the lesbian, gay, bisexual, transgender, and queer and/or questioning (LGBTQ) community? Ignatavicius and Workman (2018) offer several interviewing questions about gender identity and sexual activity that nurses can use in their practice (Box 21.4).

Strategies for Providing Culturally Competent Care

The solutions to the challenges posed by health care disparities are complex and are still being discovered (Critical Thinking Box 21.1). Some solutions involve increasing the diversity of health care providers; ensuring that all people have access to affordable, high-quality health care; promoting wellness

---

BOX 21.4 RECOMMENDED PATIENT INTERVIEW QUESTIONS ABOUT SEXUAL ORIENTATION, GENDER IDENTITY, AND HEALTH CARE

- Do you have sex with men, women, both, or neither?
- Does anyone live with you in your household?
- Are you in a relationship with someone who does not live with you?
- If you have a sexual partner, have you or your partner been evaluated regarding the possibility of acquiring sexually transmitted infections?
- If you have more than one sexual partner, how are you protecting both of you from infections, such as hepatitis B, hepatitis C, or HIV?
- Have you disclosed your gender identity and sexual orientation to your health care provider?
- If you have not, may I have your permission to provide that information to members of the health care team who are involved in your care?
- Who are your closest family members?

From Ignatavicius, D. D. (2018). Introduction to medical-surgical nursing practice. In D. D. Ignatavicius & L. M. Workman (Eds.), *Medical-surgical nursing* (9th ed., p. 10). St. Louis, MO: Elsevier.

and a healthy lifestyle; strengthening provider–patient relationships; and augmenting the cultural and linguistic competency of all health care providers.

? CRITICAL THINKING BOX 21.1

What components of cultural competence do you feel might influence health disparities? Can you think of ways to decrease disparities in health and health care in your community? What projects could you do as a nursing student to make a positive impact?

Many organizations are involved in improving cultural and linguistic competency in the health care industry by offering continuing education and training for health care personnel. The OMH provides extensive continuing education on cultural competency for health care professionals (US Department of Health and Human Services Office of Minority Health [HHS OMH], 2018). Through a web resource (https://www.thinkculturalhealth.hhs.gov/) and other offerings, this organization offers online interactive courses on cultural competency to health care providers, nurses, first responders, and oral health professionals from all points of care, helping them to deliver respectful, understandable, and effective care to patients of all ethnicities and cultural backgrounds. This sort of education is crucial because of the increasing diversity of the health care population. An additional measure for providing culturally and linguistically competent care is by increasing the diversity of the nursing workforce, as nurses comprise the largest group of healthcare professionals.

A Culturally Diverse Workforce

To meet the health care needs of an increasingly diverse society, it would be beneficial to have such diversity represented in the nursing profession. Unfortunately the diversity of the nursing workforce does not mirror that of the US population (AACN, 2015). For instance, in 2010, the US Census Bureau reported that just over one-third of the American population was from a minority background (US Census Bureau, 2011). Moreover, the US Census Bureau projects that minorities will comprise 57% of the US population in 2060 (US Census Bureau, 2012). However, in 2017, the National Council of State Boards of Nursing conducted the *National Nursing Workforce Survey*. Findings from the survey showed that minorities accounted for 19.3% of registered nurses (Smiley et al., 2018). It is also important to ensure cultural and ethnic diversity among nursing faculty who teach in nursing programs across the nation, since only 15.8% of nursing faculty are from groups underrepresented in the nursing profession (AACN, 2018).

The American Hospital Association (AHA) (2012) recommends that exposure to health careers begin early in the education of minority populations, as well as of males, to reach out to those who are currently underrepresented in nursing and who will account for an increasing share of the labor pool. The AHA states, "In addition to training all staff on cultural competency, look for opportunities to employ bicultural clinical and administrative staff to improve education, care delivery, and ultimately, outcomes" (p. 12). See Box 21.1 for information about culturally diverse nurse–patient interactions, and see the end of this chapter for additional relevant websites and online resources.

What Is the Meaning of Spirituality?

One of the challenges for the nurse providing spiritual care is that there is as yet no clear definition of spirituality (Gijsberts et al., 2011). Health care professionals recognize the important relationship between patient well-being and spirituality, but many feel underprepared to help patients incorporate this aspect of their lives into the health care setting (Blaber, Jones, & Willis, 2015). Many people confuse religion with spirituality when, in fact, they can be separate entities. Pesut et al. (2008)

BOX 21.5 COMPONENTS OF SPIRITUALITY

- Spirituality is a universal concept relevant to all individuals.
- The uniqueness of the individual is paramount.
- Formal religious affiliation is not a prerequisite for spirituality.
- An individual may become more spiritually aware during a time of need.

From McSherry, W. (2006). *Making sense of spirituality in nursing practice: An integrative approach* (p. 48). Edinburgh: Churchill Livingstone.

---

contend that current trends in health care tend to define religion as a set of institutionalized beliefs and rituals, whereas spirituality can be defined "as an individualized journey characterized by experiential descriptors such as meaning, purpose, transcendence, connectedness and energy" (p. 2804).

McSherry (2006) presents several components of spirituality with relevance to nursing; this is a helpful framework for understanding the spirituality concept (Box 21.5). At times a spiritual advisor or chaplain may be called on to serve a patient's or family's spiritual needs.

A definition of *spiritual nursing care* is "an intuitive, interpersonal, altruistic, and integrative expression that is contingent upon the nurse's awareness of the transcendent dimension of life but that reflects the patient's reality" (Sawatzky & Pesut, 2005, p. 23). It is important for nurses to refrain from imposing their spiritual beliefs on patients, as spirituality is a subjective experience and differs from one person to another. Spiritual distress is a NANDA-approved nursing diagnosis (Ackley, Ladwig, & Flynn Makic, 2017). It is essential to include the subjective spiritual assessment of patients' spiritual needs to make sure that there is a plan for providing ongoing interventions and evaluation of effectiveness. Examples of spiritual nursing interventions include prayer, presence, scripture reading, a peaceful environment, meditation, music, pastoral care, the inspiration of hope through positive affirmations, active listening, validation of patients' thoughts and feelings, values clarification, sensitive responses to patients' beliefs, and developing a trusting relationship (Callister et al., 2004). To that end, nurses have many resources available that can help them to improve the spiritual care of their patients so that the benefits of this important aspect of patient care can be realized.

Some challenges that nursing students and nurses may encounter include a lack of knowledge about a spirituality unlike their own and strong convictions regarding their own beliefs. Providing spiritual care often requires the nurse to compartmentalize his or her own beliefs and allow the patient's beliefs to prevail. For example, it may not be appropriate to provide empathy by referring to one's own source of spiritual strength. Should you be in doubt or unsure of how to provide spiritual support, it will be appropriate to ask or verify what would be meaningful to the patient and family.

Free online services allow patients to listen to religious works such as the Bible. This is useful for the patient who is too ill to read or for family members who would like to offer this service to their loved ones (www.biblegateway.com/resources/audio).

CULTURAL AND SPIRITUAL ASSESSMENT

What Are Cultural and Spiritual Beliefs Regarding Illness and Cures?

Patients' responses to illness may vary based on their cultural and spiritual beliefs. It is vital for the nurse to assess the patient's cultural and spiritual preferences using a holistic approach and asking open-ended questions (Box 21.6).

BOX 21.6 COMPONENTS OF CULTURAL AND SPIRITUAL ASSESSMENT

Communication Style
1. Does the patient speak English fluently? If not, what language does he or she prefer?
2. What does your patient consider signs of respect or disrespect? Attentiveness or nonattentiveness?
3. Is touch part of the communication process?
4. What practices are considered appropriate greetings or farewells?
5. How is silence used in communication?
6. What is the use of nonverbal communication?
7. Is a medical interpreter needed when you communicate with your patient?

Ethnic or Religious Affiliation
1. With what particular group does the patient identify?
2. What cultural practices are important to him or her?
3. How closely does the patient adhere to the traditional beliefs of the group?
4. Are there ethnic, cultural, or religious organizations that influence the patient's approach or views of health care?
5. Are there specific times during the day when tests or procedures should be avoided because of your patient's religious or spiritual practices?

Nutrition
1. What do the patient and family like to eat?
2. Are there certain ethnic or religious preferences regarding the selection or preparation of foods?
3. How is the food prepared? Who prepares it?
4. Are there foods to be encouraged (or avoided) when a person is ill?
5. Are there some fasting periods or requirements specific to beliefs or preferences concerning food items?
6. Are there any forbidden foods based on the patient's culture or foods required for the observance of a specific ceremony?

Family Relationships
1. Is the family matriarchal or patriarchal?
2. What is the patient's role in the family?
3. What is the patient's attitude toward children and older family members (extended family)?

Health Beliefs
1. How does the patient define health and illness?
2. What does the patient most fear about the illness?
3. What problems has the illness caused for the patient?
4. Does the patient rely on folk medicine or complementary and alternative therapies—for example, acupuncture, healing touch, Ayurveda, etc.?
5. Has the patient recently been treated by any traditional healers?
6. Does the patient take any herbal supplements or over-the-counter (OTC) medications?
7. Are there health topics that may be sensitive areas or considered taboo to discuss?

Health Practices
1. What are the strategies the patient uses to maintain health—for example, hygiene and self-care?
2. Whom does the patient contact when ill?
3. Does the patient prefer to have a health professional of the same gender, age, ethnic, and/or racial background?
4. Are there any restrictions related to modesty that must be respected?
5. What examination procedures are considered immodest?
6. What is the patient's way of responding to life events—for example, birth, puberty, marriage, death? Are special events or ceremonies associated with various life events?

Time Orientation
1. What is the patient's orientation to time? Is he or she future-oriented, present-oriented, or past-oriented?
2. What are the patient's views regarding being punctual and wasting time?

Continued

BOX 21.6 COMPONENTS OF CULTURAL AND SPIRITUAL ASSESSMENT—CONT'D

Personal Space Preferences

1. What is the patient's personal space preference?
   a. Territoriality or personal space is the distance that a patient prefers to maintain from another person. Large personal space is usually more than 18 inches.
   b. Various cultural groups vary widely in in their perception of appropriate personal space.
2. What is the patient's degree of comfort when talking or standing near others?

End-of-Life Care

1. What are the spiritual and religious practices that may ease the patient during end-of-life care?
2. Are there any garments, religious items, or rituals that are important to the patient during end-of-life care?
3. What are the practices of the patient's culture regarding care of the body after death? How should the body be treated?
4. Would the patient welcome a visit from a religious leader or member of the clergy?

NOTE: The Joint Commission has a publication divided into two sections: cultures and religions, which is detailed and can be a handy resource for health care providers. (Galanti, G. A. [2018]. *Cultural and religious sensitivity: A pocket guide for health care professionals* [3rd ed.]. Oakbrook, IL: Joint Commission.)
Adapted from Zerwekh, J. (2019). *Illustrated Study Guide for the NCLEX-RN® Exam* (10th ed.). St. Louis, MO: Elsevier, pp. 79–80.

> The nurse must be careful not to stereotype a patient based on generalizations of his or her cultural or spiritual background.

People of many cultures may use complementary, alternative, or integrative modalities that can affect their health status (Box 21.7). Complementary and alternative therapies are often grouped together using the acronym CAM. The National Center for Complementary and Integrative Health (NCCIH, 2019) defines complementary medicine as non-mainstream practices that are used together with conventional medicine, whereas alternative medicine is the use of non-mainstream practices in place of conventional medicine. Because the public is increasingly using complementary and alternative health approaches in the United States (Kachan et al., 2017), it is vital that the nurse have a basic understanding of these types of therapies as well as their benefits and risks (Fig. 21.1). For instance, a patient with diabetes may be ingesting ginger for general health or to address a concern (e.g., nausea). However, the nurse should know that ginger may decrease blood glucose levels. It is possible that such a patient's ingestion of ginger could influence the dosage of an oral antidiabetic agent that the patient is taking. The nurse will also have to consider that ginger could increase bleeding times if the patient is taking an anticoagulant (Lilley, Collins, & Snyder, 2017). The NCCIH has developed an app called HerbList for research-based information about the safety and efficacy of herbal products; consumers can easily access this app from their mobile devices. For additional information about the HerbList app, go to the following link: https://nccih.nih.gov/Health/HerbListApp/.

BOX 21.7 DEFINITIONS OF TERMS

Complementary therapies: therapies that are used in conjunction with conventional medicine
Alternative therapies: therapies that are used in place of conventional medicine
Integrative health: the use of complementary therapies and conventional medicine in a coordinated approach to provide holistic patient-focused care

From National Center for Complementary and Integrative Health [NCCIH]. (2018). *Complementary, alternative, or integrative health: What's in a name?* Retrieved from https://nccih.nih.gov/health/integrative-health.

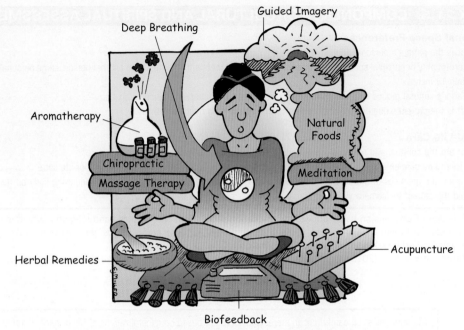

Deep Breathing

Guided Imagery

Aromatherapy

Natural Foods

Chiropractic

Massage Therapy

Meditation

Herbal Remedies

Acupuncture

Biofeedback

FIG. 21.1 Integrative health care is on the rise.

The American Holistic Nurses Association (AHNA) says that holistic nursing is defined as "all nursing practice that has healing the whole person as its goal" (AHNA, 2018). Holistic nursing is an attitude, a philosophy, and a way of being; it is not just something a person or a nurse does. Vital components of a holistic nursing assessment are the identification of cultural and spiritual practices (AHNA, 2018). Nurses must be aware of all aspects of a patient's life throughout each step of the nursing process. Having access to a comprehensive assessment tool will help them to identify important transcultural variations as they work with their patients (Fig. 21.2).

The Joint Commission (2018) acknowledges a patient's right to receive care that respects his or her cultural and spiritual values, including a spiritual assessment as a component of the regulatory standards found in the accreditation manual. It is imperative that nurses perform a spiritual assessment to determine each patient's specific needs (Critical Thinking Box 21.2).

> ### ⍰ CRITICAL THINKING BOX 21.2
>
> How much knowledge do you have regarding various complementary and integrative health therapies, such as acupuncture, Reiki, yoga, herbal medicine, and aromatherapy? Use the NCCIH website https://nccih.nih.gov/health/atoz.htm to enhance your knowledge base. Identify possible referral sources for integrative therapies and clinics in your community. You never know when a patient may ask you for information and/or a referral regarding integrative therapies.

How Do You Assess Spiritual Need?

Specific spiritual assessment tools can be used by the nurse as guides. Aspects of these tools may also be integrated into an agency assessment document or into the electronic health record.

Box 21.8 includes several areas to assess in gathering spiritual data from patients. Each spiritual area lists corresponding assessment questions. These questions can help the nurse to determine a patient's spiritual needs.

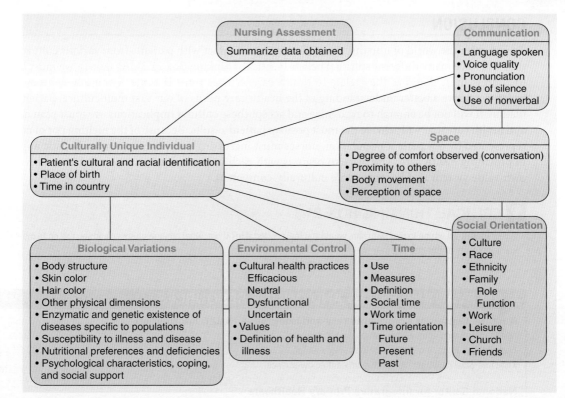

FIG. 21.2 Giger and Davidhizar's transcultural assessment model. (From Giger, J. N. [2013]. *Transcultural nursing: Assessment and intervention* (6th ed.). St. Louis, MO: Mosby/Elsevier.)

BOX 21.8	**THE FICA SPIRITUAL HISTORY TOOL**

SPIRITUAL AREAS TO ASSESS	QUESTIONS TO ASK THE PATIENT
Faith and belief	Do you have spiritual beliefs that help you cope with stress/ difficult times? Do you consider yourself spiritual or religious?
	If the patient responds in the negative, the health care provider might ask, What gives your life meaning?
Importance	What importance does your spirituality have in our life?
	Has your spirituality influenced how you take care of yourself and your health?
	Does your spirituality influence you in your health care decision making (e.g., advance directives, treatment)?
Community	Are you part of a spiritual community? Communities such as churches, temples, and mosques or a group of like-minded friends, family, or yoga practitioners can serve as strong support systems for some patients.
	Can explore further: Is this of support to you, and if so, how?
	"Is there a group of people you really love or who are important to you?"
Address in bare	How would you like me, your health care provider, to address these issues in your health care?

Reprinted with permission from The George Washington Institute for Spirituality and Health. The FICA Spiritual History Tool©™. Retrieved from https://smhs.gwu.edu/gwish/clinical/fica/spiritual-history-tool

CONCLUSION

As you enter the world of nursing, you will come into contact with patients from various cultures, and they will have many different spiritual beliefs (Critical Thinking Box 21.3). As nurses, we must be able to address these issues as they relate to health care. Nurses must become "culturally competent" in order to achieve a better understanding of the health care needs of our vast multicultural patient population. It will not be enough to recognize and accept these cultural implications; we must plan nursing and health care that will achieve the most positive patient results. Because of the melting pot of cultures represented by our patient population, nurses must increasingly implement a more holistic approach in providing health care. The place to begin is with each individual nurse, who must assess his or her own value system and become more culturally competent.

? CRITICAL THINKING BOX 21.3

If your patient asked you to pray with him, would you feel comfortable? If not, what other resources could you call on to meet the spiritual needs of this patient?

🌐 RELEVANT WEBSITES AND ONLINE RESOURCES

National Center for Complementary and Integrative Health Information
Health information. https://nccih.nih.gov/health/integrative-health
HerbList App. https://nccih.nih.gov/Health/HerbListApp
Know the Science. https://nccih.nih.gov/health/know-science

National Center for Integrative Primary Healthcare
Resources for patients and the public. https://nciph.org/public.html

National Institutes of Health Office of Dietary Supplements [NIH ODS]
Dietary supplements: What you need to know. https://ods.od.nih.gov/HealthInformation/DS_WhatYouNeedToKnow.aspx

The Office of Minority Health
Center for linguistic and cultural competency in health care. https://www.minorityhealth.hhs.gov/omh/browse.aspx?lvl=2&lvlid=34

The National CLAS Standards
https://www.thinkculturalhealth.hhs.gov/

Transcultural Nursing Society
Transcultural nursing resource links. https://tcns.org/resources/

U.S. Department of Health and Human Services
Office of Disease Prevention and Health Promotion. https://www.healthypeople.gov/
Office of Minority Health. https://www.minorityhealth.hhs.gov/

BIBLIOGRAPHY

Ackley, B. J., Ladwig, G. B., & Flynn Makic, M. B. (2017). *An evidence-based guide to planning care* (11th ed.). Maryland Heights, MO: Mosby.

Agency for Healthcare Research and Quality (AHRQ). (2013). What is cultural and linguistic competence? Retrieved from https://www.ahrq.gov/professionals/systems/primary-care/cultural-competence-mco/cultcompdef.html.

Agency for Healthcare Research and Quality (AHRQ). (2018). 2017 National Healthcare Quality and Disparities Report. Rockville, MD: AHRQ Pub. No. 18-0033-EF. Retrieved from https://www.ahrq.gov/research/findings/nhqrdr/nhqdr17/index.html.

American Association of Colleges of Nursing. (2015). Fact sheet: Enhancing diversity in the nursing workforce. Retrieved from https://www.aacnnursing.org/News-Information/Fact-Sheets/Enhancing-Diversity.

American Association of Colleges of Nursing. (2018). New minority nurse faculty scholars selected by AACN and the Johnson & Johnson campaign for Nursing's future. Retrieved from https://www.aacnnursing.org/News-Information/Press-Releases/View/ArticleId/21347/2018-minority-nurse-faculty-scholars.

American Holistic Nurses Association. (2018). What is holistic nursing? Retrieved from https://www.ahna.org/About-Us/What-is-Holistic-Nursing.

American Hospital Association. (2012). Eliminating health care disparities: Implementing the national call to action using lessons learned. Retrieved from http://www.hpoe.org/resources/ahahret-guides/809.

American Nurses Association. (2015). Code of ethics for nurses with interpretive statements. Silver Springs, MD: ANA. Retrieved from http://www.nursingworld.org/mainmenucategories/ethicsstandards/codeofethicsfornurses.

Blaber, M., Jones, J., & Willis, D. (2015). Spiritual care: Which is the best assessment tool for palliative settings? *International Journal of Palliative Nursing, 21*(9), 430–438.

Callister, L. C., et al. (2004). Threading spirituality through nursing education. *Holistic Nursing Practice, 18*, 160–166.

Dovidio, J. F., & Fiske, S. T. (2012). Under the radar: How unexamined biases in decision-making processes in clinical interactions can contribute to health care disparities. *American Journal of Public Health, 102*(5), 945–952.

Giger, J. N. (2013). *Transcultural nursing: Assessment and intervention* (6th ed.). St. Louis, MO: Mosby/Elsevier.

Gijsberts, M. J., Echteld, M. A., van der Steen, J. T., et al. (2011). Spirituality at the end of life: Conceptualization of measurable aspects—a systematic review. *Journal of Palliative Medicine, 14*(7), 852–856.

Greer, T. M., Brondolo, E., & Brown, P. (2014). Systemic racism moderates effects of provider racial biases on adherence to hypertension treatment for African Americans. *Health Psychology, 33*(1), 35–42.

Healthy People 2020. (2018a). HealthyPeople.gov. Washington, DC: U.S. Department of Health and Human Services. Retrieved from https://www.healthypeople.gov/.

Healthy People 2020. (2018b). 2020 topics and objectives. Washington, DC: U.S. Department of Health and Human Services. Retrieved from https://www.healthypeople.gov/.

Kachan, D., Olano, H., Tannenbaum, S. L., Annane, D. W., Mehta, A., Arheart, K. L., et al. (2017). Prevalence of mindfulness practices in the US workforce: National health interview survey. *Preventing Chronic Disease, 14*. https://doi.org/10.5888/pcd14.160034.

Leininger, M. (2007). Theoretical questions and concerns: Response from the theory of culture care diversity and universality perspective. *Nursing Science Quarterly, 20*, 9–15.

Lilley, L. L., Colllins, S., & Snyder, J. (2017). *Pharmacology and the nursing process* (8th ed.). St. Louis, MO: Elsevier.

Mazanec, P., & Tyler, M. K. (2003). Cultural considerations in end-of-life care: How ethnicity, age, and spirituality affect decisions when death is imminent. *American Journal of Nursing, 103*, 50–58.

McGibbon, E., Etowa, J., & McPherson, C. (2008). Health-care access as a social determinant of health. *Can Nurse, 104*(7), 22–27.

McSherry, W. (2006). *Making sense of spirituality in nursing practice: An integrative approach.* Edinburgh: Churchill Livingstone.

National Center for Complementary and Integrative Health [NCCIH]. (2019). What is complementary, alternative, or integrative health? Retrieved from https://nccih.nih.gov/health/integrative-health.

Ogbolu, Y., Scrandis, D., & Fitzpatrick, G. (2018). Barriers and facilitators of care for diverse patients: Nurse leader perspectives and nurse manager implications. *Journal of Nursing Management, 26*, 3–10. https://doi.org/10.1111/jonm.12498.

Pesut, B., et al. (2008). Conceptualizing spirituality and religion for healthcare. *Journal of Clinical Nursing, 17*(21), 2803–2810.

Project Implicit. (2018). What are implicit and explicit stereotypes? Retrieved from https://implicit.harvard.edu/implicit/faqs.html.

Sawatzky, R., & Pesut, B. (2005). Attributes of spiritual care in nursing practice. *Journal of Holistic Nursing, 23*, 19–33.

Smiley, R. A., Lauer, P., Bienemy, C., Berg, J. G., Shireman, E., Reneau, K. A., et al. (2018). The National Council of State Boards of Nursing (NCSBN) 2017 national nursing workforce survey [supplement]. *Journal of Nursing Regulation, 9*(3), 4–88.

The Joint Commission. (2018). Standards FAQ details. Retrieved from https://www.jointcommission.org/standards_information/jcfaqdetails.aspx?StandardsFaqId=1492&ProgramId=46.

U.S. Census Bureau. (March 24, 2011). 2010 Census shows America's diversity. Retrieved from https://www.census.gov/newsroom/releases/archives/2010_census/cb11-cn125.html.

U.S. Census Bureau. (December 12, 2012). U.S. Census Bureau projections show a slower growing, older, more diverse nation a half century from now. Retrieved from https://www.census.gov/newsroom/releases/archives/population/cb12-243.html.

U.S. Department of Health and Human Services Office of Minority Health [HHS OMH]. (2016). What is cultural competency? Retrieved from https://www.minorityhealth.hhs.gov/omh/content.aspx?ID=2804.

U.S. Department of Health and Human Services Office of Minority Health [HHS OMH]. (2018). Think cultural health. Retrieved from https://www.thinkculturalhealth.hhs.gov/.

van Ryn, M., Burgess, D. J., Malat, J., & Griffin, J. (2006). Physicians' perceptions of patients' social and behavioral characteristics and race disparities in treatment recommendations for men with coronary artery disease. *American Journal of Public Health, 96*(2), 351–357.

White-Means, S., Dong, Z., Hufstader, M., & Brown, L. T. (2009). Cultural competency, race, and skin tone bias among pharmacy, nursing, and medical students. *Medical Care Research and Review, 66*, 436–455.

22

Quality Patient Care

Stephanie Tippin, RN, MSN, NP-C*

ⓔ http://evolve.elsevier.com/Zerwekh/nsgtoday/.

Anyone who has never made a mistake has never tried anything new.
Albert Einstein

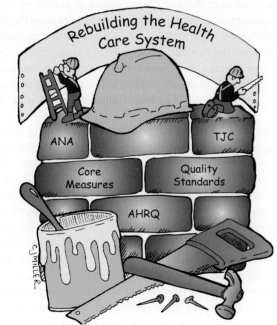

By working together using Improvement Science, we can rebuild our health care system.

After completing this chapter, you should be able to:

- Define quality standards in health care management.
- Describe the history and evolution of quality in health care.
- Define and discuss core measures.
- Define and discuss health literacy and the nurse's role.
- Identify the role of regulatory agencies in health care quality.
- Discuss the use of key indicators to measure performance.
- Describe your role in quality and performance improvement.
- Identify tools and processes for continuous quality improvement.
- Identify the role of regulatory standards and agencies.
- Incorporate successful process improvement strategies.
- Consider the value and requirements of quality credentialing.
- Synthesize understanding of the QSEN Initiative, *Healthy People 2020* and The Joint Commission National Patient Safety Goals in developing a safe patient care environment.

*We would like to acknowledge **Susan Ahrens, PhD, RN**, for her past contributions to this chapter.

Y ou may wonder why nurses need to know about quality issues to provide patient care. All nurses know that an important part of their professional life is to provide high-quality care. However, many new graduates soon discover that not all nurses do the right thing all the time for the patient and family. In fact, a landmark study in 1999, called *The Quality Chasm,* estimated that the impact of poor-quality care results in almost 100,000 deaths annually in acute care settings alone (Institute of Medicine, 2001). More current studies suggest that deaths from fatal medical errors in the United States may be as high as 250,000 (Makary & Daniel, 2016), whereas others have reported a lower number at 25,000 deaths (Shojania & Dixon-Woods, 2017). In either case, because of the costly effects of poor care, nurses must understand their important role in ensuring optimal patient care and the actions they can take to ensure excellence. According to the Institute of Medicine (2011), the Affordable Care Act requires nurses to play a key role in transforming health care to provide higher quality and safer care than ever before and to be involved at every level to redesign the system toward that end. As managers and providers of care, nurses can be a large part of changing health care delivery to be safer and more efficient.

> Look at almost any news show or sensational tabloid and you will find health care errors featured. Today more than ever, these incidents seem to have become the focus of news stories. Who or what is making this happen?

Issues on the forefront of news will take precedence over those that are routine or commonplace. Recently medical errors have become of primary concern. Quality assurance departments have the job of helping nurses and their team members avoid errors by implementing various preventive methods. They also ask for the help of nurses in mobilizing process improvement teams that work to identify risk areas and develop prevention plans. Ensuring optimal care can be likened to fire prevention as opposed to firefighting. Illegible handwriting continues to contribute to errors and has led to regulations about what medical abbreviations are appropriate to use. (See Table 11.1, The Joint Commission's official "do not use" list of abbreviations.)

Hospital leaders began to implement quality improvement (QI) programs starting in the early 1980s, with the inception of the National Demonstration Project on Quality Improvement in Healthcare, which we know today as the Institute for Healthcare Improvement (IHI, 2018). In the late 1980s, the topics of human immunodeficiency virus (HIV) and hepatitis B virus led to an increased use of gloves to prevent the transmission of infection. This led to the need to produce gloves more quickly, which resulted in the introduction of foreign supplies of latex gloves. As a result, more latex allergies surfaced. In the 1990s, more emphasis was placed on using needle-less systems to prevent needle-stick injuries, resulting in legislation to increase the number of needle-less devices used. In the 2000s, there has been concern and controversy regarding the nursing shortage and access to health care. In the 2010s, increasing demands will continue for all health care providers, with the expectation of high-quality care. As knowledge development increases, new technologies and treatments mean that health care providers will have to develop initiatives to ensure that patients receive the most effective and efficient care.

STANDARDS OF HIGH-QUALITY HEALTH CARE MANAGEMENT

Several agencies have established standards that guide quality in health care. Some of these include the American Nurses Association (ANA) Standards of Nursing Care, accrediting group standards such as those of The Joint Commission (TJC), which accredits health care organizations, and the Agency for Healthcare Research and Quality (AHRQ), which has established clinical practice guidelines designed to improve patient outcomes and reduce costs. In addition, another national program to ensure high-quality health care for the country is the Healthy People initiative. The current version of the initiative is called *Healthy People 2020*.

First introduced in 1979, a report by the US Surgeon General outlined the needs of the nation for improved health. *Healthy People 2020* contains more than 1200 objectives, with each objective having a reliable data source, baseline measures, and a specific target for improvement by 2020. The objectives were prepared by experts from multiple federal agencies and made available for public comment. Agencies that support health care research often use these objectives to identify research priorities. Funding for nursing intervention research using the *Healthy People 2020* objectives is often more likely to be awarded if all other aspects are equal.

Based on the population objectives, 12 leading health indicators were identified. These are used to determine whether or not objectives are being met. The data are collected over 10 years and used to update and improve the objectives for the upcoming 10 years. The midcourse review of Healthy People 2020 found that objectives related to occupational safety and health, genomics, and vision were doing well. Although not all findings were equally encouraging, the knowledge of what targets have yet to see positive change can help to inform decision makers involved in Healthy People 2030 (Office of Disease Prevention and Health Promotion, 2018).

TJC is an accrediting agency that evaluates care in an organization and then determines whether the overall care meets its standards of quality. TJC requires hospitals to submit error reports identifying key sentinel events that have the potential for great harm, and it publishes a monthly sentinel event alert. A sentinel event is an unexpected occurrence involving death or loss of limb or function. Such events are called *sentinel* because they sound a warning of the need for immediate investigation and response (Fig. 22.1) (The Joint Commission, 2018a).

> *Without continual growth and progress, such words as improvement, achievement, and success have no meaning.*
>
> **Benjamin Franklin**

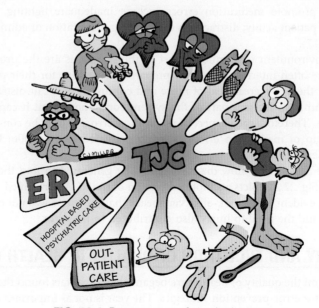

FIG. 22.1 Root-causes of sentinel events.

What Is Root-Cause Analysis?

When errors occur, the primary cause must be determined so that a solution can be found. Root cause analysis (RCA) is a process designed for use in investigating and categorizing the root causes of events. In the health care setting, there are many factors that can contribute to the cause of errors. Rather than placing blame on any one person or thing, RCA, when conducted appropriately, can identify all factors leading to the error. A hospital's risk management department often conducts an RCA, and the results are presented to the QI department for follow-up action. The role of the QI department is to be proactive at finding ways to prevent similar incidents from occurring.

Imagine an occurrence during which a nurse administers the wrong dose of a medication instead of the correct dose. In the past, the nurse (who was viewed as the last person between the medication and the patient) had sole responsibility for medication delivery. RCA has demonstrated that errors are often the result of a complex, broken system. Remedies in the past for "nurse" errors was education and sometimes discipline. RCA has shown the health care industry that medication delivery is a very complex process, and there are many things that contribute to a medication error. System issues, which are often a cause for errors that affect the delivery of medication, can be detected using the RCA process. A systems approach takes the view that most errors reflect predictable human failings in the context of poorly designed systems. Rather than focusing corrective efforts on punishment or remediation, the systems approach seeks to identify situations or factors likely to give rise to human error. Changes in the underlying systems of care in order to reduce the occurrence of errors can minimize the impact on patients and improve patient safety and outcomes (AHRQ, 2018).

As nurses encounter problems within the system, work-design problems, or human and environmental factors, many things can contribute to medication errors. Considering this, getting medications to the nursing unit or medication labeling may pose medication delivery challenges.

Researchers have found that many of the problems leading to medication errors are systemic and cultural. Common causes of medication errors include look-alike and sound-alike medication names, look-alike packaging, error-prone abbreviations, poor communication, poor procedures or techniques, patient misuse due to lack of education, distractions, and interruptions. Environmental factors that can promote medication errors include inadequate lighting, cluttered work environments, increased patient acuity, distractions during drug preparation or administration, and caregiver fatigue (FDA, 2017).

The environment is as much a part of the system as are the processes within the organization. Nurses are often interrupted as they prepare medications for their patients. Sometimes the lighting is bad, or there is a great deal of noise and confusion that can distract a nurse. Technology can be helpful and is an integral part of the system components, but it cannot address the human factors and issues. Therefore each aspect of medication errors should be considered when a cause-and-effect relationship of medication errors is being evaluated (Pape, 2006; US Department of Health and Human Services, 2018).

A root-cause factor-flow diagram should be generated to find the real origin of the error. As an example, Fig. 22.2 depicts a simplified version of the RCA performed. As the investigation proceeded, it became evident that a look-alike vial meant that the nurse was not entirely at fault. In addition, distractions and the need to hurry also contributed to the error.

HISTORY AND EVOLUTION OF QUALITY IN HEALTH CARE

Research on the quality of health care began when hospitals found the need to look outside their own expertise for error-prevention strategies. The year is not as important as the fact that health care organizations found a need to borrow from other industries that were successful at managing risk.

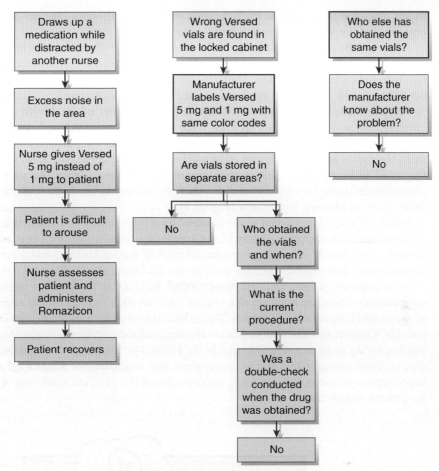

FIG. 22.2 Root-cause factor-flow diagram.

Manufacturing industries began focusing on error prevention in the early 1920s, whereas the improvement of quality in health care did not become a major issue until the 1960s, and QI techniques are still evolving.

Historically quality-improvement efforts have focused on controlling processes by inspection, so that errors were prevented. Later, the emphasis changed from inspection to proactive approaches, including the monitoring of processes.

Who Are Edward Deming, Joseph M. Juran, and Philip Crosby?

Edward Deming is often considered the father of QI, although quality concepts have developed and improved throughout several decades. What once began simply as a method for discovering how to prevent defects has evolved into highly complex methods for tracking and improving quality today. Deming's teachings embraced the philosophy that quality within an organization is everyone's responsibility.

Another valuable forefather of quality initiatives is Joseph M. Juran, who emphasized the meaning of the Pareto principle which states that 80% of problems are caused by 20% of sources, people, or things. Therefore, if you can fix the 20%, you can fix almost the entire system. Juran's work marked the beginning of the idea of *total quality management* (TQM).

Philip Crosby is considered the father of *zero defects*. He often proposed simplifying things so that everyone could understand. He also believed in the importance of communicating QI efforts and their results to the entire organization. Thereafter, ideas such as "lean" manufacturing, "just in time" product delivery, and "Six Sigma" methods crossed over into health care.

Recently there has been a real change in how members of the health care team view quality improvement within health care settings. What once was considered work only for the QI department is now brought to the frontline workers, who can best affect the outcomes. By frontline workers, we mean the nurses at the bedside and other workers in direct patient care areas who know the problems that need to be resolved. This is also termed *improvement science*. An ongoing commitment to improvement strategies supports an atmosphere of teamwork. The focus is on the process and systems rather than on blaming individuals (Fig. 22.3).

Still, health care is regulated at the national level by various governmental bodies. These agencies are responsible for approving many of the licenses for those institutions that educate personnel. For example, state boards of nursing regulate the work of nurses. Institutional accreditation is also regulated by some government agencies, such as the US Public Health Service.

As mentioned earlier, TJC, previously called JCAHO, is the primary agency used for hospital accreditation. The mere mention of a visit by TJC can elicit feelings of fear and anxiety in the minds of nurses and hospital administrators. This is because hospitals must meet certain quality standards to pass TJC's inspections and maintain accreditation, and accreditation is required to receive government funding for the provision of health care. In the 1990s, TJC first began to mandate the use of *continuous quality improvement* (CQI) and to recommend that organizations adopt a QI model for all process improvement activities. TJC typically endorses use of the *plan, do, study, act* (PDSA) cycle as a tool for process improvement.

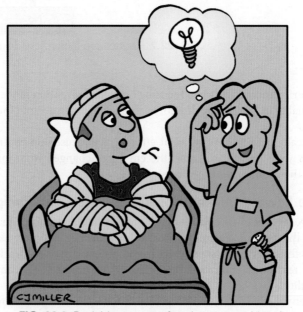

FIG. 22.3 Bedside nurses often have great ideas!

Some hospital QI departments have combined newer strategies with PDSA, including *define, measure, analyze, improve, control* (DMAIC) and *rapid cycle changes* (RCCs), which further incorporate a team focus. These are components of CQI, but more discussion of these methods will come later. TJC has also mandated specific quality outcome measures for all hospitals. Outcome measures involve looking for real patient results to determine whether an organization's goals are being achieved. TJC wants to know if the care that patients receive is meeting standards or is improving.

WHAT ARE CORE MEASURES?

Core measures include those for patients admitted with a diagnosis of acute myocardial infarction, heart failure, community-acquired pneumonia, surgical infections, pregnancy-related conditions, deep vein thrombosis, and whether specific best practices were implemented within the health care setting. These measures are those that the consumer considers important for choosing one hospital over another.

Hospitals must continue to assess the core measures that were developed by TJC. There are 12 core measure sets (acute myocardial infarction, children's asthma care, venous thromboembolism, stroke, emergency department, immunization, hospital-based inpatient psychiatric services, tobacco treatment, substance use, perinatal care, hospital outpatient, early hearing detection and intervention) as defined by TJC (2018b). The goal is to improve the quality of health care by implementing a national standardized performance measurement system. Key actions are listed in each category defining the best research-based care process appropriate for that category. By tracking these core measures, hospitals improve patient care by focusing on the results of that care.

In 2011, the Centers for Medicare and Medicaid Services (CMS) launched the Medicare Shared Savings Plan as a requirement of the Patient Protection and Affordable Care Act, to assist all health care providers across health care settings (hospitals, doctor's offices, long-term care) in coordinating care for Medicare patients. Under the Medicare Shared Savings Plan, Accountable Care Organizations (ACOs), consisting of health care providers, agree to collaborate in providing patient care versus working independently. This was an effort to control costs and provide quality patient care. In order for an ACO to receive financial compensation for services rendered to a Medicare patient from CMS, the ACO must demonstrate that it has met the performance standards set forth by the CMS (Centers for Medicare & Medicaid Services, 2018a, p. 1). There are currently 31 quality measures divided into four categories. The four quality domains include patient/caregiver experience, care coordination/patient safety, preventive health, and at-risk populations. This information is available from the CMS website at cms.gov (Centers for Medicare & Medicaid Services, 2019).

WHAT IS HOSPITAL CONSUMER ASSESSMENT OF HEALTH CARE PROVIDERS AND SYSTEMS?

HCAHPS refers to the Hospital Consumer Assessment of Healthcare Providers and Systems. It is a national program for collecting and providing health care information from the consumer's perspective, and the results are used to improve health care services. The patient survey was developed for public reporting as a way of comparing hospitals across the continuum of patient care and garnering information about the overall quality of care received from the patient's viewpoint. The HCAHPS contains ratings of communication, responsiveness, pain management, discharge information, cleanliness of the hospital environment, quietness of the hospital environment, and if patients would recommend the hospital (HCAHPS, 2017).

WHAT IS "HOSPITAL COMPARE"?

The Hospital Compare website is designed so that consumers can compare how well selected hospitals serve to provide the care recommended to their patients. This information is provided through the efforts of Medicare and the Hospital Quality Alliance and enables consumers to make informed decisions about their care. The performance measures that can be compared include information related to heart attack, heart failure, pneumonia, surgery, and other conditions (Centers for Medicare & Medicaid Services, 2018b). Consumers can go to www.hospitalcompare.hhs.gov/ and search by zip code to compare hospitals and prescribers.

JUST WHAT IS THE JOINT COMMISSION?

TJC is the major accrediting body for health care institutions that are funded by Medicare and Medicaid. The CMS is a part of the U.S. Department of Health and Human Services (HHS). Both organizations set the standards for safe practice and evaluate compliance. Having TJC accreditation symbolizes the organization's commitment to quality. This means that nearly all hospitals must be TJC-accredited to stay in business.

In the past, TJC standards have directly addressed patient safety in many areas. Beginning on July 1, 2001, additions to these standards required hospitals to develop a systematic approach to error reduction and to design patient care processes with safety in mind. For CQI initiatives, TJC recommends using things such as flowcharts, Pareto charts, run charts or line graphs, control charts, and histograms to display data. We call these "tools" or "instruments" because they help depict the measurements and track the problems and improvements. After the data have been collected, these tools enable the visualization of results of performance improvement as understood by most nurses. Other valuable tools are discussed later in this chapter.

What Are Patient Safety Goals?

A primary driving force for CQI activities is TJC's National Patient Safety Goals (NPSG). In 2001, TJC began instituting annual patient safety goals intended to improve the quality of health care. The hospital national patient safety goals are summarized in Box 22.1 (The Joint Commission, 2018c).

TJC's Board of Commissioners approved the first NPSGs in July 2002. TJC established these goals to help accredited organizations address specific areas of concern regarding patient safety. Each goal includes brief, evidence-based recommendations. *Evidence-based* means that the goals are based on real-world research and/or expert opinions. Each year, the goals and associated recommendations are reevaluated; most are continued and others may be replaced because of emerging new priorities or evidence from research studies. New goals and recommendations are announced in July and become effective on January 1 of the following year (TJC, 2018c); for more information on the NPSGs for specific organizations, see TJC's website.

MONITORING THE QUALITY OF HEALTH CARE

It is important for nurses to know how to design and conduct simple quality improvement projects to improve processes within their nursing units. Nurses need to know the basics of collecting and analyzing data and what to do with the results. They must be able to educate other nurses about performance improvement as well.

BOX 22.1   THE JOINT COMMISSION'S 2019 NATIONAL HOSPITAL PATIENT SAFETY GOALS

Goal 1: Use at least two ways to identify patients, such as using the patients' names and dates of birth. Make sure that the correct patient receives the correct blood during a blood transfusion. For newborn patients: Use distinct methods of identification for newborn patients.

Goal 2: Improve the effectiveness of communication among caregivers. Get important test results to the right staff person on time.

Goal 3: Use medications safely. Before a procedure, label medicines that are not labeled, for example, medicines in syringes, cups, and basins. Do this in the area where medicines and supplies are set up. Take extra care with patients who take medicines to thin their blood. Record and pass along correct information about a patient's medicines. Find out what medicines the patient is taking. Compare those medicines to new medicines given to the patient. Make sure the patient knows which medicines to take when he or she is at home. Tell the patient it is important to bring an updated list of medicines every time he or she visits a provider.

Goal 4: Use alarms safely. Make improvements to ensure that alarms on medical equipment are heard and responded to on time.

Goal 5: Prevent infection. Use the Centers for Disease Control and Prevention (CDC) hand hygiene guidelines or the current World Health Organization (WHO) hand hygiene guidelines. Set and use the goals for improving hand cleaning. Implement evidence-based practices to prevent health care–associated infections (HAIs) and infections caused by multidrug-resistant organisms that are difficult to treat, infection of the blood from central lines, after surgery, and urinary tract infections.

Goal 6: Identify patient safety risks. Find out which patients are most likely to try to commit suicide.

Goal 7: Prevent mistakes in surgery. Make sure that the correct surgery is done on the correct patient and at the correct place on the patient's body. Mark the correct place on the patient's body where the surgery is to be done. Pause before the surgery to make sure that a mistake is not being made.

Universal Protocol for Eliminating Wrong Site, Wrong Procedure, Wrong Person Surgery

The universal protocol applies to all surgical and nonsurgical invasive procedures. For more information on the Universal Protocol, visit The Joint Commission website: http://www.jointcommission.org/standards_information/up.aspx.

From https://www.jointcommission.org/hap_2017/npsgs/.
For more information on the National Patient Safety Goals, visit The Joint Commission website: www.jointcommission.org/PatientSafety/NationalPatientSafetyGoals/

What Is Quality Improvement?

QI refers to the process or activities that are used to measure, monitor, evaluate, and control services, which will lead to measurable improvement to health care consumers. It includes reports that must be generated to track progress. Incidence reports are sometimes referred to as QI reports or variance reports. These help guide the hospital risk management (RM) department and QI department to make system improvements (Box 22.2).

How Do We Monitor Quality?

As stated earlier, someone must monitor quality care compliance to continuously maintain and improve standards of practice. The QI department is typically the department that receives data, analyzes trends, and recommends actions to facilitate improvement in the organization. However, there should also be a CQI council as a primary decision-making nursing team as well as *quality circles* (QCs) that function along service lines, collaborating to improve care for a group of patient types.

Examples of service lines include surgical, medical, neurologic, rehabilitation, and outpatient units. These teams of nurses and other staff review specific problems or indicators each month to determine whether high-quality care is being delivered. The goal is to keep patients safe by encouraging everyone to practice according to established standards. Each service line provides an annual QI plan for the following year based on recent problem areas or identified hot topics. Because it is impossible to track everything that nurses consider important to quality care, QCs use various methods to prioritize or target their reviews. They establish unit-specific *quality indicators* for tracking problems on the nursing unit using questions with measurable answers that provide data for trending improvements.

BOX 22.2   COMMON QUALITY TERMS

Audit: A formal periodic check on quality measures to verify correctness of actions.

DMAIC: A Six Sigma process for improving existing processes that fall below institutional goals or national norms. DMAIC stands for *define, measure, analyze, improve, control.*

Key indicators: Selected data based on TJC mandates or on specific problem areas that may show the need for more extensive data collection or remedial action to resolve an identified problem (e.g., fall rates, medication error rates).

Key performance indicators (KPIs): Reflect the things that the team wants to change. These are a part of the DMAIC and RCC process. Typical KPIs are time, costs, distance, numbers of incidents, or items.

Metric: A measurement to determine the rate of compliance or noncompliance with an indicator.

Monitor: Similar to auditing; checking or verifying that an established practice has been retained.

Operational definition: A statement detailing the thing or event using specific identifiable and measurable wording with written inclusion and exclusion criteria.

Outcome or core measures: Measures that the public consumer considers important for choosing one hospital instead of another.

Pareto principle: Some 80% of the problems are caused by 20% of sources, people, or things. If you can fix the 20%, you can fix the system.

Patient safety goals: Annual goals established by TJC that highlight problematic areas in health care and describe evidence- and expert-based solutions to these problems. Goals are derived primarily from informal recommendations made in TJC's safety newsletter *Sentinel Event Alert.*

Performance improvement: A plan and documentation method to demonstrate the procedures that have been used in the past and those that will be implemented for changes in the quality of services based on this previously collected data.

Plan, do, study, act (PDSA): Contained within an RCC for planning, doing, studying, and performing actions intended to drive and maintain change.

Quality assurance: Activities that are used to monitor, evaluate, and control services to provide some measure of quality to consumers.

Quality indicators: Data that indicate whether high-quality care is being maintained. Items of concern that have arisen because of a nursing practice problem (e.g., Foley catheter securing).

Quality measures: Tools used to measure health care functions, outcomes, patients' overall health care experience, and organizational systems associated with providing quality health care.

Rapid cycle changes (RCCs): A strategy for process improvement as a part of DMAIC where changes are tried for very short time frames (3–7 days).

Six Sigma: A measurement standard in product variation that began in the 1920s when Shewhart showed that three sigma from the mean is the point where a process requires correction.

Stakeholders: Key people who will be affected by change and who can either positively or negatively influence the improvement.

Total quality management (TQM): A management style where the goal is producing quality services for the customer and where the customer defines what *quality* means.

What Is an Indicator and a Metric?

A *quality indicator* is an item of concern that has arisen because of a nursing practice problem. It is often an RM as well. For example, a quality team may have identified a problem with securing urethral catheters properly. This seems to be a recurrent issue. Perhaps several patients had urethral catheters that were inadvertently pulled out. After some investigation and collecting baseline data, the problem was identified as having to do with not securing the catheters properly. Thus the team will collect data for a specific time and will track the nurses' practices. They would count the number of urethral catheters not secured correctly and divide that by the total number of urethral catheters during a specific time frame to obtain the average rate of compliance. The metric or measure is the actual rate of urethral catheters that are secured properly (Table 22.1). The correct practice would be clarified with all nurses according to an established policy. Later, when most of the nurses were securing urethral catheters correctly, there may not be a need to monitor this particular practice any longer. In essence, the indicator is the problem, and the metric is the measurement of that problem.

TABLE 22.1 INDICATOR AND METRIC DESCRIPTORS

INDICATOR	METRIC DESCRIPTORS
Admission documentation	Metric 1—Rate of patients' identified learning needs not documented within 24 h of admission. Metric 2—Rate of skin assessment (Braden scale) not documented within 24 h of admission. Metric 3—Rate of patients' identified spiritual needs not documented within 24 h of admission.
Foley securing	Metric 1—Rate of Foley catheters not secured in place according to the procedure described in Potter and Perry's textbook.
Intravenous tube labeling	Metric 1—Rate of continuous flow intravenous tubing that has not been labeled with the date and time it needs to be changed. Metric 2—Rate of intermittent flow tubing (IVPB) that has not been labeled with the date and time it needs to be changed.
Skin care	Metric 1—Rate of high-risk patients, as defined by the Braden scale (<17), who have pressure ulcers within 2–4 days of admission. Metric 2—Rate of those patients with pressure ulcers who are • Stage 1 • Stage 2 • Stage 3 • Stage 4 Unstageable Suspected of having deep tissue injury
TORAV/VORAV Telephone or verbal orders	Metric 1—Rate of telephoned physician's orders that did not contain read-back verification by using *telephone order read-back and verified* (TORAV) documentation with the signature of person taking the order on the first two charts of each odd-numbered day.

A unit-based QI nurse is usually assigned the responsibility to audit charts or to verify a procedure by direct observation to determine compliance with a specific nursing practice. The results are compiled and sent to the QI department. After nurses are reeducated about the correct practice and the same indicator is tracked for several months to see whether there has been an improvement. This is done until noncompliance reaches preestablished criteria (e.g., below 5%) and/or compliance is 95%.

Indicators are sometimes selected based on an RM issue. For example, a patient may have suffered an injury because a catheter was not secured correctly. The critical thinking exercise (Critical Thinking Box 22.1) can help you to discover another example of how important chart auditing can be.

? CRITICAL THINKING BOX 22.1

An audit review committee composed of the quality coordinator, three nurses, two case managers, a physical therapist, and a pharmacist was charged with reviewing the care of patients undergoing total hip replacement. The patients' care did not seem to conform with the expected length of stay (LOS) as established by Medicare diagnosis related group (DRG) reimbursement charts. As committee members reviewed the chart and discussed the care of all 20 patients, they noted that Mr. Garcia had been ready for discharge at 10:00 a.m. on Tuesday but the case manager for that nursing unit was not able to place him in a rehabilitation unit until 48 h later. Many of the other 19 charts depicted similar scenarios. As a result, the hospital was not reimbursed for the entire LOS at a loss of approximately $4000 per incident.

1. Who is responsible for the error?
2. What do you think should be done in this situation?
3. What steps can be taken to prevent this situation from recurring in the future?

Table 22.1 shows some examples of metrics. Metric descriptors contain more detailed information about what is to be measured and not measured. For example, if bedside nurses were measuring the rate of intravenous tubing labeled according to policy, they would further define what type of tubing is being used. Further exploration would determine whether data should include only primary intravenous lines or both primary and piggyback lines. Most likely the metrics would include both, but it is always best to be specific about what is to be counted. TJC surveyors typically look at these details.

Of primary importance, metrics and key indicators are developed after baseline data have been collected and careful consideration has been given to how things really exist before any actions toward improvement are implemented. Improvement should not be based on hearsay or what someone *thinks* the problems are. When baseline data are being collected, the QI nurse does not tell anyone what indicator is being measured. In this way, the true patterns of clinical practice can be discovered. Otherwise the results will not be as accurate or would be skewed.

The data are analyzed on a monthly or quarterly basis by the QI department. They are tracked and trended with graphic displays, such as run charts or graphs or bar graphs. Written committee reports are prepared to explain the graphs and to keep a record of the findings. Based on the results over time, new processes may need to be developed or more education done. The QI department personnel generally develop the final reports for major hospital committees, for the Chief Nursing Officer, and for other councils. Such reports are usually reviewed at each TJC visit. Thus we see that the contributions of each bedside nurse and the unit QI nurse are quite valuable in TJC survey process. TJC often commends hospitals based on their QI efforts.

What Are Core Measure Sets?

TJC mandates that organizations continuously track certain core measures to monitor quality care. Currently, there are 12 core measure sets. Each core measure includes certain performance measures that health care institutions track for reporting. Some of these include advance directives, autopsy rates, leaving against medical advice (AMA) and elopement rates, blood product use rates, blood transfusion reaction rates, conscious sedation complication rates, fall rates, medication error rates, mortality rates, pain management effectiveness, tobacco treatment rates, influenza vaccine administration rates, restraint use, perinatal care, rates of deep vein thrombosis, and surgical site infection rates. Simply put, these remain a part of TJC accreditation standards. Core measure sets are selected based on TJC problem areas that tend to recur. These may show the need for more extensive data collection or remedial action to resolve an identified problem. Regardless of whether there is improvement, TJC core measures must be continually tracked.

What Is Performance Improvement?

Performance improvement (PI) is synonymous with QI, and the terms are used interchangeably. Today, *improvement science* is the term often used, because the process has become very data driven. PI is a plan and documentation method that demonstrates what the standard procedures will be for nurses and others within the hospital. It includes changes that have been implemented based on previous data collection. PI is similar to the nursing process (assess, diagnose, plan, implement, and evaluate). Often QI nurses are called on to conduct small data collection processes and provide reports. Critical Thinking Box 22.2 provides a sample scenario so you can try out these skills.

? CRITICAL THINKING BOX 22.2

Metrics and Indicators

Your nursing unit has experienced a problem with the intravenous tubing not being labeled to show when it had to be changed. You are the quality improvement (QI) nurse who must collect data for a process improvement project. The nurse manager has asked you to determine baseline data for a month and report your findings to her.

1. How would you go about doing this?
2. What would be the indicators?
3. What would be the metrics?
4. How would you present the results tabulated for a month to the stakeholders or managers?

After the RM and QI departments assess performance within the hospital system regarding the patient care services rendered, a diagnosis of sorts is made that demonstrates where standards are not being met. We often use the Pareto principle by looking for the 20% of sources that caused 80% of the problems. Planning involves fixing the 20% that contributed to the problem. Implementation occurs as new strategies are put into place to resolve the problems or errors. Evaluation takes place as data are collected through time, demonstrating compliance or noncompliance with the new technique. If noncompliant, in-service education may be conducted to emphasize the problem areas, and the measurement process continues.

The US Pharmacopeial Convention (USP) has played a major role in collecting and trending medication error rates related to patient deaths. This organization has existed since 1820 to promote quality standards for medication use. In 1991, the USP began more intense investigation on the prevention of medication errors. With the increased use of herbal and dietary supplements by consumers, the USP has contributed to ongoing efforts in setting standards for dietary supplements. This organization has been instrumental in focusing on problems with both the product and the system where medications and dietary supplements are prescribed, dispensed, administered, and used (United States Pharmacopeia, 2018).

One important quality initiative started by the USP and now licensed to Quantros is the MEDMARX study, in which hospitals can enter their medication error data in an effort to help other hospitals understand why errors occur (Quantros, 2009). MEDMARX reports help hospital QI departments and nurses avoid similar errors in the future.

What Are the Barriers to Quality Improvement?

One of the primary barriers to implementing effective QI programs is cost. The cost of providing high-quality services within the health care organization has increased greatly during the past few decades. This is because of decreased payments from health insurance companies, including Medicare and Medicaid, as well as the increased costs of doing business. Health care organizations continue to look for ways to cut expenses by reducing the high cost of supplies or reducing staff. However, with the continuing shortage of qualified registered nurses, reducing the number of nurses is neither advisable nor acceptable, especially when we think about the errors that can occur as a result. Nevertheless, improving quality can help offset many of the internal costs of care. When quality is high, liability costs are typically low, and vice versa. Liability risks are often reduced as quality initiatives prevent problems from happening. Soon, the organization begins to reap the rewards of "fire prevention" rather than constant "firefighting." After the hospital organization realizes that the cost of a lawsuit for each death or disability related to a medication error far outweighs the cost of nurses, quality becomes critical. Other barriers to QI are nurses' loyalty to old practices and failure to recognize that changes based on evidence are needed.

Nurses are often unaware of the need to change or are unwilling to change their practice from the way they have always done things. Many practicing nurses remain resistant to change because it seems threatening and because it requires effort, retraining, and restructuring of habits. However, if we always do things the same old way, we will always receive the same results, which might not be good.

Many nurses have learned about how evidence-based practice (EBP) can help them in evaluating current practice. By looking into research studies about hospital issues and using EBP, nurses can make process changes that are tested in practice. This new knowledge provides the confidence nurses need when telling patients, physicians, and other nurses why they used specific practices. In addition, it is important to remain a lifelong learner of new information, especially because there is always uncertainty in decision making.

WHAT ARE SOME OTHER AGENCIES INFLUENCING PATIENT SAFETY?

The National Patient Safety Foundation (NPSF) is a nonprofit organization that for years has demonstrated a commitment to patient safety in health care by providing resources for both health care providers and consumers. Part of their mission is to promote understanding among caregivers and consumers. The NPSF holds an annual conference where patient safety knowledge is shared and research results are presented. The organization also funds research to improve safety and quality care (National Patient Safety Foundation, 2018).

The Institute for Healthcare Improvement (IHI) is another nonprofit organization that is highly involved in patient safety initiatives. Founded in 1991, the IHI works to advance QIs and conducts seminars and conferences on patient safety topics. Their website has free open school courses in quality, and anyone can take these minicourses. The IHI is also involved in helping organizations implement patient safety ideas. They offer learning modules in their "open school," where continuing education units or credits are offered (Institute for Healthcare Improvement, 2018).

The Quality and Safety Education for Nurses Institute (QSEN) site was developed to help prepare future nurses who will be needed in their health care environments to improve patient safety. The idea is to teach student nurses to always be thinking about how to improve care for patients. It began in 2005 when the American Association of Colleges of Nursing (AACN) emphasized the importance of QI system thinking in nursing education. They took the stance that nurses today ought to begin their nursing careers with knowledge about how to create and continuously improve systems of care.

Funded by the Robert Wood Johnson Foundation, the QSEN project group came up with six competencies for teaching QI (Table 22.2). These six core competencies include patient-centered care, teamwork and collaboration, evidence-based practice, QI, safety, and informatics. Within each category are specifics about knowledge, skills, and attitudes (KSAs).

TABLE 22.2 QSEN CORE NURSING COMPETENCIES
Obtained from: http://qsen.org/competencies/
• Patient-centered care
• Teamwork and collaboration
• Evidence-based practice
• Quality improvement
• Safety
• Informatics

In 2012, the QSEN project transitioned into the Case Western Reserve University QSEN Institute. A textbook entitled *Quality and Safety in Nursing: A Competency Approach to Improving Outcomes*—designed to have a lasting impact on nursing education—has been published. The continued focus of the institute's important work will be on educating faculty in graduate programs to teach quality and safety competencies (Quality and Safety Education for Nurses, 2018).

The Institute of Medicine (IOM) was established in 1970 as a nonprofit organization whose goal is to supply unbiased health care information so health care providers could make informed health decisions by providing reliable research evidence. In July 2016, the name was changed to the National Academy of Medicine (NAM) (2018).[1] This organization is responsible for several patient safety publications, including *To Err Is Human: Building a Safer Healthcare System; Keeping Patients Safe: Transforming the Work Environment of Nurses; Crossing the Quality Chasm: A New Health System for the 21st Century;* and *The Future of Nursing: Leading Change, Advancing Health* (NAM, 2018). In *The Future of Nursing* report, the IOM stresses the importance of nursing in ensuring high-quality health care for the nation. The report identifies the barriers that prevent nurses from practicing effectively. In conclusion, the report identifies eight recommendations that will reduce barriers to improving the nation's health care system (Table 22.3). For each recommendation, the research team identifies actions for educators, legislators, administrators, and nurses to ensure that these important changes are made. Most states have established "action coalitions" to support the initiation of these steps.

It is important to note that the report identifies nurses as key figures in promoting needed changes to support health, prevent illness, and care for patients with diverse and complex health care needs. Based on current research related to nursing care outcomes, the report stresses that a successful and safe health care system rests on advances in the education and autonomy of nurses.

The rationale for supporting the value of nurses is that they have specific strengths in such areas as care coordination, health promotion, and QI. Nurses can fill new and expanded roles in a redesigned health care system. This will require that they be allowed to practice in accordance with their professional training; they will also need higher levels of education, which will better prepare them to deliver patient-centered, equitable, safe, high-quality health care. They must be able to engage with physicians and other health care professionals to improve care and assume leadership roles in the redesign of the health care system. In this new system, primary care and disease prevention are the drivers. Payment is

TABLE 22.3 THE INSTITUTE OF MEDICINE'S RECOMMENDATIONS FOR THE FUTURE OF NURSING

- Remove scope of practice barriers.
- Expand opportunities for nurses to lead and diffuse collaborative improvement efforts.
- Implement nurse residency programs.
- Increase the proportion of nurses with a baccalaureate degree to 80% by 2020.
- Double the number of nurses with a doctorate by 2020.
- Ensure that nurses engage in lifelong learning.
- Prepare and enable nurses to lead change to advance health.
- Build an infrastructure for the collection and analysis of interprofessional health care workforce data.

Obtained from: http://iom.nationalacademies.org/Reports/2010/The-Future-of-Nursing-Leading-Change-Advancing-Health/Recommendations.aspx.

[1]Reports issued prior to June 30, 2015 will continue to be cited as IOM reports in perpetuity. Reports after that date will be located at this URL: http://nationalacademies.org/hmd/Reports.aspx

based on value, not quantity of services performed, which should slow the increasing costs of health care (IOM, 2011).

The IOM recommendations are available at the NAM website along with an abbreviated version of the entire report (http://nationalacademies.org/HMD/Reports/2010/The-Future-of-Nursing-Leading-Change-Advancing-Health.aspx).

Change is vital, improvement the logical form of change.

James Cash Penney

QUALITY IMPROVEMENT METHODS

There are several methods that serve to improve QI. Whatever approach is used, the values of the institution will be evident in the QI plan. For example, if an organization places emphasis on the prevention of worker injury, their CQI program will include this idea. Leadership personnel must be genuinely committed to CQI or it will not work. They must empower nurses and other employees to help plan and implement the needed strategies for change. Data must be collected systematically—not sporadically or on a whim. Blaming previous personnel for making mistakes does nothing to improve things. The work involves examining system issues with a proactive approach rather than always being reactive. This means anticipating risks and preventing them.

Many organizations use quality teams, working groups, or QCs to conduct much of the data collection and improvement techniques. These groups need to have a sense of collaboration and appreciation for the value and ideas each person brings to the table. They must be committed to being a part of the solution, not a part of the problem.

Some problems we typically encounter in hospitals are delays in room assignments, delays in medication delivery, delays in treatments or other care, and internal system delays (e.g., dietary, linen). All of these time delays ultimately cost us more. Yet efficient people may not even realize these time traps are occurring because they are so accustomed to developing and using "work arounds" to eliminate them (Pape, 2006). Work arounds are a safety threat, because working around something means getting around the problem instead of solving it. This can leave patients vulnerable to medication errors. An example of a work around is the habit of borrowing medications from another patient in the interest of saving time. This type of practice is dangerous and does nothing to solve the systemic problem. Perhaps the pharmacy technician missed placing the medication in the patient's drawer or put it in the wrong one.

Other people simply ignore these time traps or delays in getting their work done. Instead, they just put in their 8 or 12 hours and go home, hoping that perhaps tomorrow will be better. This is also not a productive way to solve problems on the nursing unit.

> Everyone wins when nurses join others who are willing to make things work well. Thus it is critical to know about current CQI methods.

TOOLS AND PROCESSES FOR CONTINUOUS QUALITY IMPROVEMENT

Tools for CQI include forms, methods, and analytic techniques that help to clarify a problem. Quality tools are more specific because they include tools applied to solving organizational or unit-specific problems. This discussion does not include all the tools that can be used for CQI but provides an overview of the more up-to-date tools used today (Fig. 22.4).

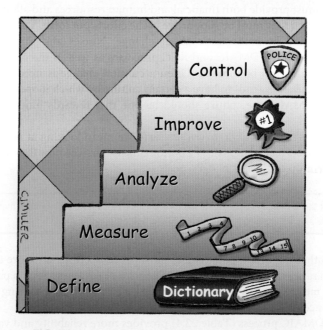

FIG. 22.4 Stair steps to high-quality health care.

What Is Six Sigma?

Six Sigma (SS) quality improvement methods are one approach taken to create a culture of safety management at the institutional level.

Sigma is a measurement standard that reflects how well a product or process is performing. In the 1920s, Walter Shewhart showed that three sigma from the mean is the point where errors start to occur. Shewhart was one of Edward Deming's teachers and is responsible for the PDSA cycle of process improvement. Credit for coining the term *Six Sigma* (SS) goes to Bill Smith of Motorola. SS uses statistics to improve the efficiency of business processes. The primary goal of SS is to increase profits and reduce problems by improving standard operating procedures, reducing errors, and decreasing misuse of the system.

SS methodology is used with improvement science and involves reducing variation in practice through the application of DMAIC. In other words, after a protocol has been found to be effective, everyone is trained to do it the same way. The SS DMAIC process is used primarily for improving existing processes that do not meet institutional goals or national norms. DMAIC can save companies thousands of dollars per project. SS means having no more than 3.4 defects per million opportunities, or 99.99966% accuracy. The idea is to focus on the voice of the customer (VOC), whether internal or external, and to reduce risks associated with high-volume, high-risk, problem-prone areas of practice. Internal customers are nursing staff that we work with and personnel from other departments. External customers include patients and visitors. This means that even the bedside nurse has a voice as an internal customer of the system. From the time DMAIC is adopted, nursing administrators must be supportive and trained in RCCs as a part of process improvement.

They must provide both financial and human resources and allow sufficient time for project teams to work. Then they must be supportive of the efforts put forth. The entire organization must be behind the effort and be enthusiastic about change. Nurses and other health care providers must be educated about the DMAIC and RCC processes as well. If the organizational culture is too resistant to change, this will be difficult. Often a cultural change is needed before the process can succeed. Every organization tends to have a certain culture by which it operates. When an organization is dealing with DMAIC, the culture should be one that rewards innovative ideas and is not resistant to change.

When referring to *data-driven methods,* we mean looking at real results that have been measured using numbers (calculations). The bottom line is that we know that we are not perfect, but we can strive to perform up to this 99.99966% goal.

> Let's put this goal into perspective. If you take a million blood pressure readings, there should be no fewer than 3.4 that are incorrect.

Another important point is that most processes function more effectively if they are kept within a certain range of error. The intent is to control peaks and valleys in performance (those things that are way off target). In this instance, a flat line is a good thing as long as it is near the 100% mark of compliance.

The DMAIC process (Table 22.4) provides more reliability and validity than other QI models and has become a national trend in QI strategies. Many companies will do business only with those who are using DMAIC.

RCTs of change are part of DMAIC. Recent use of the DMAIC model was found helpful in improving medication administration and reducing medication errors for several hospitals. As a result of a medication administration checklist, nurses' focus was improved and there was less variation in practice. Signs with the words "Do Not Disturb During Medication Administration" reminded other people of the process. The protocol checklists and signs remained as reminders to reduce distractions; they were simple, inexpensive tools that helped to keep patients safe. Nurses also liked them because they helped them to expedite their work (Pape, 2013; Pape et al., 2005).

In another QI project, an operating room team improved patient outcomes from postoperative hypothermia by using the DMAIC model. Because of the DMAIC team approach and the use of real data, patients' temperatures showed improvement in the postanesthesia care unit (PACU) because patients were warmed in the preoperative holding area before surgery (Bitner et al., 2007) (Research for Best Practice Box 22.1).

TABLE 22.4 DEFINE, MEASURE, ANALYZE, IMPROVE, CONTROL

DMAIC is pronounced *DUH-MAY-ICK* which includes:	
DEFINE	Define the issue, possible causes, and goals
MEASURE	Measure the existing system with metrics
ANALYZE	Analyze the gap between the existing system and goal
IMPROVE	Improve the system with creative strategies
CONTROL	Control and sustain the improvement

🔍 RESEARCH FOR BEST PRACTICE BOX 22.1

Nurse-Physician Rounding

Practice Issue

One of the most important steps for reducing error and improving efficiencies is in improving nurse-physician relationships. This quality improvement study considered the impact of nurse-physician rounding on making improvements to their practice and patient care (Burns, 2011).

   The study showed that using nurse-physician rounds in this 350-bed hospital did improve communication and efficiencies. The researchers began with a desire to improve patient satisfaction by having their medical needs met. Riegel and colleagues (2018) noted that rounding increased patient perception of communication with physician and nurse and decreased the number of telephone calls needed to clarify patient care. Another study by Brosey and March (2015) identified that structured hourly nurse rounding was an effective method to improve patient satisfaction and clinical outcomes and found that patient falls and hospital-acquired pressure ulcers decreased during the research project time period. Sharma and Klocke (2014) surveyed nursing staff before and after implementation of a patient-centered interprofessional (hospitalist-nurse) rounding process for patients. There was a substantial improvement in nursing staff satisfaction related to the improved communication and rounding by hospitalist providers. Patient-centered rounding also positively affected nursing workflow, nurses' perceptions of value as team members, and job satisfaction. Patient-centered rounding positively contributed to a transformation of a team-based collaborative model, thus enhancing interprofessional relationships.

Implications for Nursing Practice

- Nurse–physician relationships can improve through collaborative care.
- Of importance are frequent input and communication in planning and implementation of nurse-physician rounding projects.
- Support from management is critical to the success of physician–care provider–nurse rounding. The nurse manager needs significant coaching and intervention.
- Physician/care provider support is also critical to the success of the rounding process.
- Daily communication between physicians and nurses will promote the success of the process.
- A standardized rounding tool or checklist can assist patients, nurses, and physicians in communicating effectively (Johnson & Conner, 2014).
- The use of a simple inexpensive door sign can promote positive change in communication among health care professionals (Riegel, Delp, & Ward, 2018).
- Collaborative rounds between physicians and nurses can improve patient satisfaction scores.

Considering This Information

What would you do to promote collaborating with physicians or other health care providers?

References

Brosey, L. A., & March, K. S. (2015). Effectiveness of structured hourly nurse rounding on patient satisfaction and clinical outcomes. *Journal of Nursing Care Quality*, *30*(2), 153–159. https://doi.org/10.1097/NCQ.0000000000000086.

Burns, K. (2011). Nurse-physician rounds: A collaborative approach to improving communication, efficiencies, and perception of care. *Medsurg Nursing*, *20*(4), 194–199.

Johnson, B. T., & Conner, B. T. (2014). What works: Physician and nurse rounding improves patient satisfaction. *American Nurse Today*, *9*(12). Retrieved from http://www.americannursetoday.com/nurse-physician-rounding-patient-satisfaction/.

Pritts, K., & Hiller, L. G. (2014). Implementation of physician and nurse patient rounding on a 42-bed medical unit. *Medsurg Nursing*, *23*(6), 408–413.

Riegel, N., Delp, S., & Ward, C. W. (2018). Effects of nurse-physician collaborative rounding. *Medsurg Nursing*, *27*(3), 149–152.

Sharma, U., & Klocke, D. (2014). Attitudes of nursing staff toward interprofessional in-patient-centered rounding. *Journal of Interprofessional Care*, *28*(5), 475–477. https://doi.org/10.3109/13561820.2014.907558.

HOW DO WE USE DMAIC

The DMAIC flow diagram (Fig. 22.5) provides an overview of the DMAIC process. The framework shows how the process flows from start to finish and on to the next project. However, depending on the project, the steps may not always follow the path directed by the arrows. Depending on the situation, teams may sometimes have to change direction.

Sometimes the process may have to stop at the measure phase and go back to the design phase to develop formats for measuring. For example, the team may want to do some brainstorming or conduct RCCs to develop the best data collection format before moving on. Other times the format that was developed may not have worked, forcing the team to try using a different one. Now we see that the PDSA cycle also fits well with DMAIC (Fig. 22.6). The PDSA is a way to examine change by developing a strategy to test the change (*plan*), complete a test of the plan (*do*), review the results (*study*), and determine what modifications may be needed (*act*).

PDSA is used to plan and conduct RCCs although there is no "one size fits all" for organizations using DMAIC. Nevertheless, the organization must standardize the DMAIC process somewhat so that everyone can understand their roles and functions during each step. As indicated, the PDSA cycle is contained within the RCC; thus each project will be done slightly differently. The main focus is to keep on track with the goal in mind and to use real data, not guesswork or gossip, to direct decisions. As they say, if you do not measure it, you cannot fix it.

The Define Phase

In the define phase, a charter is developed as a written document of the work the team will accomplish. A charter is usually developed and agreed on among the team members as to what they see as the problem and where they want to go. First, they identify the business case, main goals, team leaders, and team responsibilities or roles. The business case is a statement about why it is important to consider resolving the problem in terms of cost, injury, or standards.

When team members are chosen, it is important to include only those who want to be part of the solution and not part of the problem. This is no place for whiners or complainers. Then set team rules (attendance, absence, how decisions are made). During meetings, ask that only one conversation go on at a time (no sidebars). Determine what the limits are on resources (financial, personal, time), and plan to discuss those.

Allow brainstorming during meetings. *Brainstorming* is a process by which a group of people think about, talk about, and list many solutions to a given problem. Some ideas may sound crazy at first, but group members should not ridicule them. The oddest ideas can often become very useful ones. Although this may cause some delays in meeting goals, it is a valuable part of the process. That is how great innovative ideas start. During meetings, identify who the stakeholders are and how they will be affected. Stakeholders are key people who will be affected by change and those who can either influence or derail the improvement. Consider how to sell ideas to the stakeholders. Also, identify support resources and supportive people. Who will provide the money and/or support the recommended changes?

Next, write the problem and goal statements. The problem statement will be similar to the business case. Write down the cost of doing nothing differently (firefighting) versus the cost of improving. These costs can be in dollar amounts or lost time, injury, errors, or dissatisfaction, for example. Set the goal in terms of how much saving is planned—10%? 25%? By what date?

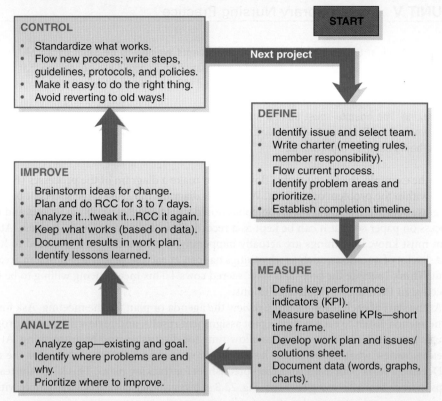

FIG. 22.5 This flow diagram provides an overview of the define, measure, analyze, improve, control (DMAIC) process using rapid cycle changes *(RCCs)*. The framework depicts the flow from the starting point, *define*, through *control*, and then to the next project. However, depending on the project, the process may not always follow the path directed by the arrows. Depending on the situation, teams may sometimes have to change direction.

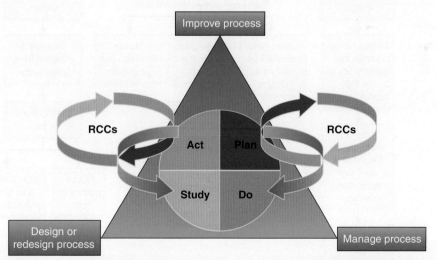

FIG. 22.6 The "Six Sigma" engine depicts the parts of define, measure, analyze, improve, control (DMAIC) to (1) improve processes, (2) design or redesign processes, and (3) manage processes. This diagram, designed by Dr. Tess Pape, depicts how the plan, do, study, act (PDSA) and rapid cycle changes (RCCs) tie into DMAIC. The most powerful difference between Six Sigma's DMAIC and other improvement methods is the precision used in finding and maintaining solutions to problems. The PDSA cycle also fits well with DMAIC. PDSA is used to plan and conduct RCCs tests of change. There is no "one size fits all" for organizations using DMAIC to move toward Six Sigma.

Example: Problem Statement—The number of patients waiting to be seen by an MD in the emergency department (ED) is excessive, and patients are dissatisfied. Controls are needed so that there will be a limited number of minutes between bed placement and MD arrival to bedside. Patients must be cared for efficiently so that they can get through the system in a timely manner, thus making room for more patients who are waiting. The hospital must contain costs and improve patient satisfaction.

Example: Goal Statement—There will be a 25% decrease in amount of time patients must wait in the ED before being seen by a physician.

In the example, the team would "flow out," or make a diagram of the processes (Fig. 22.7) that take place within the problem or the unit. When flow diagramming, use large sheets of paper or write on a dry erase board. If a board is used, someone should still take notes or obtain images and record the flow process on paper so that it can be kept as a record. Flow the current "as is" process. At this point, the team must know how things are actually happening, not how they are supposed to happen.

Ask a lot of questions, such as why things happen at each step. Identify problem areas for improvement. Think "outside the box" and slay "sacred cows"! This means being willing to be innovative and objective in thinking of possible solutions.

At the start of each team meeting, review the agenda or plan for the meeting. Ask for any additions to the agenda, listen to each person's past assignment results, and review the overall progress that individuals have made. It is important to allow time for discussion and brainstorming. At the end of the meeting, review what major points have been presented and set assignments for the next meeting.

Develop a work plan using an Excel spreadsheet for tracking plans. This keeps the team focused and helps to track brainstorming sessions. Fig. 22.8 shows another flow process example with a medication delivery process diagrammed systematically.

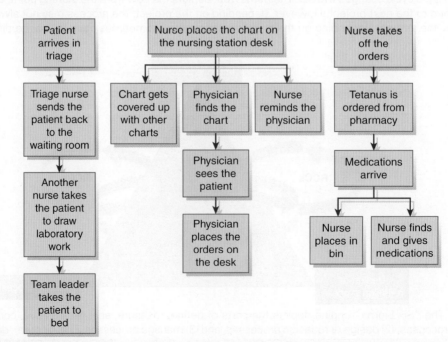

FIG. 22.7 This is a process-flow example of patient wait time. There are inputs, processes, and outputs in a typical flow diagram.

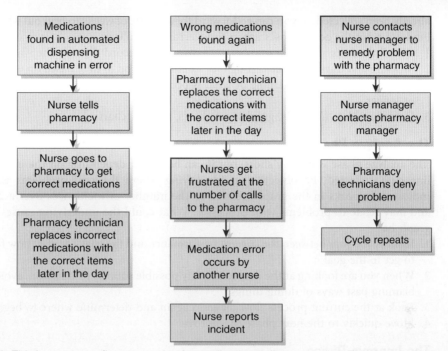

FIG. 22.8 This is a process-flow example of a medication delivery process. There are inputs, processes, and outputs in a typical flow diagram.

The Measure Phase

Everyone within the team must agree on what is to be measured. These are called *key performance indicators* (KPIs). KPIs should reflect the things that the team sees as problem areas. Typical KPIs are time, costs, distance, number of incidents, or items. It is best to use whole numbers (with decimals) and measurable facts. Never use what someone *thinks* is a problem. Measure the problem first. It is also important to identify who will be responsible for data collection, retrieval, and analysis. Ultimately, if the team fails to document everything, things will fall apart quickly.

Identify what specifically will be measured to determine improvements and what will not be measured. Operational definitions for the KPIs detail the thing or event using specific wording with written inclusion and exclusion criteria. These are similar to the metric descriptors discussed earlier. They define in detail what is to be measured and also what is not going to be measured. This helps get everyone in agreement on what is identifiable and measurable.

For example: KPI #1—The number of near-miss medication incidents on the nursing unit because of wrong medications found in the automated dispensing machine. We are including only those kept in the automated dispensing machine and are excluding any kept in other areas.

Begin by measuring baseline numbers. That is, start with what exists currently before any changes are made. In other words, do not meddle with things until you know how bad the problem is. Do not tell anyone what is being investigated or measured. Otherwise it could skew the measures, and you will not see any true changes when you do RCCs. Baseline measures can be retrospective if data have already been collected, or you can go forward for a couple of weeks to find out what the real data show. Find out what the actual losses are in time, errors, or dollars.

1. Get all the facts about the numbers of errors first. Record them in the work plan.
2. Measure and track the issue throughout a defined period of time based on what would be a realistic time frame to obtain a sample of what is occurring. This may have to be done for 2 to 4 weeks or longer.
3. Document data in words, graphs, pie charts, and bar charts.

The Analyze Phase

The analyze phase is usually short, but it can be longer depending on the issue. Analyze the baseline data collected. Be objective in identifying where the real problems exist. These may be indicated by peaks in the graphs related to the number of incidences over a 2- to 4-week period and may relate to problems with processes. What could the underlying causes of the peaks in the graph be?

1. Identify the *gaps* between the current performance and the goal. Identify how far you need to come to get to the goal.
2. When you are looking at the data to identify possible sources of variation, avoid blaming people or blaming past ways of doing things.
3. Look at the current process flow diagram again and determine where to begin making a change.
4. Move quickly to the next phase to improve.

The Improve Phase

The improve phase is a good place to determine whether measures reflect the true problems. The problem and goal statements may have to be revised based on the findings. The data collected may have shown that no real problem exists or that the problem involves other issues.

Now use the PDSA cycle (Table 22.5) to plan and implement some RCCs. The idea is to think of creative ways to improve things. Brainstorm ideas for the RCCs that you might try based on a problem

TABLE 22.5	**THE PLAN, DO, STUDY, ACT (PDSA) CYCLE WITHIN RAPID CYCLE CONTROL (RCC)**
PLAN	State the goal of the RCC cycle. Make predictions about what will be expected to happen. Who will be responsible, at what time, and where? When will it occur? Where will it take place first? What are we trying to accomplish? How will we know when we get there? Roughly, how far do we expect to come (percentage, minutes)? Use only data that are reflective of the key performance indicators (KPIs). For example, you would not measure the time it takes to do something if you were looking at the number of incidents. What change can we feasibly make that will result in improvement? Be realistic about what can be changed. How long should it take? How many days should you run the RCC to see a result? Keep it as short as possible; for example, 7–10 days.
DO	First, carry out the RCC on one or two nursing units for 3–7 days. If it needs tweaking, make a small change, and RCC again for 3–7 days or longer, depending on the issue. Then move to another nursing unit.
STUDY	Compare the resulting data to your predictions, to baseline, and contrast it to previous time frames. For example, what was the improvement in time compared with last week?
ACT	Act on what was discovered after the initial RCC. What are the new changes the team can make based on results? What might the next cycle be? Go on to do another RCC to improve the process further.

process step within the flow diagram and the baseline metrics. Brainstorming is the process where all team members spontaneously contribute and gather ideas without excluding any idea given. It is usually performed rapidly, with all ideas considered and recorded. Be clear about what the target is and play off of each other's suggestions.

The group may consider using a fair voting method or writing out RCC ideas, so that all ideas can be obtained without factors that might influence unbiased sharing. The collective ideas can then be reviewed by the group leader and presented to the group.

1. Ask yourself "Can a step in the process be eliminated?" Simplifying steps and deleting steps in a process can often eliminate big defects.
2. Can a new method be tried?
3. Next, conduct the RCC using the PDSA cycle (see Table 22.5) for 3 to 7 days. Include staff education before starting the RCC so that everyone understands what is expected.
4. Conduct the RCC and study the results. Document everything in the work plan.
5. Analyze the data with percentage calculations for improvements over baseline for the previous week.
6. Document all brainstorming sessions.

Use data to determine whether there were improvements or a lack of improvement. What percentage of improvement was there this week compared with last week? Compared with the baseline measure? How many minutes difference is there? Make decisions based on fact, not assumptions. Small improvements still mean improvement, and they help determine whether you are on the right track or not.

Small changes may have to be made in the process that was tried, so tweak it and test it again with a change in the RCC over 3 to 7 days. Compare percentages again (against baseline or the previous week) and determine whether there was any improvement.

Market the solutions to the people whose cooperation is needed. If frontline people have been involved at the outset, this part is easier. Prepare for possible objections to the implementation of the change, and plan to overcome them.

The Control Phase

Now you are ready to establish controls to keep things going in the right direction. Controlling and sustaining the improvement is not easy and requires the development, documentation, and implementation of an ongoing monitoring plan.

1. Standardize the steps in the new process and detail new flow diagrams. Write standard operating procedures, protocols, steps, guidelines, or policies so that it will be easier for people to do the right thing and more difficult for them to do the wrong thing.
2. Educate everyone about the new practice. Distribute the information in a systematic manner so that everyone in the organization has an equal chance of being informed. Educate new employees in correct procedures and be an example for them to follow.
3. Keep people informed of any changes.
4. Prevent reversion back to old ways or breaks in the "critical links" in the process by developing a process to monitor that changes have stuck, and gains are sustained. Keep the process on its new course and maintain the new practices you worked so hard to develop. Backsliding can occur easily because people tend to return to old habits. Change can be difficult when people are faced with an unfamiliar or new situation.
5. Continue to measure KPIs routinely to see whether solutions are still working. If slipping occurs, reinforce the new change or do more RCCs.

BOX 22.3   AN EXAMPLE OF DEFINE, MEASURE, ANALYZE, IMPROVE, CONTROL (DMAIC) IN THE EMERGENCY DEPARTMENT

Problem statement: A physician does not see emergency department patients in a timely manner.

Define

The team *defined* the cause of the problem as having to do with where the charts were placed.

   Goal: Get the charts to the physicians sooner.

   Business case: Cost of doing nothing different = Unhappy patients, possible patient complications, lack of bed space, and bottlenecks throughput.

Measure

Key performance indicator (KPI) #1 = Time between patient bed placement and being seen by physician.

   The team *measured* the actual average baseline data (KPI #1) during a 2-week period. Baseline = 90 min (15 min).

   Target = Patients should be seen within 30 min of bed placement (a 50% improvement) within a month.

Analyze

The team *analyzed* the gap between the existing situation and the goal of 30 min (gap = 60 min). The gap also depended on which physician was on duty.

   Can something be done about which physician is on duty? Not really.

   The team brainstormed for other ideas. Could something be done about where charts were placed? Yes.

Improve

The team *improved* by doing rapid cycle changes (RCCs).

   KPI #1 = Time of patient bed placement to seen by physician.

   RCC #1: For the next 5 days, the team members who were involved placed charts in a separate bin and measured KPI #1.

   Result = The physician saw patients on time 34% of the time. So the team tweaked the plan and did more RCCs.

   RCC #2: For the next 5 days they placed charts on a separate bedside table (the deck) and set up a log book of times when the charts were placed and picked up.

   Still measured KPI #1 = Time of patient bed placement to time seen by physician and added another KPI.

   KPI #2 = Time between charts placed on deck and picked up from deck.

   Result = Physician saw patients on time 20% of the time.

   The team again brainstormed, tweaked the plan, and did more RCCs.

   Next 5 days, one physician was assigned as deck officer to oversee the process.

   Result = physician saw patients on time 99% of the time within 30 min.

Control

The team *controlled* and sustained the improvement by establishing a standard practice.

   They wrote a protocol and announced the new practice.

   The protocol was always to place charts on deck and to assign a deck officer to monitor the timeliness of chart retrieval.

   The department director monitored effectiveness of the protocol and watched for slippage into the old ways.

Box 22.3 provides a simplified example of DMAIC used successfully in one emergency department. Many of the important details have been left out because of limited space. However, the basic process can be seen. Now see what you can do with the DMAIC process on a small scale using the scenario in Critical Thinking Box 22.3.

> ### ? CRITICAL THINKING BOX 22.3
>
> A retrospective review of several charts showed that documentation for 40% of prn medications was lacking a previous assessment of pain. About 50% of the charts did not have documentation that the pain was evaluated according to policy within 30–45 min after the prn medication was administered. You have been asked to lead a team to resolve the problems that occurred mainly on your nursing unit.
> 1. What standard of practice has been violated?
> 2. How would you go about conducting your problem resolution using the DMAIC approach for process improvement?
> 3. Who would you include on your team?
> 4. Who will develop the work plan and issue solutions sheet?
> 5. When will meetings be held? What are the ground rules?
> 6. What is the business case?
> 7. What are the goals and targets?
> 8. What are the KPIs?
> 9. What RCC can be performed?
> 10. Imagine that you have some excellent RCC results. What will you do to control the improvement?

KPI, Key performance indicator; *RCC*, rapid cycle change.

> Practice improves results with time, and it can be a lot of fun.

HEALTH CARE PROVIDER CREDENTIALING FOR QUALITY IMPROVEMENT

Some larger health care organizations require that an individual obtain a certification in health care quality within a certain period after the hire date. Persons can become a *Certified Professional in Healthcare Quality* (CPHQ) after taking a certification test to determine their knowledge of quality management, QI, case/care/disease/utilization management, and risk management at all employment levels and in all health care settings.

Although there is no longer a minimum education requirement, those who test should have worked in quality management for a minimum of 2 years and should review testing requirements before investing money into taking the examination. Approximately 75% of those who apply to test actually achieve certification.

HEALTH LITERACY

Health literacy is a key issue in today's health care. It is addressed in Healthy People 2020 and is a common thread in health care programs. The HHS defines health literacy as the degree to which individuals have the capacity to obtain, process, and understand the basic health information needed to make appropriate health decisions (HHS, 2019). A goal of health literacy in to improve a person's ability to be accountable for his or her health as well as the health of his or her family. Some examples of poor health literacy include not being able to understand prescription labels or health-related materials, inability to locate needed services or manage chronic health problems, or poor communication with providers. In addition, health literacy is not just the result of individual abilities but also the health literacy–related demands of a very complex health care system. Low health literacy may lead to a variety of negative outcomes for the patient. For example, communication barriers between a provider and the patient have been associated with increased hospitalizations, the inability to make health-related decisions, and failure to adhere to a treatment regimen (ODPHP, n.d.).

Nurses play an important role in improving health literacy. It is important to identify patients' specific health literacy levels and make simple communication adjustments. These may include providing assistance with completing complex forms, using simple language and defining technical terms, using mixed media such as video, models or illustrations, and being culturally sensitive. Health care professionals must work together to ensure that health information and services can be understood and used by all their patients. We must engage in skill building with health care consumers and health care providers. Nurses can be productive partners in reaching adults with limited literacy skills (HRSA, 2017).

CONCLUSION

Quality is about fire prevention, not firefighting, and accountability for one's actions is critical in nursing. We must provide quality of care that is cost-effective and meets the health needs of our patients. We do not have the luxury of giving a patient all the time we would like or using any equipment and supplies we might want. That is why it is important to find safe solutions that save time and money. Nurses must be accountable to both the quality of care and the economics of providing that care. In QI, the organization must first consider the voice of the customer, whether internal or external. The "squeaky wheel" issues sometimes occur where organizations start implementing improvements. However, action should be taken first on matters associated with high-volume, high-risk, problem-prone practices and where errors frequently occur. Proven methods for QI should be emphasized in all health care settings.

DMAIC is one method for improving quality, and it should be taught as a standard process so that everyone in the organization understands the roles and functions during each step. PDSA is used to plan and conduct rapid cycle tests of change. Certainly, each organization must evaluate using DMAIC to move toward Six Sigma. The future of quality and patient safety is promising, as more and more health care providers and organizations are committed to investing time, education, and resources for safety changes. Improvement is everyone's business, as cost savings are realized with improved processes and reduced liability. Increasingly, nurses are required to know about QI processes as soon as they begin their careers. See the end of this chapter for relevant websites and online resources that will serve as great resources for you while you are in nursing school and in your professional practice, so be sure to check them out! The future of health care will demand more vigilance as the Affordable Care Act takes the nursing profession in new directions.

> Change is inevitable; it is the one thing you can always count on. Things will never be exactly as they once were. So, if you want to prevent other people from making changes for you, you have to get involved in the process. Rather than resist change, embrace it and make it yours! He who fails to invent change is at the mercy of those who will! Regardless of what is going on around you, remember that as a nurse you have a responsibility to provide care in a way that is research-based and follows best practices. It means that nurses must monitor the health care delivery process and evaluate outcomes to ensure high-quality care.

RELEVANT WEBSITES AND ONLINE RESOURCES

Agency for Healthcare Research and Quality (AHRQ)
AHRQ Innovation exchange. http://www.innovations.ahrq.gov/.
AHRQ Innovation exchange—checklists with medication vest or sash reduce distractions during medication administration.
  https://innovations.ahrq.gov/profiles/checklists-medication-vest-or-sash-reduce-distractions-during-medication-administration
AHRQ's mistake-proofing the design of health care processes. http://archive.ahrq.gov/professionals/quality-patient-safety/
  patient-safety-resources/resources/mistakeproof/index.html
AHRQ's patient safety network. https://psnet.ahrq.gov/

Centers for Medicare & Medicaid Services (CMS)
http://www.cms.gov/.

HCAHPS
HCAHPS: Patients' perspectives of care survey. https://www.cms.gov/Medicare/Quality-Initiatives-Patient-Assessment-Instruments/
  HospitalQualityInits/HospitalHCAHPS.html

Health Resources & Services Administration (HRSA)
https://www.hrsa.gov/
Health literacy. https://www.hrsa.gov/about/organization/bureaus/ohe/health-literacy/index.html

Institute for Healthcare Improvement (IHI)
http://www.IHI.org/.
IHI Open School. http://www.ihi.org/education/ihiopenschool/overview/Pages/default.aspx
Transforming care at the bedside. http://www.ihi.org/offerings/Initiatives/PastStrategicInitiatives/TCAB/Pages/Materials.aspx

Institute for Safe Medication Practices (ISMP)
http://www.ismp.org/.

Institute of Medicine (now the National Academy of Medicine (NAM)
http://nationalacademies.org/hmd/About-HMD.aspx

Little K
Creating run charts. http://www.youtube.com/watch?v=03-8vtwCW9c.

National Patient Safety Foundation (NPSF) (combined with IHI in May 2017)
https://www.npsf.org/page/aboutus

Office of Disease Prevention and Health Promotion (ODPHP)
Health literacy. https://www.healthypeople.gov/2020/topics-objectives/topic/social-determinants-health/interventions-resources/
  health-literacy

Press Ganey
Nursing Database of Nursing Quality Indicators (NDNQI). http://www.pressganey.com/solutions/clinical-excellence/nursing-quality

Quality and Safety Education for Nurses Institute (QSEN)
http://qsen.org/.

The Joint Commission (TJC)
http://www.jointcommission.org/.
2019 National patient safety goals. http://www.jointcommission.org/standards_information/npsgs.aspx.

The Joint Commission Center for Transforming Healthcare
Safety culture. http://www.centerfortransforminghealthcare.org/projects/detail.aspx?Project=6.

World Health Organization (WHO)
http://www.who.int/en/.

BIBLIOGRAPHY

Agency for Healthcare Research and Quality (AHRQ). (2018). Systems approach. Retrieved from https://psnet.ahrq.gov/primers/primer/21.

Bitner, J., et al. (2007). A team approach to the prevention of unplanned postoperative hypothermia. *AORN Journal, 85*, 921–929.

Centers for Medicare & Medicaid Services. (2018a). 2018 Reporting—ACO measures narrative. Retrieved from https://www.cms.gov/Medicare/Medicare-Fee-for-Service-Payment/sharedsavingsprogram/Downloads/2018-reporting-year-narrative-specifications.pdf.

Centers for Medicare & Medicaid Services. (2018b). Hospital compare. Retrieved from https://www.cms.gov/medicare/quality-initiatives-patient-assessment-instruments/hospitalqualityinits/hospitalcompare.html.

Centers for Medicare & Medicaid Services. (2019). Quality measures and reporting specifications. Retrieved from https://www.cms.gov/Medicare/Medicare-Fee-for-Service-Payment/sharedsavingsprogram/Quality-Measures-Standards.html.

Federal Drug Administration (FDA). (2017). Medication error reporting. Retrieved from https://www.fda.gov/Drugs/DrugSafety/MedicationErrors/ucm080629.htm.

HCAHPS. (2017). *HCAHPS:* Patients' perspectives of care survey. Retrieved from https://www.cms.gov/Medicare/Quality-Initiatives-Patient-Assessment-instruments/HospitalQualityInits/HospitalHCAHPS.html.

Institute for Healthcare Improvement. (2018). History. Retrieved from http://www.ihi.org/about/pages/history.aspx.

Institute of Medicine. (2011). The future of nursing: Leading change, advancing health. Committee on the Robert Wood Johnson Foundation initiative on the future of nursing, at the Institute of Medicine (pp. 1–620). National Academy of Sciences. Retrieved from *http://nationalacademies.org/HMD/Reports/2010/The-Future-of-Nursing-Leading-Change-Advancing-Health.aspx.*

Institute of Medicine. (2001). Crossing the quality chasm: A new health system for the 21st century. Retrieved from http://www.nationalacademies.org/hmd/Reports/2001/Crossing-the-Quality-Chasm-A-New-Health-System-for-the-21st-Century.aspx.

Makary, M. A., & Daniel, M. (2016). Medical error—the third leading cause of death in the US. *BMJ, 353,* Retrieved from http://www.bmj.com/content/353/bmj.i2139.long.

National Academy of Medicine (formerly Institute of Medicine). (2018). About the NAM. Retrieved from https://nam.edu/about-the-nam/. http://nationalacademies.org/hmd/about-hmd/division-name.aspx.

National Patient Safety Foundation. (2018). About us. Retrieved from https://www.npsf.org/page/aboutus.

Office of Disease Prevention and Health Promotion. (2018). Midcourse review. Retrieved from https://www.healthypeople.gov/2020/data-search/midcourse-review.

Pape, T. M. (2013). The effect of a five-part intervention to decrease omitted medications. *Nursing Forum, 48,* 211–222. https://doi.org/10.1111/nuf.12025.

Pape, T. M. (2006). Workaround error, AHRQ WebM&M cases and commentaries. Retrieved from https://psnet.ahrq.gov/webmm/case/118.

Pape, T. M., et al. (2005). Innovative approaches to reducing nurses' distractions during medication administration. *Journal of Continuing Education in Nursing, 36,* 33–39.

Quality and Safety Education for Nurses Institute. (2018). Quality and safety education for nurses (QSEN) Institute. Retrieved from http://qsen.org/.

Quantros. (2009). MEDMARX: Adverse drug event reporting. Retrieved from https://www.medmarx.com/docs/about.pdf.

Shojania, K. G., & Dixon-Woods, M. (2017). Estimating deaths due to medical error: The ongoing controversy and why it matters. *BMJ Quality and Safety, 26,* 423–428.

The Joint Commission. (2018). Sentinel event alert. Retrieved from http://www.jointcommission.org/topics/hai_sentinel_event.aspx.

The Joint Commission. (2018). Core measure sets. Retrieved from http://www.jointcommission.org/core_measure_sets.aspx.

The Joint Commission. (2018). 2019 National Patient Safety Goals. Retrieved from http://www.jointcommission
.org/standards_information/npsgs.aspx.

U.S. Department of Health and Human Services, Office of Disease Prevention and Health Promotion. (2019).
Health literacy. Retrieved from https://health.gov/communication/about.asp.

U.S. Department of Health and Human Services. (2018). Medication errors and adverse drug events. Retrieved
from https://psnet.ahrq.gov/primers/primer/23/medication-errors.

United States Pharmacopeia. (2018). Retrieved from http://www.usp.org/.

23

Nursing Informatics

Cheryl D. Parker, PhD, RN-BC, CNE, FHIMSS

ⓔhttp://evolve.elsevier.com/Zerwekh/nsgtoday/.

*If we cannot name it [nursing practice], we cannot control it, finance it,
research it, teach it, or put it into public policy.*
Norma M. Lang, PhD, RN, FAAN, FRCN

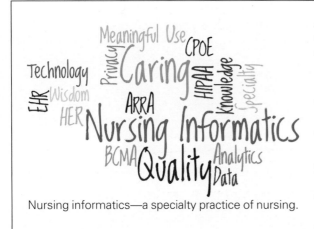

Nursing informatics—a specialty practice of nursing.

After completing this chapter, you should be able to:
- Define nursing informatics.
- Discuss the necessity of using recognized taxonomies and standardized nursing languages in nursing documentation.
- Discuss laws and regulations impacting nursing informatics.
- Discuss trends associated with the computerized electronic record, e-health, and mobile devices.
- Describe what a nurse specializing in nursing informatics might do.
- Review the steps in evaluating the validity of a website.
- Discuss future trends in nursing informatics.

At the crossroads of technology and patient care stand the nurses who have chosen nursing informatics (NI) as their specialty. Nursing informatics is a well-established specialty within nursing, which today has evolved to be an integral part of health care delivery and a differentiating factor in the selection, implementation, and evaluation of health IT that supports safe, high-quality, patient-centric care.
Healthcare Information Management Systems Society (HIMSS) Position Paper: Transforming Nursing Practice through Technology & Informatics, June 17, 2011

Computer technology is pervasive today. Everywhere we turn, technology is in evidence. The neighborhood grocery store has automated scanners and checkout lines. Your bank has automated tellers, check scanners, wire transfers, and online services. The school and local libraries have automated catalogs, interlibrary lending, and online books. From our homes and smartphones, we can access the world through the Internet. We can research any question, text, e-mail, watch streaming videos, and purchase just about anything. You can complete an advanced degree without ever stepping foot on a campus with a faculty and fellow students who can be literally half a world away. A litany of computerized marvels could fill volumes.

Technology has impacted our culture in multiple ways. When answering machines were first introduced, many people considered their use to be quite rude. Now, just the opposite is true—it is rude if your voice mailbox is full. Sending handwritten invitations with an RSVP has been replaced with online invites and automatic tracking of accepts and declines.

The explosion of new technology since the early 1980s that makes all this possible is truly phenomenal. What is even more incredible, and perhaps a bit frightening to some, is this seems to be just the beginning. The time will come when the thoughts, communications, creations, manuscripts, learning material, and financial assets of the civilized world exist primarily in electronic form. If the lights went out, civilization as we know it would cease to exist, as most of the modern society depends on the electrical and information infrastructure.

Health care is not immune. Some of the most complex automated systems, and certainly some of the most complex requirements for these systems, can be found in the health care environment. Systems to serve the diverse needs of the health care industry—from the administration and financial departments to the many clinical disciplines—need to be implemented and integrated across the continuum of care within modern health care organizations. As a result, the demand for health care professionals who are knowledgeable in the application of this technology is growing rapidly.

Even with technology all around us, some users do not always feel comfortable with it, especially in the patient care environment where everything may be new and seem ever-changing. Even so, there are some relative constants that make the field less confusing and easier to manage. The goal of this chapter is not to make you a computer guru or even an entry-level informatics nurse (IN), but, given that technology touches almost every patient encounter, you do need to know the basics of how to use and troubleshoot it. Consider the use of glucometers; few of us understand exactly how they analyze the blood sample from a technical level, but we need to know how to use them, how to change batteries or charge them, and how to figure out what an error code means and what to do about it.

The goal of this chapter is to explore how nursing and health care are embracing, harnessing, and using technology to increase the quality of patient care in all health care settings.

> Always remember that technology is only a tool to help us care for our patients. It should never replace our critical thinking and nursing judgment!

NURSING INFORMATICS

Nursing Informatics: Why Do I Care?

In the back of your mind you may be thinking, "So why do I care about nursing informatics and technology? I'm still learning to take care of patients." Well, in today's world, technology and patient care are completely interwoven. From the electronic medical record (EMR) to the devices you will use to monitor and care for your patients to the accumulation of data that will allow you to provide care most effectively, technology and informatics are a part of our daily nursing practice whether we realize it or not. Look at Fig. 23.1 and see how many technology-enabled items you can pick out. And who knows? Maybe someday you will decide that nursing informatics (NI) is the specialty for you. However, even if you don't see yourself in an informatics role in the future, information management and application of patient care technologies are part of the American Association of Colleges of Nursing (AACN)

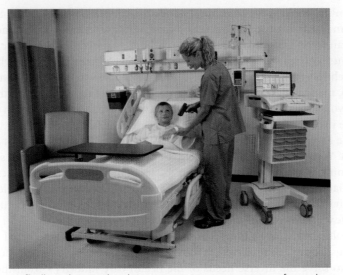

FIG. 23.1 Nurses are finding that technology supports many areas of nursing practice. (Courtesy Rubbermaid Healthcare, Huntersville, NC). Now owned by Capsa Healthcare. https://www.capsahealthcare.com/contact-us.

Essentials of Baccalaureate Education for Professional Nursing Practice (2008). Those who are in more advanced nursing roles at the Master's and DNP levels also have informatics included in their AACN Essentials (AACN, 2006; AACN, 2011).

What Is Nursing Informatics?

In 1994, the American Nurses Association (ANA) recognized the field of NI. In 2015, the ANA updated the definition of NI as "the specialty that integrates nursing science with multiple information management and analytical sciences to identify, define, manage, and communicate data, information, knowledge, and wisdom in nursing practice" (ANA, 2015, p. 1).

The ANA further identified two distinct roles in NI: the IN and the informatics nurse specialist (INS). The IN has experience in NI but does not have an advanced degree in the specialty. The INS has graduate-level education in informatics or a related field (ANA, 2015). Nurses in both IN and INS roles "support nurses, consumers, patients, the interprofessional health care team, and other stakeholders in their decision-making in all roles and settings to achieve desired outcomes. This support is accomplished through the use of information structures, information processes, and information technology" (ANA, 2015, p. 2).

With the advent of both specialty and integrated clinical information systems (CIS), the longitudinal electronic health record (EHR) has become the goal of health care organizations and is now supported by federal mandate. The EHR will reflect a record of patients' health care throughout their lives. Although this realization of 100% integrated patient data in one longitudinal electronic record is becoming more technologically feasible, few organizations have reached this goal. There are still outstanding issues regarding how to handle outside information that comes into a facility; for example, old systems may not be able to interface with new ones, corrupt data may be received from old systems, and resources may be unavailable to enter all the data from old paper charts. Although solutions are being developed to solve some of these problems, it will take time to reach the ultimate goal.

Information is power. The extensive clinical background of the IN/INS is invaluable to the success of the implementation of the hardware and software applications needed to transform health care.

Nurses have a unique understanding of workflow, the hospital and clinical environment, and the specific procedures that are necessary for effective health care information infrastructure. Moreover, the IN/INS roles are critical members of the team when translating information into practical models that can be applied to improve the health care systems and patient outcomes.

The 2015 Healthcare Information Management Systems Society (HIMSS) Informatics Nurse Impact Survey asked organizational leaders to provide input on the roles and impact of INs in their organizations. Organizations responding to this survey included hospital or health systems (75%), vendor or consulting firms (4%), and other organizations such as home health, ambulatory care facilities, and academic or government facilities. Nearly all respondents noted that INs play a significant role in user education. INs are also widely involved in workflow analysis, patient safety, compliance with policies and regulations, quality outcomes, system implementation, user support, and gaining buy-in from end users (HIMSS, 2015). In short, the focus of NI is to improve patient care with health care technology that encourages clinicians to make more accurate and timely decisions.

So how does one become an expert in this unique field of nursing? What does a nurse specializing in NI do on a daily basis? How does informatics impact the work of a clinical nurse? Let's explore the answers to all of these questions.

Experience and Education

In the past, many nurses in informatics roles did not have formal education beyond their nursing preparation. They were "recruited" by their employers to help build and implement an EMR application. These nurses learned on the job, and advanced degrees were not required; however, this is no longer true. According to the 2017 HIMSS Nursing Informatics Workforce Survey, "fifteen percent have received on-the-job training and more than half of the 2011 respondents reported having a postgraduate degree (56 percent), which includes Masters in Nursing or other field/specialty and PhD in Nursing or other field/specialty."

INs who want to hold leadership roles in NI will need graduate-level preparation. A student who held a leadership role in NI and was enrolled in a NI master's program once said that she thought she knew all about NI, but she learned that she only knew about it at her own organizational level. Her graduate-school education had broadened her perspectives and introduced her to new concepts and ways of thinking (C. Parker, 2011, personal communication).

Role of the Informatics Nurse/Informatics Nurse Specialist (IN/INS)

The IN/INS must have a basic knowledge of how computers and networks work as well as an understanding of system analysis, design principles, and information management (IM). It is important for the IN/INS to converse with both the clinical staff and the technology staff regarding hardware, software, communications, data representation, and security. An IN/INS will be comfortable with software and hardware implementation, training, testing, presenting, and facilitating knowledge (Critical Thinking Box 23.1).

? CRITICAL THINKING BOX 23.1

What has been your experience and exposure to the use of technology in the hospital? Your school? At home? Think of ways to become more familiar with the use of computers and other technology.

Currently, the majority of IN/INSs are working with EMRs/electronic health care records (EHR) development and implementations. Typical job responsibilities consist of (1) product evaluation; (2) system implementation, including preparing users, training, and providing support; (3) system development and quality initiatives, including system evaluations/problem solving and quality improvement/patient safety; and (4) other duties as assigned (HIMSS Nursing Informatics Workforce Survey, 2017).

It is important to note that not all nurses in IN/INS roles work on implementation of the EMR/EHR. Some work for health care product vendors in both the hardware and software areas. They help inform the next generation of existing products, and they work with engineers/design teams to create new products, always bringing the patient care viewpoint and the needs of the end user to the design process. Others work for consulting firms and specialize in workflow improvement using technology, whereas others still work for government, third-party payers, and educational institutions (HIMSS Nursing Informatics Workforce Survey, 2017). The variety is seemingly endless.

The Certification Process

In 1994, the American Nursing Credentialing Center (ANCC) provided a method for nurses to become certified in this specialty. The baccalaureate degree is the minimum requirement needed to take the certification exam. Nurses can obtain RN-BC certification in informatics nursing through the ANCC.

PROFESSIONAL PRACTICE, TRENDS, AND ISSUES

What Are Regulatory and Accreditation Requirements?

Although there are many regulatory and governmental agencies instituting health care policy, the Health Insurance Portability and Accountability Act (HIPAA) and The Joint Commission (TJC) impact the daily work of every clinician and organization. The nurse must have a clear understanding of HIPAA regulations and of TJC requirements to be able to provide safe nursing care.

Privacy and Confidentiality

Every health care organization has a responsibility to itself, to its patients, and to the community at large to maintain control of its information systems. Because the internal workings of health care rely on accurate and current data and information, personal data about employees and patients must be kept safe and confidential. A corporate security plan is essential to all health care organization. Maintaining confidentiality implies a trust of the individuals who handle that data and information. These health care workers ensure the privacy of this information and use it only for the purposes for which it was disclosed.

Security policies must be explicit and well defined. Confidentiality agreements should be reviewed and signed when starting employment and yearly thereafter. Breaches of security, confidentiality, or privacy should be addressed and resolved quickly, and the offender should be charged accordingly. Every lapse should be treated openly and used as an example for others to take note of. The IN may be involved in the investigation process and the writing of the policies and procedures.

Health Insurance Portability and Accountability Act of 1996

In 1996, the HIPAA of 1996 was signed into law. The law defines the standards that were developed to ensure that health care organizations collect the right data in a common format so that the data can be shared as well as protect the privacy and security of patient data. The major impact from this regulatory legislation is in these areas are as follows:

- Health information privacy law
- Data security standards
- Electronic transaction standards

To comply with many requirements, health care entities must adopt written privacy policies and procedures that define how they intend to abide by the highly complex regulations and how they will protect individually identifiable health information. It is the responsibility of health care organizations to ensure that all staff members who have access to patient information understand the consequences of noncompliance with HIPAA.

In 1998, it was proposed that all health plans, health plan providers, and health care clearinghouses that maintain or transmit health information electronically be required to establish and maintain responsible and appropriate safeguards to ensure the integrity and confidentiality of the information. Although this seems logical, it is a very difficult and time-consuming task when using automated systems that did not previously meet these requirements (Critical Thinking Box 23.2).

? CRITICAL THINKING BOX 23.2

How have your clinical facility and/or school made changes to accommodate the Health Insurance Portability and Accountability Act (HIPAA) requirements?

The year 2013 brought another wave of "sweeping change" to the HIPAA Privacy, Security, Enforcement, and Breach Notification Rules according to Leon Rodriguez, director of the HHS Office for Civil Rights. HHS Secretary Kathleen Sebelius stated, "The new rule will help protect patient privacy and safeguard patients' health information in an ever expanding digital age." According to the January 17, 2013, press release issued by the US Department of Health and Human Services:

> The changes in the final rulemaking provide the public with increased protection and control of personal health information. The HIPAA Privacy and Security Rules have focused on health care providers, health plans and other entities that process health insurance claims. The changes announced today expand many of the requirements to business associates of these entities that receive protected health information, such as contractors and subcontractors. Some of the largest breaches reported to HHS have involved business associates. Penalties are increased for noncompliance based on the level of negligence, with a maximum penalty of $1.5 million per violation. The changes also strengthen the Health Information Technology for Economic and Clinical Health (HITECH) Breach Notification requirements by clarifying when breaches of unsecured health information must be reported to HHS.
>
> Individual rights are expanded in important ways. Patients can ask for a copy of their electronic medical record in an electronic form. When individuals pay by cash they can instruct their provider not to share information about their treatment with their health plan. The final omnibus rule sets new limits on how information is used and disclosed for marketing and fundraising purposes and prohibits the sale of an individual's health information without their permission.
>
> The final rule also reduces burden by streamlining individuals' ability to authorize the use of their health information for research purposes. The rule makes it easier for parents and others to give permission to share proof of a child's immunization with a school and gives covered entities and business associates up to one year after the 180-day compliance date to modify contracts to comply with the rule. (U.S. Department of Health & Human Services, 2013a)

Violation of HIPAA standards carries serious consequences. Violations of health information privacy can lead to termination of employment and even indictment and prison time. In 2010, a former researcher at the UCLA School of Medicine was sentenced to 4 months in federal prison and was fined $2000 for violations of the HIPAA privacy rule. He accessed 323 confidential patient records of high-profile actors, without a valid reason or authorization but without profiting from it through the sale or use of the information (Dimick, 2010).

Although criminal penalties are rare, they can happen. Civil penalties in the form of fines to individuals and organizations are more common. If a data breach affects more than 500 individuals, Section 13402 (e) (4) of the HITECH Act requires that the secretary of the US Department of Health and Human Services post notification of the covered entity on the HHS website found at https://www.hhs.gov/hipaa/for-professionals/breach-notification/index.html.

HIPAA and the Use of Mobile Computing Devices

Patient privacy and HIPAA compliance in the clinical area are becoming more important than ever, especially because of the growing use of laptops, tablet PCs, and cell/smartphones that take pictures and record videos (Critical Thinking Box 23.3). According to a research study by Ponemon Institute (2014) on patient privacy and data security, top threats to patient records are criminal attacks, employee negligence regarding unsecured mobile devices (smartphones, laptops, and tablets), and third parties' attacks.

❓ CRITICAL THINKING BOX 23.3

Do you know your clinical facility's policies on cell/smartphone use in patient care areas? How about picture taking, Internet use, Internet access policy, information security access, and user-ID/password agreement?

You can violate an organization's Health Insurance Portability and Accountability Act policies and not even realize it!

The influx of mobile computing technology, such as tablet computers or smartphones, is creating new implications for protection of privacy and security. How to protect confidential information is something that we learn at the beginning of our nursing careers; however, protecting that same information on a mobile device may not be so easily understood. The following is a list of some simple precautions to take to help secure patient information that may be stored on a mobile device. These recommendations should be followed as standard practice:
■ Keep careful physical control of the device at all times.
■ Use a password or other user authentication and a time-out to reactivate the authentication.
■ Install and enable encryption.
■ Install and activate remote wiping and/or remote disabling.
■ Disable and do not install or use file-sharing applications.
■ Disable the infrared ports and Wi-Fi except when they are actually being used.
■ Do not send infrared or Wi-Fi transmissions in public locations.
■ Keep your security software up-to-date.
■ Research mobile applications (apps) before downloading.
■ Use adequate security to send or receive health information using public Wi-Fi networks.
■ Delete all stored health information before discarding or reusing the mobile device.

With the use of new technologies, there is a potential to improve patient safety and outcome as well as to reduce potential injury; however, at the same time, there is an increased risk for exposing confidential patient information. A cautionary approach along with assuming the responsibility for safeguarding the confidentiality of information should be used if you download patient information into a mobile device.

The Joint Commission

TJC wrote the IM standards in the mid-1990s. These 10 standards outline the need for IM regulation. Since then, IM has been woven throughout various standards and the National Patient Safety Goals. An example of this is noted in Standard IM.02.01.03 of the revised requirements for the Laboratory Accreditation Program, where the lab must have a "written policy addressing the integrity of health information against loss, damage, unauthorized alteration, unintentional change, and accidental destruction" (TJC, 2014, p. 1).

TJC sends out a team of experts for a review of every health care organization that wishes to be certified. This team inspects and reviews a variety of areas within each organization. The IN/INS may be called on to lead the effort for preparing for a TJC visit and for maintaining ongoing compliance (Critical Thinking Box 23.4).

❓ CRITICAL THINKING BOX 23.4

Have you had the opportunity to be in clinical during a visit by The Joint Commission? If so, what did you observe? How was the staff prepared for the visit?

Cybersecurity

Health care is a primary and lucrative target for cybercriminals, costing health care organizations an average of over $11 million per year (Landi, 2017). Whole books are devoted to the topic of cybercrime and cyberthreats, but let's cover a few highlights.

Cyberthreats include the following:

- Unpatched software—out-of-date software, which has not had updates and patches applied
- Ransomware—malware that prevents authorized users from accessing data until ransom is paid
- Phishing (pronounced "fishing")—using e-mail, telephone, or text message posing as a legitimate institution to lure individuals into providing sensitive and usable data
- Loss of data stored on mobile device
- Insider fraud and misuse of data

The two technology trends that are driving cybercrime are the Internet of Things (IoT) and the proliferation of data sources. From phones, tablets, PCs, our fitness devices, and the cloud, data are everywhere.

Models and Theories

Nomenclature, Classification, and Taxonomy

The quote from Dr. Lang at the beginning of the chapter has never been more true. Traditionally, nurses documented care using personal preference, unit standards, or facility policy. Standardized nursing languages, sometimes called *nomenclatures*, offer a recognized, systematic classification and consistent method of describing nursing practice. Nomenclatures act as descriptors or labels, classifications are group or class entities, and taxonomy is the study of classifications.

In 2018, the ANA updated its position statement on the inclusion of recognized terminologies to support nursing practice within health care information technology (HIT) systems to recommend the following:

- When exchanging data with another setting for problems and care plans, Systematized Nomenclature of Medicine—Clinical Terms (SNOMED CT) and Logical Observation Identifiers Names and Codes (LOINC) should be used for exchange. LOINC should be used for coding nursing assessments and outcomes and SNOMED CT for problems, interventions, and observation findings (ONC, 2018).

- Health information exchange between providers using the same terminology does not require conversion of the data to SNOMED CT or LOINC codes.
- Development of a clinical data repository that includes multiple recognized terminologies should be based on the national recognized terminologies of ICD-10, CPT, RxNorm, SNOMED CT, and LOINC (American Nurses Association, 2018).

The ANA recognized terminologies/data sets as listed in the 2018 revised position statement continue to include the following:

1. NANDA—Nursing Diagnoses, Definitions, and Classification
2. Nursing Interventions Classification System (NIC)
3. Nursing Outcomes Classification System (NOC)
4. Nursing Management Minimum Data Set (NMMDS)
5. Clinical Care Classification (CCC) (formerly Home Health Care Classification [HHCC])
6. Omaha System
7. Perioperative Nursing Dataset (PNDS)
8. SNOMED CT
9. Nursing Minimum Data Set (NMDS)
10. International Classification of Nursing Practice (ICNP)
11. ABC Codes for billing
12. LOINC

The need for consistency causes problems for software vendors as they attempt to produce unique and robust software packages that still use the recognized labels and groupings of nursing practice elements. So what happens?

Currently, each software vendor uses a unique, possibly patented naming convention for their specific functionality and then must "explain and define" these names and labels in their literature or presentations by relating them back to recognized nursing practice or data elements. This causes confusion to the user community.

Learning about and working with standardized nursing languages will ensure nursing contributions are an integral part of any EMR. Understanding those contributions through research and teaching will help further define the scope of nursing practice. Until complete standardization occurs, nurses must be prepared to use different classification systems at different facilities or even with systems from different vendors within the same facility (Critical Thinking Box 23.5).

? CRITICAL THINKING BOX 23.5

What has been your experience or exposure to these different standardized nursing languages? What does your clinical agency use?

Theories

Although there are multiple theories that are applicable to NI practice, the three most common are as follows:

- General systems theory—This theory organizes interdependent parts working together to produce a product that none used alone could produce. Key elements are input, process, output, control, and feedback.
- Rogers' diffusion of innovation theory—A five-step process of an individual's decision to adopt an innovation, which includes knowledge, persuasion, decision, implementation, and confirmation (Rogers, 2003).
- Change theory—Kurt Lewin's change theory is discussed in Chapter 10.

ELECTRONIC HEALTH RECORDS

Every day, nurses encounter technology, and this technology is changing the ways that health care is delivered in the hospital, physician's office, or patient's home. EHR have replaced pencil-and-paper charting. Florence Nightingale expressed a desire for medical records that were standardized, organized, and legible, and these goals are equally valid today.

> *In attempting to arrive at the truth, I have applied everywhere for information, but in scarcely an instance have I been able to obtain hospital records fit for any comparison.*
> **Florence Nightingale (Notes on a Hospital, 1873)**

EHRs are essential for health care to leverage state-of-the-art technology to deliver the highest-quality, lowest-cost patient care. Two other terms coming into vogue are the *comprehensive health record* and the *connected health record*. These terms describe two different visions of the next generation of the EHR. These visions include social determinants of health and more into nontraditional sources of data, including families/caregivers, school clinics, senior centers, and community health facilities. Other experts see the next step in EHR development to include shared care planning, genomics and personalized medicine, population health and public health, and remote monitoring and sensors (Zieger, 2018).

The e-World Is Coming…Wait, It's Here

Although most "e-words" come from the commerce or business sector, the term *eHealth* is generally understood, despite its lack of precise definition, because of the dynamic environment of the Internet. E-health has come to characterize not only a technical development but also a state of mind, a way of thinking that focuses on improvement of health care via information and communication technology.

The World Health Organization (WHO) provides the following definition for eHealth: "the use of information and communication technologies (ICT) for health" (2018a).

WHO (2018b) goes on to define *mHealth* as "a component of eHealth and involves the provision of health services and information via mobile technologies, such as mobile phones, tablet computers, and Personal Digital Assistants (PDAs)." However, despite its appearance in 2000, by 2015 there was no single consensus definition, nor is it included in MeSH taxonomy (https://meshb-prev.nlm.nih.gov/search).

Eysenbach (2001) feels that eHealth stands not only for "electronic" but implies a lot of other *e*'s, which he feels represent what e-health is all about (Box 23.1). He states that it should also be **e**asy to use, **e**ntertaining, **e**xciting, and most of all, it should **e**xist (Critical Thinking Box 23.6)!

? CRITICAL THINKING BOX 23.6

A 2012 survey from the Pew Internet & American Life Project found that one in three American adults have accessed the web for information about a medical condition (Pew Research Center, 2013). How have you (or your family) used the Internet for your own health or medical care? What about your patients? How will you help them use the Internet to better their understanding of their health?

Electronic Medical Record and Electronic Health Record

There is still some debate about whether an EHR and an EMR are the same or different. HealthIT.gov defines EMR as "a digital version of the paper charts…. An EMR contains the medical and treatment history of the patients in that office, clinic, or hospital" (HealthIT.gov, 2018a, para 1).

BOX 23.1   THE 10 E'S IN "E-HEALTH"

1. **Efficiency** leading to decreasing costs by avoiding duplicate or unnecessary diagnostic or therapeutic interventions, through enhanced communication possibilities among health care establishments, and through patient involvement.
2. **Enhancing quality of care** by allowing comparisons among different providers, involving consumers as additional power for quality assurance, and directing patient streams to the best quality providers.
3. **Evidence-based** intervention effectiveness and efficiency should not be assumed but proven by rigorous scientific evaluation.
4. **Empowerment** of consumers and patients by making the knowledge bases of medicine and personal electronic records accessible to consumers over the Internet; e-health opens new avenues for patient-centered medicine and enables evidence-based patient choice.
5. **Encouragement** of a new relationship between the patient and health professional, toward a true partnership where decisions are made in a shared manner.
6. **Education** of physicians and health care providers through online sources (continuing education) and consumers (health education, tailored preventive information for consumers).
7. **Enabling** information exchange and communication in a standardized way among health care establishments.
8. **Extending** the scope of health care beyond its conventional boundaries.
9. **Ethics** e-health involves new forms of patient–physician interaction and poses new challenges and threats to ethical issues such as online professional practice, informed consent, privacy, and equity issues.
10. **Equity** to make health care more equitable is one of the promises of e-health, but at the same time there is a considerable threat that e-health may deepen the gap between the "haves" and "have nots," deepening the "digital divide."

Adapted from Eysenbach, G. (2001). What is e-health? *Journal of Medical Internet Research, 3*(2). Retrieved from www.jmir.org/2001/2/e20/.

Further description of EHRs focuses on the total health of the patient—going beyond standard clinical data collected in a single event such as a provider's visit or hospitalization. They provide a broader view on a patient's care. EHRs are designed to reach out beyond the health organization that originally collects and compiles the information. They are built to share information with other health care providers so they contain information from all the clinicians involved in the patient's care (HealthIT.gov, 2018a, para 2).

Figs. 23.2 and 23.3 illustrate screenshots from a patient's EMR.

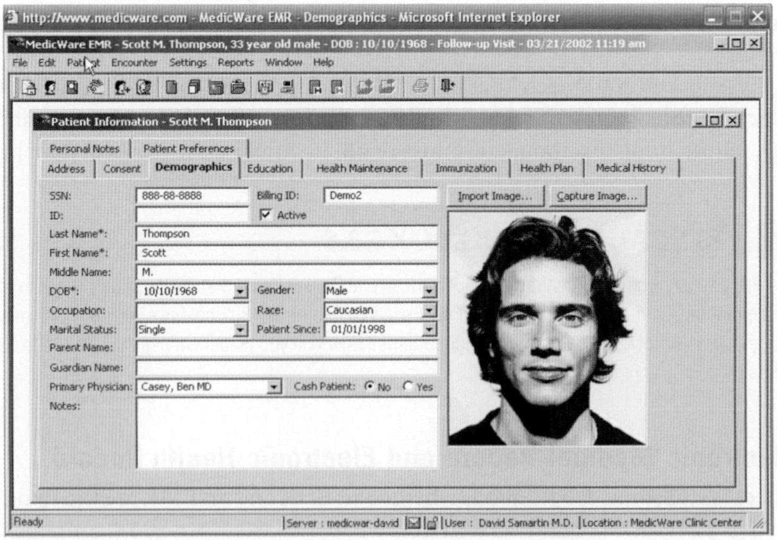

FIG. 23.2 Patient information screen. (Courtesy Medicware, Irwindale, CA.)

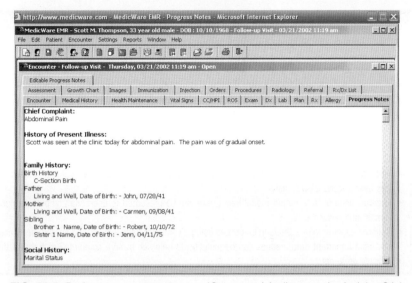

FIG. 23.3 Patient encounter screen. (Courtesy Medicware, Irwindale, CA.)

For example, a patient is seen in a primary care provider (PCP) office for complaints of indigestion. The PCP completes a history and physical, does an electrocardiogram (ECG), and runs basic lab studies. All data are in the computer at the office comprising one EMR for that patient. The patient is sent home with instructions. Later that evening, the patient feels worse and goes to the emergency department (ED). Using standalone EMRs, the following would occur: because it is after hours, the data in the patient's EMR at the PCP office are not available. A new EMR is begun. The next day the PCP would have no idea that the patient was seen in the ED.

Using an integrated EHR, the ED would be able to access the information from the PCP's system, and the next day the PCP would be notified that the patient was seen in ED and would have access to all the data collected during the ED visit.

Advantages of the EHR are listed in Box 23.2. This patient-centric approach to documentation of care is becoming the new standard of care.

As mentioned in the IOM report, *Key Capabilities of an Electronic Health Record System* (2003), a listing of essential features of the EHR (Box 23.3) must be addressed for our outdated health care system model to take advantage of the potential benefits of the "e-revolution." With federal initiatives pushing the adoption of EHRs throughout all health care institutions by 2014, how nursing is practiced has already significantly changed. Nurses are regularly interacting with informatics tools and systems to ensure safe and quality care. In a recent survey conducted by Zebra Technologies, 65% of nurses currently use mobile devices for accessing health data and patient information. It is anticipated that by 2022, 97% of nurses will use some type of mobile device at the bedside for patient care (Zebra Technologies, 2018).

Nursing informatics leaders are reporting that we are seeing more and more nurses who have never documented in a paper record or know how to use a paper medication administration record.

BOX 23.2   ADVANTAGES OF ELECTRONIC HEALTH RECORDS

- Simultaneous, remote access to patient from many locations
- Legibility of record—no handwriting
- Safer data—backup and disaster recovery system, so less prone to data loss
- Patient data confidentiality—authorized use can be restricted and monitored automatically
- Flexible data layout—can recall data in any order (chronologically or in reverse chronological order)
- Integration with other information resources
- Incorporation of electronic data—can automatically capture physiological data from bedside monitors, laboratory analyzers, and imaging devices
- Continuous data processing—check and filter the data for errors, summarize and interpret data, and issue alerts and/or reminders
- Assisted search—can search free-text or structured data to find a specific data value or to determine whether a particular item has been recorded previously
- Greater range of data output modalities—data can be presented to users via computer-generated voice, two-way pagers, e-mail, and smartphones
- Tailored paper output—data can be printed using a variety of fonts, colors, and sizes to help focus the clinician's attention on the most important data; images can be included to help see a more complete "picture" of the patient's condition
- Always up-to-date

BOX 23.3   EIGHT CORE FUNCTIONS OF THE ELECTRONIC HEALTH RECORD

A committee of the Institute of Medicine of the National Academies has identified a set of eight core care delivery functions that electronic health record (EHR) systems should be capable of performing to promote greater safety, quality, and efficiency in health care delivery.

These eight core functions are:

1. Health information and data
2. Result management
3. Order management
4. Decision support
5. Electronic communication and connectivity
6. Patient support
7. Administrative processes and reporting
8. Reporting and population health

Data from Institute of Medicine. (2003). Key capabilities of an electronic health record system. *Data Standards for Patient Safety*. Retrieved from http://www.nationalacademies.org/hmd/Reports/2003/Key-Capabilities-of-an-Electronic-Health-Record-System.aspx.

Personal Health Record

There is movement toward inclusion of data collected by the patient into the EHR. This is called the personal health record (PHR) and "is an electronic record of an individual's health information by which the individual controls access to the information and may have the ability to manage, track, and participate in his or her own health care" (HHS.gov, n.d.). PHRs are available from several sources. A health care provider may provide them as an extension of an EMR. Insurance providers may have PHRs for their clients. Online services such as WebMD and Microsoft Health Vault are also available. These data could include family history, real-time blood glucose readings, or exercise information sent directly from a fitness device to the PHR. Then, with permission of the patient, these data elements could be uploaded into the patient's PCP's EMR. Sounds good? Well, yes and no. The concepts of a PHR raise some interesting questions concerning data ownership, how to move data from one EMR to another, the rights of the patient to withhold data from a health care provider, and what happens if an online PHR provider ceases operation, such as when Google Health terminated services as of January 1, 2013. The coming few years will bring many changes in the concepts of a PHR. What the successful PHR model will be has yet to be determined.

Technology Changing Workflow for the Better—Medication Fulfillment

Another IOM study, *Preventing Medication Errors* (2006), recommends a greater use of information technologies in prescribing and dispensing medications (medication fulfillment), such as point-of-care (POC) reference information (handheld devices). Having detailed information about a medication at your fingertips addresses the issue of trying to keep up with all of the relevant information needed for the nurse to administer, and the physician or health care provider to prescribe a medication safely (Fig. 23.4).

Computerized Provider Order Entry and Clinical Decision Support

Computerized provider order entry (CPOE) completely changes the workflow of writing orders. CPOE is a technology-enabled process that allows providers such as physicians, nurse practitioners, and pharmacists to enter patient care orders directly into a computer system that transmits these orders directly to the receiving department (pharmacy, radiology, dietary, etc.) without intervening steps such as RN review for clarity and completeness. The true benefits of CPOE come with implementing clinical decision support systems (CDSSs) at the same time (Connelly & Korvek, 2018).

Clinical decision support (CDS) is a type of health information technology that provides health care providers, nurses, patients, and other individuals with relevant person-specific information that is presented at the right time for the health care provider to make a clinical decision about the patient's plan of care. Computerized alerts, reminders, diagnostic support, potential drug interactions, and clinical guidelines are a few CDS tools that assist health care providers and nurses with clinical decision-making and improving workflow (ONC, 2018). The Office of the National Coordinator for Health Information Technology adds that the CDS can operate exclusively as a stand-alone system; however, the majority of CDS applications are integrated into the EHR system (ONC, 2018).

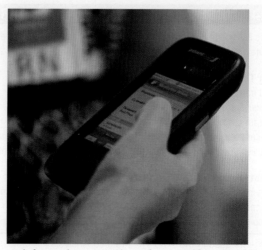

FIG. 23.4 Accessing patient information at point of care. (Courtesy PatientSafe Solutions, San Diego, CA.)

Barriers to Health Information Technology Still Remain

There still remain major barriers to the complete integration of health information technology. These barriers include the following:

- Lack of standardization across care areas—the need for laboratory data and pharmacy systems to be integrated with the patient's EHR, and the ED systems need to share data with the inpatient systems.
- Siloed data—hospital data, provider practice data, and long-term care facility data may all be in separate systems with steep fees for building interfaces to allow for exchange of data.
- Cost and funding—information technology is costly, and often the major costs are borne by hospitals rather than shared by other providers, payers, and employers.
- Privacy and security concerns—a single set of privacy laws is needed to simplify the task of communicating across facilities, agencies, and local, state, and federal governments.
- Lack of a uniform approach (number) to match patients to their record—a single authentication number is needed to reduce safety risks and provide a uniform access to patient data (Christodoulakis, Asgarian, & Easterbrook, 2017).

TRENDS

When the first edition of this textbook was published in the early 1990s, the section on computer technology was new and innovative. It was the cutting edge of technology that sent many nurse educators, students, and practicing nurses scrambling to make sense of how the computer might affect them. The explosion of knowledge and technology has visibly changed our mind-set on the use of computer technology to the extent that computer literacy is integrated within nursing education. Being faced with devices, equipment, computer sensors, "smart" body parts, and EHRs that involve technological skills, information technology impacts the way that nursing is practiced and delivered. Technology and informatics skills are spread throughout the 2019 NCLEX-RN Test Plan (NCSBN, 2019; Box 23.4).

BOX 23.4   NCSBN TEST PLAN FOR NCLEX-RN EXAMINATION

The following is an excerpt from the *2019 NCLEX-RN Test Plan* regarding the content area of Information Technology on the NCLEX-RN exam:

Information Technology
- Receive and transcribe health care provider orders[a]
- Apply knowledge of facility regulations when accessing client records
- Access data for client through online databases and journals
- Enter computer documentation accurately, completely and in a timely manner
- Utilize resources to enhance client care (e.g., evidenced-based research, information technology, policies, and procedures)[a]

Confidentiality/Information Security
- Assess staff member and client understanding of confidentiality requirements
- Maintain client confidentiality and privacy[a]
- Intervene appropriately when confidentiality has been breached by staff members

[a]Activity Statements used in the 2017 RN Practice Analysis.
Data from National Council State Board of Nursing. (2019). *2019 NCLEX-RN Test Plan*. Retrieved from https://www.ncsbn.org/2019_RN_TestPlan-English.htm.

Although there are numerous trend areas, using the Internet to communicate and to provide patient self-care, evaluating Internet resources, and using mobile computing devices are certainly in the forefront.

THE NEXT GENERATION OF HEALTH CARE DELIVERY

Undoubtedly, the Internet has transformed our ability to locate health information and to connect via e-mail and social networking such as Facebook, Twitter, or Pinterest with other individuals who have similar interests. Websites such as PatientsLikeMe.com allow people with chronic illnesses to share their feelings, disease progression, and responses to treatments with others in similar situations.

The federal government recognizes the importance of having access and quality information and has established a series of goals in the *Healthy People 2020 Topics and Objectives* (US Department of Health & Human Services, 2018). Health information on the Internet can dramatically improve patients' abilities to manage their own health care conveniently. Of course, not all web-based information is accurate, which raises concerns about the quality of information individuals are using and the impact this information has on the overall health of an individual.

> Internet users must still proceed with caution when seeking health care information online because there is a plethora of incomplete and inaccurate information that can be dangerous.

As nurses, we need to have a better understanding of how consumers find health information on the Internet, how to evaluate the quality of this information, and how to help our patients critically evaluate and manage the information (ANA, 2011; Greenberg et al., 2004).

A 2001 study by RAND for the California Healthcare Foundation showed that the information on health websites is often incomplete or out of date and highly commercialized, and this has not improved much. This might be of little concern if consumers routinely consulted health care professionals about the information. However, the Pew Internet and American Life Project (Pew Research Center, 2002) found that just 37% of consumers discussed the information they found online with a physician or nurse, and considering that most health information on the Internet is written in a style that is above the ninth-grade reading level, many individuals come away from the source of information confused, especially the underserved populations who need the information the most. Considering this, it is important for nurses to educate the public on how to distinguish credible and evidence-based health-related information from unreliable and inaccurate information found on the Internet.

The US National Library of Medicine and National Institutes of Health provides an excellent website on Evaluating Health Information at http://www.nlm.nih.gov/medlineplus/evaluatinghealthinformation .html, including some resources in Spanish.

> Imagine having access to your complete EHR no matter where you are in the world and being able to download portions of whatever documentation you need to a CD-ROM or removable drive (thumb drive) or safely store on a cloud-based server.

Patient Engagement

Many of you may have heard of the term *patient engagement*, but what is it and how does technology play a role? To be engaged, patients must use the resources available to maximize their health. When we add health information technology to the concept of patient engagement, we get the definition from the Office of the National Coordinator for Health Information Technology, "The ability of individuals to easily and securely access and use their health information electronically serves as one of the cornerstones of nationwide efforts to increase patient and family engagement and advance person-centered health" (HealthIt.gov, 2018b).

Practically everyone is familiar with e-mail. Your instructor may require you to complete assignments and submit your work via e-mail attachment instead of submitting a hard copy. You probably send e-mail to family and friends on a daily basis. Although more than 88% of people in the United States now use the Internet and e-mail daily (and many access health information), few physicians communicate with their patients through e-mail (Antoun, 2015; Internet World Stats, 2017). Patients are demanding health care to employ the technologies they use in other areas of life. Patients now want to make health care appointments the same way they book an airline flight or make a reservation at a restaurant. They want to communicate with their health care provider directly via electronic means rather than leaving a message with a receptionist (Deloitte, 2016). Considering the popularity of e-mail and despite its potential for rapid, asynchronous, and documentable communication to improve both the quality and efficiency of health services delivery, the use of e-mail communication has not been widely adopted by many physicians. There are several reasons for this, ranging from HIPAA concerns to billing issues; however, the demand from consumers is breaking down the objections. HIPAA does not prohibit e-mail but calls for reasonable safeguards, policies, and approaches (Hook, 2017).

Classes are moving online and may be 100% asynchronous or may be combined with video conferencing. Many of you may complete your next degree without ever stepping into a traditional classroom. In 2017 and beyond, patient engagement must be reported on to the Center for Medicare and Medicaid Services (CMS) and can be a key factor in value-based reimbursement for facilities and providers.

Telemedicine, Telehealth, and Health Monitoring

If you were asked how long telecommunication has been used in the US health care, would you select (a) the Civil War, (b) WWI, (c) WWII, or (d) Korean War? The answer is (a) the Civil War. Okay, it was a bit of trick question, since telecommunication in those days was the telegraph. But in the 1900s, physicians were one of the first professions to adopt the telephone in their practice (Zundel, 1996).

Today, the use of telecommunication technologies to provide health care is expanding at a phenomenal rate. Surprisingly, it's not just the under-30 population who is embracing this technology. Long labeled as technology-adverse, the senior population is proving just the opposite, especially since telemedicine visits via two-way video reduces the burden of travel to a provider's office.

School nurses are using technology linking PCPs and mental health professionals directly to both urban and rural settings, providing care without having to take children out of school or parents from work. Using technology to monitor chronic conditions such as Type 1 diabetes has shown to be effective in both the pediatric and adult populations.

Telemedicine has also expanded in the emergency and acute-care settings. Telestroke, telepsychiatry, and teledermatology programs are bringing needed expertise to underserved areas. Imagine you are a new ICU nurse, and rather than being on your own, you have a team of experienced ICU nurses who may be hundreds of miles away yet can see and hear everything you do. If you are tied up with one patient, they can monitor the other for you or help you assess a complex patient situation.

Health-related applications for smartphones are appearing everywhere. People are monitoring their heart rates, sleep patterns, and blood glucose readings. There are attachments for smartphones that can diagnose an ear infection or take a diagnostic-quality 12-lead ECG. In development now are devices for checking pulmonary edema and contact lenses that monitor glucose levels or intraocular pressure to help manage diabetes and glaucoma. New applications are even helping to diagnose a person's mental state by evaluating vocal inflections, facial expressions, vital signs, galvanic skin responses, and even the frequency and content of electronic communications.

Cloud Computing

Cloud computing has become a very real disrupter in the business world. But what is it? It is "the delivery of computing services—servers, storage, databases, networking, software, analytics, and intelligence and more—over the Internet ('the cloud') to offer faster innovation, flexible resources, and economies of scale" (Microsoft Azure, 2018). Think of it this way: instead of buying a CD with an application on it, then installing in your home computer, you buy a subscription to the software, then either use it online or download a copy to your computer. But you do not own the software and you don't have to pay for upgrades as long as you pay your subscription. For a health system, this means they don't have to have a massive IT organization but can outsource to a cloud computing service at a significantly lower cost (Raza, 2017).

Big Data

Another concept you may hear and wonder about is "big data." The following is a simplistic explanation but provides an idea of what big data is. Think about all the data we collect on a single patient during a 4-day hospital stay. Now add all the data we collect on all the patients in that hospital during that same 4 days. Now add to that all the data we collect on all the patients in all the hospitals in the United States during those 4 days—that is a lot of data (i.e., Big Data!). All of this data is too much to do anything with using traditional data management. So people working in informatics have developed and continue to develop ways of using the massive amounts of data to look for patterns and trends that may help us identify early warning signs, predisposing factors, and other patterns to improve health and health care.

Robotics in Patient Care

Robotics is a growing area for melding technology into patient care. While things like surgical robots have been in use since the 1900s when the FDA approved the first robotic intervention device, the applications of robotics have widened significantly. Japan, which has a rapidly growing percentage of elders and a chronic shortage of professional care workers, is focusing on robotics to help with direct patient care. From robots who greet and respond to verbal responses, to direct care robots, which can lift patients or lead patients in exercise activities to therapeutic robots—robotics are becoming part of the health care environment. Therapeutic robots built to look like cute animals such as a dog or baby harp seal deliver emotional responses based on sensors and produce the benefits of animal therapy without the problems live animals bring (Fig 23.5).

Artificial Intelligence in Health Care: The Time Is Almost Here

There has been a great deal of speculation about when artificial intelligence (AI) will have a significant impact on health care. But first, what is artificial intelligence? It is when a machine can learn from experience, change its actions based in new inputs, and then perform human-like tasks. The term was first used in 1956 but is widely used today especially since the advent of Watson—the IBM supercomputer. While Watson is really good at playing Jeopardy, the computer uses AI and sophisticated analytical software to answer questions posed using natural language (i.e., questions phrased the way humans ask them). Watson is being used in several areas of health care already, including the following:

- Managing care of complex patients
- Accelerating drug discovery by being able to manage the volume of drug research data far better than humans can
- Identifying appropriate cancer treatments in studies
- Matching patients with clinical trials (Speights, 2018)

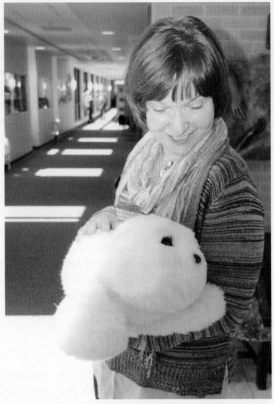

FIG. 23.5 Robotic harp seal. (Dr. Sandra Petersen, DNP, APRN, FNP/GNP-BC, PMHNP-BE, FAANP uses a robotic harp seal in her research on dementia.)

Health care experts picked the top 12 ways AI will revolutionize the delivery and science of health care (Bresnick, 2018):
1. Unifying mind and machine through brain–computer interfaces
2. Developing the next generation of radiology tools—without the need for biopsies
3. Expanding access to care in underserved or developing regions
4. Reducing the burdens of electronic health record use
5. Containing the risks of antibiotic resistance
6. Creating more precise analytics for pathology images
7. Bringing intelligence to medical devices and machines
8. Advancing the use of immunotherapy for cancer treatment
9. Turning the electronic health record into a reliable risk predictor
10. Monitoring health through wearables and personal devices
11. Making smartphone selfies into powerful diagnostic tools
12. Revolutionizing clinical decision-making with AI at the bedside

But there are ethical issues to consider as well. Shannon (2018) raises the following questions about the use of AI: Do we treat data or do we treat patients? Where could genetic testing lead? Think of movies such as *Gattaca*, where children are the products of prenatal genetic engineering. There is much to consider as technology advances at a rapid pace.

PATIENTS AND THE INTERNET

What Do I (and Patients) Need to Know to Evaluate an Internet Resource?

In her classic article, McGonigle (2002) suggests a five-step plan to evaluate websites (Box 23.5).

> Remember that anybody can publish anything on the web. Make sure you critically evaluate the source of the information.

This is more important than ever as a lot of people use the Internet to search for health-related topics. It is important to encourage patients to focus their Internet searching endeavors to well-known and reputable sites. For example, the US Surgeon General's Family History Initiative is a great place to start with promoting the importance of a well-documented family health history. In addition to the Office of the Surgeon General, other US Department of Health and Human Services (USDHHS) agencies involved in this project include the National Human Genome Research Institute (NHGRI), the Centers for Disease Control and Prevention (CDC), the Agency for Healthcare Research and Quality (AHRQ), and the Health Resources and Services Administration (HRSA). A downloadable free tool

---

BOX 23.5 HOW TO EVALUATE WEBSITES

Step 1: Authority

Who is/are the author(s)? Describe each author's authority or expertise. Are professional qualifications listed? How can you contact the author(s)? Who is the site's sponsor? What does the URL tell you? What type of domain does it come from (.gov, .mil, .edu, .org)? Is the site copyright protected? If the website is offering medical information, is the website HONcode certified? To learn more about Health on the Net Foundation Code of Conduct (HONcode), visit: https://www.hon.ch/HONcode/Pro/.

Step 2: Timeliness and Currency

When were the site materials created? When did it become active on the Web? When was it last updated/revised? Are the links up-to-date? Are the links functional? When were data gathered? What version/edition is it?

Step 3: Purpose

Who is the targeted audience? What is the purpose of the website? Are the goals/aims/objectives clearly stated? Does the website present facts or opinions? Does the website offer an area for consumers and another one for health care professionals?

Step 4: Content Accuracy and Objectivity

Does the information provided meet the purpose? Who is accountable for accuracy? Are the cited sources verifiable and published within the last 5 years? What is the value of the content of this site related to your topical needs? How complete and accurate are the content information and links? Is the site biased? Does it agree with other expert sources? Does it contain advertisements?

Step 5: Structure, Design, and Access

What is the appearance of the site? Does the site load quickly? Do multimedia, graphics, and art used on the page serve a purpose, or are they just decorative or fun? Is there an element of creativity? Is there appropriate interactivity? Is the navigation intuitive? Are there icons? Is it a secured site? Is an index with links available?

McGonigle, D. (2002). How to evaluate websites. *Online Journal of Issues in Nursing, 6,*2.
Medical Library Association. (2016). *Find good health information.* Retrieved from http://mlanet.org/resources/userguide.html.
Thomason, C. J. (2017). *Expert advice: How to evaluate the credibility of an online website.* Retrieved from https://nursingeducationexpert.com/expert-advice-online-website-evaluation/.
U.S. National Library of Medicine. (2015). *MedlinePlus guide to healthy web surfing.* Retrieved from https://www.nlm.nih.gov/medlineplus/healthywebsurfing.html.
University of Maryland. (2018). *Evaluating websites.* Retrieved from https://myelms.umd.edu/courses/1195203/pages/evaluating-web-sites.

entitled "My Family Health Portrait" is available at http://www.genome.gov/27527640. This tool helps patients organize their family trees and identify common diseases that may run in their families. After completing the required information, the tool will create and print out a graphic representation of the patient's family generations and the health disorders that may have moved from one generation to the next. This is a powerful tool for predicting illnesses (USDHHS, 2016) and can be brought by the patient to a health care provider appointment.

The CARS Checklist

Acronyms are always helpful in remembering important key features. The CARS checklist (Credibility, Accuracy, Reasonableness, and Support), developed by Harris in 1997 and updated in 2007, is designed to help evaluate a website. Although few sources will meet the majority of the criteria, the checklist will help in separating the high-quality information from the poor-quality information.

✓ Credibility—An authoritative source, which includes author's credentials and evidence of quality control such as peer review.
✓ Accuracy—A source that is correct today (not yesterday) and is comprehensive.
✓ Reasonableness—Look at the information for fairness, objectivity, moderateness, consistency, and worldview.
✓ Support—A source that provides convincing evidence for the claims made and which can be triangulated (find at least two other sources that support it).

Harris (2007) notes that you will also need a little "café" advice to live with the information you obtained from your Internet search.

■ Challenge the information and demand accountability.
■ Adapt and require more credibility and evidence for stronger claims—it is okay to be skeptical of the information.
■ File new information in your mind rather than immediately believing or disbelieving it.
■ Evaluate and reevaluate regularly. Recognize the dynamic, fluid nature of the information.

Patient Portals

HealthIT.gov (2017) defines a patient portal as a secure online website that gives patients convenient, 24-hour access to personal health information from anywhere with an Internet connection. Using a secure username and password, patients can view health information such as the following:

■ Recent doctor visits
■ Discharge summaries
■ Medications
■ Immunizations
■ Allergies
■ Lab results
  Some patient portals also allow you to:
■ Securely message your doctor
■ Request prescription refills
■ Schedule non-urgent appointments
■ Check benefits and coverage
■ Update contact information
■ Make payments
■ Download and complete forms
■ View educational materials

DATA ACCESS AT THE POINT OF CARE

POC documentation has surfaced as a need in health care because of the interruption in workflow created by electronic documentation. Thirty years ago, patients' flow sheet documentation was kept on a clipboard at the bedside. The nurse walked into a room, collected vital data, wrote it on the flow sheet, and went on to the next patient. While this was an excellent workflow for the clinical nurse, it made aggregating data across patient visits or across groups of patients a monumental task. Picture the ED nurse, with an unconscious patient, who is confronted with a stack of paper records that have been rolled to the ED in a wheelchair by a medical records person—trying to put together a concise, cohesive picture of the patient's history would be next to impossible.

Computers in the Nurses' Station

Enter electronic clinical documentation. This made it easier to review patient data from previous visits and to do research across patient populations, and it completely changed the workflow of the clinician at the bedside. We went from patient to patient collecting data until we finally had time to sit down in front of a computer to enter the data into the patient's chart. We then attempted to regurgitate all the data we had either scribbled on a piece of paper or, worse yet, tried to commit it to memory. And even worse than that, we had multiple person-to-person conversations, telephone calls, and alerts between gathering data and documentation, all of which interfered with our recall of the details of care given to a patient in the previous hours.

Research has shown that POC documentation reduces data latency and data errors. A variety of POC devices are now available to return documentation back to the POC and to help us handle the vast amount of data that we receive every day.

Mobility in the Clinical World

To free clinicians from computers at the nurses' station, computers were put on carts—first desktops, then laptops. The next generation of workstations on wheels added medication storage to improve workflow. While tablet computers have been "the thing" for providers since the introduction of the iPad in 2010, there has not been widespread adoption by nurses at the bedside. Mobile application development has focused on the providers, and nurses have been reluctant to give up a keyboard and large monitor because of the design of the clinical applications they use. Expect this trend to change in the next 5 years as software applications continue to evolve (Fig. 23.6).

Smartphones

Just as personal digital assistants, aka PDAs, and mobile phones merged to become the smartphone, now smartphones and tablet computers are rapidly merging. By the time you read this chapter, the differences between the two devices will be almost imperceptible if they not have vanished altogether—in fact, some of you may not have ever heard the term PDA (Critical Thinking Box 23.7).

> **? CRITICAL THINKING BOX 23.7**
>
> Do you have a smartphone? If so, how do you use it? If not, do you anticipate purchasing one in the near future? Do you find nurses in the hospital or clinic setting using smartphones on a regular basis? What programs do they or you use?

Smartphones can run applications that can perform cardiac monitoring, monitor blood glucose levels, blood pressure, diet, and activity, as well as allow users to check for drug interactions, calculate dosages, analyze lab results, schedule procedures, order prescriptions, and automate other clinical

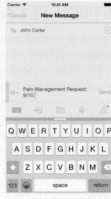

FIG. 23.6 Smartphone communication application using text messaging. (Courtesy PatientSafe Solutions, San Diego, CA.)

tasks, thus reducing the probability of errors and increasing patient safety. However, smartphones can also be used for multiple modes of communication. We just have to be careful not to violate HIPAA when using our personal phones! Check Chapter 19 for tips on effectively using social media and other virtual environments in both your profession and personal life.

Applications are now being developed to aid in managing the constant influx of information using multiple modes of communication such as text messaging, voice messages and calls, and alarms (Figs. 23.7 and 23.8). However, because of their limited memory and scaled-down operating systems, it is still impossible to access the entire scope of the patient's electronic record on a smartphone.

Using Data to Improve Care at the Bedside

Companies are now taking data and using it to help the bedside nurse care for patients. For example, gathering real-time patient satisfaction scores and combining them with clinical documentation give clinicians a different view of the care process and how the patient might perceive it (Fig. 23.9).

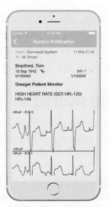

FIG. 23.7 Smartphone communication application text messaging templates. (Courtesy Voalte, Sarasota, FL.)

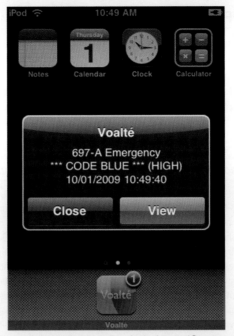

FIG. 23.8 Smartphone communication application alarm. (Courtesy Voalté, Sarasota, FL.)

Activity for 4th Floor – 411 - Bailey

▼ **Patient**

Joan Sharon Bailey	LeadIt Goal Score	Care team		Hospital Visit Indicares	
Age: 12 years (6/14/2002)		Physicians:	Attending - **Magee**	Patient Request Rate:	**0.73** / hr
	At Goal		Admitting - **Magee**	Interaction Wait Time:	**122** secs
		Caregivers:	**Howard Bailey**	Critical Request Rate:	**0.61** / hr
			Ruby Mendoza	Interruption Rate:	**2.12** / hr

▼ **IndiCare® and Activity** (Previous 24 hours)

Patient Request Rate	Patient Interaction Wait Time	Critical Request Rate	Interruption Rate
0.83 / hr	**85.63** secs	**0.25** / hr	**1.79** / hr

411 → | 18:00 20:00 22:00 0:00 2:00 4:00 6:00 8:00 10:00 12:00 14:00 16:00 |
       | 19:00 21:00 23:00 1:00 3:00 5:00 7:00 9:00 11:00 13:00 15:00 17:00 |

• Normal	▣ Water OT	▣ Pain OT	▢ Toilet Asst OT	▢ Toilet OT	✕ Shower OT	★ Staff Assist	☆ Admit	◁ Transfer Out
▢ Normal OT	○ Pain	○ Toilet Asst	▲ Toilet	✦ Shower	✹ Bed Exit	✵ Code Blue	▷ Transfer In	▢ Discharge
• Water								

Inpatient Survey   **Disqualify Patient**

Patient Response

25% ▼   Has a caregiver been in to check on you every hour?   [+ Notes]
             ○ Yes ○ No
Responses : 4
Goal : 78%

86% ▲   Has our staff responded to your requests in a timely manner?   [+ Notes]
             ○ Yes ○ No
Responses : 7
Goal : 76%

100% ▲   Have we done an excellent job in managing your pain?   [+ Notes]
             ○ Yes ○ No
Responses : 5
Goal : 82%

[Save Answers]

FIG. 23.9 Leadit-patient-activity. (From sphere3consulting.com.)

NURSING INFORMATICS AND YOU

Do you see now how your practice will involve informatics on a daily basis? From electronic documentation to using technology-laden equipment such as smart IV pumps and beds, barcode medication administration, and a variety of POC diagnostics equipment to communication tools such as smartphones and use of CDSSs, technology will touch every part of your patient care (Research for Best Practice Box 23.1).

RESEARCH FOR BEST PRACTICE BOX 23.1
Use of Technology Improves Safety of Medication Administration

Practice Issue

Approximately 7000–9000 people die each year because of a medication error. Medication errors in the inpatient setting cost the health system well over $40 billion per year (Bhimji & Scherbak, 2018).

Most nurses have heard of the case of the newborn twins of actor Dennis Quaid and his wife Kimberly receiving 10,000 units of heparin instead of 10 units. Although not all adverse drug events (ADEs) are preventable, using bar-code technologies can prevent those that are the result of a breakdown in the Five Rights of Medication Administration. But the technology only works when nurses use it. In a study by Koppel and colleagues (2008), nurses were found to use a work-around instead of using barcode medication administration (BCMA) in more than 10% of the medications delivered. Five years later, Rack, Dudjak, and Wolf (2012) found that more than half of nurses surveyed indicated that they used a work-around rather than the BCMA. They concluded that understanding why work-arounds occur and taking steps to prevent them will help achieve the goal of making the use of BCMA technology easier than developing a work-around. Bowers and colleagues (2015) found that the implementation of the BCMA increased the use of the workstation on wheels at the bedside and the use of the MAR at the point of care, which helped ensure that current orders were being implemented. The 2017 Leapfrog Group Report showed that while facilities have the technology to safely administer medication, it is not being used effectively.

Implications for Nursing Practice

Don't use a work-around as a quick-fix solution to a bigger problem. If technology is hampering your work, tell your manager. Don't try to save time by bypassing the BCMA process.

Many of the medication errors were made unknowingly by nurses—BCMA can help ensure that the Five Rights are followed every time.

The Institute for Safe Medication Practices (2019) recommends that electronic communication systems, "display patient identification information containing at least two unique identifiers in a prominent area (e.g., upper left hand corner) of all screens/windows in a consistent order so that users can efficiently and accurately find and verify patient identity" (p. 8).

Considering This Information

Have you used BCMA yet? Has anyone taught you a work-around? Why would you want to bypass a BCMA alert and when? What type of electronic health record (EHR) safety design feature have you observed in the clinical setting?

References

Bowers, A. M., Goda, K., Bene, V., et al. (2015). Impact of bar-code medication administration on medication administration best practices. *CIN: Computers, Informatics, Nursing, 33*(11), 502–508. https://doi.org/10.1097/CIN.0000000000000198.

Institute for Safe Medication Practices. (2019). Guidelines for safe electronic communication of medication information. Retrieved from https://www.ismp.org/resources/guidelines-safe-electronic-communication-medication-information.

Koppel, R., Wetterneck, T., Telles, J. L., et al. (2008). Workarounds to barcode medication administration systems: Their occurrences, causes, and threats to patient safety. *Journal of American Medical Informatics Association, 15,* 408–423.

Rack, L., Dudjak, L., & Wolf, G. (2012). Study of nurse workarounds in a hospital using bar code medication administration system. *Journal of Nursing Care Quality, 27*(3), 232–239. https://doi.org/10.1097/NCQ.0b013e318240a854.

The Leapfrog Group. (2017). Latest report: First-ever data on bedside bar coding shows hospitals have the technology to safely administer medication, but fall short on using it effectively. Retrieved from http://www.leapfroggroup.org/news-events/latest-report-first-ever-data-bedside-bar-coding-shows-hospitals-have-technology-safely.

In addition, you may become part of the implementation team for a new software application as a super user. Super users are individuals who have been through additional training for a software application and who are responsible for helping others on their unit. You may be a subject-matter expert (SME) at some point in your career and help design the data input screens of an application.

Basic computing and information literacy skills are essential for all nurses, whether working directly with patients in any environment, teaching, or any of the other varied positions held by nurses today.

CONCLUSION

Nursing informatics is a specialty grounded in the present while planning for the future. Nursing informatics nurses face many challenges in their daily activities, because they are in a position to wear many hats and bear many responsibilities. The next challenge after EHR implementation will be using the data in a meaningful way to improve patient care and lower costs. Computing devices and applications will continue to evolve and improve point-of-care access. Touch screens and voice input are already beginning to have an impact. Change is the only constant. At the end of this chapter are relevant websites and online resources on the concepts that have been presented.

The challenge will be for informatic nurses and informatics nurse specialists to assume leadership roles in informatics, while the nurse educator, manager, and practicing nurse prepare to embrace the generalized applications of working within a computerized environment. No longer will it be sufficient to turn on a computer and complete a simple task. A nurse will need to be able to use technology in all the forms found in health care organizations, access information, as well as access and use data and evaluate the content of the information provided to the patient population. Wishing will not make technology go away, so savvy nurses will focus on the benefits that technology brings to patient care, learn the skills they need, and embrace the future with all the changes it will bring.

🌐 RELEVANT WEBSITES AND ONLINE RESOURCES

American Health Information Management Association (AHIMA)
What Is a Personal Health Record (PHR)? http://www.myphr.com/StartaPHR/what_is_a_phr.aspx

American Medical Informatics Association (AMIA)
AMIA NI Working Group. http://www.amia.org/programs/working-groups/nursing-informatics

American Nursing Informatics Association (ANIA)
https://www.ania.org/

Centers for Medicare & Medicaid Services (CMS)
Promoting Interoperability (PI). http://www.cms.gov/Regulations-and-Guidance/Legislation/EHRIncentivePrograms/index.html?
    redirect=/ehrincentiveprograms/

HealthIT.gov
Privacy, Security, and HIPAA. http://www.healthit.gov/providers-professionals/ehr-privacy-security

HIMSS
Impact of the Informatics Nurse Survey Final Report
    https://www.himss.org/library/2017-nursing-informatics-workforce-survey-full-results

Nursing Informatics
    https://www.himss.org/library/nursing-informatics/%3FnavItemNumber%3D16520

Continued

🌐 RELEVANT WEBSITES AND ONLINE RESOURCES—CONT'D

Medicare.gov
Manage Your Health. https://www.medicare.gov/manage-your-health/

Microsoft
Microsoft Health Vault. https://www.healthvault.com/en-us/

U.S. Department of Health & Human Services (HHS)
Health Information Privacy (2018). http://www.hhs.gov/ocr/privacy/

WebMD
WebMD Personal Health Record. http://www.webmd.com/phr

Your Mobile Device and Health Information Privacy and Security
http://www.healthit.gov/providers-professionals/your-mobile-device-and-health-information-privacy-and-security

BIBLIOGRAPHY

American Association of Colleges of Nursing. (2006). Essentials of Doctoral Education for Advanced Nursing Practice. Retrieved from https://www.aacnnursing.org/Portals/42/Publications/DNPEssentials.pdf.

American Association of Colleges of Nursing. (2008). Essentials of Baccalaureate Education for Professional Nursing Practice. Retrieved from https://www.aacnnursing.org/Portals/42/Publications/BaccEssentials08.pdf. https://www.aacnnursing.org/Portals/42/Publications/BaccEssentials08.pdf.

American Association of Colleges of Nursing. (2011). Essentials of Master's Education in Nursing. Retrieved from https://www.aacnnursing.org/Portals/42/Publications/MastersEssentials11.pdf.

American Nurses Association. (2011). Fact sheet: Navigating the world of social media. Retrieved from https://www.nursingworld.org/~4af5ec/globalassets/docs/ana/ethics/fact_sheet_-_navigating_the_world_of_social_media_web.pdf.

American Nurses Association. (2015). *ANA scope and standards of nursing informatics practice.* (2nd ed.). Washington, DC: ANA.

American Nurses Association. (2018). Inclusion of recognized terminologies supporting nursing practice within electronic health records and other health information technology solutions. Retrieved from https://www.nursingworld.org/practice-policy/nursing-excellence/official-position-statements/id/Inclusion-of-Recognized-Terminologies-Supporting-Nursing-Practice-within-Electronic-Health-Records/.

Antoun, J. (2015). Electronic mail communication between physicians and patients: A review of challenges and opportunities. *Family Practice, 33*(2), 121–126.

Bhimji, S. S., & Scherbak, Y. (2018). Medication Errors. [Updated 2018 Oct 27]. In *StatPearls [Internet]*. Treasure Island (FL): StatPearls Publishing. Jan. Retrieved from https://www.ncbi.nlm.nih.gov/books/NBK519065/.

Bresnick, J. (2018). Top 12 Ways Artificial Intelligence Will Impact Healthcare. *HealthITAnalyticscom.* Retrieved from https://healthitanalytics.com/news/top-12-ways-artificial-intelligence-will-impact-healthcare.

Christodoulakis, C., Asgarian, A., & Easterbrook, S. (2017). Barriers to adoption of information technology in healthcare. In *Paper presented at the ACM CASCON conference, Toronto, CA.* Retrieved from http://www.cs.toronto.edu/~christina/documents/ACM_CASCON2017.pdf.

Connelly, T. P., & Korvek, S. J. (2018). Computer provider order entry (CPOE). Retrieved from https://www.ncbi.nlm.nih.gov/books/NBK470273/.

Deliotte. (2016). Deloitte's 2016 consumer priorities in health care survey. Retrieved from https://www2.deloitte.com/us/en/pages/life-sciences-and-health-care/articles/us-lshc-consumer-priorities-promo.html.

Dimick, C. (2010). Californian sentenced to prison for HIPAA violation. *Journal of AHIMA.* Retrieved from http://journal.ahima.org/2010/04/29/californian-sentenced-to-prison-for-hipaa-violation/.

Eysenbach, G. (2001). What is e-health? *Journal of Medical Internet Research*, 3(2). Retrieved from www.jmir.org/2001/2/e20/.

Harris, R. (2007). Evaluating Internet research sources. Retrieved from http://www.niu.edu/facdev/programs/handouts/evaluate.htm.

HealthIT.gov. (2017). What is a patient portal? Retrieved from https://www.healthit.gov/faq/what-patient-portal.

HealthIT.gov. (2018a). EMR vs EHR – What is the difference? Retrieved from https://www.healthit.gov/buzz-blog/electronic-health-and-medical-records/emr-vs-ehr-difference/.

HealthIT.gov. (2018b). Patient engagement. Retrieved from https://www.healthit.gov/playbook/patient-engagement/.

HHS.gov. (n.d.). Personal health records (PHRs) and the HIPAA privacy rule. Retrieved from http://www.hhs.gov/sites/default/files/ocr/privacy/hipaa/understanding/special/healthit/phrs.pdf.

HIMSS. (2015). 2015 impact of the informatics nurse survey final report. Retrieved from https://www.himss.org/sites/himssorg/files/FileDownloads/2015%20Impact%20of%20the%20Informatics%20Nurse%20Survey%20Full%20Report.pdf.

HIMSS. (2017). Nursing informatics workforce survey. Retrieved from https://www.himss.org/sites/himssorg/files/2017-nursing-informatics-workforce-executive-summary.pdf.

Hook, J. (2017). HIPAA and e-mail: There are rules. Retrieved from https://www.foxgrp.com/hipaa-compliance/hipaa-and-e-mail-rules/.

Institute of Medicine. (2003). Key capabilities of an electronic health record system. Data standards for patient safety. Retrieved from http://www.nationalacademies.org/hmd/Reports/2003/Key-Capabilities-of-an-Electronic-Health-Record-System.aspx.

Institute of Medicine. (2006). Preventing medication errors: Report brief. Retrieved from http://www.nationalacademies.org/hmd/~/media/Files/Report%20Files/2006/Preventing-Medication-Errors-Quality-Chasm-Series/medicationerrorsnew.ashx.

Internet World Stats. (2017). Internet usage and population statistics for North America. Retrieved from http://www.internetworldstats.com/stats14.htm#north.

Landi, H. (2017). Report: Healthcare organizations spend 12.5 million a year on cybersecurity. Retrieved from https://www.healthcare-informatics.com/news-item/cybersecurity/report-healthcare-organizations-spend-125-million-year-cybersecurity.

McGonigle, D. (2002). How to evaluate websites. Online Journal of Issues in Nursing, 6,2.

Microsoft Azure. (2018). What is cloud computing? A beginner's guide. Retrieved from https://azure.microsoft.com/en-us/overview/what-is-cloud-computing/.

National Council of State Boards of Nursing. (2019). NCLEX-RN® detailed test plan candidate version. Retrieved from https://www.ncsbn.org/testplans.htm.

Office of the National Coordinator for Health Information Technology [ONC]. (2018). Clinical decision support. Retrieved from https://www.healthit.gov/topic/safety/clinical-decision-support.

Pew Research Center. (2002). Vital decision: A Pew internet health report. Retrieved from http://www.pewinternet.org/2002/05/22/vital-decisions-a-pew-internet-health-report/.

Pew Research Center. (2013). Health online, *2013*. Retrieved from http://www.pewinternet.org/2013/01/15/health-online-2013/.

Ponemon Institute. (2014). Third annual benchmark study on patient privacy & data security sponsored by ID experts. Retrieved from http://www.ponemon.org/blog/fourth-annual-benchmark-study-on-patient-privacy-and-data-security.

RAND Corporation. (2001). Proceed with caution: A report on the quality of health information on the Internet. San Francisco, CA. Sponsored by the California Health Care Foundation. Retrieved from http://www.chcf.org/~/media/MEDIA%20LIBRARY%20Files/PDF/PDF%20P/PDF%20ProceedWithCautionCompleteStudy.pdf.

Raza, K. (2017). How the cloud is transforming healthcare. Retrieved from https://www.forbes.com/sites/forbestechcouncil/2017/06/13/how-the-cloud-is-transforming-healthcare/#71b83cfa1fd7.

Rogers, E. M. (2003). *Diffusion of innovation* (5th ed.). New York: Free Press.

Shannon, P. (2018). Researchers say use of artificial intelligence in medicine raises ethical questions. Stanford Medicine. Retrieved from https://med.stanford.edu/news/all-news/2018/03/researchers-say-use-of-ai-in-medicine-raises-ethical-questions.html.

Speights, K. (2018). 4 Ways IBM Watson's artificial intelligence is changing healthcare. Retrieved from https://www.fool.com/investing/2018/01/12/4-ways-ibm-watsons-artificial-intelligence-is-chan.aspx.

The Joint Commission (TJC). (2014). Information management. Retrieved from https://foh.psc.gov/tjc/im/standards.pdf.

U.S. Department of Health and Human Services. (2013a). New rule protects patient privacy, secures health information. Retrieved from http://www.hhs.gov/news/press/2013pres/01/20130117b.html

U.S. Department of Health and Human Services. (2013b). How can you protect and secure health information when using a mobile device? Retrieved from https://archive.healthit.gov/providers-professionals/how-can-you-protect-and-secure-health-information-when-using-mobile-device.

U.S. Department of Health and Human Services. (2016). U.S. Surgeon General's family history initiative. Retrieved from www.hhs.gov/familyhistory/.

U.S. Department of Health and Human Services. (2018). Healthy People 2020. Retrieved from https://www.healthypeople.gov/.

World Health Organization (WHO). (2018a). eHealth at WHO. Retrieved from http://www.who.int/ehealth/en/.

World Health Organization (WHO). (2018b). Key definitions. Retrieved from http://www.who.int/tb/areas-of-work/digital-health/definitions/en/.

Zebra Technologies. (2018). The Future of Healthcare: 2022 Hospital Vision Study. Retrieved from https://www.zebra.com/content/dam/zebra_new_ia/en-us/solutions-verticals/vertical-solutions/healthcare/white-paper/2022-hospital-vision-study-en-global.pdf.

Zieger, A. (2018). Comprehensive health record vs. connected health record. *EMR & EHR*. Retrieved from https://www.emrandehr.com/2018/03/26/comprehensive-health-record-vs-connected-health-record/.

24

Using Evidence-Based Practice and Nursing Research

Peter G. Melenovich, PhD, RN, CNE

http://evolve.elsevier.com/Zerwekh/nsgtoday/.

The new challenge is for nurses to use research methods that can clearly explicate the essential nature, meanings, and components of nursing so that nurse clinicians can use this knowledge in a deliberate and meaningful way.
Madeline Leininger

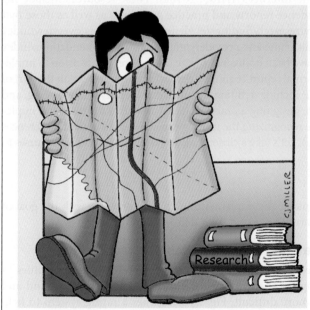

Nursing research is the road map to interprofessional practice.

After completing this chapter, you should be able to:
- Define evidence-based practice.
- Understand the importance of evidence-based practice.
- Identify the steps in evidence-based practice.
- Explore the process of research utilization.
- Identify the steps in the process of research utilization.
- Discuss the difference between conducting research and research utilization.
- Identify resources for evidence-based nursing practice.
- Identify the characteristics of your practice context.
- Explore the steps for conducting research.
- Describe ways in which nursing research can be used to guide your nursing practice.
- Describe the function of the National Institute of Nursing Research.

WHAT IS EVIDENCE-BASED PRACTICE?

Evidence-based practice (EBP) "is a problem solving approach to clinical practice that integrates a systematic search for and critical appraisal of the most relevant evidence to answer a burning clinical question, one's own clinical expertise, and patient preferences and values" (Melnyk & Fineout-Overholt, 2005, p. 6). Historically health care—and more specifically, nursing care—was based on tradition. In other words, we simply replicated what had been previously done in nursing, without question to the support of evidence for what we were doing or the impact on patient outcomes. As nursing has evolved and the expectation for continually improving patient outcomes has come to the forefront, a greater emphasis has been placed on implementing nursing care that is supported through the use of the best research available. EBP incorporates many additional sources of data that may contribute to improved nursing care.

EBP goes beyond nursing research in considering other sources of documentation that may improve nursing care. Research published by other disciplines is included (e.g., medical research and social research), as well as nonresearch data that may contribute to practice (e.g., financial data and clinical experts). This is prudent at a time when the complexity of health problems is increasing and the discovery of new data is more rapid than ever before (Research for Best Practice Box 24.1).

The US Department of Health and Human Services has established EBP centers and clinical practice guidelines that are available through the Internet (AHRQ, 2018a). These resources include the most current information on completed evidence reports and practice guidelines as well as those that are in progress (see http://www.ahrq.gov/research/findings/evidence-based-reports/overview/index .html and http://www.ahrq.gov/professionals/clinicians-providers/guidelines-recommendations/index .html). However, not all aspects of practice have been evaluated to date. Therefore, the decision to implement an EBP protocol that does not have a formal report requires a dedicated commitment on the part of all those involved. The steps in applying EBP include defining the problem; identifying, reviewing, and evaluating the data applicable to the problem; designing a practice change based on the data; and implementing the change in nursing practice while recognizing the nurse's experience and patient preferences (see Relevant Websites and Online Resources). Let's take a closer look at the steps that will assist nurses to integrate EBP into their practice.

Step 1: Define the Problem

As nursing professionals who will be responsible for implementing an EBP protocol with the goal of improving patient outcomes, we must first recognize and fully define the problem.

Step 2: Identify, Review, and Evaluate the Data Applicable to the Problem

Most nurses use their own clinical experience with patients and patient preferences and values in planning nursing care. However, searching for the evidence to address the question at hand and critically evaluating the evidence may be more difficult. Fig. 24.1 outlines a rating system to help you know how strong the evidence from research or other sources might be with Level I representing the most rigorous research studies. Keep in mind that as you move up the pyramid, fewer research studies are available; it's important to recognize that high levels of evidence may not exist for your clinical question. Nurses must be able to locate and evaluate research studies that will serve as the foundation of any potential EBP protocol. The specific nursing practice that will be changed, in addition to the practice context, will determine the types of data included for review.

🔍 RESEARCH FOR BEST PRACTICE BOX 24.1

Wound Care

Practice Issue

The increased acuity of patient needs, combined with advances in wound care, have the potential to create frustrating situations for the new graduate nurse. It is essential for the new graduate to prevent pressure injuries and provide wound and ostomy care that reflects current best practice measures and the newest advances in technology.

Implications for Nursing Practice

1. Approximately 2.5 million pressure ulcers occur each year in the United States, adding an estimated burden of more than $11 billion in expenditures, with reported estimated costs of between $500 and $150,000 per individual pressure ulcer (AHRQ, 2014; NPUAP, 2014).
2. Approximately 60,000 patients die annually from complications of pressure injuries (AHRQ, 2014).
3. Wound and ostomy care has emerged as a specialty practice for RNs (Wound Ostomy and Continence Nursing Certification Board [WOCNCB], 2019).
4. Wound and ostomy care needs and procedures can vary significantly across practice settings (de Leon et al., 2016).
5. New graduate RNs are more competent in patient care and less competent in clinical reasoning, recognizing limits, and seeking help.
6. New graduate RNs are more likely to use written information, care guidelines, and agency-specific policies to guide their practice.
7. New graduate RNs are more competent with using technology to seek answers and specific information related to current patient care practices.

Considering This Information

What can you do to keep up-to-date on wound and ostomy care guidelines and treatments?

References

Agency for Healthcare Research and Quality (AHRQ). (2014). *Preventing pressure ulcers in hospitals. A toolkit for improving quality of care*. In Retrieved from https://www.ahrq.gov/professionals/systems/hospital/pressureulcertoolkit/index.html.
de Leon, J., Bohn, G. A., DiDomenico, L., Fearmonti, R., Gottlieb, H. D., Lincoln, K., et al. (2016). Wound care centers: Critical thinking and treatment strategies for wounds. *Wounds, 28*(10), S1–S23.
National Pressure Ulcer Advisory Panel (NPUAP). (2014). *European Pressure Ulcer Advisory Panel and Pan Pacific Pressure Injury Alliance*. In E. Haesler (Ed.), *Prevention and treatment of pressure ulcers: Clinical practice guideline*. Osborne Park, Western Australia: Cambridge Media. Retrieved from *http://www.npuap.org/resources/educational-and-clinical-resources/prevention-and-treatment-of-pressure-ulcers-clinical-practice-guideline/*.
Wound Ostomy and Continence Nursing Certification Board (WOCNCB). (2019). *Certification*. Retrieved from http://www.wocncb.org/.

Step 3: Design a Practice Change Based on the Data While Incorporating the Clinical Expertise of the Nurse and Patient Preferences

Prepare a *written plan* for the new nursing practice. The plan needs to be consistent with your practice context to be effective. For maximum benefit, the plan will also require the consensus of those who will implement it.

Step 4: Implement the Change in Nursing Practice

Move the new plan into nursing practice on a *defined schedule*. Staff in-services may be required so that those involved can fully understand the change. Monitor and evaluate the implementation process. Moreover, as noted by Melnyk and Fineout-Overholt (2005), EBP must recognize the great experience

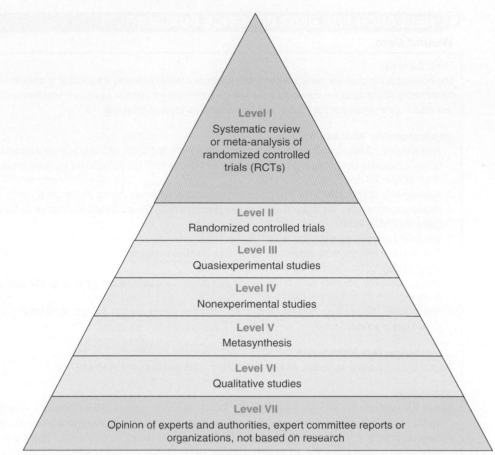

FIG. 24.1 Levels of evidence; evidence hierarchy for rating levels of evidence associated with a study design. (From Lo-Biondo-Wood, G. L., & Haber, J. [2018]. *Nursing research: Methods and critical appraisal of evidence-based practice* [9th ed.]. St. Louis: Mosby/Elsevier, p. 13).

that nurses bring to the practice setting and patient input and preferences if successful implementation is to be realized (Fig. 24.2).

Now let's consider using the EBP process in a hypothetical situation.

Mario works in an intensive care unit in which many of the patients require mechanical ventilation. At a recent staff meeting, Mario and his coworkers learned that their unit's rate of ventilator-associated pneumonia (VAP) was greater than rates in many other hospitals. Concerned by this, Mario volunteered to work on this project. He began with a review of the literature. Using a nursing literature database, Mario was able to find a number of research studies conducted in the past few years that examined the same issue. In addition, he found that multiple professional organizations had issued evidence-based guidelines to reduce the occurrence of VAP. After reading these articles, Mario drafted a set of clinical practice guidelines based on these articles that reflected the unique needs of his unit and its patient population. Mario then presented his guidelines to the nursing staff and provided short educational in-service sessions on their application. The staff agreed to adhere to these new practice guidelines for a period of 3 months. At the end of that time, they would compare their incidence of VAP using the new clinical guidelines with the incidence of VAP using the old clinical guidelines.

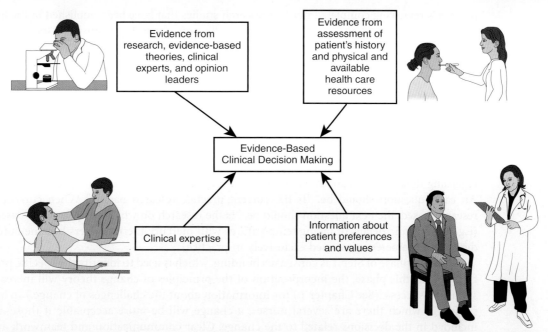

FIG. 24.2 Model of evidence-based clinical decision making. (Reprinted with permission from Potter, P. A., Perry, A. G., Stockert, P. A., Hall, A. M., & Ostendorf, W. R. [2017]. *Fundamentals of nursing* [9th ed.]. St. Louis: Elsevier, p. 53.)

At the end of the 3-month period, Mario and his coworkers were pleased to find a significant decrease in the occurrence of VAP among their patients. Working with nursing administration, Mario's proposed clinical practice guidelines became the new standard of care on his unit.

THE NEED FOR NURSING PRACTICE BASED ON RESEARCH

In the recent past, there has been a continuing increase in costs associated with the delivery and receipt of health care in the United States. At the same time, there has been more and more scrutiny of how those health care dollars are spent. The decision of which health care treatments receive funding from health care insurance is now based primarily on documentation of favorable patient outcomes. In addition, patients want to know that the dollars they spend on health care will help them to get well and feel better—they want to purchase something that works for them. Nurses must be able to demonstrate that the nursing care they provide is cost-effective and improves the health of patients. As we continue to move to a health care setting that recognizes the importance of patient care that utilizes the most current and appropriate evidence, we must understand how research utilization will assist us in meeting the goal of improving patient outcomes through EBP.

WHAT IS NURSING RESEARCH UTILIZATION?

The ability to transfer research into clinical practice is essential for ensuring quality in nursing. The process of research utilization involves transferring research findings to clinical nursing practice. In the process of research utilization, the emphasis is on using *existing* data (findings or evidence) from previous nursing research studies to evaluate a current nursing practice. A major component of the process is reviewing completed nursing research studies that have been published in the literature. In contrast, conducting new research involves the collection of *new* data to answer a specific clinical practice question. Nursing research utilization is a step-by-step process incorporating critical thinking and decision making to ensure that a change in practice has a sound basis in nursing science.

What Are the Steps for Nursing Research Utilization?
Step 1: Preutilization
The first step in the application of nursing research to nursing practice is the recognition that some aspect of nursing practice could be done in a safer, more efficient, more beneficial, or simply a different way. This begins an exploratory phase in which nursing colleagues in the practice setting are consulted regarding their opinions about the need to find a new approach for some aspects of nursing practice. An early question should be, "Is the current practice research based?" When current practice is research based, the next question should be, "Is the research on which the practice is based current?" (e.g., the specific details of taking temperatures with mercury thermometers became outdated when digital thermometers were used exclusively in practice).

A second phase of Step 1 is consensus building, which is used to identify the specific practice to be changed. In this phase, the incorporation of the principles of change theory will increase the possibility of success. (See Chapter 10 for information about the challenges of change.) In any practice setting in which there are several nurses, a change will be more acceptable if those affected are included in the decisions related to the change. Clear communication and teamwork are essential elements of this process. Group consensus is crucial for the successful application of research findings.

The third and final phase of Step 1 delineates the aspect of nursing practice that will be changed into a concise statement of the *practice problem*. This statement will answer the question, "In our current nursing practice, what do we want to change, improve, or make more efficient?" The narrower and more specific the statement of the practice problem, the easier your task will be in Step 2.

Step 2: Assessing
The second step in research utilization is the identification and critical evaluation of published research that is related to the practice problem you have identified (Fig. 24.3). Nursing literature is searched to identify those studies that address your practice problem. Although some studies may have explored the exact practice problem that you are examining, it is likely that most researches will have approached the problem from a different point of view. Your task will be to analyze and critically evaluate the research reports to determine which findings are adaptable to your practice problem and context.

While reviewing the literature for research reports that have examined your practice problem, it is essential that the research reports you are reviewing are peer-reviewed to ensure credibility. Peer-reviewed or refereed research studies are different from popular sources and non–peer-reviewed research reports, wherein the research manuscript is submitted to a scholarly journal where it is reviewed by a panel of experts (peer reviewers or referees) in that respective field or area of study. An editorial board that is not expert in the content area under study typically reviews non–peer-reviewed reports (e.g., editorials, newsletters, opinion statements). In addition, peer-reviewed articles have a designated manuscript format, which includes an abstract, research problem/objective, methodology, data collection, discussion, conclusion, and references, whereas non–peer-reviewed or popular/trade journals do not ascribe to a specific formatting style (NCSU Libraries, 2014). So, you might be asking yourself, "What does the peer-review process involve and what are my chances of

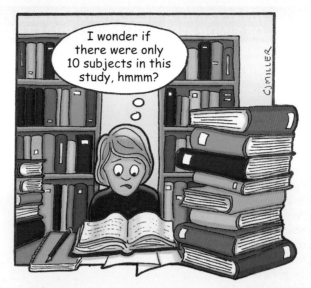

FIG. 24.3 Nine out of ten nurses recommend…

publishing a research report in a peer-reviewed journal?" North Carolina State University (NCSU) offers an overview of the peer-review process via an online video available at http://www.lib.ncsu .edu/tutorials/peerreview/.

Organizing and summarizing adaptable findings into an outline format will provide you with your primary working document where you can quickly access research reports that are applicable to your practice problem (Box 24.1). Reading a nursing research article can feel daunting, especially if you are unsure of how to conduct a critical appraisal of the findings presented in the research. Suggestions for analyzing and evaluating a research article are provided in Box 24.2.

The use of the Internet and electronic databases has made a thorough search of the current literature easier. However, the enormous volume of materials now available also increases the complexity of a review of literature. For example, the keywords used in a search can either return no articles or hundreds of articles. When you are conducting an electronic search, a valuable technique is to begin searching within the most recent year and then move back one year at a time until an adequate research base is identified. Limiting your searches to the use of nursing-oriented database and peer-reviewed journals may also help you find pertinent literature. The Cumulative Index to Nursing and Allied Health Literature (CINAHL) is an excellent place to start your search. In addition, you may wish to limit your search to journal articles only; otherwise the online database may return reports from magazine articles and newspapers. Listed at the end of this chapter are Relevant Websites and Online Resources to use in locating and reviewing peer-reviewed journals as well as online EBP resources.

There are times, however, when an electronic search is not adequate. Keep in mind that many of the classic research studies were published before electronic formats were widely used, and these classic studies may not be available online. Also, there may be valuable studies that are available in hard copy only. Because of these limitations of electronic sources, you may need to make a trip to the stacks in the library if you are looking for historical research. See Box 24.3 for hints on conducting a literature search.

BOX 24.1   ANALYZING A RESEARCH ARTICLE FOR POTENTIAL USE OF FINDINGS IN NURSING PRACTICE

1a. The Purpose of the study is:
1b. The importance of this study to nursing practice is:
 2. The Research Question/Hypothesis is:
(If the question/hypothesis is not stated, it could be):
3a. The Independent Variable(s) is/are:
3b. The Dependent Variable(s) is/are:
(If there are no independent and dependent variables, the Research Variable[s] is/are):
3c. Definition(s) of the variable(s) of interest to me is/are:
 4. The Conceptual Model/Theoretical Framework linked with this study is:
5a. The content areas in the Review of Related Literature are:
5b. The review does/does not evaluate both supporting and nonsupporting studies:
6a. The Research Design used for the study is:
6b. The design is/is not appropriate for the research question:
6c. The control(s) used in this study is/are:
6d. The Study Setting is:
7a. The Target Population is:
7b. The Sampling Method is:
7c. The Sampling Method is/is not appropriate for the design:
7d. The criteria for participants are:
7e. The sample included _____ participants.
 7f. The sample is/is not representative of the population:
8a. The Study Instrument(s) is/are:
8b. Instrument validity and reliability information is presented and is of adequate levels for confidence in using the results:
9a. The Data Collection Method(s) is/are:
9b. The Data Collection Method(s) is/are (is not/are not) appropriate for this study:
10. Steps were taken to protect the Rights of Human Subjects:
11a. The Data Analysis Procedure(s) is/are:
11b. The Data Analysis Procedure(s) is/are appropriate for the level of data collected and the research question/hypothesis:
11c. The Research Question/Hypothesis is/is not supported:
12. The author(s) major Conclusions and/or Implications for Nursing Practice are:

Step 3: Planning

Planning for research utilization is accomplished in three phases. The first phase involves determining the new approach, or *innovation*, that will be used on the basis of the findings from the review of the literature. Previous research findings will be used to design the innovation in the context of your practice setting (e.g., intensive care unit, ambulatory care, home care). The expected *practice outcomes* should also be determined based on the literature and may need to be adjusted according to the characteristics of your particular practice.

Phase two of planning is the establishment of a systematic method for implementing the new approach. A *specific plan* should be established and followed so that the new approach is applied appropriately. Policies and procedures for implementation may need to be written. This phase may include staff training for the new approach.

The third phase of planning involves establishing a *method for evaluating* the practice outcomes or effects of the new approach. The outcomes are usually some specific improvements in patient care. Ideally, your evaluation will indicate both the quality and the quantity of the change in the outcome.

BOX 24.2 HOW TO READ A NURSING RESEARCH ARTICLE

A research article should answer the following:

What?
Read the problem statement, purpose, research question, and results/findings.

Is the content of the article related to my question?

Why?
Read the problem statement or the review of literature.

Why was the research done?

When?
Do more recent findings provide a better answer?
Read the date of publication.

When was the study done? Is it classic, current, or outdated?

How?
Read the method and design sections.

What research method was used? Is it a quantitative, qualitative, or mixed-methods approach?

Who?
Read the method section.

Who were the subjects? What was the sample?

Where?
Read the method section.

In what setting was the research done?

So What?
Read the findings and discussion.

Are the findings helpful to my problem and me?

Do Not:

Do not automatically accept what you read; critically evaluate the content. You can only evaluate what is written and reported; do not assume anything about what is not written.

What to Do When
When the statistical procedures are beyond your level of understanding:
- Read the results section, being alert for specific phrases that will tell you the answer to the research question. For example, "the hypothesis was not supported."
- Look at the tables; tables should be understandable without the narrative.
- Assume that the appropriate statistical analysis was performed correctly and that the researcher has interpreted the results correctly.
- Have someone who understands the statistics read the article and ask his or her opinion, or get a consultant.

BOX 24.3 HINTS FOR CONDUCTING A LITERATURE SEARCH

1. Do some narrowing before you go to online databases. Think about some key terms or alternative terms for your problem. Be prepared to narrow or expand your search, depending on what you find.
2. Plan to spend time conducting your literature search, but do not waste valuable time. Query the online database "help" menu to assist you with getting started.
3. Begin by identifying the major professional nursing journals that publish nursing research. Determine if those journals are available in the database, and start your literature review with those. If your problem is in a specialty area, review specialty journals.
4. If you find an article related to your problem, look at *that* author's reference list for other current articles and journals.
5. Read the abstract of the article first; this will give you a quick overview of the article to determine if it is relevant to your topic under study.
6. Know the limitations of the databases where you do your search.
7. Carefully appraise information obtained from the Internet that is not part of an established online database, such as Journals-@Ovid; EBSCOhost; ProQuest; Thomson Gale PowerSearch.

Step 4: Implementing

This step involves the implementation or application of the new approach, along with the collection of the evaluation data. By following the specific plan that you established in Step 3, the new approach will be introduced into practice. It is important that you begin collecting your evaluation data at the same time so that you can clearly determine the effect of the new approach.

Step 5: Evaluating

Step 5 involves the evaluation of the implementation (Step 4) to determine whether the new approach improved practice outcomes. Whether or not you will continue using the new approach in the practice setting may also be determined based on new technology, economic considerations, or changes in staffing. If there is no change in outcomes, you may want to return to the previous practice, or the evaluation phase may lead to another research utilization project. For example, if the practice problem is significant and the practice outcomes were not improved, another new approach may be tried.

Research Utilization: What Is It Not?

Research utilization does *not* entail simply taking the findings of a single research study and using those findings in nursing practice. Research studies are replicated to rule out chance findings and validate previous studies. Similar studies with different populations are conducted to determine the applicability of findings to different groups of people. For these reasons, research utilization encompasses the findings of many studies to develop the new approach that will be put into practice.

Data are collected in the process of research utilization. However, research utilization is not the collection of data to answer a research question, as is the case when conducting research. The data collected in research utilization are needed for evaluation to determine whether there is some advantage to the new approach in the practice setting. The data collected must be carefully considered in light of your specific setting.

Research utilization should not be confused with a review of nursing practice. Practice review involves a quality control/risk management process to evaluate the appropriate use of resources related to a specific treatment. As with research utilization, practice review use does not entail the use of nursing research findings during the process of evaluation.

When you review the nursing research literature for research utilization, as mentioned previously, there is no assurance that you will find studies that are directly applicable to your practice situation. Your specific question may not have been the topic of previous research studies. In this case, you may have to either adapt the findings from the literature, conduct your own research, or both.

RESEARCH UTILIZATION COMPARED WITH NURSING RESEARCH AND THE CONDUCT OF RESEARCH

How Is the Use of Research in Practice Different From Conducting Research?

As illustrated in Table 24.1, the major steps involved in both conducting and utilizing research are the same. Both are problem-solving processes involving critical thinking. For example, a clinical practice problem may provide the impetus to conduct and use research. However, there are differences. Conducting research taps into the "ways of knowing," whereas using research taps into the "ways of doing."

TABLE 24.1 COMPARISON OF PROCESSES

An Overview of the Nursing Process, Conducting Research, and Research Utilization

NURSING PROCESS	CONDUCTING RESEARCH	RESEARCH UTILIZATION
Preprocess Establish a nurse–patient relationship	**Preplanning** Identify the need for a research study Determine feasibility	**Peruse** Identify a practice problem that needs a new approach
Scan the literature	Obtain consensus	
Assessing Gather data	**Assessing** Identify the problem State research purpose Begin to formulate the research question Review the literature	**Assessing** Identify and critically evaluate published research related to your practice problem Identify the findings that are adaptable to your problem and your context
Planning Diagnose Set goals	**Planning** Identify and define the variables Select a conceptual or theoretical model	**Planning** Determine the new approach and the desired outcomes Establish a systematic method for implementing the new approach
Prioritize Determine nursing interventions	Select research design Finalize research question Plan data analysis Write research proposal	Establish a method for evaluating the outcomes of the new approach
Formulate care plan Negotiate a site for data collection Complete human subjects review		
Implementing Initiate the plan Train data collectors Obtain subject sample Collect the data Prepare data for analysis	**Implementing** Prepare questionnaires Collect data about the outcomes of the new approach	**Implementing** Begin using the new approach
Evaluating Determine the patient response	**Evaluating** Analyze the data Organize the data	**Evaluation of the Implementation** Determine whether the practice changes improved the patient outcomes
Answer the research question Interpret the results Report the findings Plan next project	Decide whether to continue using the new approach	

Steps for Conducting Research

Step 1: Identify the Problem
    Identify potential issues within the setting and work with authorities in the practice area to define the problem.

Step 2: Establish What Is Already Known About the Problem

Perform extensive literature searches, within scholarly article databases, to determine what is known about the topic and if any research has been previously been conducted in relation to the established problem.

Step 3: Establish a Plan for Conducting the Research

Explore the various research methodologies to determine the best approach for attaining information as it relates the established problem, using research. Identify the question(s) to be answered or the hypothesis to be tested. Consider using the PICOT format, where **P** represents the population of interest, **I** represents the intervention of interest, **C** represents the comparison of interest, **O** represents the outcome of interest, and **T** represents the time frame. The T element may or may not be applicable (Fig. 24.4). Explore the best methods for collecting the research data. Determine the best approach for analyzing the research data.

Step 4: Implement the Research Study

Attain the necessary approvals for the study. Enlist study participants. Perform the research study and collect the data.

Step 5: Examine the Data

Evaluate the data collected from the research study. Apply the results of the data to the research study question(s) or hypothesis. Examine the outcomes of the research study.

Step 6: Utilize the Findings

Determine the strengths and weaknesses of the research study. Apply the results of the research study the established problem. Make recommendations for future research on the topic. Implement the findings, if applicable. Share the findings of the research study with other professionals within the field.

Let us consider the application of the steps for conducting research utilizing a case study.

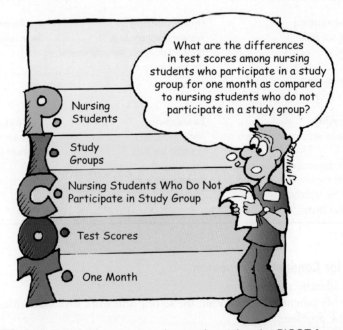

FIG. 24.4 Developing a research question using the PICOT format.

The nursing unit that Mary works on has observed an increase in the number of catheter-acquired urinary tract infections (CAUTIs) in their medical surgical unit. The problem was discussed at length in the monthly nursing staff meeting. Mary and a few of her colleagues have decided to discuss the issue with the clinical nurse specialist (CNS) on the unit. The CNS on the unit worked with the nurses to conduct a thorough literature search to determine what research had already been completed in regard to CAUTIs. After review of the literature, a PICOT was created and the research team identified a few research questions to be addressed in the upcoming research study. Moreover, the team decided that a quantitative, experimental, research design would best assist the team in gathering the best data to answer the questions of the study. The team attained the necessary approvals to conduct the study and patient participants were recruited for the study. The data collected from the research study was analyzed by the research experts within the hospital and the results were applied to the study research questions. The results of the study were discussed and applied to practice. The effectiveness of the findings was evaluated on multiple occasions and the team was pleased to see a decrease in the number of CAUTIs at the end of 2 months.

The team shared the positive results of the research study that yielded a reduction in the number of CAUTIs with the hospital administration, and the results were utilized throughout the hospital system. In addition, the research team wrote up the results of their study, including the strengths and weaknesses of the CAUTI research study, and published them is a research article with goal of improving patient outcomes on a larger scale.

The *utilization of research* involves the systematic process of integrating the findings of completed nursing research studies into clinical nursing practice.

Research utilization also entails reviewing research that has already been completed to develop a new approach to nursing practice. In reviewing research studies, pay particular attention to the type of research methodology employed—quantitative, qualitative, or mixed methods (Table 24.2). All three processes—research utilization, nursing research, and the nursing process—have the same five major steps. However, the specific tasks for each process are different.

What Is the Relationship Between Nursing Theory and Research Utilization?

Nursing theory used as the theoretic framework of a research study is essential for the continued development of nursing theories; new research findings will support theory or will suggest the modification of theory. In contrast, when a specific nursing theory is used as the framework for nursing practice, the focus is on the intervention. The intervention that is designed in the planning phase of research utilization must be consistent with the theory. For example, if Orem's theory of self-care requisites were used for nursing practice, a successful intervention would be one that emphasizes self-care rather than care received from others. There is a close relationship between nursing research and research utilization because of the focus of both on nursing practice.

DEFINING YOUR PRACTICE CONTEXT

Your practice context will determine to what degree you can apply the findings from nursing research to your practice problem. A *practice context* entails a blending of all those factors and systems that contribute to the delivery of nursing care. This blend includes the health, social, and cultural characteristics of the patient population served: the type of practice setting, the economic resources of the setting, the type of health care delivery system, the existing policies and procedures, the staffing pattern, and the administrative structure. Each factor or system can be either enabling or inhibiting, but it is the practice context as a whole that is evaluated to determine the applicability of nursing research findings.

TABLE 24.2 COMPARISON OF QUANTITATIVE, QUALITATIVE, AND MIXED-METHODS RESEARCH DESIGNS

RESEARCH DESIGNS	QUANTITATIVE RESEARCH	QUALITATIVE RESEARCH	MIXED-METHODS RESEARCH
Philosophical paradigm	• Examination of a cause-and-effect relationship • Deductive approach	• Acquire understanding of phenomena by observing behaviors, reactions, statements of study participants • Inductive approach	• Involves aspects of quantitative and qualitative philosophical frameworks. Blending of both deductive and inductive approaches
Purpose of study	• Study focuses on supporting or refuting the null hypothesis • The research variables are discussed and examined in detail to determine if a relationship or causality exists	• Study typically focuses on central concept or aspect for further exploration	• Provides rationale for why both quantitative and qualitative methods are warranted in the study
Research question	• Closed-ended questions • Questions ask, "What differences exist," "What is the effect," "What is the relationship … ?" • Null hypothesis is either supported or refuted based on study findings	• Open-ended questions • Questions ask, "How" or "Why"? • Broad questions that seek to explore perceptions, beliefs, attitudes of a particular phenomenon of interest	• May include both closed-ended and open-ended questions
Data collection	• Follows specific sequence • Similar to scientific method; numeric data collected through questionnaires, surveys, established instruments • Large sample size	• Data collected through observing, interviewing, audio/video recording • Small sample size • Study participants are typically selected by researcher	• Dependent on the type of mixed-method design employed
Data analysis	• Statistical analysis; numeric data reported • Data analyzed is unbiased and objective	• Researcher interprets data by developing themes based on participants' views and observations • Data analyzed is subjective in nature; may include words, artifacts, images, anecdotal statements	• Dependent on the type of mixed-method design employed

What Are the Health, Social, and Cultural Characteristics of the Patient Population Being Served?

To begin defining your practice context, you will need to identify any characteristics that are specific to the group of people who will be receiving nursing care. Is there some particular health characteristic that should be considered? For example, if you teach prenatal classes, the health characteristic will be pregnancy. Are there some particular social and cultural characteristics that need to be considered? If your prenatal classes are for pregnant teenagers who are single, then social characteristics require special consideration. Be as thorough and as specific as possible in identifying these characteristics.

What Are the Health Care Delivery Characteristics of Your Setting?

As you continue to define your practice context, specify the type of practice setting, the economic constraints of the setting, the type of health care delivery system, the existing policies and procedures, the staffing patterns, and the administrative structures. In other words, include all the characteristics of the care setting that will either contribute to or inhibit the process of applying research findings. If your practice setting were in a hospital where there is a limit to the length of stay for a particular surgery, then a new approach that would increase that length of stay would not be an appropriate one for implementation. Furthermore, when implementing a new approach in practice, care must be taken to preserve or improve the current health care delivery standards.

What Are the Motivators and Barriers for Incorporating Nursing Research into Your Practice?

Identify your bridges (motivators) and roadblocks (barriers) in the practice setting (Critical Thinking Box 24.1). The more individuals in the practice setting from whom you can attain consensus on the new approach to practice, the easier it will be to implement. Those who understand the need for making a change in practice will be more likely to support the change. (See Chapter 10 for information on change theory.) Those who feel they had a part in the decision making surrounding the new approach are also more likely to promote it. In both instances, these colleagues become motivators for the implementation of innovation and change.

> ### ⍰ CRITICAL THINKING BOX 24.1
>
> Think about…
> * What are the barriers that might inhibit your use of research findings?
> * Are these findings applicable to your practice setting?
> * How would you go about minimizing the barriers?

As with any change process that involves a group of people, it is very likely that some individuals in the practice setting will be resistant to the new approach. Those who are resistant may present barriers that prevent the full implementation of the new process. They may complain about a lack of time to learn the new approach, for example, in an effort to avoid being a part of what they do not support. These colleagues, as well as budgetary and personnel constraints, are examples of barriers.

In addition, the research literature may present barriers to implementing a new approach. For example, if there are only a few research studies reported in the nursing literature that are related to your practice problem, then the lack of replication of the findings may prevent you from developing a research-based approach for your particular practice problem. Another barrier is the time lag from the completion of a research project until the project report is published. This time lag, which may be a few years, may make the research findings obsolete. For example, research related to glass oral thermometers would be obsolete, because your practice setting now uses electronic ear thermometers. When reviewing the literature, try to limit your search criteria to studies published within the previous 5 years, unless it is a classic study that will substantiate the need for conducting research on your practice problem.

THE NATIONAL INSTITUTE OF NURSING RESEARCH

What Is Its Function?

The National Institute of Nursing Research (NINR) is a branch of the National Institutes of Health (NIH), which is under the jurisdiction of the U.S. Department of Health and Human Services. Each institute within the NIH focuses on a specific area of health care research; the NINR is a major source of federal funding for nursing research. The NINR also supports education in research methods, research career development, and excellence in nursing science.

Other functions of the NINR are to establish a National Nursing Research Agenda. This agenda is composed of priority topics for nursing research and may be related to a national health need, or they may be in an area that requires research for the advancement of nursing science. Many nurses have received funding to support clinical and basic research on health and illness across the lifespan. Funded research includes health promotion and disease prevention, quality-of-life issues, health disparities, end-of-life and palliative care, symptom management research, data science, global health, and genomic science. For more information, visit the NINR website (http://www.ninr.nih.gov/).

THE AGENCY FOR HEALTHCARE RESEARCH AND QUALITY

What Is Its Function?

As part of the Omnibus Budget Reconciliation Act of 1989, the Agency for Health Care Policy and Research (later renamed the Agency for Healthcare Research and Quality [AHRQ]) was established to enhance the quality and effectiveness of health care services. The AHRQ conducts and supports general health services research, develops clinical practice guidelines, and disseminates research findings and guidelines to health care providers, policy makers, and the public. As mentioned previously, one arm of the AHRQ supports the EBP Centers Program (AHRQ, 2018b), which develops reports about interventions that are based on published scientific studies related to health care. For more information about AHRQ, visit their website (www.ahrq.gov/).

CONCLUSION

Nursing has a growing body of evidence on which we can support our practice. Moreover, research utilization is a key component of effectively implementing EBP protocols aimed at improving patient outcomes. Whether you are a new graduate or an experienced nurse, there are ample opportunities for you to apply research in your area of clinical practice. When areas of practice need to be changed, it is important to have valid information and data to support the need for change. Check out your hospital resources, establish networking and colleague support, and participate in EBP in your workplace setting.

🌐 RELEVANT WEBSITES AND ONLINE RESOURCES

American Nurses Association
Research toolkit. https://www.nursingworld.org/practice-policy/innovation-evidence/improving-your-practice/research-toolkit/

American Speech-Language Hearing Association
Evidence-based practice tutorials and resources. http://www.asha.org/Research/EBP/Evidence-Based-Practice-Tutorials-and-Resources/

California State University, Chico
What is a scholarly article? https://www.csuchico.edu/lins/handouts/scholarly.pdf

Duke University Medical Center Library & Archives
Resources for EBP. http://guides.mclibrary.duke.edu/nursing/ebp

Indiana Center for Evidence-Based Nursing Practice
http://ebnp.org

National Institute of Nursing Research
Building the scientific foundation for clinical practice. https://www.ninr.nih.gov/

North Carolina State University
Anatomy of a scholarly article. http://www.lib.ncsu.edu/tutorials/scholarly-articles/
Peer review in five minutes. http://www.lib.ncsu.edu/tutorials/pr/
Scholarly vs. popular materials guide. http://www.lib.ncsu.edu/guides/spmaterials/

The Academy of Medical-Surgical Nurses
Evidence-based practice. https://www.amsn.org/practice-resources/evidence-based-practice

University of North Carolina
Evidence-based nursing introduction. http://guides.lib.unc.edu/c.php?g=8362&p=43029

BIBLIOGRAPHY

Agency for Healthcare Research and Quality (AHRQ). (2018a). Clinical guidelines and recommendations. Retrieved from http://www.ahrq.gov/professionals/clinicians-providers/guidelines-recommendations/index.html.

Agency for Healthcare Research and Quality (AHRQ). (2018b). Evidence-based practice centers (EPC) program overview. In Retrieved from http://www.ahrq.gov/research/findings/evidence-based-reports/overview/index.html.

Melnyk, B. M., & Fineout-Overholt, E. (2005). *Evidence-based practice in nursing & healthcare. A guide to best practice.* Philadelphia: Lippincott Williams & Wilkins.

NCSU Libraries. (2014). Peer review in 3 minutes. Retrieved from http://www.lib.ncsu.edu/tutorials/peerreview/.

Potter, P. A., Perry, A. G., Stockert, P. A., & Hall, A. M. (2017). *Fundamentals of nursing* (9th ed.). St. Louis, MO: Elsevier.

25

Workplace Issues

*Mary Boyce, MSN, RN, CCRN, CNE**

ⓔhttp://evolve.elsevier.com/Zerwekh/nsgtoday/.

Fear is the father of courage and the mother of safety.
Henry H. Tweedy

The safety of the people is the supreme law. (Salus populi suprema lex.)
Cicero (106–143 BC)

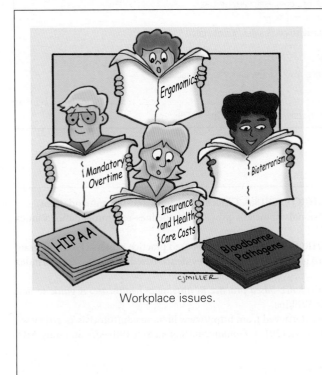

Workplace issues.

After completing this chapter, you should be able to:

• Determine your risk for encountering a workplace issue that can affect your health or well-being.
• Understand ergonomics and ways to protect self from workplace injury.
• Strategize ways to recognize errors and minimize further harm or injury.
• Know the risk of exposure to hazardous substances.
• Recognize the risk for violence at work and how to reduce your risk.
• Analyze workplace bullying and harassment.
• Create a personal plan to handle workplace problems such as staffing shortages and being assigned (floating) to an unfamiliar workplace.
• Identify useful internet sites to remain up to date with potential workplace issues (e.g., Occupational Safety and Health Administration [OSHA], Centers for Disease Control and Prevention [CDC], American Nurses Association [ANA]).

*We would like to thank Susan Ahrens, PhD, RN, for her previous contributions to this chapter.

Ahospital, nursing center, clinic, or physician's office can present potential hazards to your future health and well-being. *This is especially true if you are not informed.* Many nurses are aware of the risk of exposure to infection, but they are not aware of other hazards that exist in health care organizations. Nurses in a health care organization have an increased risk for injury, toxic chemicals, bioterrorism, and violence. How well a health care organization plans and protects workers from occupational hazards is a measure of how safe you can expect to be and what safety measures you need to take as you work. This chapter addresses workplace issues that could potentially affect your health and well-being and provides strategies to avoid injury, occupational exposure, and illness.

QUESTIONS TO ASK WHEN STARTING A NEW POSITION

As a nurse, when you are preparing to start a new position, ask your employer to answer the following questions to evaluate the impact workplace issues will have on your health and well-being:

- Is the hospital latex-free? If not, what latex will I be exposed to?
- Will patient safety equipment such as lifts, transfer boards, and gate belts be available? How much will I be lifting, pulling, and tugging? Does the hospital use lift teams?
- Ask to see a common patient room. Think about moving around in the room, and ask how much moving of furniture, stretchers, or equipment you will be doing. Will I be using a computer? Is it wall mounted so that I need to stand to type, or will there be a desk to sit at when I need to type?
- What is the nursing injury rate for the unit I will be working on?
- Who is the contact person for worker's compensation in the organization? Would I be able to return to work in a light-duty capacity if I am injured? For how long? What are the rules of the state?
- Does the organization have an antiviolence program? How does the organization address bullying behaviors and other hostile work situations such as sexual harassment?
- Is the organization needleless? If not, what is my exposure risk?
- What is the organization's policy for exposure to infectious agents? Does it include testing, medication, counseling, and follow-up? What is the process for this? (This information can often be found in the employee handbook.)
- What is the organization's tuberculosis (TB) prevention plan? Does the plan adhere to Occupational Safety and Health Administration (OSHA) regulations? How often will I be tested?
- Does the organization have an influenza prevention plan? Does it follow the Centers for Disease Control and Prevention (CDC) guidelines?
- Is there a plan for handling potentially toxic or infectious substances such as blood, chemoprophylaxis, and suction canisters? What is my potential exposure? Will I receive training in correct handling? Will annual refreshers be offered?
- Where will I park? Is the area well lit? Is it patrolled? Have there been any serious events in the past 6 months?
- Does the organization provide vaccinations for infections I might be exposed to, such as influenza, chickenpox, and hepatitis B?
- Who is responsible at the hospital for the surveillance plan for multidrug-resistant organisms (MRSA, VRE)?
- How often will I be expected to work "off shift" (shifts other than what I normally work), on-call, or mandatory overtime?
- How often will I need to work on a unit other than my assigned unit? How will I be oriented?

ERGONOMIC HAZARDS FOR HEALTH CARE WORKERS

Nurses have chosen a profession that places them at risk for serious musculoskeletal injuries. In 2016, registered nurse (RN) injury and illness incidence rates were 104.2 cases per 10,000 full-time employees compared with 91.7 cases in all other occupations. The most prevalent injuries were related to physical effort resulting in sprains, strains, or tears. RN injuries primarily affected the back (Dressner & Kissinger, 2018). Unfortunately, these types of injuries are the most debilitating. Imagine if you could not raise your arms or reach for things without severe pain. What if you needed help to dress yourself because you lost flexibility in your shoulder joint? What would happen if every step you took resulted in pain in your back and down your leg? What if sitting or lying down did not relieve your distress? These are potential health-related problems of nurses that can be minimized by following safety standards and protocols.

Back Injury

So, what is your risk? That is somewhat unclear because studies investigating work-related injuries in nursing vary. One study reported that 90% of nurses complain of back pain (Kyung Ja & Sung-Hyun, 2011). Master, Serranheira, and Loureiro (2017) found that 89% of primary care nurses suffered a work-related musculoskeletal disorder, of which 63% were lower back injuries. The risk for injury increases if the nurse provides direct patient care such as turning, toileting, and providing for activities of daily living. Lifting, repositioning, and transferring are actions associated with work-related injuries (OSHA, 2015). On average, nurses and other health care workers manually lift an estimated 3600 pounds per shift (American Nurses Association [ANA], n.d.). In addition, the configuration of a patient's room and the placement of furniture, monitors, and equipment can require the nurse to reach and stretch in nonergonomic positions. These factors increase the risk of injury. Back-related injuries reduce the already short supply of nurses, and when there are fewer nurses, the risk for back-related and other musculoskeletal injuries increases. It becomes a vicious cycle.

In the past, it was believed that use of proper body mechanics with safe lifting techniques could prevent back and shoulder injuries. However, the ANA (2016) suggests there is no safe way to lift or turn a physically dependent patient manually. Many of the situations in which nurses are injured involve patients making sudden, quick changes in position. Therefore proper body mechanics are not enough to safeguard against injury, because the nurse cannot adjust in a way that fully protects the back. *Teaching nurses to use proper body mechanics to lift and turn patients does not result in fewer injuries* (ANA, 2016). Because of the dangers associated with manual patient handling, the current recommendations by the ANA include eliminating manual lifting and using assistive patient-handling devices for lifting, transferring, and turning patients (ANA, 2016).

It is important that nurses take care of their backs, even when they are young, flexible, and strong, because aging contributes to the risk for a career-ending injury. In addition, as people age, there is a loss of flexibility and increased musculoskeletal instability. Repetitive stress on the structures of the spine, shoulders, and hips can cause small repeated muscle and tendon damage that could manifest in serious debilitating injury. Consider what happened to Sandy.

Sandy was a strong, flexible, and healthy nurse. She could lift patients in bed, turn them, bathe them, and ambulate them without help. Very seldom did she ask for help. She could stand, walk briskly, and work for 16 hours without a break. She was proud of her abilities and the fact that she was everything to her patient. She was the nurse on the unit everyone loved to work with because of her independence and willingness to help others.

Today at age 50, things are much different. She sits in an office all day wishing for her bedside job. She changed jobs because she could no longer work at the bedside. Her shoulders, knees, back, and hips were damaged from the chronic stress of repetitive lifting, straining, and reaching during her career.

Safe Patient Handling and Mobility

What could have been done? Implementation of a safe patient handling and mobility (SPHM) program would be a current solution to an age-old problem. The ANA has endorsed H.R. 4266/S.2408, the Nurse and Health Care Worker Protection Act of 2015, which is proposed legislation to improve the quality of patient care and protect nurses by addressing SPHM (ANA, n.d.). Currently the legislation is still under review at the federal government.

Prompted by the ANA, 12 states—California, Illinois, Maryland, Minnesota, Missouri, New Jersey, New York, Ohio, Rhode Island, Texas, Washington, and Hawaii—have enacted "safe patient handling" legislation (ANA, 2016).

Even though federal legislation is under review and even if your state has not enacted legislation to support safe patient handling, many organizations and facilities have instituted SPHM programs. According to ANA Factsheet (n.d.), successful SPHM programs have reduced the incidence of injury, in some cases up to 95%. In addition, the cost savings in injury prevention and nurse turnover due to injury could save $27,000 and $103,000 per nurse, respectively. SPHM programs must be supported by management and administration who are willing to make a commitment to safety for patients and health care providers. An interprofessional committee, involving front-line health care providers, would create policies and procedures specific to the facility needs. As a nurse hired at the facility, you would be trained to assess each patient to determine mobility needs per shift or daily. Hands-on training by SPHM champions would give you a chance to learn to use the equipment to provide safe transfers. You might learn to use ceiling track lifts in a bariatric unit. Those same champions are experts available to answer questions and reinforce adherence to standards. Documentation of patient mobility assessment and utilization of appropriate techniques is essential. SPHM is often discussed at preshift huddles and staff meetings to evaluate how well the program is working and if revisions are needed.

So, what can a nurse do to reduce the risk of serious back injury? First, be aware of the potential risk by assessing each patient's dependency needs and abilities when deciding what assistive devices to use. Do not move, lift, or turn a dependent person without an appropriate assistive device or help (Fig. 25.1). Next, know what assistive devices are available to you, and learn how to use them properly. If your organization does not have devices readily available, become an advocate for a safe patient-handling program. If an injury occurs, report the injury according to policy and follow through with your health care provider (HCP) advice for medical treatment. For more information on ways to promote safe patient handling and start a SPMH program in your facility, visit https://www.nursingworld.org/practice-policy/work-environment/health-safety/handle-with-care/

Although no specific strategies have been statistically proven to prevent or treat low back pain in nurses, stretching exercises may be beneficial (VanHoof et al., 2017). Nurses should consider developing a practice for "warming up" and stretching before they start their workday. This is to be followed by stretching again at the end of a day. Another strategy to maintain a limber, flexible body core is to enroll in a yoga or Pilates program.

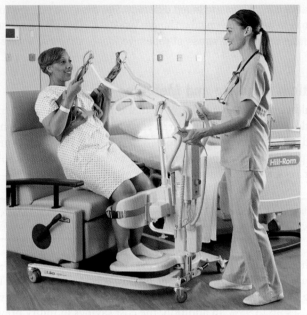

FIG. 25.1 Mechanical lift system.

Ergonomic Workstations

Currently, many jobs are performed at a computer work area, often in a "shared" area. This is the case in a hospital setting, where nurses, physicians, and ancillary caregivers frequently use the workstation 24 hours a day. Change, variation, and adjustment to fit an individual worker are basic to the well-being of each worker. Workstations should be adjustable to accommodate users of many different heights, weights, and individual needs. Computer vendors must keep in mind that the "typical" nurse is in his or her mid-40s, so letter size and font, as well as proper lighting and the avoidance of shadows, are vitally important to aid in viewing computer screens.

The successful ergonomic design of an office workstation depends on several interrelated parts, including the task, the posture, and the work activities. The three activities alone can be difficult to handle, but these activities must also interact properly with existing furniture, equipment, and the environment. The combination of the aforementioned makes the picture more complicated. Important parts of the workstation are the chair, desk, and placement of the computer (CPU), keyboard, and monitor.

The chair should be padded appropriately, be easily adjustable, and have strong lumbar support. Usually, wheels allow easy movement, and armrests may or may not be used because they sometimes cause more problems, depending on the individual needs of the user. Therefore armrests should be fully adjustable to accommodate the user.

The desk must be wide and deep enough to accommodate the computer's monitor, keyboard, and mouse, with ample space around the machine to write, use the phone conveniently, and perform all other desktop activities. Keep the area clear of clutter and crowding.

Ideally, the placement of the monitor, keyboard, and mouse would be adjustable for every worker, but because this is rarely possible, the monitor height should be approximately 18 to 22 inches above the desk surface, causing most users to view the screen with slightly lowered eyes.

The keyboard should be placed directly in front of the user and the mouse on the user's dominant-hand side of the machine. Some nursing stations designate certain machines as left-handed mouse machines so that the mouse will not need to be switched numerous times during a shift. Be sure to use a mouse pad to ensure traction, lessening the frustration and continual long movements of the mouse (Critical Thinking Box 25.1). Workstations on wheels (WOWs) or wireless computers on movable stations provide the nurse with accessibility to patients while administering medications and completing assessments. However, they often clutter small rooms and need to be plugged in frequently. If the stations are not properly locked when in use, they may present a fall or slip risk. Some individuals wearing glasses need "computer lenses" to make reading the monitor easier and screen out blue light, which is associated with a higher incidence of cataracts and macular degeneration (Wood, 2014).

? CRITICAL THINKING BOX 25.1

What is your workplace environment like? What lift equipment do you have? Have ergonomics been considered? How could you make it better?

Repetitive Motion Disorders

Poor workplace design is often the major source for repetitive motion disorders (RMDs) or cumulative trauma disorders (CTDs). RMDs have been associated with users who work for long periods at poorly constructed or poorly arranged workstations.

Ergonomic design of work tasks can reduce or remove some of the risks. Other solutions may include

- Information and training to workers about body positions that eliminate the opportunity for repetitive stress injuries to occur
- Frequent switching between standing and sitting positions, reducing net stress on any specific muscle or skeletal group
- Routine stretching of the shoulders, neck, arms, hands, and fingers

> Having a thorough understanding of ergonomic principles can help to prevent injuries.

WORKPLACE VIOLENCE: A GROWING CONCERN IN HEALTH CARE

Witnessing the aftermath of a violent attack on a nurse colleague is a powerful realization that the potential for being harmed by another person at work is very real. As a nurse, you are at risk for harm from coworkers, patients, and families. No matter what the occupation, workplace violence is an ongoing concern in the United States. For RNs in 2016, 12.2% of all injuries were violent events, which reflected an incidence rate 3 times greater than for all other occupations (Dressner & Kissinger, 2018). The nature of health care workers' jobs puts them at risk for workplace violence, which can result in injury or death (Foley & Rauser, 2012).

Workplace violence is defined by the United States Department of Labor as "an action (verbal, written, or physical aggression) which is intended to control or cause, or is capable of causing, death or serious bodily injury to oneself or others, or damage to property. Workplace violence includes abusive behavior toward authority, intimidating or harassing behavior, and threats" (n.d.). Nurses often fail to report acts of violence because of a lack of understanding or a belief that "nothing can be changed" (McNamara, 2010). Failure to report can contribute to escalation of the situation until physical violence occurs. In some cases, nurses have never encountered a hostile person before, and they do not understand how to recognize and deescalate the situation. In other situations a nurse can have a history of violence and the experience can bring forth images and memories, called post-traumatic stress disorder (PTSD). Anyone who has experienced violence is at risk for experiencing this phenomenon wherein the individual can experience intense emotions such as anxiety, depression, anger, and flashbacks (reexperiencing the initial event) in response to verbal or physical violence.

Recently, a nurse in a large urban hospital was working with a young man who had been hospitalized with chest pain. He had denied any drug use; however, it was found that he habitually used cocaine and also consumed large amounts of alcohol on a regular basis. Once the physician discharged him, the patient grew increasingly agitated waiting for the paperwork for his discharge. He wanted to leave the facility to resume his drug-related behaviors.

The nurse had been working on the unit less than a year after graduation and did not recognize the patient's increasing agitation. He used the call light to repeatedly summon the nurse to the room asking when he could leave. When she entered the room in response to his fifth call and told him it would be another 30 minutes before she could complete the paperwork for his discharge, he attacked her. Before she was able to call for help, she was assaulted and seriously injured, requiring surgical repair of lacerations and a head injury. The nurse recovered fully from a physical standpoint but suffered severe PTSD and was not able to return to her chosen profession. All the nurses on the unit suffered emotionally. Some were fearful that a similar event could happen to them.

In response to incidents such as this, along with other events occurring in the community, the hospital administration developed a crisis intervention program. This program taught nurses and other hospital staff how to recognize signs of escalating anger that could result in a violent attack and strategies to deescalate the situation. Nurses were also taught how to protect themselves during an attack (e.g., keeping the door between you and the patient for easy escape). Knowing how to recognize an escalating situation and how to defend against an attacker helped these nurses to believe they could manage future situations that put them at risk for harm.

In addition, the hospital instituted a "code white" program. A code white or in some facilities a "code gray" alerts all staff of a potentially violent situation. Anyone could initiate the code if *any* person became loud or abusive, made threats, or acted in a physically threatening and harmful manner. A code white ensured that resources were available to help deescalate the situation and that no nurse or any other staff member would be alone with someone who was acting out. Trained volunteers and other staff from the hospital, including security staff, responded to a code white, which would be announced over the hospital's public announcement system. It was emphasized to nursing staff members that any time they felt unsafe, a code white should be called. The code could be implemented by using the phone system or by pushing a strategically placed alarm button. After instituting the program, there were no further incidents in which nurses were harmed over the ensuing years.

So, what do you need to do when you start your first job? First, be familiar with your organization's policies regarding workplace violence. Next, consider taking a crisis intervention course to become familiar with the signs of escalating violence, such as pacing, using foul language, raising one's fist, or using threats. Learn strategies to deescalate anger. Finally, do not ever try to handle a potentially violent person on your own. Use whatever procedures your organization has put in place to defuse situations; for example, call security or call a code white (Fig. 25.2).

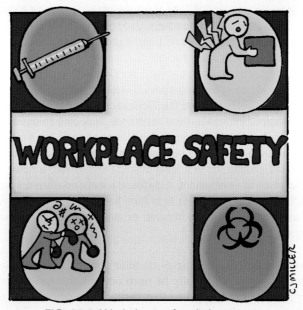

FIG. 25.2 Workplace safety is important.

Lateral Violence (Bullying) and Other Forms of Workplace Harassment

As a nurse and individual, it is easy to recognize overt violence. Most hospitals have procedures and policies to handle violent events. Less common is recognition and action related to *horizontal or lateral violence*, which is often called *bullying* in the workplace; however, these terms are different. Lateral violence refers to violence directed to an individual by another individual who is considered a colleague or equal in terms of job scope, whereas bullying is defined by Kirchner (2009) as "the purposeful exertion of power that is perceived by the victim as physically or emotionally threatening" (p. 177). Most of us believe that the backyard bullies of our childhood will disappear in adulthood. Unfortunately, recent evidence has proven otherwise. Our bullies of childhood tend to grow into the bullies of our adulthood. Consider what happened to Judy:

Judy was excited to start work in the critical care department. She was pleased that the manager had selected her to start there, because she understood the criteria for working in that department as a new graduate were very strict. She had chosen a preceptor from the nurses she knew.

Soon, she found herself to be totally stressed out by work. Always optimistic, she was now nervous and had an onset of migraine headaches. She was not sleeping or eating normally. Her family was very concerned.

At the request of her family, Judy went to see a counselor at the employee assistance program. The counselor helped her to identify that nurses on the unit were bullying her by targeting and isolating her by their responses to the things she did or said. For example, during shift report, if she asked a question, the nurses at the report table would put down their pens and stare at her or roll their eyes. If she asked for help lifting a patient, everyone would ignore her. The nurse who was the leader of the bullying would yell at her in front of everyone for minor transgressions (if she dropped a pill or forgot to write her blood glucose readings on the report board). If Judy made a mistake, everyone knew about it, and the story of the event would grow as it was passed on to others. Judy overheard these comments and was often angry. The anxiety caused by knowing she would be treated unfairly every day was impairing Judy's ability to grow and develop as a new nurse. It was also having a negative effect on her patient care and personal health.

Judy needed to understand better what was happening to her so that she could recognize the signs if she was ever the victim of bullying again. She also needed to develop a plan to manage her current situation. She found a website called the Workplace Bullying Institute (www.bullyinstitute.org) that provides a wide array of helpful information and assistance, including coaching and current legislation. With the help of her counselor, Judy developed an action plan to address her situation. After time off to contemplate her work life and after she realized the bullying behavior would not be addressed at her current place of employment, Judy found another job in a local hospital and started a new position.

At her new place of employment, Judy found a wonderful mentor and was soon growing as a nurse. Her physical health improved, and with help from her counselor and coach, she was once again a mentally healthy person. Judy had learned from her experience and was determined never to allow a bully to have such an impact on her again.

You may have heard that "nurses eat their young." Mild forms of hazing activity are common in many professions and can usually be overcome by those who are victims of these behaviors. New nurses may feel the need to prove that they can be counted on to provide safe patient care. They may find their work ethic, values, and skills are being "tested" by other nurses. This type of activity usually lasts for the first weeks of a new position and gradually improves as a new nurse becomes integrated into the work life of the unit.

In contrast, lateral violence goes beyond this initial struggle and has serious physical and psychological consequences for the victim as well as negative patient safety outcomes, which has been documented in the research literature (Blair, 2013; McNamara, 2010). In nursing practice, Kirchner (2009) defined lateral violence as a type of workplace abuse that occurs between individuals who are on the same level or equal in terms of their job responsibilities (i.e., nurse to nurse). Bullying is not a single event—it occurs over time.

Lateral violence can occur in any workplace setting. Health care environments are particularly situated to foster bullies, because they are hierarchical in nature and tend to involve a great deal of change. In addition, the underlying culture of health care has tended to foster the idea that certain rites of passage must be endured by all new staff. Many of our health care organizations are fear driven and feel pressured to raise productivity standards higher and higher to improve profits. According to the Workplace Bullying Institute (2015), these factors can create a culture that fosters bullying. A manager, supervisor, physician, or coworker can be a potential bully. The signs that you may be experiencing bullying are identified by individuals who had been targets at the workplace (Box 25.1).

For most nurses, the idea that another person would deliberately target them for lateral violence and bullying is difficult to comprehend. We often have a naïve belief that bullying is a part of childhood but not a part of adulthood. As a result, the person being bullied can experience a multitude of psychological and physical reactions. The target of lateral violence may even believe that the bullying is his or her fault.

Research has indicated that many psychological and physical effects can result from lateral violence. Lateral violence and bullying create anxiety, fear, and anger in most adults. Because lateral violence is unrelenting and often severe in nature, the victimized individual has a heightened stimulation of the sympathetic nervous system. As a result, the target of a bully can develop psychological and physical symptoms, including vomiting, anxiety disorders, chest pain, and abdominal pain. Depending on the bullying situation, the signs and symptoms of PTSD may follow (Matthiesen & Einarsen, 2004).

BOX 25.1   SIGNS OF BEING BULLIED

Experiences Outside Work

- You feel like throwing up the night before the start of your work week
- Your frustrated family demands that you stop obsessing about work at home
- Your doctor asks what could be causing your skyrocketing blood pressure and recent health problems and tells you to change jobs
- You feel too ashamed of being controlled by another person at work to tell your spouse or partner
- All your paid time off is used for "mental health breaks" from the misery
- Days off are spent exhausted and lifeless; your desire to do anything is gone
- Your favorite activities and fun with family are no longer appealing or enjoyable
- You begin to believe that you provoked the workplace cruelty

Experiences At Work

- You attempt the obviously impossible task of doing a new job without training or time to learn new skills, but that work is never good enough for the boss
- Surprise meetings are called by your boss with no results other than further humiliation
- Everything your tormenter does to you is arbitrary and capricious, working a personal agenda that undermines the employer's legitimate business interests
- Others at work have been told to stop working, talking, or socializing with you
- You are constantly feeling agitated and anxious, experiencing a sense of doom, waiting for bad things to happen
- No matter what you do, you are never left alone to do your job without interference
- People feel justified screaming or yelling at you in front of others, but you are punished if you scream back
- HR tells you that your harassment isn't illegal, that you have to "work it out between yourselves"
- You finally, firmly confront your tormentor to stop the abusive conduct and you are accused of harassment
- You are shocked when accused of incompetence, despite a history of objective excellence, typically by someone who cannot do your job
- Everyone—coworkers, senior bosses, HR—agrees (in person and orally) that your tormentor is a jerk, but there is nothing they will do about it (and later, when you ask for their support, they deny having agreed with you)
- Your request to transfer to an open position under another boss is mysteriously denied

From Workplace Bullying Institute (http://www.workplacebullying.org/individuals/problem/early-signs/).

Because most of us are unprepared to deal with a bully in the workplace, it can be difficult to determine what actions to take to address it. The Workplace Bullying Institute website (http://www.workplacebullying.org/individuals/solutions/wbi-action-plan/) has an excellent plan to follow. Drs. Namie and Namie (2003) suggest taking the following three steps if you are the target of a bully:

1. *Name it.* Say, "I am being bullied!" "I have a bully at work!" "Jackie is a backyard bully." Other ways to validate it for your own sense of self is to say, "I did not ask for this! Jackie targeted me to bully." This type of self-talk will help to validate your experience.

2. *Seek respite.* From their work, Drs. Ruth and Gary Namie believe that if you are being bullied, you need to take time off from work to "BullyProof" yourself. During your time off from work, you need to accomplish five things: (a) check your mental health, (b) check your physical health, (c) research state and federal legal options, (d) gather data regarding the economic impact the bully has had on your unit, and finally (e) start a job search for a new position, because this will give you more options as you address your current work situation.

3. *Expose the bully.* Most people who are being bullied are not willing to expose the bully. However, for your mental and physical health, you need to consider giving your employer an opportunity to address the situation (Workplace Bullying Institute, 2015).

Consider the following:

Mary was a confident nursing student who expressed her superiority to fellow students. She was the first to answer questions and correct others if she thought they made mistakes. While in nursing school, the faculty avoided her and did not address her behaviors or the effect those behaviors were having on other students and the learning environment. Mary graduated from nursing school and was hired as a medical-surgical nurse in a busy metropolitan facility. She carried her behaviors from nursing school to employment. She belittled colleagues and expressed disgust with their lack of organization and poor time management skills. Mary's colleagues went to the unit manager to report her behaviors and attitude. The unit manager, Jennifer, had recently attended a seminar about creating a culture of civility. Jennifer was aware of some of the consequences of incivility, such as employee dissatisfaction and turnover, increased illness and sick days, and poor patient care. Jennifer provided training and reinforced the standards expected on the unit. Staff nurses were empowered to have strategic, planned conversations with Mary. Mary did not expect the confrontation, because no one had ever questioned her communication and behaviors before. She did not consider herself to be a bully or an instigator of lateral violence. She agreed to practice communication strategies and shared that she felt insecure about her abilities as a new graduate but was determined to never let it show. Jennifer reinforced to the unit staff that all team members should report bullying or incivility. Remaining silent is the worst response. Further training and role-playing sessions were provided to the staff.

Bullying and incivility can begin when a nursing student is socialized into the profession. It may occur between students or with a student and faculty member. Altmiller (2012) reported that students felt justified to behave uncivil if faculty behaved with incivility towards them. So, from students, to nurses, to leaders, and administrators, a culture of civility in needed. Nurses are called to be role models of civility. How civil are you? Take the Clark (2013) Workplace Civility Index. Visit http://stopbullyingtoolkit.org/Clark-Workplace-Civility-Index.pdf.

Given the devastating impact that workplace violence and bullying have on nurses and patient outcomes, the ANA issued a position statement indicating that the nursing profession has initiated a zero-tolerance policy for workplace violence and bullying and charged all nurses and health care professionals to implement measures for creating a culture of respect (ANA, 2015).

OTHER WORKPLACE ISSUES

Needlestick and Sharps Safety

In addition to the workplace issues already identified, latex allergy, severe acute respiratory syndrome (SARS), human immunodeficiency virus (HIV), TB exposure, and needlestick injuries are issues that can affect your health if you are not aware of how to prevent exposure and injury (Box 25.2). The OSHA has established guidelines that organizations must follow to protect workers. The Needlestick Safety and Prevention Act (P.L. 106-430), which became law on November 6, 2000, provides important protections for health care workers regarding needlestick injuries. Advocating for workplace safety, the ANA was instrumental in having this piece of federal legislation passed. This act amends the Blood-Borne Pathogen Standard (administered by OSHA) to require the use of safer devices to protect from sharps injuries. It also requires that employers solicit the input of nonmanagerial employees who are responsible for direct patient care regarding the identification, evaluation, and selection of effective engineering and work-practice controls (Fig. 25.3).

In addition, the act requires employers to maintain a sharps injury log to document, at a minimum, the type and brand of device involved in each incident, the department or work area in which the exposure occurred, and an explanation of how the incident happened. The information

---

| BOX 25.2 | **NEEDLESTICK AND SHARPS-RELATED INJURIES** |

- Needlestick and sharps-related injuries expose all health care workers to potential bloodborne pathogens (hepatitis B virus, hepatitis C virus, and human immunodeficiency virus).[1]
- It is estimated that 385,000 needlestick injuries occur in hospitals annually.[2]
- The majority of needlestick injuries occur in surgical settings such as the operating room and at the patient's bedside.[3]
- The Food and Drug Administration, Centers for Disease Control and Prevention, National Institute for Occupational Safety and Health, and the Occupational Safety and Health Administration (OSHA) issued a statement in 2012 encouraging all health care workers in surgical settings to use only blunt-tip suture needles when suturing muscle and fascia.[1]
- All sharps and needlestick injuries must be recorded by the employer as required under OSHA's Recordkeeping Standard.[3]

Data obtained from:

[1]Centers for Disease Control [CDC]. (2012). FDA, NIOSH, & OSHA Joint safety documentation: Blunt-tip surgical suture needles reduce needlestick injuries and the risk of subsequent bloodborne pathogen transmission to surgical personnel. Retrieved from http://www.cdc.gov/niosh/topics/bbp/pdfs/Blunt-tip_Suture_Needles_Safety.pdf.
[2]Centers for Disease Control [CDC]. (2013). Sharps injuries. Retrieved from http://www.cdc.gov/niosh/stopsticks/sharpsinjuries.html.
[3]Occupational Safety and Health Administration [OSHA]. (2016). *Healthcare wide hazards: Needlestick/sharps injuries*. Retrieved from https://www.osha.gov/SLTC/etools/hospital/hazards/sharps/sharps.html.

---

is to be recorded and maintained in a way that protects the confidentiality of injured employees. The log serves as an important data source to help determine the relative effectiveness and safety of currently used devices and to guide the development of future products. You need to be familiar with these requirements, as well as any additional guidelines that have been established by your local or state health departments. In some states the guidelines established by health departments are more strict than those established by OSHA. Currently, every organization that uses needles or sharp devices should have policies covering needlestick and sharps exposures/injuries to protect and treat their employees.

Handling Staffing Shortages

The shortage of experienced nurses has created many challenges and changes in the health care environments in which we work. Many of these changes are just beginning. We will see many more in the years to come as the supply does not meet the demand and the need for nursing grows. As a nurse, you need to understand these issues, how to find the best place to work, and how to cope with situations such as high nurse-to-patient ratios and mandatory overtime.

An organization (hospital, clinic, nursing center) that provides an environment that is conducive to good nursing care is the best place to be. It does not need to be the newest and most technologically advanced hospital in a large city.

Finding a good place to work can be challenging and requires a solid evaluation of the potential work environment. For years, many health care organizations have ignored the needs of nursing (Duclos-Miller, 2002). To attract nurses, many health care organizations use incentives rather than making substantial changes to the environment for nursing (workloads, autonomy). Of course, the lure of higher salaries, benefits, sign-on bonuses, and tuition repayment programs can be highly appealing for new nurses; however, these incentives can distract new nurses from investigating other issues that will have a greater effect on long-term job satisfaction. As a new nurse looking for a position, it may be challenging to find the best fit. Fortunately, there are research-based criteria that can help you determine whether an organization provides a good environment for nursing.

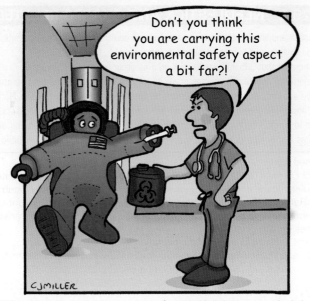

FIG. 25.3 Nurses must be aware of potential threats to their health.

In the early 1980s, the American Academy of Nursing (AAN) commissioned a study to determine what hospital characteristics attract nurses. Characteristics such as nursing autonomy, low nurse–patient ratios, and collaborative relationships with physicians were attractive to nurses. From this work, Magnet hospitals were identified that embodied these essential characteristics that promoted nursing. In our current nursing shortage, hospitals actively seek Magnet status to attract nurses. In addition, Magnet hospitals are known to have better patient outcomes. The American Nurses Credentialing Center (ANCC) is responsible for judging whether hospitals achieve this status. A hospital awarded a Magnet Recognition Program would be a good place to work for most nurses (Critical Thinking Box 25.2). To find the magnet hospitals in your state visit this website: https://www.nursingworld.org/organizational-programs/magnet/find-a-magnet-facility/.

? CRITICAL THINKING BOX 25.2

To find out more about the characteristics of the Magnet model, see https://www.nursingworld.org/organizational-programs/magnet/why-become-magnet/benefits/. Determine the benefits of being employed in a magnet facility.

Currently, no matter where you work, you may need to cope with a situation in which the number of patients under your care, their needs, and acuity may be greater than what you are able to provide. What should you do?

First, it is important to understand the chain of command for your organization. In other words, who do you report your concerns to, and what are your next steps if you feel the issue is not resolved? For example, perhaps the supervisor is the person approach, and if that does not resolve the situation, according to the chain of command, you contact your manager, then the director for the department, then the chief nursing officer. With each step in the process of reporting, remain focused on the issues, present the facts, offer suggestions for resolution, and remain respectful and professional. Here are some things to consider:

- How many patients do you have? What is going on with each of them? What nursing tasks do you need to accomplish? What are your priorities (safety issues)? What tasks would be "nice to do if you are able and have the time"?
- What are your resources? Do you have someone to whom you can delegate tasks? What support do you have from patients' families (e.g., to help watch a confused patient)?
- Are you aware of a nurse colleague who might be able to come and help (e.g., someone who was not considered by those who worked on staffing the unit)? What about someone who works on another similar unit who might be willing to pick up time?
- Is there anyone who can help out for a few hours to cover the gap and make sure there are no safety issues?
- Is there any other way to deliver care? For example, working together as a team to take care of patients can be a more efficient way to function for a particular shift, even though it is not ideal and can result in fragmented care.
- What are your hospital's policies for high-census or high–patient-load situations? For example, can you decrease the frequency of assessment from every 4 hours to every 6 to free up some time?
- Consider how sick your patients are. Is there anyone who might be discharged to lighten the load?

Gather your facts and present your concerns to the next person in authority—a charge nurse or a supervisor. Do not threaten to leave or make rash statements; just present your facts. Ask for whatever assistance is available. Tell this person what your concerns are and what you can and/or cannot accomplish in your shift based on the high patient load. Use a concise, clear outline of the situation and what you need from that individual.

Document Your Concerns

If the response you receive does not result in satisfaction, then you need to calmly tell your charge nurse or supervisor that you are going to report your concerns to the next person in charge. Again, do not threaten. If the situation is continuous rather than intermittent, use the notes you have documented to figure out the pattern of what is happening.

> Remember that difficult situations tend to be in the forefront of your mind, whereas reality might be different. This is human nature.

Consider the following example:

Some nurses told their nurse manager that they were always getting patients from surgery who did not meet criteria to be discharged from the recovery room. The examples that they gave were very disturbing to the new manager, so she asked them to keep a log of patients who were unstable when they reached the unit. In the next month, instead of a large number of patients coming back from the recovery room unstable, they experienced only two. In both situations the patients became hypotensive and required a significant amount of care to stabilize their condition. What the staff and the manager realized after looking at the data was that those two situations were so stressful that they "forgot" the 50 patients who came back without a problem. The other important thing that happened was that a solution was found to prevent the hypotensive events. The nursing staff worked with the surgical providers and made certain that patients received adequate fluids in the recovery room. During the following months, the nurses had no further events. Improved patient care was the result of the careful and diligent documentation and the nursing staff's willingness to work toward finding a solution. This is why documentation of events is so important.

If your notes tell you that poor staffing occurs more often than not, and you are not able to get your patient care done, then you need to work with your manager to determine the reasons. Is your unit understaffed for the needs of your patients? Does your unit have many vacancies? Does your unit have a lot of sick calls? Are assignments being done correctly? Are nurses performing frequent nonnursing functions such as phlebotomy, running errands, or transcribing orders? Does your unit need someone to help with nonessential nursing duties such as bathing or feeding patients? Many organizations involve staff nurses to help solve these problems. Volunteer to work with a group to make changes. If your organization or unit is not willing to work with you to make the workload easier, then you may need to consider a job change. Working together as a team and being able to solve staffing issues with creative solutions is the goal of any discussions with leadership. Consider this unit's experience:

Nurses on the telemetry unit on the 7 AM to 7 PM shift were exhausted. They had a large unit of patients with high acuities. Their patients were generally elderly and had heart failure, and many had multiple chronic health problems. The unit had been approved for an additional RN position, but it had been vacant for more than a year because there was a serious nursing shortage in their area. Everyone felt deflated, and people were beginning to feel that the situation was never going to improve. They enjoyed the challenges of the unit, but they were tired and experiencing burnout. The manager held a staff meeting seeking solutions to their staffing difficulties.

After intense discussions with few solutions, one of the nurses stated, "Most of the time, I just need someone to help me with morning care and making sure my patients get turned and fed before their meals get cold!" The other nurses on the unit agreed with her comments. After discussions, a solution to their short staffing was found.

The manager was able to hire a nursing student to help on the unit for 6 hours in the morning by assisting with hygiene care, turning, feeding, and ambulating patients. The relief of having this help accomplished what they needed, and the morale on the unit significantly improved. As an added bonus, the nursing student soon graduated and decided to stay on the unit because of her positive experience. She started out as a new RN, and her orientation was shortened because of the time she had spent on the unit before her graduation. Everyone won—the patients, staff, and health care facility.

Mandatory Overtime

Unfortunately, mandatory overtime is another way that hospitals deal with poor staffing. Mandatory overtime creates a loss of control for the nurse regarding the ability to schedule nonwork activities, including essential family functions. Mandatory overtime may also put safe patient care at risk because of nurse fatigue and subsequent loss of the ability to concentrate, critically think, and make good judgments. Bae (2012) found 60% of nurses surveyed in the United States worked overtime. Of the sample, approximately 17% reported it was the norm to work more than 40 hours per week. The study also found that long hours worked by nurses were a combination of both mandatory and voluntary overtime hours. Mandating overtime is a major concern of our professional associations (e.g., ANA; American Association of Critical Care Nurses).

Although it is our professional duty to ensure that nursing services are continued until the patient's care is transferred to another nurse, our duty to ensure that patients receive safe treatment may be in conflict if mandatory overtime results in fatigue and the possibility of a serious error occurring. According to Duclos-Miller (2002), all nurses need to recognize that by accepting a nursing position, they have made a commitment to the organization to provide nursing care at specified intervals. After we accept responsibility for a patient assignment, we have that responsibility either until our services are no longer needed or until we transfer the responsibility to someone else. Does this mean we need to work beyond our capacity?

> Many states have enacted legislation prohibiting mandatory overtime. Is your state one of them? You can go to the ANA website to find out whether your state has mandatory overtime legislation.

Legislation opposing mandatory overtime is a priority of the ANA. Legislating overtime of nurses may not be the only answer. Health care organizations must be able to provide care to their patients, and legislation will not be sufficient to alleviate the workloads imposed if there are not enough nurses to take care of patients.

In addition to the previous discussion related to developing a good work environment for nursing, creative solutions can be developed by management and nursing staff to handle shortages without resorting to mandatory overtime. Some ideas include the following:

- Develop an on-call system that provides one or two extra nurses per shift.
- Develop policies that limit mandatory overtime and ensure rotation among all staff.
- Provide incentives to encourage part-time nursing staff to pick up extra time.
- Develop creative shifts for high-activity, high-volume times (e.g., perhaps a special 11 AM to 2 PM shift to provide staff for admissions and transfers and to reduce the workload for the rest of the staff).
- Develop processes to identify shortages with enough time to arrange coverage.
- Reward nurses who do put forth extra effort for the organization. For example, one hospital provides a bonus of $100 for every 100 hours of on-call time (in which an individual agrees to be available to come in if needed).
- Improve the workplace environment in ways that are advocated by the American Association of Critical Care Nurses, and institute recommendations from the "Healthy Work Environment" campaign and by the ANCC Magnet program. These recommendations have proven that better environments draw nurses and can alleviate shortage situations.

What should you do if you are mandated to stay over your scheduled shift because of a staffing shortage? First, you should be familiar with your organization's policy regarding mandatory overtime *before* this happens. If the policy is unacceptable to your life circumstances, you probably should not be working in the facility. If you find yourself in a situation in which you believe you are too fatigued to stay over your shift, you need to follow the chain of command in asking for assistance with your situation. Again, you need to assess your situation and provide the charge nurse, supervisor, or manager with the facts of your situation. You need to document your concerns and follow up as needed after the event. If you believe your organization policy regarding mandatory overtime can be improved or eliminated, work with your manager and others to change it.

> Most causes of medical errors relate to system problems:
> 1. Communication problems
> 2. Inadequate information flow
> 3. Human problems
> 4. Patient-related issues
> 5. Organizational transfer of knowledge
> 6. Staffing patterns/work flow
> 7. Technical failures
> 8. Inadequate policies and procedures (Agency for Healthcare Research and Quality [AHRQ], 2003)

Assigned to a Unit That Is Unfamiliar (Floating)—What Do I Do Now?

One interesting phenomenon about health care is that it has a cyclic nature to some extent. What this means is that during certain times of the year, there may be fewer or greater numbers of patients needing any one service at any given time. Thus sometimes on a particular unit you may have more and sometimes fewer patients. It would be great to have a break when your patient volumes are lower; however, it does not work this way in most situations, because there are always units that need help. No one would want patients to suffer from lack of care when there is a nurse available on a unit that has fewer patients. For both economic and logistical reasons (e.g., another unit is very busy), nurses who are less busy are often instructed to work on a unit that is not their "home unit." The question becomes, "What will I do if this happens?" Consider the following situation and imagine what you might do.

Denise was finished with her orientation and had been working on her own for approximately 6 months. She was told about the floating policy on her unit—how everyone took turns if help was needed on another unit. The unit had been very busy since she had started working, so she did not often think of the issue of floating until this evening. When she came to work, the unit was very quiet, and she was told to report to the surgical unit. Because Denise normally worked on a medical unit, she was naturally anxious about this assignment. The nurses on her unit were sympathetic, but they reminded her of the unit's policy and that it was her turn to go to another unit (float).

When Denise arrived on the surgical unit, she was given an assignment of five patients with a variety of surgical problems (gallbladder to colon resection). Most of her patients had tubes, dressings, and a variety of comorbidities such as diabetes and hypertension that complicated their recovery. Two hours into her shift, she was completely overwhelmed. The nurses she was working with were very kind, but they were also busy, and Denise did not want to bother them with ongoing questions about the location of items and the policies for dressing changes and management of nasogastric tubes. Denise managed to get through the night without any mishaps; however, she was charting until 8 AM (she was supposed to be off duty at 7 AM).

Denise continued to be angry and upset about the floating for many days. She was hostile toward the charge nurse, supervisor, fellow nurses, and even her manager for making her do this. Because her unit did not become busy right away, she worried about having to float again. She felt she could handle it occasionally but not repeatedly. She began to think about leaving. Denise's manager, Joyce, approached her after several days and asked to discuss the situation. Joyce said she had some thoughts and ideas that might help. Denise reluctantly sat down with Joyce to hear her ideas.

Issues surrounding floating are some of the most concerning and intensely felt by nurses, managers, and administrators. Some journal articles and nursing newsletters recommend that nurses agree to float and always take an assignment. Other sources advise nurses to agree to go but to only do basic nursing care and not to take an assignment. The ethical issue involved in floating is that if you are not on your assigned unit, there will be a disproportionately high number of patients to nurses, which would increase errors, or there is the risk of having a less skilled nurse on a unit, which can also lead to problems. Studies have not demonstrated that the risk of a less skilled nurse has contributed to patient harm, whereas studies of nursing workload have indicated that the greater the workload, the greater the risk for harm to patients (Kane-Urrabazo, 2006).

Data are available that support the more patients a nurse has, the more likely that an error will occur (Kane-Urrabazo, 2006); however, there are no data that tell us how many—if any—patients experience adverse outcomes by floating nurses. Although many nurses passionately believe that if they go to another unit the likelihood of an error occurring is very high, there are no data to support this contention.

Therefore some argue that it is unethical for a nurse to refuse an assignment if it is reasonable. Refusing an assignment to float could result in harm to a patient because of unreasonable workloads on the other unit. On the other hand, the organization owes its nurses, and patients, an orientation session on all the units to which they may be assigned. This notion is based on the ideas of distributive justice (Kane-Urrabazo, 2006). Many states, such as Iowa and Texas, have written guidelines or position statements on floating, as have many nursing organizations such as the American Association of Colleges of Nursing (AACN) and the American Organization of Nurse Executives (AONE). Regulatory agencies such as The Joint Commission (TJC) have stated that leaders in organizations must define the qualifications and competencies necessary to provide patient care. Hospitals need to have floating policies and plans to orient staff to units where they may be assigned. Again, what should conscientious nurses do to ensure the safety of their patients and to protect their ability to practice?

As Denise met with her manager, the manager first thanked her for floating and not making a big deal about it at the time. Her manager acknowledged that floating was very unsettling, and she asked Denise what would have made the change in assignment better. Denise told her manager that she was glad to have been able to help on the other unit, because it was very busy, and she did not know what they would have done had she not been there. However, Denise felt it would have been better if she had been given orientation to that unit and to surgical patients before being asked to float there. She added that it would have helped to know where supplies were located and to know what patient care standards were used to help them recover from surgery.

As a result of Denise's conversation with the manager, an orientation program was developed to help nurses who were floating to other unfamiliar units. To make this successful, the hospital was divided into "pods" of similar units. Nurses would only float within their pod. A support system was built into floating situations by assigning a manager or supervisor "buddy" to check on the floating nurse periodically throughout the shift to see whether there were any issues or problems. A debriefing session was held with each nurse who floated to determine ways to make the experience better.

Several months later, Denise was pulled to help another unit. Although she did not like being off her normal unit, she tolerated the experience much better than she did the first time. She made sure she had a resource person to help her with problems and questions. She was able to leave at her normal time. Overall, she felt good about helping out another unit.

If you are assigned to float, don't panic! Remain professional in all of your actions! It might be helpful to remember first that you are going to help another unit that does not have enough staff to care for their patients. If nothing else, focus on the patients and what you would want for someone you love if he or she were a patient on the busier unit.

Then, think of the other unit, and consider what types of patients are on the unit. When you arrive, ask for any overflow patients who might have needs similar to patients on your normal unit (e.g., any overflow medical patients if you have a medical background). Ask for a quick tour of the unit and the unit standards of care (e.g., how to manage care of the postoperative mastectomy patient). Ask to be assigned to patients who are less complex because you will be learning as you go along. Ask for help as you need it. Ask whether a nursing assistant can be assigned with you.

If you arrive at the assigned unit and things do not go well, report the experience to your supervisor as soon as possible. Document your conversations. Try to enjoy your patients and appreciate what you have learned during your shift. If it is available to you, use the internet to investigate unfamiliar patient-care issues. Remember, regardless of your experience, you are doing what is best for the patient.

Making a Mistake—What Do I Do Now?

Every year, thousands of medication errors are made in hospitals (Institute of Medicine [IOM], 1999). In addition to medication errors, other errors compound to contribute to many serious effects on patients every year, including death. The IOM was chartered in 1970 as the advisor for the U.S. health care system regarding the quality of care (www.iom.edu). In 2003, Congress mandated that the IOM perform a comprehensive study regarding drug safety and recommendations for a system-wide change. The landmark 1999 IOM report on errors in health care stated that 44,000 to 98,000 people die every year from errors (IOM, 1999).

Karen was a conscientious person and a cautious nurse. As a new nurse, she was constantly worried that she would make a mistake. Every day, throughout her orientation, she would breathe a sigh of relief at the end of her shift that she had not made a mistake. In fact, a year went by without any event. One very busy day as she charted her last medications for the day, she had the awful realization that she had given an intravenous medication to the wrong patient. She went into the room hoping that somehow the medication (an intravenous piggyback) had not gone through the pump. Unfortunately, the patient had received a dose of medication that she was not ordered to receive.

Karen quickly checked the patient's allergies; then she went about assessing the patient for any untoward effects. Fortunately, the patient did not seem to be experiencing any adverse effect at this time. Through checking, Karen determined that the medication did not have any interaction with any other drug the patient was receiving. The medication was rather benign (Pepcid), and a case could be made that the patient would benefit from the medication, even though it was not ordered.

Karen had to decide what to do. She thought of herself as the "perfect" new graduate. She had not made a mistake in the year since she had been out of school. What would happen to her image with her colleagues? What about her manager, who had just last week praised Karen for her "careful attention to detail." Now she thought, "Could I be fired?"

Fortunately for Karen, her patient did not suffer adverse effects from the medication; however, the fact that a very cautious nurse made such an error demonstrates a gap in medication safety. What might have contributed to this event? The only way that this event can contribute to the understanding of what happened is if Karen reports it. Karen did not necessarily realize this because she was thinking mainly of the implications for the patient and for her practice of nursing.

To meet regulatory agency standards, hospitals must have a process for reporting and analyzing errors. Karen remembered that she was shown the process for reporting medication and other errors or events (including injury to herself). She also remembered that there was a policy for how to do this and how to document the event. She went to the policy manual online and looked it up.

As she read the policy, Karen learned that she needed to complete the online report for medication error, which included all aspects of what happened. The form also asked her to report her feelings regarding the event, because her hospital was trying to understand what it was like to experience an event and what kept nurses from reporting. She learned from reading the policy that the leadership of the hospital appreciated her taking time to complete the form and report the event. She also learned that unless she was deliberately harming the patient, she would not receive disciplinary action; however, her peers would review the event to determine what she could have done to prevent it.

Another step in the process was for Karen to notify the charge nurse, supervisor (or her manager), and the physician. This was difficult for her to do; however, Karen followed through on completing these steps of the process. To her surprise, the physician, charge nurse, and supervisor were all professional and understanding when she notified them of the event.

Karen's manager thoroughly discussed the medication error with her the following day. Karen was glad she had taken notes and had thought through what had happened, because this enabled her to provide her manager with a lot of detail about what had happened. Her manager was very matter of fact about the situation and did not berate or otherwise demean Karen in any way. She also suggested (strongly) that Karen see a counselor at the employee assistance program because she assumed that Karen would have a lot of feelings about what had happened, and these feelings could potentially affect her self-confidence. Karen followed through on this advice as well. She was glad that she did because she eventually realized that even though her medication error did not have an adverse event on the patient, it had indeed shaken her confidence and was affecting her ability to care for her patients (Research for Best Practice Box 25.1).

RESEARCH FOR BEST PRACTICE BOX 25.1
Medication and Practice Errors

Practice Issue

As the care of patients becomes more complex, the delivery of medications also becomes more complex. Currently, nurses are frequently faced with interruptions during the delivery of medications. Adding to interruptions, other factors such as inadequate communication, medication storage, and failing to follow the six rights of medication administration (right patient, medication, dose, route, time, documentation) can contribute to medication errors (Institute for Safe Medication Practices, 2010). The problem is that, at a time when the reporting of all errors is extremely important, not all are reported (Ulanimo et al., 2006). Nurses fear retribution or disciplinary action, despite the fact that most organizations do not punish nurses in any way for errors that occur (unless they are committed deliberately).

Implications for Nursing Practice

* Nurses need to be aware of potential errors by examining the complexity of their work flow and reporting near misses.
* Nurses need to follow standards of care and avoid shortcuts to care (i.e., have a second nurse verify all high-alert medications prior to giving to your patient)
* During the delivery of medications, nurses must take steps to avoid interruptions (e.g., don't page a physician, don't start a procedure, don't start a conversation with another person, don't answer the phone unless it is absolutely necessary).
* Nurses need to know their hospital policy and procedure for handling and reporting errors.
* Nurses need to read back and verify for accuracy all incoming telephone orders.
* If a nurse is involved in an error, that nurse should seriously consider counseling to manage the strong feelings that result from making a mistake in a nurse–patient relationship. Nurses often experience posttraumatic stress disorder following an event in which an error is made.
* Nurses should be actively involved in finding solutions to prevent errors in the future. This might include using barcode-assisted medication technologies in conjunction with an electronic medication administration record (Seibert et al., 2014).

Considering This Information

Knowing that you could be involved in an error someday, how can you prepare yourself to prevent this from happening and to be able to handle an error if it does happen?

References

Institute of Medicine. (1999). *To err is human: Building a safer health system*. Washington, DC: National Academies Press. Retrieved from http://iom.nationalacademies.org/reports/1999/to-err-is-human-building-a-safer-health-system.aspx.

Institute for Safe Medication Practices. (2010). *ISMP medication safety alert! Nurse advise-ERR [Newsletter]*. Retrieved from http://www.ismp.org/Newsletters/nursing/default.asp.

Institute for Safe Medication Practices. (2016). *Targeted medication safety best practices to hospitals*. Retrieved from https://www.ismp.org/Tools/BestPractices/Default.aspx.

Lilley, L., Collins, S. R., & Snyder, J. S. (2016). *Pharmacology and the nursing process* (8th ed.). St. Louis, MO: Elsevier.

Seibert, H. H., Maddox, R. R., Flynn, E. A., & Williams, C. K. (2014). Effect of barcode technology with electronic medication administration record on medication accuracy rates. *American Journal of Health-System Pharmacy, 71*(3), 209–218. https://doi.org/10.2146/ajhp130332.

Ulanimo, V., O'Leary, C., & Connolly, P. (2006). Nurses' perceptions of causes of medication errors and barriers to reporting. *Journal of Nursing Care Quality, 12*, 28–33.

Wood, G. W. (2014). *Light and eye damage. American Optometric Association*. Retrieved from www.aoa.org/light-and-eye-damage.

CONCLUSION

As you stand at the door, your new license in hand, the greatest human adventure awaits you. Nursing is one of the most difficult and most rewarding professions that exist. As a nurse, you have the opportunity to be part of and witness the most intimate moments in the lives of individuals and families. You have the ability to change people and be changed forever.

Nurses in the hospital need to become more involved in the design, management, and environment of their units. Too often, nurses yield their responsibility and power to the nurse manager and lose out on this opportunity. Nurses need to speak up in nonemotional (but passionate) voices to correct situations that put them and their patients at risk. There are solutions to mandatory overtime, floating, work-related injuries, and workplace violence. At the end of this chapter is a list of relevant websites and online resources related to current workplace issues. Nurses need to be at the forefront of developing demonstration projects and research on ways to improve the work and healing environment. With the critical thinking and problem-solving skills nurses have, we can make a difference.

🌐 RELEVANT WEBSITES AND ONLINE RESOURCES

American Association of Colleges of Nursing
https://www.aacnnursing.org.

American Association of Critical Care Nurses Healthy Work Environment
https://www.aacn.org/nursing-excellence/healthy-work-environments.

American Nurses Association
www.nursingworld.org.
Safe Patient Handling. https://www.nursingworld.org/practice-policy/work-environment/health-safety/handle-with-care/.
Violence, Incivility, & Bullying. https://www.nursingworld.org/practice-policy/work-environment/violence-incivility-bullying/.

American Nurses Credentialing Center Magnet Status Certification
https://www.nursingworld.org/organizational-programs/magnet/.

American Organization of Nurse Executives
www.aone.org.

Institute of Medicine
http://iom.nationalacademies.org/.

Occupational Health and Safety Administration
www.osha.gov.

The Joint Commission
www.jointcommission.org.

United States Department of Labor
www.dol.gov.

BIBLIOGRAPHY

AHRQ's Patient Safety Initiative. (2003). *Building foundations, reducing risk. Interim Report to the Senate Committee on Appropriations.* AHRQ Publication No. 04–RG005. Rockville, MD: Agency for Healthcare Research and Quality.

Altmiller, G. (2012). Student perceptions of incivility in nursing education: Implications for educators. *Nursing Education Research, 33*(1), 15–20.

American Nurses Association. (2015). ANA sets "zero tolerance" policy for workplace violence, bullying. Retrieved from http://nursingworld.org/MainMenuCategories/WorkplaceSafety/Healthy-Nurse/bullyingworkplaceviolence/ANA-Sets-Zero-Tolerance-Policy-for-Workplace-Violence-Bullying.html.

American Nurses Association. (n.d.). Factsheet. Nurse and healthcare worker protection act. Retrieved from https://www.nursingworld.org/~4af9f9/globalassets/practiceandpolicy/work-environment/health–safety/nursehealthcareworkerprotectionact-factsheet.pdf.

American Nurses Association. (2016). Safe patient handling and mobility (SPHM). Retrieved from http://nursingworld.org/MainMenuCategories/Policy-Advocacy/State/Legislative-Agenda-Reports/State-SafePatientHandling.

American Nurses Association. (2018). Safe staffing. Retrieved from https://ana.aristotle.com/SitePages/safestaffing.aspx.

Bae, S. (2012). Nursing overtime: Why, how much, and under what conditions? *Nursing Economics, 30*(2), 60–72. Retrieved from https://www.nursingeconomics.net/ce/2014/article30026071.pdf.

Blair, P. L. (2013). Lateral violence in nursing. *Journal of Emergency Nursing, 39*(5), e75–e78. https://doi.org/10.1016/j.jen.2011.12.006.

Clark, C. M. (2013). *Creating and sustaining civility in nursing education.* Indianapolis, IN: Sigma Theta Tau International Publishing.

Dressner, M., & Kissinger, S. (2018). Occupational illnesses and injuries among registered nurses. *Monthly Labor Review,* 1–8. Retrieved from https://www.bls.gov/opub/mlr/2018/article/occupational-injuries-and-illnesses-among-registered-nurses.htm.

Duclos-Miller, P. (2002). Mandatory overtime: Is it really necessary? *Connecticut Nurse News,* March–May 2002.

Foley, M., & Rauser, E. (2012). Evaluating progress in reducing workplace violence: Trends in Washington state workers' compensation claims rates, 1997–2007. *Work, 42,* 67–81.

Institute of Medicine. (1999). To err is human: Building a safer health system. Washington, DC: National Academies Press. Retrieved from http://iom.nationalacademies.org/reports/1999/to-err-is-human-building-a-safer-health-system.aspx.

Institute of Medicine. (2005). Identifying and preventing medication errors. Retrieved from http://iom.nationalacademies.org/activities/quality/medicationerrors.aspx.

Kane-Urrabazo, C. (2006). Management's role in shaping organizational culture. *Journal of Nursing Management, 14,* 188–194.

Kirchner, B. (2009). Safety: Addressing inappropriate behavior in the perioperative workplace. *AORN Journal, 90*(2), 177–180. https://doi.org/10.1016/j.aorn.2009.07.003.

Kyung Ja, J., & Sung-Hyun, C. (2011). Low back pain and work-related factors among nurses in intensive care units. *Journal of Clinical Nursing, 20*(3/4), 479–487. https://doi.org/10.1111/j.1365-2702.2010.03210.x.

McNamara, S. (2010). Workplace violence and its effect on patient safety. *AORN Journal, 92*(6), 677–682. https://doi.org/10.1016/j.aorn.2010.07.012.

Master, T., Serranheira, F., & Loureiro, H. (2017). Work related musculoskeletal disorders in primary health care nurses. *Applied Nursing Research, 33,* 72–77. Retrieved from https://doi.org/10.1016/j.apnr.2016.09.003.

Matthiesen, S. B., & Einarsen, S. (2004). Psychiatric distress and symptoms of PTSD among victims of bullying at work. *British Journal of Guidance and Counseling, 32,* 335–356.

Namie, G., & Namie, R. (2003). *The bully at work: What you can do to stop the hurt and reclaim your dignity on the job.* Naperville, IL: Sourcebooks.

Ulanimo, V., O'Leary, C., & Connolly, P. (2006). Nurses' perceptions of causes of medication errors and barriers to reporting. *Journal of Nursing Care Quality, 12,* 28–33.

United States Department of Labor. (n.d.). DOL workplace violence programs—appendices. Retrieved from http://www.dol.gov/oasam/hrc/policies/dol-workplace-violence-program-appendices.htm.

Wood, G. W. (2014). Light and eye damage. American Optometric Association. Retrieved from www.aoa.org/light-and-eye-damage.

Workplace Bullying Institute. (2015). The WBI 3-step target action plan. Retrieved from http://www.workplace bullying.org/individuals/solutions/wbi-action-plan/.

VanHoof, W., O'Sullivan, K., O'Keefe, M., Verschueren, S., O'Sullivan, P., & Dankaerts, W. (2017). The efficacy of interventions for low back pain in nurses: A systematic review. *International Journal of Nursing Studies, 33,* 222–231. Retrieved from https://ac.els-cdn.com/S002074891730247X/1-s2.0-S002074891730247X-main.pdf?_tid=393e9eaf-18ef-4480-b8b6-275c957a6296&acdnat=1546405589_86ebba5e8200432c441f83eba7eaa1c6.

Emergency Preparedness

Tyler Zerwekh, BA, MPH, DrPH, REHS and JoAnn Zerwekh, EdD, RN

ⓔhttp://evolve.elsevier.com/Zerwekh/nsgtoday/.

> *Preparation through education is less costly than learning through tragedy.*
> **Max Mayfield, Meteorologist and Director of the National Hurricane Center, circa 2006**

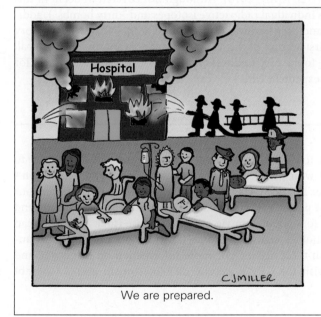

We are prepared.

After completing this chapter, you should be able to:
- Identify various acute community health threats to which the medical community is susceptible.
- Identify regulatory initiatives undertaken to prevent and respond to future emergencies.
- Discuss the variety of diseases/agents that are likely to be involved in a biologic, chemical, or radiologic terrorism attack in addition to the clinical and community health consequences of each.
- Discuss the importance of personal protective equipment and when to implement its use.
- Recognize the concept of triage and apply basic treatment principles therein.
- Identify approaches to enhance personal and family preparedness for emergencies.

Terrorism alarms millions of people every year. It is a violent and deadly form of intimidation with the intent to debilitate governmental function and create a climate of hysteria. Terrorists take advantage of people's panic to achieve their goals. To the terrorist, an event that results in mass fatalities, disruption, and overconsumption of vital resources is a profitable outcome. Since the events of September 11, 2001, and subsequent anthrax mail attacks, terrorism on U.S. soil is a reality. From September 2001 to February 2018, there have been 437 events of terrorism within the United States (Roser, Nagdy, & Ritchie, 2018). Preparation for responding to acts of terrorism and other disasters, both natural and technological, has increased immensely, both in the community and on health care fronts. Community health nurses and clinical nurses have been assigned new responsibilities and roles in the wake of massive federal, state, and local efforts to prepare for public health emergencies. This chapter highlights the various public health threats to which the medical community is susceptible, regulatory initiatives undertaken to prevent future emergencies, and recent public health preparedness efforts bestowed to the nursing profession as the shift to an all-hazards clinical response is integrated throughout the medical and nursing community.

WHAT IS PUBLIC HEALTH PREPAREDNESS?

Public health preparedness, as it relates to the nurse, can be divided into two major categories: (1) clinical preparedness and (2) community-based approaches. The clinical aspects of public health preparedness will focus on agent identification and education for various threats, administrative and regulatory efforts to increase preparedness, and epidemiologic clues that may indicate a public health event has occurred.

The basis for public health preparedness is focused on the concept of preparing for chemical, biologic, radiologic, nuclear, and explosive threats—or CBRNE events. The term *CBRNE* originates from previous military and emergency response organizations such as the U.S. Marine Corps, the U.S. Army, and the Canadian Military Services (U.S. Army, 2016). Although not covered in detail in this chapter (because emphasis will be placed on individual radioactive isotopes and "dirty bombs"), additional information about nuclear weapons and preparedness can be found at the Nuclear Regulatory Commission website (www.nrc.org). The first section of this chapter focuses primarily on chemical, biologic, and radiologic events as they relate to the preparedness and response measures necessary for the licensed nurse to provide efficient and expedient care.

CLINICAL PREPAREDNESS

What Are Biologic Agents?

Given the importance of responding rapidly to a bioterrorism-related event, nurses need to be able to recognize the major syndromes associated with the Centers for Disease Control and Prevention's (CDC's) defined "high-risk" agents. Anthrax, botulism, plague, and smallpox are considered the four top agents for potential bioterrorism because plague and smallpox can be spread person to person and botulism and anthrax can be disseminated to a population via airborne release (they are not spread person to person). Table 26.1 discusses the etiology, signs/symptoms, transmission, and isolation/standard precaution in the care of patients with these agents. For more information on diagnostic and medical management of biologic agents, visit the CDC's website on bioterrorism agents (www.bt.cdc.gov/bioterrorism).

What Are Chemical Agents?

The use of chemical weapons poses an array of problems for the clinical nurse, including contamination, decontamination, and personal protection within the health care facility. Chemical agents can be divided into major classifications based on the makeup of the chemical agent and its clinical presentation. The following section focuses on the primary chemical agents most likely to be used in a terrorist event, along with their symptoms, diagnosis, and treatment options.

Of all the chemical agents of concern for the registered nurse, whether in the clinical or public health sector, nerve agents present the greatest challenge in providing expedient recognition, treatment, and response to a chemical weapon release and subsequent mass casualty event. The nerve

TABLE 26.1 BIOTERRORISM AGENTS

DISEASE/ AGENT	DESCRIPTION PATHOLOGY	SIGNS AND SYMPTOMS	TRANSMISSION	CLINICAL MANAGEMENT
Anthrax *Bacillus anthracis*	Pulmonary: Bacterial spores Toxins cause hemorrhage and obstruction of alveoli in lungs. Cutaneous: Spore enters skin through existing cuts or abrasions in 1–7 days after contact. Gastrointestinal: Ingestion of contaminated, undercooked meat Causes inflammatory lesions in the ileum or cecum	Pulmonary: Flulike Respiratory failure Hemodynamic collapse Usually fatal Cutaneous: Local skin—head, forearms, hands Localized itching followed by a papular lesion that turns vesicular and develops a black eschar in 2–6 days Responds well to antibiotics Gastrointestinal: Abdominal pain, nausea, vomiting, fever within 3–5 days Bloody diarrhea, emesis Usually fatal	Anthrax is a durable spore that lives in the soil; transmission by inhalation of the spore, contact with the spore, and the ingestion of contaminated food No person-to-person contact	Vaccine is available. (This vaccine is not traditionally given to health care workers; has limited availability.) Standard isolation precautions Ciprofloxacin—treatment of choice Postexposure antibiotic prophylaxis for 60 days, if vaccine not available; otherwise 30 days
Botulism *Clostridium botulinum*	A spore-forming anaerobe found in the soil that produces a lethal neurotoxin Neurologic symptoms occur 12–36 h after foodborne botulism and 24–72 h after aerosol exposure.	No fever Drooping eyelids, weakened jaw clench, difficulty swallowing or speaking Blurred vision and double vision Arm paralysis followed by respiratory and leg paralysis Respiratory depression Recovery may take months	Ingestion of toxin-contaminated food; the toxin can be made into an aerosol and inhaled (manmade) Improperly canned foods Contaminated wound No person-to-person contact	Antitoxin available with investigational vaccines being studied Standard precautions Careful clean-up of contaminated food Toxin can be inactivated by heating food or beverage to 212°F (100°C) for at least 10 min. Interdisciplinary planning for nutrition, respiratory and neurologic support, and rehabilitation during long recovery period
Plague *Yersinia pestis*	Bacteria found in rodents and fleas Types: Bubonic	Bubonic: Fever, chills, painful lymphadenopathy (bubo—usually in inguinal, axillary, or cervical lymph nodes)	Direct person-to-person spread Flea bites In a bioterrorist event, most likely to be aerosolized	There is no proven vaccine for the pneumonic plague, which is the most likely version in a bioterrorist event, although vaccines are under development.

Continued

TABLE 26.1 BIOTERRORISM AGENTS—CONT'D

DISEASE/ AGENT	DESCRIPTION PATHOLOGY	SIGNS AND SYMPTOMS	TRANSMISSION	CLINICAL MANAGEMENT
	• Most common • Occurs 2–8 days after bite • 50% fatality if not treated Pneumonic • Occurs 1–3 days after inhalation of organism • Survival unlikely if not treated within 18 h of symptom onset Septicemic (most deadly)	Pneumonic: • Fever, cough, chest pain • Bloody sputum • Sputum can be thick and very purulent or watery with gram-negative rods • Bronchopneumonia and respiratory failure		Antibiotics only effective if administered immediately (streptomycin or gentamicin) Droplet isolation precautions and contact precautions until decontamination is complete, when gross contamination is suspected and when incising and draining buboes Respiratory support
Smallpox Variola major virus	Vaccine created in late 1700s Routine vaccination ceased in the United States with eradication of smallpox in 1979.	Prodrome of fever, myalgia Lesions progress from macules to papules, to pustular vesicles Vesicles on the distal limbs (hands, feet) as opposed to truncated vesicles with chickenpox	Incubation period 10–17 days Highly contagious Direct person-to-person contact, air droplets, and handling contaminated material	Standard, contact, and airborne/droplet precautions (negative pressure room with high efficiency particulate air [HEPA] filtration) for containment One case is a public health emergency due to the high communicability. No known cure Vaccine available and should be given within 2–3 days of exposure Vaccinia immune globulin (VIG) available
Tularemia Francisella tularensis	Bacterial infectious disease of animals Mortality 35% without treatment	Sudden onset of high fever, sore throat, headache, swollen lymph nodes Skin ulcer from tick bites Progresses to pneumonia, pleural effusion with weight loss	Incubation period 1–21 days No person-to-person spread Spread by rabbits and ticks Ingestion of contaminated water, aerosols, or agricultural dusts	Standard precautions Gentamicin treatment of choice Vaccine under development
Viral hemorrhagic fevers Marburg virus Ebola virus Lassa fever	Carried by rodents and mosquitos Virus can be aerosolized	Fever, conjunctivitis, headache, malaise, prostration, nausea, vomiting Hemorrhage of tissues and organs Hypotension Organ failure	Direct person-to-person spread by bodily fluids Marburg: 5–10 day incubation Ebola: 2–21 day incubation Lassa fever: 1–3 weeks' incubation	No vaccine or drug therapy available; however, ribavirin effective in some cases Isolation for containment Use standard, contact, and droplet precautions, including PPE Supportive treatment and care

PPE, Personal protective equipment.

agents, also known as *organophosphate esters*, are the most severe, most incapacitating, and most likely to be implemented of all chemical agents (Wetter et al., 2001). Sarin, soman, tabun, and VX gases are the major chemicals in this group that inhibit acetylcholinesterase. The most well-known use of nerve agents in terrorism occurred in March 1995 when the Japanese cult Aum Shinrikyo attacked a Tokyo subway with 1.3 L of sarin, causing 5510 casualties (Olson, 1999). These agents are liquid at room temperature, but in vapor form they penetrate the cornea, dermis, and respiratory tract. VX gas presents a unique threat because of its markedly greater toxicity and lower volatility, which translates into greater concern for secondary contamination among stricken patients. The effects of these agents are the result of unopposed action of acetylcholine at muscarinic and nicotinic receptors. Initial effects are related to the muscarinic effects, including rhinorrhea, salivation, miosis, and headache. With severe poisoning, nicotinic effects can be observed. The muscarinic and nicotinic effects are manifested by bronchospasm, vomiting, incontinence, muscle fasciculation, convulsions, respiratory failure, and death (Wetter et al., 2001). The antidotes for nerve agent poisoning include atropine at fairly high doses—several milligrams to hundreds of milligrams in some cases—and pralidoxime (2-PAM), up to 8 mg.

The choking, or pulmonary, chemical agents are similar to the blister agents; however, in the choking agents the mechanism of action takes place primarily in the respiratory system. The agents of note in this category are chlorine gas and phosgene (Wetter et al., 2001).

In chlorine gas the majority of exposures occur by inhalation and lead to symptoms of ocular, nasal, and respiratory irritation. The most notable use of chlorine gas occurred at the Battle of Ypres in World War I, where German troops released 160 tons of chlorine gas, exposing nearly 50,000 Allied forces in battle (Szinicz, 2005). Common signs and symptoms of exposure can include eye redness and lacrimation, nose and throat irritation, cough, and suffocation. For cutaneous exposures, burning and blistering of the dermal layer are possible. Currently, there is no available biologic marker for chlorine exposure (CDC, 2018a).

Another choking chemical agent, phosgene gas, has often been described as smelling like freshly cut grass. The majority of exposures to phosgene occur by inhalation. Phosgene exposure has clinical presentation/symptom patterns similar to those of chlorine gas (CDC, 2018a). See Critical Thinking Box 26.1.

? CRITICAL THINKING BOX 26.1

What personal protective equipment (PPE) is available to you at your clinical facility? How does your facility handle exposure to hazardous or toxic material (e.g., blood, bacteria, radioactive)?

Does the use of PPE change with the type of threat presenting at a health care facility (chemical vs. biologic vs. radiologic)?

What Are Radiologic/Radioactive Agents?

The clinical or emergency department (ED) nurse is aware of another concept, which is the potential for patients entering the hospital exposed with radiation. The concept of dirty bombs is relatively new to the field of emergency preparedness, coming to prominence after the 9/11 World Trade Center attacks. A dirty bomb is a radiologic dispersal device (RDD) that combines an explosive such as dynamite with a radioactive material. In the field, the explosion itself would be of greater concern in terms of damage to property and human life; however, the concern in the hospital ED would be the arrival of patients contaminated with radioactive material. The extent of local contamination would depend on a number of factors, including the size of the explosive, the amount and type of radioactive material used, the means of dispersal, and weather conditions. Those closest to the RDD would be the most likely to sustain physical trauma injuries caused by the explosion. As radioactive material spreads, it becomes less concentrated and less harmful (U.S. Nuclear Regulatory Commission, 2018). Acute radiation syndrome (ARS) is an acute illness caused by irradiation of the entire body (or most of the body) by a high dose of penetrating radiation in a very short period (usually a matter of minutes). The major cause of this syndrome is depletion of immature parenchymal stem cells in specific tissues (CDC, 2018a). See Table 26.2 for a listing of syndromes associated with ARS. An excellent website to learn more about radiation syndromes and radioactive agents can be found at https://emergency.cdc .gov/radiation/arsphysicianfactsheet.asp. Also see Critical Thinking Box 26.2.

> ### ❓ CRITICAL THINKING BOX 26.2
>
> What is your organization's policy for managing CBRNE events? Who is the designated safety officer? Where is a copy of the organization safety plan and emergency situation's response plan?

What Is a Pandemic?

In April 2009, public health and medical professionals around the country experienced the first wave of an influenza pandemic on U.S. soil in more than 40 years. Not since the Hong Kong pandemic flu strains of 1968 to 1969 had the medical and scientific community seen such a rapid and expansive surge of H1N1 influenza cases both in the United States and worldwide (CDC, 2018d).

A traditional influenza pandemic can be distinguished from regular seasonal flu epidemics in two major facets: (1) widespread, worldwide cases of the same strain and (2) a novel strain of influenza virus unexpected or previously unidentified in the human population (CDC, 2018d). Typical influenza pandemics often work in waves, which are periods of 6 to 8 weeks between spikes in case totals that can be attributed to primary public health prevention (vaccination), a mutation in virus strain, or a new host susceptibility.

The World Health Organization (WHO) has developed a global pandemic influenza preparedness plan that categorizes various events of a pandemic into different phases (Fig. 26.1). Each phase requires both the clinical and public health nurse to execute specific preparedness and responsive measures to mitigate the influenza pandemic threat. It can be expected during phases 5 and 6, health care facilities will begin "cohorting" influenza patients. Cohort nursing (staff cohorting) is defined as the use of a dedicated team of health care staff to care for patients infected with a single infectious agent. Evidence suggests that this approach may be beneficial when control methods have been unsuccessful and/or an outbreak is continuing. There is some evidence to suggest cohort nursing is an effective intervention to further minimize the risk of cross contamination and should be implemented if there are adequate resources to do so.

For nurses, pandemic influenza planning and response presents a unique and novel approach to clinical and evidence-based practice. It can be expected during pandemic influenza operations that in the onset of mass vaccinations in the general population, the availability of influenza vaccine will be limited as vaccine manufacturers rush to create and fill vaccine orders. When this occurs, federal health authorities, such as the CDC and U.S. Department of Health and Human Services (USDHHS), recommend prioritizing population groups to receive the initial limited supplies of influenza vaccine. These priority groups are identified based on individual medical fragility (i.e., immunosuppression) and susceptibility to the pandemic influenza virus. The astute nurse must be aware of the variability of influenza virus from season to season and must consider priority options when vaccinating selected populations based on these factors. The CDC Influenza website is an excellent source to locate current influenza vaccine priority groups and useful information regarding clinical identification and medical screening (www.cdc.gov/flu/).

TABLE 26.2 ACUTE RADIATION SYNDROMES

SYNDROME	DOSE[a]	PRODROMAL STAGE	LATENT STAGE	MANIFEST ILLNESS STAGE	RECOVERY
Hematopoietic (bone marrow)	Above 0.7 Gy (above 70 rads) (mild symptoms may occur as low as 0.3 Gy or 30 rads)	Symptoms are anorexia, nausea, and vomiting. Onset occurs 1 h to 2 days after exposure. Stage lasts for minutes to days.	Stem cells in bone marrow are dying, although patient may appear and feel well. Stage lasts 1–6 weeks.	Symptoms are anorexia, fever, and malaise. Drop in all blood cell counts occurs for several weeks. Primary cause of death is infection and hemorrhage. Survival decreases with increasing dose. Most deaths occur within a few months after exposure.	In most cases, bone marrow cells will begin to repopulate the marrow. Full recovery is probable for a large percentage of individuals; recovery process may last from a few weeks up to 2 years after exposure. Death may occur in some individuals at 1.2 Gy (120 rads). The LD50/60[b] is about 2.5–5 Gy (250–500 rads).
Gastrointestinal (GI)	Above 10 Gy (above 1000 rads) (some symptoms may occur at as low as 6 Gy or 600 rads)	Symptoms are anorexia, severe nausea, vomiting, cramps, and diarrhea. Onset occurs within a few hours after exposure. Stage lasts about 2 days.	Stem cells in bone marrow and cells lining GI tract are dying, although patient may appear and feel well. Stage lasts less than 1 week.	Symptoms are malaise, anorexia, severe diarrhea, fever, dehydration, and electrolyte imbalance. Death is caused by infection, dehydration, and electrolyte imbalance. Death occurs within 2 weeks of exposure.	The LD100[c] is about 10 Gy (1000 rads).
Cardiovascular (CV)/central nervous system (CNS)	Above 50 Gy (5000 rads) (some symptoms may occur at as low as 20 Gy or 2000 rads)	Symptoms are extreme nervousness and confusion; severe nausea, vomiting, and watery diarrhea; loss of consciousness; and burning sensations of the skin. Onset occurs within minutes of exposure. Stage lasts for minutes to hours.	Patient may return to partial functionality. Stage may last for hours but often is less.	Symptoms are return of watery diarrhea, convulsions, and coma. Onset occurs 5–6 h after exposure. Death occurs within 3 days of exposure.	No recovery is expected.

[a]The absorbed doses quoted here are "gamma equivalent" values. Neutrons or protons generally produce the same effects as gamma, beta, or x-rays but at lower doses. If the patient has been exposed to neutrons or protons, consult radiation experts on how to interpret the dose.
[b]The LD50/60 is the dose necessary to kill 50% of the exposed population in 60 days.
[c]The LD100 is the dose necessary to kill 100% of the exposed population.
From Centers for Disease Control and Prevention. (2016). CDC emergency preparedness and response. Retrieved from www.cdc.gov/nceh/radiation/factsheets/ars.doc

WHO Pandemic Influenza Phases (2009)	
Phase	**Description**
Phase 1	No animal influenza virus circulating among animals have been reported to cause infection in humans.
Phase 2	An animal influenza virus circulating in domesticated or wild animals is known to have caused infection in humans and is therefore considered a specific potential pandemic threat.
Phase 3	An animal or human-animal influenza reassortant virus has caused sporadic cases or small clusters of disease in people but has not resulted in human-to-human transmission sufficient to sustain community-level outbreaks.
Phase 4	Human-to-human transmission of an animal or human-animal influenza reassortant virus able to sustain community-level outbreaks has been verified.
Phase 5	The same identified virus has cuased sustained community-level outbreaks in two or more countries in one WHO region.
Phase 6	In addition to the criteria defined in Phase 5, the same virus has caused sustained community-level outbreaks in at least one other country in another WHO region.
Post Peak Period	Levels of pandemic influenza in most countries with adequate surveillance have dropped below peak levels.
Post Pandemic Period	Levels of influenza activity have returned to the levels seen for seasonal influenza in most countries with adequate surveillance.

FIG. 26.1 World Health Organization *(WHO)* pandemic phases. (Adapted from WHO. [2009]. *Pandemic phase descriptions and main actions by phase.* World Health Organization. Retrieved from http://www.who.int/influenza/resources/documents/pandemic_phase_descriptions_and_actions.pdf)

The critical component for the community and public health nurse is the careful medical screening and identification of these priority groups to receive the pandemic influenza vaccine. The nurse must be cognizant of different criteria that make the recipient eligible or deferred for a pandemic influenza vaccine. Many times the deferral list for pandemic influenza vaccination is similar to the same deferral groups for seasonal influenza. Some of the maladies and conditions that could defer pandemic influenza vaccination include (1) severe allergy to eggs or egg products, (2) life-threatening allergic reaction to a previous influenza vaccination dose, (3) Guillain-Barré syndrome, and (4) sick or ill or symptoms of illness at the time of vaccination (CDC, 2018c).

What Is Personal Protective Equipment in Disaster Response?

In discussing the previously mentioned CBRNE agents, the nurse must be prepared to manage and treat patients affected by any of these agents. It is important to understand that the first line of defense in clinical care for disaster medicine is personal protective equipment (PPE). PPE provides a barrier and protective layer against exposure to the various agents implicated in an event. Different levels of

PPE are necessary for different agents. To understand the correct level of PPE needed in clinical response, it is important to identify the different levels of PPE.

Level D is primarily a work uniform and is used for nuisance contamination only. It requires only coveralls and safety shoes/boots. Other PPE is based on the situation (types of gloves, etc.). It should not be worn on any site where respiratory or skin hazards exist. Level C protection should be selected when the type of airborne substance is known, concentration measured, criteria for using air-purifying respirators met, and skin and eye exposure is unlikely. Level B protection should be selected when the highest level of respiratory protection is needed but a lower level of skin and eye protection is necessary. Level B protection is the minimum level recommended on initial site entries until the hazards have been further identified and defined by monitoring, sampling, and other reliable methods of analysis, and equipment corresponding with those findings has been placed into use. Level A protection should be worn when the highest level of respiratory, skin, eye, and mucous membrane protection is needed. Occasionally, there will be instances where PPE levels will need to be upgraded to a higher level (level D to A) and/or downgraded to a lower level (level A to D). The reasons for these changes can include suspicion of presence of increased dermal and airborne hazards or hazard analysis information that has confirmed a lower risk threat. *It is imperative to state that only safety officers and/or incident commanders can make the determination and decision to increase or decrease PPE levels.* Fig. 26.2 demonstrates common PPE equipment and practices at the different levels. After the proper PPE is chosen and donned, specific instructions for maintenance, sanitization, replacement, and care must be considered. These specific instructions should be listed in the facility's all-hazards plan or can be found at the CDC Emergency Response Resources website: http://www.cdc.gov/niosh/topics/emres/ppe.html.

To protect:	Level D	Level C	Level B	Level A
Skin (dermal)	**Inner barrier:** Street clothes **Outer barrier:** Coveralls, scrubs or other protection	**Inner barrier:** Environmental temperature dependent Street clothes/scrubs to insulated coveralls **Outer barrier:** Hooded chemical-resistant clothing		**Inner barrier:** Totally encapsulating chemical-protective suit **Outer barrier:** Disposable protective suit (if warranted)
Skin— specifically hands	**Disposable gloves** **Cut-resistant gloves, if warranted**	**Disposable, chemical-resistant inner and outer gloves** **Cut-resistant gloves, if warranted**		**Chemical-resistant outer gloves over encapsulating suit** **Cut-resistant gloves, if warranted**
Respiratory		**Air purifying respirator (APR)** • Full mask for unknown hazards and some zoonoses • Half-mask for non-zoonotic	**Self-contained breathing apparatus (SCBA)**	
Eyes		**Goggles, face shield**	**(SCBA)**	
Footwear	**Boots or shoes appropriate to perform duties**		**Chemical-resistant steel toe boots**	**Chemical-resistant steel toe boots over encapsulating suit**

Known hazard **No risk of skin contamination** **No risk of inhalation** **No risk of hazardous material contact**   **Unknown hazard** **Skin contamination imminent** **Respiratory exposure imminent** **Eye exposure imminent**

FIG. 26.2 Equipment to provide protection based on personal protective equipment level. (Adapted from http://www.epa.gov/emergency-response/personal-protective-equipment)

What Is Disaster Nursing?

> As witnessed by the 2005 Hurricane Katrina and Indonesian tsunami events, natural disasters are a reminder of the critical role that emergency and public health nurses play in disaster response.

Disaster nursing integrates a wide range of nursing-specific knowledge and practices that facilitate the promotion of health while minimizing health hazards and peripheral life-damaging factors. Disaster nursing can be further subdivided into two major components: (1) implementation of the public health levels of prevention and (2) emergency triage and response.

In community health nursing, the role of the nurse in disaster response is to effectively promote the three levels of public health prevention. In *primary public health prevention* during disasters, the community health nurse must emphasize the components and principles of preparedness in both the non-disaster stage (before disaster occurs) and in the predisaster stage (disaster is pending). According to Nies and McEwen (2015), "preventive actions during the nondisaster stage include assessing communities to determine potential disaster hazards; developing disaster plans at local, state, and federal levels; conducting drills to test the plan; training volunteers and health care providers; and providing educational programs and information to the community regarding effective disaster preparedness" (p. 561). Community health nurses will be required to maintain strong physical and mental health dispositions during a disaster to provide a concerted response to their patients. This includes knowledge of the disaster plans of the community and the facility, inclusive of staff and patients. Nurses also need to educate their patients in the awareness and implementation of disaster kits and family emergency response plans in anticipation of a potential natural disaster. In the next stage—*secondary public health prevention*—the disaster has occurred and the nurse must emphasize the components and principles of response with a focus on preventing further injury or destruction. The response stage is one of the most important aspects of natural disasters because it requires efficient execution of nursing practice while maintaining professionalism and mental support to the afflicted community and patients, with safety being considered before search and rescue. As the scale of disaster increases, the role and responsibilities of the nurse increase proportionately (Nies & McEwen, 2015).

The last stage of *public health prevention—tertiary*—focuses on recovery and integrates the community health nurse's operations after the disaster has occurred to restore the community to its previous level of functioning and its residents to their maximum functioning (Nies & McEwen, 2015). In the recovery stage, the nurse is confronted with unexpected or sudden loss of key personnel and patients, in addition to the management of mental health issues in individuals related to the disaster. In addition to preventing a recurrence or minimizing the effects of future disasters, the nurse will be involved with debriefing meetings to identify problems with the disaster plan and make revisions.

What Are the Levels of Disasters?

During small natural disasters, also known as level I disasters, the community health nurse works in cooperation with local emergency medical systems and the community to provide medical support. Examples of level I disasters include auto accidents and house fires. Level II disasters require the community health nurse to respond in a greater capacity using larger casualty practices in coordination with regional response agencies (such as state health and emergency management agencies). Examples of level II disasters include train derailments, building collapses, and tornadoes. Level III disasters exhaust the most resources (including both the physical and mental resources of the community health nurse). Level III disasters consume local, state, and federal resources to the fullest extent and require an extended response time by the community health nurse that can last weeks and even months. Examples of level III disasters include earthquakes, tsunamis, hurricanes, and mass casualty events.

WHAT IS TRIAGE?

The core concept that ED nurses face is *triage*. Triage is a system of sorting patients according to medical need when resources are unavailable for all persons to be treated. For example, a patient presenting to the ED with chest pain will take priority in receiving intervention over a patient coming in with nausea and diarrhea. Remember ABCs when triaging patients! Although the genesis of triage has been documented in hospitals back to the mid-20th century, the concept was brought to wide attention by the California emergency medical services in response to earthquakes in the 1990s. In disaster triage a mass casualty incident causes a surge of patients in the ED requiring emergency assessment. In addition, disaster patients' needs are usually categorized by the placement of printed triage cards/tags. Fig. 26.3 depicts

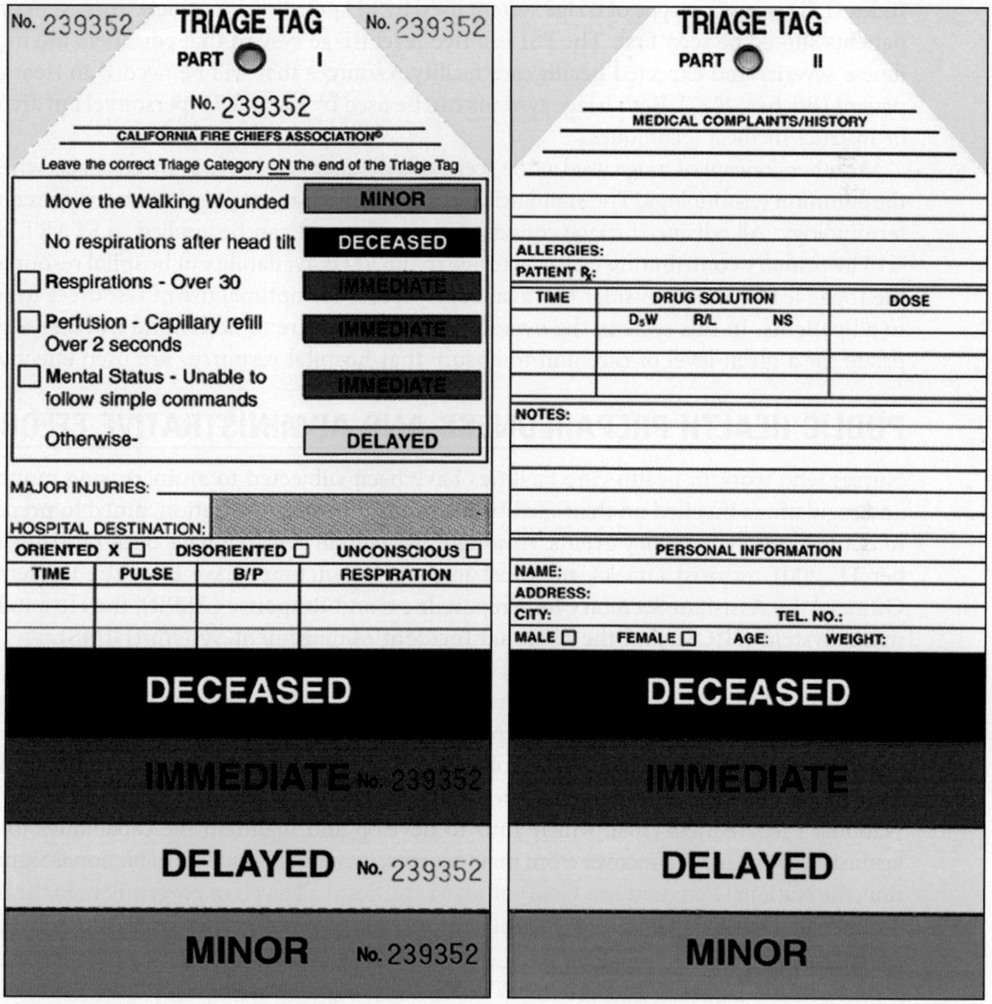

FIG. 26.3 An example of a triage tag.

BOX 26.1   START SYSTEM OF TRIAGE

The START system divides injured personnel into four separate groups:

- Deceased (Black)—Injured persons who are beyond the scope of medical assistance. Persons are tagged "Deceased" only if they are not breathing and attempts to resuscitate have been unsuccessful.
- Immediate (Red)—Injured persons who can be assisted or their health aided by advanced medical care immediately or within 1 h of onset.
- Delayed (Yellow)—Injured persons who can be assisted after "Immediate" persons are medically cared for first. "Delayed" persons are medically stable but require medical assistance.
- Minor (Green)—Injured persons who can be assisted after "Immediate" and "Delayed" persons have been attended to medically. Persons tagged "Minor" will not need medical care for at least several hours and can usually walk with assistance (usually consisting of bandages and first aid).

a sample triage card. The START (Simple Triage and Rapid Treatment) system is the most common type of disaster triage used by ED personnel (Box 26.1). In nondisaster instances, the Emergency Severity Index (ESI) is another type of triage system used by ED personnel routinely to assist in prioritizing which patients should be seen first. The ESI is a five-level triage system that considers the incoming patient's illness severity and expected health care facility resources that will be needed to treat and stabilize the patient (Bucher, 2017). Both triage systems can be used by trained ED personnel but are not to supersede or instruct medical techniques.

Another concept of triage used at the scene of a disaster is that of advanced triage, where colors replace the common terminology. The standard colors used in advance triage have been paired with the START terminology. All advanced triage concepts are similar and can be applied to START concepts.

The primary contributing factor to triage in the ED is availability of hospital resources. For example, the triage leader must consider bed availability issues for optimal use of resources to provide safe care to all patients. In this system, the overall goals of triage are to determine whether a patient is appropriate for a given level of care and to ensure that hospital resources are used effectively.

PUBLIC HEALTH PREPAREDNESS AND ADMINISTRATIVE EFFORTS

Nurses who work in health care facilities have been subjected to an increasing number of standards and regulations invoked on their facility by federal and state legislation aimed to prepare and respond to public health emergency events. Among those federal acts that have been ratified since the September 11, 2001 terrorist attacks, the most important outcomes have been the implementation of the Office of the Assistant Secretary for Preparedness and Response (ASPR), the Hospital Incident Command System (HICS), and the National Incident Management System (NIMS).

Under the federal administration of ASPR, the development of the Hospital Preparedness Program has witnessed a shift toward enhancement of the ability of hospitals to prepare for and respond to public health emergencies. Hospitals and outpatient care facilities have initiated coordination with EMS and other health care partner agencies to collaborate with local and state public health agencies in receiving funding for public health emergency preparedness (USDHHS, 2005). This funding is applied toward the National Preparedness Goal, which aims to develop and maintain the capabilities to prevent, protect against, respond to, and recover from major events, including Incidents of National Significance. In addition, the National Preparedness Goal will assist entities at all levels of government in the development and maintenance of the capabilities to identify, prioritize, and protect critical infrastructure (USDHHS, 2005).

The National Preparedness Goal has shifted from a sole bioterrorism preparedness effort to *all-hazards preparedness* collaboration.

The key areas of focus under the National Preparedness Goal for 2018 include comprehensive planning, public information and warning, operational coordination, forensic preparedness, access control, cybersecurity, and physical protective measures. Also included are streamlined delivery of medical countermeasures to exposed populations, triage and initial stabilization of casualties and commencement of definitive care for those likely to survive their injuries and illness and returning medical surge resources to preincident levels while identifying the recovery process. In addition, all hospitals and health care facilities must incorporate NIMS, education and preparedness training, and evaluations for corrective actions (based on preparedness training) to reach all capabilities established under the Hospital Preparedness Program (USDHHS, 2015).

As mentioned earlier, hospitals receiving ASPR and other federal preparedness funds must comply with the application of the NIMS developed by the Federal Emergency Management Agency (FEMA). NIMS provides a consistent nationwide template to establish federal, state, tribal, and local governments and private sector and nongovernmental organizations to work together effectively and efficiently to prepare for, prevent, respond to, and recover from domestic incidents, regardless of cause, size, or complexity, including acts of catastrophic terrorism. NIMS benefits include a unified approach to incident management; standard command and management structures; and emphasis on preparedness, mutual aid, and resource management (FEMA, 2015; FEMA, 2019).

> Hospitals and health care facilities were required by The Joint Commission to be NIMS compliant by the end of calendar year 2007, to confirm successful training of hospital staff under NIMS, and to implement the HICS emergency response command structure during hospital emergency responses. The health care agency's Emergency Management Plan should indicate specific responses to the types of disasters likely to be encountered by the organization. The organization needs to identify the potential emergencies that could occur in the defined service territory and how the disaster might affect the ability to continue to provide care and treatment to individuals (The Joint Commission [TJC], 2018).

Other specific criteria regarding emergency management for health care facilities under The Joint Commission's requirements include annual review and revision of the Emergency Management Plan, Policies and Procedures, Communication Plan, and Training (TJC, 2018).

One component of NIMS is for hospitals and health care facilities to execute HICS during hospital emergencies. HICS is a comprehensive incident management system intended for use in both emergent and nonemergent situations. It provides hospitals of all sizes with tools needed to advance their emergency preparedness and response capability—individually and as members of the broader response community. HICS is designed to be implemented for all routine or planned hospital events, regardless of size or type; this helps establish a clear chain of command and standardizes response processes. This standardized response allows entities from different organizations to be integrated under one common structure that can address response issues and delegate responsibilities (California Emergency Medical Services Authority, 2014). Additional information regarding HICS can be found online at https://emsa.ca.gov/disaster-medical-services-division-hospital-incident-command-system-resources/.

COMMUNITY HEALTH NURSE ISSUES AND PUBLIC HEALTH PREPAREDNESS

Epidemiologic Aspects

The epidemiologic response to a terrorist event plays a pivotal role in public health, both related and unrelated to biologic terrorism. Epidemiologists and infection control nurses must recognize and act on rapid determination that an unusual event has occurred. These nurses must be able to perform surveillance for additional case identification and tracking, and they must prevent the spread of disease through the implementation of effective intervention methods. This component of emergency response, when executed correctly and expeditiously, can significantly reduce morbidity and mortality in exposed populations (Zerwekh & Waring, 2005).

A critical component of an effective epidemiologic response to an emergency—both in the health care facility and in the community—is the acute identification and recognition of epidemiologic clues that could signal a biologic event. Early recognition of these clues can be achieved through surveillance (passive and active) and monitoring of patients presenting to health care facilities (Zerwekh & Waring, 2005). Two major clues that a biologic terrorism event has occurred are a clear differential diagnosis and the formation of an epidemiologic curve. Additional epidemiologic indicators of a biologic event are listed in Box 26.2.

It is possible that none of the listed clues will occur during a given bioterrorism event. However, the presence of one or more indicators on the list should alert infection control nurses, ED nurses, or community health nurses of such an event.

Another practice in both the health care facility and public health realms at the forefront of biologic terrorism early detection is the concept of *syndromic surveillance*. Syndromic surveillance applies health-related data, such as trends in patient symptomatology or disease presentation that precedes clinical diagnosis to indicate a substantial probability of an outbreak that would warrant further investigation and public health response (Zerwekh & Waring, 2005). For example, investigation of ICD-10-CM codes, chief complaint, similar signs and symptoms exhibited by patients in the ED, and frequency of antibiotic/prophylactic therapy prescribed can all be applied and integrated into a successful syndromic surveillance network. In the public health setting, monitoring inventory of over-the-counter medications (e.g., cough/cold medicines) and identification of excessive absenteeism of students at a school or employees in the workplace setting are other trends surveyed to detect the possibility of an outbreak or bioterrorism event before clinical diagnosis has been made. Different frameworks (such as the Outbreak Management System) are currently being developed to determine the most efficient approach to a successful syndromic surveillance network. The key concepts of a successful syndromic surveillance program are timeliness of reporting data, validity and quality of data, and system experience (Zerwekh & Waring, 2005).

BOX 26.2 EPIDEMIOLOGIC CLUES THAT COULD SIGNAL A BIOLOGIC EVENT

- Large numbers of ill persons with a similar clinical presentation, disease, or syndrome
- An increase in unexplained diseases or deaths
- Unusual illness in a population
- Higher morbidity and mortality in association with a common disease or syndrome or failure of such patients to respond to regular therapy
- Single case of disease caused by an uncommon agent, such as smallpox, Machupo hemorrhagic fever, pulmonary anthrax, glanders
- Several unusual or unexplained diseases coexisting in the same patient without any other explanation
- Disease with an unusual geographic, temporal, or seasonal distribution (e.g., influenza in the summer or Ebola hemorrhagic fever in the United States)
- Similar disease among persons who attended the same public event or gathering
- Illness that is unusual or atypical for a given population or age group
- Unusual or atypical disease presentation
- Unusual, atypical, unidentifiable, or antiquated strain of an agent
- Unusual antibiotic resistance pattern
- Endemic disease with a sudden, unexplained increase in incidence
- Atypical disease transmission through aerosols, food, or water, which suggests deliberate sabotage
- Many ill persons who seek treatment at about the same time

The epidemiologic response plays a pivotal role in public health emergencies. The implementation of surveillance, case identification and tracking, and early intervention methods can significantly reduce morbidity and mortality in exposed populations.

What Is the Strategic National Stockpile?

The Strategic National Stockpile (SNS) program stores large quantities of medicine and medical supplies to protect the citizens of the United States during a public health emergency, including (but not limited to) a terrorist attack, pandemic outbreak, or natural disaster such as an earthquake or hurricane. Effective Oct. 1, 2018, the SNS is managed by the Office of the ASPR in the USDHHS. For more information on ASPR and its role in preparing for, responding to, and recovering from natural disasters and public health threats (ASPR, 2018). This national inventory of antibiotics, chemical antidotes, antitoxins, airway maintenance supplies, and other medical equipment will support and refresh existing community resources being implemented during a public health emergency. The SNS "push-pack," once requested, will be delivered to any state or U.S. territory within 12 hours of request. Federal authorities have ensured enough medicine and equipment to supply multiple communities for an extended period during an event. In such an event, public health nurses can expect to be enlisted to assist in the evaluation and delivery of medications and equipment to every person in the affected community. Recent examples of SNS deployment in the United States occurred during the 2017 Hurricanes Harvey, Irma, and Maria, the 2016 Zika virus outbreak, and the 2014 Ebola virus event.

What Is a CHEMPACK?

The SNS CHEMPACK is a federal program designed to supplement the medical response in the event of a chemical nerve agent release. The scope of this program is specifically targeted for nerve agents classified as organophosphates (nerve agents), such as sarin and VX gases. The CHEMPACK containers, delivered to each of the 50 states and stored in geographically strategic locales, possess both emergency medical services (EMS) and hospital caches. Both caches contain such chemical antidotes as MARK-1 kits (intramuscular autoinjectors of atropine and 2-PAM), atropine injectors, PAM kits, diazepam, and sterile water.

The public health nurse must be aware of the possibility of medication administration during a chemical weapon event and must be refreshed on the proper dosage and clinical practice applications.

What Is ESAR-VHP?

The Emergency System for Advance Registration of Volunteer Health Professionals (ESAR-VHP) is a federally funded program through ASPR that forms a national system that allows efficient use of volunteer health professionals in emergencies by providing verifiable, up-to-date information regarding the volunteer's identity and credentials to hospitals or other medical facilities in need of the volunteer's services. Each state's ESAR-VHP system is built to standards that will allow quick and easy exchange of health professionals with other states, thereby maximizing the size of the population able to receive services during a public health or presidentially declared emergency (Critical Thinking Box 26.3).

> **❓ CRITICAL THINKING BOX 26.3**
>
> How do you register for ESAR-VHP in your state? What organization is responsible for coordinating the process? Who should register?

Medical Reserve Corps

The Medical Reserve Corps (MRC), initiated by the U.S. Office of the Surgeon General, is another resource developed to help communities in planning for and responding to a public health or medical emergency (MRC, 2018). Community-based MRC units function as a mechanism to organize and use volunteers who want to donate their time and expertise to prepare for and respond to emergencies on a local scale. MRC volunteers supplement existing emergency and public health resources by including medical and public health professionals such as physicians, nurses, pharmacists, dentists, veterinarians, and epidemiologists. The primary objectives of MRC units are to improve health literacy, increase disease prevention, eliminate health disparities, and, most important, improve public health preparedness (MRC, 2018).

Public health nurses need to be aware of the presence of MRC units and are encouraged to enlist in the MRC at their local jurisdiction. During times of medical emergencies, it is likely that public health nurses will be working alongside MRC units in a collaborative effort to minimize morbidity and mortality while maximizing the public health and medical response.

Disaster Medical Assistance Teams

Disaster Medical Assistance Teams (DMATs) are yet another public health preparedness and response resource with which a community health nurse might interact during a medical emergency. These teams, supported through the National Disaster Medical System, are deployable units divided by geographic region (USDHHS, 2017). The units are composed of teams of various clinical health specialties that include (but may not be limited to) communications, logistics, maintenance, and security. These teams are locally based but can be deployed federally on request. The responsibilities of DMAT teams include triage of victims at a disaster site, medical care at the site, and staging of locations outside the disaster site for transportation of patients to alternative health care facilities. DMAT teams also serve as care centers for evacuation areas, where they can set up mobile medical care facilities for injured and traumatized persons evacuating a declared disaster area.

WHAT DO I NEED TO KNOW ABOUT COMMUNITY PREPAREDNESS ISSUES?

The community health nurse has a responsibility not only in promoting public health and preventing disease but also in delivering primary prevention methodologies related to disaster and emergency preparedness. For the community health nurse, the three critical components of preparedness include mental health preparedness, individual preparedness, and family preparedness. The National Response Framework (USDHS, 2015), which aligns federal coordination structures, capabilities, and resources into a unified local and community response, is presented in Fig. 26.4. The community health nurse must also be cognizant of emerging trends and issues as they relate to disaster preparedness and response.

WHAT DO I NEED TO KNOW ABOUT DISASTER MENTAL HEALTH?

Any type of public health or medical disaster can cause a range of psychological reactions, from acute moderate symptoms to chronic severe stress-related psychological disorders. Traumatic medical emergencies can induce an array of personal stress responses, ranging from horror, helplessness, and anger to more progressive and severe reactions such as depression, substance abuse, and disconnection from society. Traumatic events affect those who witness the event, as well as survivors, rescue workers, and friends and relatives of victims. Although the prevalence of immediate emotional reactions is well

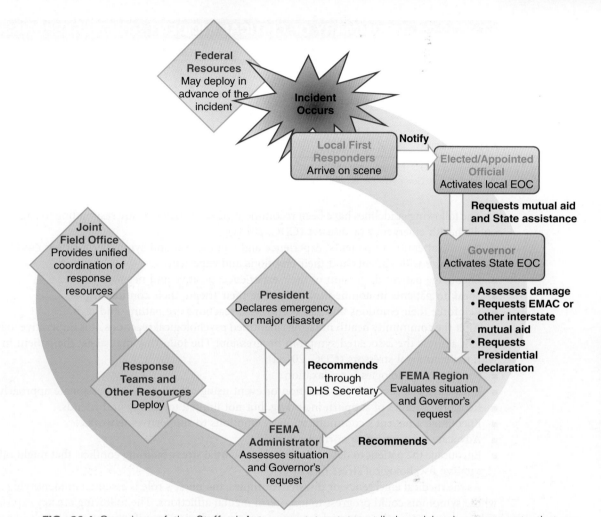

FIG. 26.4 Overview of the Stafford Act support to states, tribal, and local governments that are affected by a major disaster or emergency. *DHS,* Department of Health Services; *EMAC,* Emergency Management Assistance Compact; *EOC,* Emergency Operations Center; *FEMA,* Federal Emergency Management Agency. (From U.S. Department of Homeland Security. *National response framework.* Retrieved from www.fema.gov/pdf/emergency/nrf/nrf-stafford.pdf)

documented, the community health nurse must focus and be aware of the development of psychological reactions that persist from days to years after the public health event (CDC, 2018a).

The first practice a nurse should implement is the cognizance and awareness of the onset of psychological reactions in persons suffering from disaster mental health symptoms. When confronted with a patient suffering from such symptoms (Table 26.3), the nurse must identify concrete needs and attempt to assist—for instance, a person may ask, "How do I know if my friend is alive?" or "Are my parents OK?" or "How is my pet doing?" These concrete needs may be critical in identifying early symptom development of mental health problems.

TABLE 26.3 SUMMARY OF CRITICAL INCIDENT STRESS RESPONSES

PHYSICAL	COGNITIVE	EMOTIONAL	BEHAVIORAL
• Fatigue	• Nightmares	• Guilt	• Restlessness
• Chills	• Inattentiveness	• Fear	• Dissociation
• Unusual thirst	• Confusion	• Intense anger	• Antisocial behavior
• Nausea	• Poor memory recall	• Depression	• Alcohol abuse
• Headaches	• Poor problem-solving ability	• Irritability	• Sudden diet variations
• Disorientation		• Anxiety	

Adapted from: U.S. Department of Labor. Occupational Safety and Health Administration (OSHA). (n.d.). *Critical Incident Stress Guide*. Retrieved from https://www.osha.gov/SLTC/emergencypreparedness/guides/critical.html

The following guidelines have been recommended for nurses who are responding to patients after a public health emergency or disaster (CDC, 2018a):

- Provide attention to patients' experience and compassion and sympathy for their emotions.
- Empathize with patients and their emotions and experiences.
- Encourage patient discussion of their experience; positive and negative.
- Speak to patients in nonmedical terms—be their friend, their confidant.
- Reinforce their emotions and reactions; these reactions are natural and tacit.

After the community health nurse has identified psychological reactions, it is imperative to help the patient address the associated symptom progression. The following may assist the patient in coping with the emotional stressors (CDC, 2018a):

- Suggest methodologies for relaxation.
- Encourage discussion of the situation or event using a calm and compassionate approach.
- Reinforce sources of support, including, but not limited to, family and friends.
- Encourage a patient's communication of emotions to supportive networks.
- Advocate for a return to normal routine.
- Encourage the patient to defuse day-to-day potential stress-building conflicts that might otherwise catalyze psychological stress onset.

As the medical emergency or disaster continues, the nurse's role is essential in identifying patients whose symptoms could progress to long-term mental afflictions. The following are key exposure factors in determining the potential for long-term psychological manifestations as a result of a disaster (CDC, 2018a):

- Proximity to the event. Persons geographically closer to the event may be inclined to a greater psychological response.
- Previous psychological stability and history of past traumatic events. Patients who have experienced previous traumatic events or were experiencing psychological disorders before the event are predisposed to increased psychological reactions after the event.
- Importance and depth of the event. Patients who lose a friend or immediate family member may be inclined to greater psychological reaction development.

The nurse must be cognizant of continued progression of psychological reactions. Certain symptoms can assist the nurse in recognizing the development and onset of long-lasting psychological reactions, including the development of posttraumatic stress disorder. When such symptoms are identified, the community health nurse is recommended to do the following (CDC, 2018a):

- Refer patients for follow-up with a mental health professional (specifically trained in traumatic events, if possible) to seek additional counseling and guidance.
- Provide follow-up and guidance as needed.

Another concept the disaster response nurse must be cognizant of is the stress associated with care of these patients in this mental health and disaster capacity. It has been encouraged for the nurse to perform critical stress and critical incident debriefing after each shift. The physical and psychological well-being of those experiencing this stress, as well as their future ability to function through a prolonged response, will depend upon how they manage this stress. Signs and symptoms of incident strain and stress on a nurse can be categorized into four response types: physical, emotional, cognitive, or behavioral. As expected, each nurse will respond to a critical stress event with a different emotion, which can cause myriad reactions and emotions. Table 26.3 is a summary of potential stressor responses the disaster response nurse may face during the duties of response.

Individual and Family Preparedness Issues

In regular practice, the public health nurse must be cognizant of the concept of community and family emergency preparedness. Whether in mitigation of a previous event or in everyday practice, the promotion of community/family preparedness to the population is critical in minimizing morbidity and mortality and alleviating personal confusion and anxieties during a public health event. Special emphasis toward the promotion of family/community preparedness is encouraged each year during the month of September, which has been designated as National Preparedness Month (USDHS, 2018b).

Community preparedness can be further subclassified under efforts initiated at home, work, and school. Preparedness efforts undertaken at the home should focus on creating a disaster preparedness kit, establishing family emergency communication and evacuation plans, and recognizing potential disasters in the family's community. A family disaster preparedness kit should include enough essential supplies for each family member to last a minimum of 3 consecutive days; it is important for the family to revisit the preparedness kit every 6 months to replace expired supplies (USDHS, 2018a) (Box 26.3 and Critical Thinking Box 26.4). Fig. 26.5 provides common equipment included in a family preparedness kit.

? CRITICAL THINKING BOX 26.4

What plans have you and your family made regarding disaster preparedness?

The development of a family communications and evacuation plan will help to prepare family members to share responsibilities and work together as a team during a public health event. The public health nurse should recommend that family members discuss the types of probable disasters in their community and consider how members might respond to each scenario. Evacuation routes should include primary and secondary meeting places—it is recommended that the primary place be somewhere in the immediate vicinity around the house and that the secondary site be at a location away from the home in case family members are unable to return to the neighborhood (USDHS, 2018a). It is important that each family member know the phone number and address of the secondary site. Families should also nominate an out-of-area family friend who can serve as an emergency contact should the scale of disaster overwhelm local communication resources and local telephone calls become more difficult to make. This contact will serve as the information hub for family members not only if they are separated but also for event update information. It is important to encourage family members to practice their communication and evacuation plans regularly.

As society becomes more "connected" with internet-based devices, it is important to recognize applications that can serve as assistance to an individual or family during an emergency. The Red Cross, CDC, FEMA, and American Heart Association have apps specifically designed to inform

BOX 26.3   RECOMMENDED DISASTER PREPAREDNESS KIT

Recommended Items to Include in a Basic Emergency Supply Kit

- Water
  - One gallon of water per person per day, for drinking and sanitation
  - Children, nursing mothers, and sick people may need more water
  - If you live in a warm-weather climate, more water may be necessary
  - Store water tightly in clean plastic containers such as soft drink bottles
  - Keep *at least* a 3-day supply of water per person
- Food—at least a 3-day supply of nonperishable food
- Battery-powered or hand-crank radio and a National Oceanic and Atmospheric Administration weather radio with tone alert and extra batteries for both
- Flashlight and extra batteries
- First aid kit
- Whistle to signal for help
- Dust mask, to help filter contaminated air, and plastic sheeting and duct tape to shelter-in-place
- Moist towelettes, garbage bags, and plastic ties for personal sanitation
- Wrench or pliers to turn off utilities
- Manual can opener for food (if kit contains canned food)
- Local maps
- Cell phone with chargers, inverter, or solar charger

Additional Items to Consider Adding to an Emergency Supply Kit

- Prescription medications and glasses
- Infant formula and diapers
- Pet food and extra water for your pet
- Important family documents such as copies of insurance policies, identification, and bank account records in a waterproof, portable container
- Cash or traveler's checks and change
- Emergency reference material such as a first aid book or information from www.ready.gov
- Sleeping bag or warm blanket for each person; consider additional bedding if you live in a cold-weather climate
- Complete change of clothing including a long-sleeved shirt, long pants, and sturdy shoes; consider additional clothing if you live in a cold-weather climate
- Household chlorine bleach and medicine dropper (A solution of 9 parts water to 1 part bleach can be used as a disinfectant. Or in an emergency, you can treat water by adding 16 drops of household liquid bleach per gallon of water. Do not use scented or "color-safe" bleaches or bleaches with added cleaners.)
- Fire extinguisher
- Matches in a waterproof container
- Feminine supplies and personal hygiene items
- Mess kits, paper cups, paper plates, plastic utensils, paper towels
- Paper and pencil
- Books, games, puzzles, or other activities for children

Courtesy Department of Homeland Security (www.ready.gov). Recommended items to include in a basic emergency supply kit.

the individual of preparedness, response, and recovery activities during an emergency. Disaster Alert is another app that identifies and informs the individual of current hazards and disasters occurring in real-time and couples those events with individual preparedness and response activities related to each event (https://www.pdc.org/apps/disaster-alert/). For communication during disasters, there are two specific apps that can assist family or community members in communication during an event. Zello is an app that can be summarized as a "walkie-talkie" function to keep in communication with other

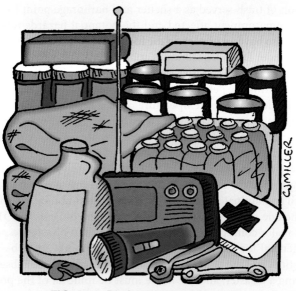

FIG. 26.5 Disaster preparedness kit.

Zello users. Nextdoor focuses more on the immediate community but also serves as a great reservoir for law enforcement and emergency officials to post updates regarding a disaster. Other apps that focus specifically on evacuation are GasBuddy and Waze. GasBuddy displays the nearest working gas pump in real time. Waze is a useful app for evacuation routes, updating in real time traffic jams, closed roads, and alternative routes to a destination.

Emerging Trends and Issues in Emergency Preparedness

The clinical and community health nursing field must be cognizant that environmental health professionals play extremely important roles in all-hazard emergency preparedness, response, recovery, and mitigation. For nurses to understand how disasters impact the environment is essential to effectively assessing, diagnosing, and treating a patient while providing heightened preventive measures to the community before, during, and after an emergency or disaster.

Carrying out the traditional functions of environmental health, such as safeguarding drinking water supplies, controlling disease-causing vectors, conducting food safety inspections, and ensuring safe and healthy building environments, may be challenging after emergency and disaster events. Clinicians must be able to anticipate, recognize, and respond to many issues. They need access to guidance, information, and resources that will assist them in preparing for, responding to, and recovering from the adverse impacts of emergencies and disasters.

During particular natural disaster emergencies, vectors and their associated diseases move to the forefront of environmental health responses. An excess of standing water, trash/rubbish accumulation, and the potential for wildlife interaction increase the opportunity for vector-borne diseases in humans. The most common of these diseases are directly related to the event that occurred: West Nile virus or other vector-borne diseases from mosquitoes and standing water, leptospirosis and typhus fever from rat harborage around trash/rubbish, and rabies, shigellosis, and other zoonoses from potential interaction and contact with wildlife displaced in the environment because of the emergency. It is important to identify the hazard and to link possible diseases related to the event. For instance, the 2011 Joplin, Missouri, tornado event created much trash/rubbish throughout the neighborhood, and this accumulation of trash served as a shelter and harborage point for rodent activity. The nurse must be astute to the environment affected and the potential hazards related to the event.

Disasters also have an impact on the food safety in an affected jurisdiction. The clinician needs to be aware of the major foodborne illnesses and circumstances that can initiate foodborne outbreaks related to an emergency event. The first concern is for persons being sheltered during an event. As shelters provide food during the person's stay, it is critical to know that food must be properly stored, prepared, cooked, and held at proper temperature during serving times. Likewise, food-service establishments and food retailers can often be impacted by events that may cause the facility to lose power for an extended period and/or be directly affected by the event. A thorough case history during work-up can assist the nurse in determining a differential diagnosis. For example, many grocery stores and restaurants were flooded by the 2012 Superstorm Sandy, causing them to lose power for days. These events compromise the integrity of the food by losing safe storage temperatures or coming into direct contact with contaminated and flooded waters. Common diseases from ingestion of these tainted food products include salmonellosis, shigellosis, *Escherichia coli* H7:O157, and noroviruses.

The last major concept of environmental health in disaster response is the notion of pollution control. This general topic has some subsets that the nurse must be aware of: hazardous materials, air/water pollution, and the building environment. Each of these subsets has unique conditions associated with it during a disaster, and the nurse must be mindful of the potential disease processes associated with each. Hazardous materials arise out of physical infrastructure destruction. The most common of these hazardous materials include household hazardous materials (bleach, ammonia, etc.), and diesel fuel/petrol products. These hazards can cause inhalational, ingestion, and dermal irritations, as well as other health issues when exposed to the human body. The nurse needs to be aware of previous exposure history when assessing the patient and be mindful of potential hazardous material exposure.

Air and water quality pollution issues have a substantial presence in the environment during emergencies. Particulate matter and other air toxics can be released from damaged infrastructure and can cause irritations and infections to those exposed to the air without proper PPE. This was never more evident than during the response to the 2001 World Trade Center attacks, when many citizens and emergency responders suffered respiratory conditions caused by the direct exposure to the particulates and dust in the environment. Water pollution issues also carry a threat to human health, primarily because of exposure from the biologic, chemical, and physical hazards within the contaminated water. Salmonellosis, hepatitis, chemical fertilizers, and diesel are some of the more common pathogens seen in contaminated water. These concerns are greatly exacerbated during flood events.

Finally, the nurse must be aware of ailments caused from the building environment. Buildings can be compromised during an emergency, whether it is taking on water from flooding, electrical hazards from electrical lines, or chemical hazards present from the physical destruction of the facility. The nurse needs to be educated on common mold exposures and treatment protocols for the exposed patient. Emergency room nurses may encounter patients who have been burned or electrocuted from the building infrastructure and must use correct burn/electrocution treatment protocols. And last, as discussed previously, there is a risk present in dermal, ingestion, and inhalational exposure to chemicals released in the building environment after a disaster. Additional information, treatment protocols, and resources regarding the clinical and community health response to environmental health related disasters can be obtained at the CDC's website at http://www.cdc.gov/nceh/. See box at the end of this chapter for more relevant websites and online resources.

Another emerging clinical and public health threat nurses must be cognizant of is the alarming increase in school and public venue shootings, also known as "active shooters." An active shooter is an individual actively engaged in killing or attempting to kill people in a populated area, and recent active shooter incidents have underscored the need for a coordinated response by public health, medical, clinical, and law enforcement professionals to save lives. Between the Sandy Hook Elementary School shooting on December 14, 2012, and June 30, 2015, there were 122 school shootings resulting in 34 total deaths and more than 94 injured. On a larger scale, there have been another 250 active shooter events outside of schools from the years 2000 to 2017, resulting in 799 deaths and 1418 wounded (Federal Bureau of Investigation, 2018). There are several agencies, in addition to health and medical, that will be involved in an active shooter incident. These agencies will vary from jurisdiction to jurisdiction but generally fall into one of the following categories: law enforcement, EMS, fire, emergency management, and public works. Health care facility nurses need to be cognizant that removal of patients' clothing should be kept to a minimum, if possible. Wounds and/or trauma to the patient, gunpowder particles on the clothing or other unique presentations can have considerable investigative value as evidence and should not be modified. Doffing of patient clothing should be done in a manner that will minimize the loss of physical evidence. If the clothing is bloody, do not allow blood and debris from one area or garment to contaminate another area or garment. Do not roll garments up in a ball. Never put wet or bloody garments in plastic bags. Carefully place garments in paper bags (one item per bag), seal, date, and initial. Label the bags with the patient's tracking tag. Handle clothing as little and carefully as possible. Pertinent items that could be considered evidence but need to stay with the patient, such as health aids, should be documented by the nurse and then notification submitted to law enforcement. All of this is best accomplished in discussions of these issues prior to an event and during review and updating of emergency protocols. The clinical and community health nurse must be aware of the risk present in active shooter events, which further underscores the need for appropriate and repeated training within the ICS and triage systems described previously (FBI, 2018).

The 2010 Institute of Medicine Report

Another issue in nursing emergency preparedness focuses around the 2010 Institute of Medicine (IOM) report titled *The Future of Nursing: Leading Change, Advancing Health*. In relation to emergency preparedness, the Emergency Nurses Association announced the endorsement of the IOM report, and the organization aims to integrate recommendations and practices in emergency care related to emergency preparedness events. Specifically, the initiatives focus around enhancement of education and training, partnerships with physicians and other health care providers, and improving workforce planning.

There are several opportunities in which the clinical and community health nurse can engage to enhance educational and training processes. Nurses can become certified in Basic and Advanced Disaster Life Support trainings aimed to develop a commonality of approach and language in the health care community, which improves the care and coordination of response in weapons of mass destruction (WMD) disasters and public health emergencies. These courses review "all-hazards" topics, including natural and accidental manmade events, traumatic and explosive events, nuclear and radiologic events, biologic events, and chemical events. The courses also discuss information on the health care professionals' role in the public health and incident management systems, community mental health, and special needs of underserved and vulnerable populations. Another opportunity for higher levels of training and education are opportunities provided by the United States Department of Homeland Security's Center for Domestic Preparedness (CDP). This federal agency clearinghouse is the primary resource for hands-on training, education, and exercises for first responders, including clinical and community health nurses. The trainings are grouped into classes in a classroom and then hands-on educational and training experience covering many topics including emergency care, mass casualty incidents, health care leadership, pandemics, and incident command, to name a few. Additional information and a listing of classes can be found at the CDP website: https://cdp.dhs.gov/training/resident/.

Enhancing partnerships with physicians and other health care providers can be accomplished through novel local best practices being implemented throughout the health care arena. For instance, hospitals, EMS, and public health have begun to use a practice known as "Triage Tuesday," where every patient delivered to the emergency room by an ambulance is triaged based on their actual symptom presentation. The patient is turned over to the hospital staff, and the emergency room must work the patient based on his or her triage tag. This practice not only increases familiarity with triage tags and with understanding the prioritization of triage skills, but it also bridges the gap between communication and collaboration among hospitals, EMS, and public health.

Last, nurses can enhance the last IOM recommendation of improving workforce planning by becoming active in membership in the groups listed previously (DMAT, DMORT, ESAR-VHP, MRC). These response groups assist in standardizing planning, response, and recovery activities as they relate to emergency preparedness and response. Another option for increasing workforce planning also centers on adding HICS and ICS courses for nurses to increase their experience. The higher-level courses refine the focus of planning and responding to disaster events where nurses will be used.

CONCLUSION

Whether in the clinical or the community environment, the role of the nurse in relation to emergency preparedness continues to expand and develop as local, state, and national preparedness efforts are executed. The nurse must continue to be aware and informed of evolving threats such as biologic, chemical, or radioactive terrorism while maintaining up-to-date training and knowledge of effective responses to public health disasters. The initiatives and programs mentioned in this chapter will ultimately aid nurses in comprehensive and efficient preparation, response, recovery, and mitigation to any public health emergency with which they may be confronted throughout their professional nursing tenure.

⊕ RELEVANT WEBSITES AND ONLINE RESOURCES

Centers for Disease Control and Prevention (CDC)
http://www.cdc.gov/.

Hospital Incident Command System (HICS)
www.emsa.ca.gov/hics/hics.asp.

United States Department of Homeland Security's Center for Domestic Preparedness (CDP)
http://cdp.dhs.gov/resident/index.htm.

BIBLIOGRAPHY

Bucher, L. (2017). Nursing management: Emergency, terrorism, and disaster nursing. In S. L. Lewis, L. Bucher, M. Heitkemper, M. M. Harding, J. Kwong, & D. Roberts (Eds.), *Medical-surgical nursing: Assessment and management of clinical problems* (10th ed., pp. 1628–1648). St. Louis, MO: Elsevier.

California Emergency Medical Services Authority. (2014). HICS overview. State of California. Retrieved from http://www.emsa.ca.gov/disaster_medical_services_division_hospital_incident_command_system_resources.

Centers for Disease Control. (2018a). CDC emergency preparedness and response. Retrieved from http://emergency.cdc.gov/ or www.cdc.gov/nceh/radiation/factsheets/ars.doc.

Centers for Disease Control. (2018b). National Center for Environmental Health. Retrieved from http://www.cdc .gov/nceh/.

Centers for Disease Control. (2018c). Persons who should not be vaccinated. Retrieved from http://www.cdc.gov/ flu/protect/whoshouldvax.htm#flu-shot.

Centers for Disease Control. (2018d). Seasonal flu. Retrieved from http://www.cdc.gov/flu/index.htm. http:// www.cdc.gov/flu/pandemic-resources/.

Center for Domestic Preparedness. (n.d.). Resident training. Retrieved from https://cdp.dhs.gov/training/ resident/.

Federal Bureau of Investigation. (2018). Active shooter incidents. Retrieved from https://www.fbi.gov/about-us/ office-of-partner-engagement/active-shooter-incidents.

Federal Emergency Management Agency. (2015). The 2015 National Preparedness Goal. Retrieved from https:// www.fema.gov/media-library/assets/documents/25959.

Federal Emergency Management Agency. (2019). The National Incident Management System (NIMS). Retrieved from http://www.fema.gov/national-incident-management-system.

Healthcare and Public Health Sector Coordinating Council. (2017). Active shooter planning and response in a healthcare setting. Retrieved from https://www.fbi.gov/file-repository/active_shooter_planning_and_ response_in_a_healthcare_setting.pdf/view.

Medical Reserve Corps (MRC). (2018). Retrieved from https://mrc.hhs.gov/HomePage.

Nies, M. A., & McEwen, M. (2015). *Community/Public health nursing* (6th ed.). St. Louis, MO: Elsevier.

Office of the Assistant Secretary for Preparedness and Response (ASPR). (2018). Strategic national stockpile. Retrieved from https://www.phe.gov/Preparedness/Pages/default.aspx.

Olson, K. B. (1999). Aum Shinrikyo: Once and future threat? *Emerging Infections Diseases, 5*(4), 513–516.

Roser, M., Nagdy, M., & Ritchie, H. (2018). Terrorism. OurWorldInData.org at the University of Oxford. Retrieved from https://ourworldindata.org/terrorism.

Szinicz, L. (2005). History of chemical and biological warfare agents. *Toxicology, 214*(3), 167–181.

The Joint Commission (TJC). (2018). Emergency management standards. Hospital and critical access hospital accreditation programs. Oakbrook Terrace, IL: The Joint Commission. Retrieved from http:// www.jointcommission.org/emergency_management.aspx.

U.S. Army Medical Research Institute of Chemical Defense. (2018). Retrieved from https://cbrnecentral.com/ category/chemical-defense/.

U.S. Department of Health and Human Services. (USDHHS). (2005). Hospital preparedness program. *Public Law,* 109–417.

U.S. Department of Health and Human Services. (USDHHS). (2017). Disaster Medical Assistance Teams (DMAT). Retrieved from https://www.phe.gov/Preparedness/responders/ndms/ndms-teams/Pages/ dmat.aspx.

U.S. Department of Homeland Security (USDHS). (2018a). Basic disaster supplies kit. Retrieved from http:// www.ready.gov/kit.

U.S. Department of Homeland Security (USDHS). (2018b). National preparedness month. Retrieved from https://www.ready.gov/september.

U.S. Department of Homeland Security (USDHS). (2015). National response framework (3rd ed.). Retrieved from https://www.fema.gov/media-library-data/1466014682982-9bcf8245ba4c60c120aa915abe74e15d/National_ Response_Framework3rd.pdf.

U.S. Department of Labor. Occupational Safety and Health Administration (OSHA). (n.d.). Critical Incident Stress Guide. Retrieved from https://www.osha.gov/SLTC/emergencypreparedness/guides/critical.html.

U.S. Nuclear Regulatory Commission. (2018). Fact sheets on dirty bombs. Retrieved from www.nrc.gov/ reading-rm/doc-collections/fact-sheets/dirty-bombs.html.

Wetter, D. C., Daniell, W. D., & Treser, C. D. (2001). Hospital preparedness for victims of chemical or biological terrorism. *American Journal of Public Health, 91,* 710–716.

Zerwekh, J. T., & Waring, S. C. (2005). The epidemiology of bioterrorism. In R. Pilch, & R. Zilinskas (Eds.), *The encyclopedia of bioterrorism.* New York: Wiley and Sons.

INDEX

Note: Page numbers followed by *f* indicate figures, *t* indicate tables, and *b* indicate boxes.

Management *(Continued)*
characteristics and theories of, 220–221
decentralization of, 419
definition of, 218
evidence-based, protocols and
interventions for, 236–238
functions of, 218–220
hierarchy of, 220
leadership *versus*, 218–227
power and authority in, 233–235
problem solving in, 235–240
problem-solving strategies in, 235–236
resources for, 246b
Management style, 221–223
autocratic, 221–222
continuum of, 222
democratic, 222
Laissez-faire, 222
Manager, 218
nurse as, 150t, 152–153
Mandatory overtime, 607, 610–611
legislation against, 611
Marburg virus, as bioterrorism agent,
621–622t
Margin (or profit), 380
Market, barriers to entry to, in marketplace
allocation decisions, 379
Marketplace allocation decisions,
378–379
Master's degree nursing program, 166–168
areas of specialty within, 168
choice of, 168–169
health care reform and, 149
nontraditional paths for, 165
Mead, Margaret, 406
Media information, for employment,
82–85
Mediation, 424
Medicaid, 456
collective bargaining and, 414
staffing requirements by, 414
Medical assistants (MAs), 324
Medical futility, 451
Medical power of attorney, advance
directives and, 490–491
Medical Reserve Corps (MRC), 634
Medical "tourism", 506
Medicare, 456
collective bargaining and, 414
insurance coverage, 385t
prospective payment system and, 346
Medicare Shared Savings Plan, 525
Medication, administration of, 483b
NCLEX-RN® examination and, 130
Medication-assisted therapy (MAT),
396–397

Medication errors, 614, 615–616b
causes of, 611
common causes of, 522
negligence and, 482–483, 483b
prevention of, 563
MEDMARX reports, 531
Meeting
action timeline for, 286f
improvement communication in, 284,
284b
Six Thinking Hats for, 284, 285b
Membership
in nursing associations, 422
sound contract and, 425
Men, communication style of, 272
Mental exercise, for self-care, 47
Mental health, disaster, 634–642
Mental potential, 48–50
Mentee
characteristics of, 65, 65t
checklist for, 65t
as follower, 61
role of, 64–65, 65b
Mentor, 60, 65b
attributes of, 68b
benefits of, 63–64, 64b
characteristics of successful, 62–63,
63–64b, 63f
different definitions for, 60
expectations of, 63f
finding, 17, 61–62
historical background of, 54
as leader, 61
need for, 63–64, 64f
preceptor *versus*, 55f
role of, 64f
time to let go and, 61
transitioning from mentee to, 66–67
Mentor power, 398
Mentoring, 53f, 54–56
benefits in, 63–64
coaching and precepting *versus*, 54
definition of, 54
e-mentoring, 67–69, 68–69b
extra mile of, 60
focus of, 60
future of, 67–70
moment, 63
as partnership, 60–61
peer, 69–70, 69–70b
process of, 61
promoting civility through, 67b
relationships, types of, 65, 66t
rewards of, 60
through reality shock, 65–66
Mentoring moment, 63

Mentoring relationship, 63–64, 64b
establishing, 62
through reality shock, 65–66
types of, 65, 66t
Mentorship, 53–72, 53f, 71b
Mercy killing, 449–450
Metaparadigms
definitions of, 181b
nursing theory definition, 178
Metric, quality patient care and, 528–530,
528b, 529t
Middle-range theories, 178
Military, mortality rate of, 138
Mindfulness, cultivating, 41–42, 42b
exercises, 42
Minor activity, 17
Misdemeanors, 471
nursing practice violations as, 492
Mission or philosophy statement, in
assessing organization, 86, 86b
Mixed-methods research design, 592t
Mobile computing devices
HIPAA and, 556, 556b
patient safety and, 556
precautions, 556
Mobility, 426
in clinical world, 571, 572f
Modeling and Role Modeling Theory,
182–183t
Monitor, 528b
Montag, Mildred, 146b, 148
Moral courage, 436b
Moral distress, 436b
Moral/ethical principles, 438–446, 438f
autonomy and, 438
beneficence, 438
decision-making approaches, 440–442
deontological, 440
situational, 441
teleological, 440
definition of, 436b
fidelity and, 439
justice and, 439
nonmaleficence and, 438
rule and, 439–440
veracity and, 439
Moral hazard, 379
Moral reasoning, 436b
Moral uncertainty, 436b
Morality, 440
Morning after pill, 448
Motivational theory, of management, 221
Motivators, nursing research, 593, 593b
Motor mouth personality, 283
Mourning, 283
Mouse personality, 283–284

Workplace *(Continued)*
  needlestick and sharps safety in, 606–607, 607*b*, 608*f*
  safety in, 603*f*
  sexual harassment in, 312–315
Workplace Bullying Institute, 603–604
  steps of handling bully, 605
Workplace Civility Index, 606
Workplace reality, 17
Workplace violence, 601–606, 603*f*
  bullying and harassment as, 603–606, 605*b*
  "code white" program for, 602

Workplace violence *(Continued)*
  definition of, 601–602
  incidence of, 602
  report of, 601–602
Workstation
  ergonomic design of, 600–601, 601*b*
  as shared, 600
  on wheels, 571, 600–601
World Health Organization (WHO), 624, 626*f*
Wound care, 581*b*
Written communication, 274–275
  guidelines for, 274–275
  patient safety and, 252–254, 252*b*

Written order
  transcribing of, 254, 254*b*
  types of, 254*t*

Y

Y2K, 147
Yellow hat, 285*b*
Yersinia pestis, 621–622*t*
Young, D.A.B, 141–142

Z

Zderad, Loretta, 182–183*t*
Zero defects, 524